Oxford Medical Publication

Malignant Pleural Mesothelioma

Malignant Pleural Mesothelioma

Edited by

Kenneth O'Byrne
and

Valerie Rusch

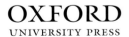
OXFORD

UNIVERSITY PRESS

OXFORD
UNIVERSITY PRESS

Great Clarendon Street, Oxford OX2 6DP

Oxford University Press is a department of the University of Oxford.
It furthers the University's objective of excellence in research, scholarship,
and education by publishing worldwide in

Oxford New York

Auckland Cape Town Dar es Salaam Hong Kong Karachi
Kuala Lumpur Madrid Melbourne Mexico City Nairobi
New Delhi Shanghai Taipei Toronto

With offices in

Argentina Austria Brazil Chile Czech Republic France Greece
Guatemala Hungary Italy Japan South Korea Poland Portugal
Singapore Switzerland Thailand Turkey Ukraine Vietnam

Oxford is a registered trade mark of Oxford University Press
in the UK and in certain other countries

Published in the United States
by Oxford University Press Inc., New York

A catalogue record for this title is available from the British Library

Library of Congress Cataloging in Publication Data
(Data available)

ISBN 0 19 852930 9   978 019 852930 9

10 9 8 7 6 5 4 3 2 1

Typeset by EXPO
Printed in China
on acid-free paper by Phoenix Offset

Contents

List of contributors

R. P. Abratt
University of Cape Town,
Cape Town, South Africa

S. H. Ahmedzai
Academic Unit of Supportive Care,
University of Sheffield,
Royal Hallamshire Hospital,
Sheffield, S10 2JF, UK

P. Baas
Department of Thoracic Oncology,
The Netherlands Cancer Institute,
Plesmanlaan 121, 1066 CX Amsterdam,
The Netherlands

S. Baka
Department of Medical Oncology,
Christie Hospital NHS Trust,
Manchester, UK

Y. I. Baris
Güven Medical Centre, and Chief of
National Mesothelioma Study Committee,
Ankara, Turkey

F. Blackhall
Department of Medical Oncology,
Christie Hospital NHS Trust,
Manchester, UK

M. Bocchetta
Loyola University,
Cardinal Bernardin Cancer Center Room 205,
2160 South First Ave,
Maywood, IL 60153, USA

D. J. Boffa
Thoracic Service,
Department of Surgery,
Memorial SloanKettering Cancer Center,
New York, NY 10021, USA

S. Broomfield
University of Western Australia,
School of Medicine and Pharmacology,
4th Floor, G Block, Queen Elizabeth II
Medical Centre, Perth, WA, Australia, 6000
and the West Australian Institute for Medical
Research, Queen Elizabeth II Medical Centre,
Perth, WA, Australia, 6009

A. Budgen
c/o Irwan Mitchell Solicitors,
Riverside East,
2 Millsands, Sheffield,
South Yorkshire, S3 8DT, UK

J. A. Burgers
Department of Thoracic Oncology,
Netherlands Cancer Institute—Antoni van
Leeuwenhoek Hospital,
Plesmanlaan 121, 1066 CX,
Amsterdam, The Netherlands

M. Carbone
Loyola University,
Cardinal Bernardin Cancer Center Room 205,
2160 South First Ave,
Maywood, IL 60153, USA

H. Clayson
Hospice of St Mary of Furness,
Ford Park, Ulverston,
Cumbria, LA12 7JP, UK

S. Danson
Department of Medical Oncology,
Christie Hospital NHS Trust,
Manchester, UK

N. H. de Klerk
Institute for Child Health Research,
Subiaco, and Centre for Child Health Research,
University of Western Australia,
Western Australia

P. A. DeLong
Pulmonary and Critical Care Medicine,
Dartmouth-Hitchcock Medical Center,
One Medical Center Drive,
Lebanon, NH 03756, USA

J. G. Edwards
Department of Thoracic Surgery,
University Hospital of Leicester NHS Trust,
Glenfield, Leicester, UK

S. Emri
Department of Chest Diseases,
Hacettepe University, School of Medicine,
and Member of National Mesothelioma
Study Commitee,
Ankara, Turkey

J. Entwisle
University Hospitals of Leicester NHS Trust,
Glenfield Hospital,
Groby Road,
Leicester, LE3 9QP, UK

D. A. Fennell
Thoracic Oncology Research Group,
Centre for Cancer Research and Cell Biology,
Northern Ireland Cancer Centre,
University Floor, City Hospital, Lisburn Road,
Belfast, BT9 7AB, Northern Ireland

K. M. Foster
University of Texas Southwestern,
5323 Harry Hines Blvd,
Dallas, TX 75390, USA

F. Galateau-Sallé
Department of Pathology,
University of Caen,
France

S. G. Gray
Trinity College Institute of Molecular
Medicine,
St James's Hospital,
Dublin 8, Ireland

P. S. Hasleton
Department of Pathology,
Clinical Sciences Building,
Manchester Royal Infirmary,
Manchester, UK

J. P. Hegmans
Erasmus MC, Department of Pulmonology,
Rotterdam, The Netherlands

C. Jackaman
University of Western Australia,
School of Medicine and Pharmacology,
4th Floor, G Block, Queen Elizabeth II
Medical Centre, Perth, WA, Australia, 6000
and the West Australian Institute for Medical
Research, Queen Elizabeth II Medical Centre,
Perth, WA, Australia, 6009

J. E. King
Department of Thoracic Surgery,
Birmingham Heartlands Hospital,
Birmingham, UK

B. Koloska
University of Western Australia,
School of Medicine and Pharmacology,
4th Floor, G Block, Queen Elizabeth II
Medical Centre, Perth, WA, Australia, 6000
and the West Australian Institute for Medical
Research, Queen Elizabeth II Medical Centre,
Perth, WA, Australia, 6009

S. Lansley
University of Western Australia,
School of Medicine and Pharmacology,
4th Floor, G Block, Queen Elizabeth II
Medical Centre, Perth, WA, Australia, 6000
and the West Australian Institute for Medical
Research, Queen Elizabeth II Medical Centre,
Perth, WA, Australia, 6009

J. N. Lipsitz
Lipsitz and Ponterio, LLL
Attorneys at Law,
135 Delaware Ave Suite 506,
Buffalo, NY 14202, USA

A. E. Martin-Ucar
Department of Thoracic Surgery,
Glenfield Hospital,
Groby Road,
Leicester LE3 9QP, UK

B. T. Mossman
Department of Pathology,
University of Vermont College of Medicine,
89 Beaumont Ave,
Burlington, VT 05405, USA

A. W. Musk
Departments of Medicine and Public Health,
University of Western Australia,
Nedlands, Western Australia, and
Department of Respiratory Medicine,
Sir Charles Gairdner Hospital, Nedlands,
Western Australia

D. J. Nelson
School Biomedical Sciences, Kent St.,
Curtin University, Bentley, WA, Australia, 6102
and the University of Western Australia,
School of Medicine and Pharmacology,
4th Floor, G Block, Queen Elizabeth II
Medical Centre, Perth, WA, Australia, 6000

J. Niklinski
Department of Thoracic Surgery,
Medical Academy of Bialystok,
Poland

M. E. R. O'Brien
Royal Marsden,
Hospital NHS Trust,
Sutton, Surrey,
SM2 5PT, UK

K. J. O'Byrne
Hope Directorate,
St James's Hospital,
Dublin 8, Ireland

M. D. Peake
University Hospitals of Leicester NHS Trust,
Glenfield Hospital,
Groby Road,
Leicester, LE3 9QP, UK

A. Powers
Cleveland Clinic Foundation,
Department of Pathology/L25,
9500 Euclid Avenue,
Cleveland, OH 44195, USA

M. Ranson
Department of Medical Oncology,
Christie Hospital NHS Trust,
Manchester, UK

A. U. Ribate
Royal Marsden, Hospital NHS Trust,
Sutton, Surrey, SM2 5PT, UK

B. W. S. Robinson
University of Western Australia,
School of Medicine and Pharmacology,
4th Floor, G Block, Queen Elizabeth II
Medical Centre, Perth, WA, Australia, 6000
and the West Australian Institute for Medical
Research, Queen Elizabeth II Medical Centre,
Perth, WA, Australia, 6009

R. M. Rudd
Mesothelioma Unit,
St Bartholomew's Hospital and
London Lung Cancer Group,
University of London,
London, UK

V. W. Rusch
Thoracic Service,
Department of Surgery,
Memorial Sloan-Kettering Cancer Center,
New York, NY 10021, USA

R. Salgado
Department of Pathology,
University Hospital Antwerp,
Wilrijkstraat 10, B-2650,
Edegem, Belgium

A. M. Smith
University of Western Australia,
School of Medicine and Pharmacology,
4th Floor, G Block, Queen Elizabeth II
Medical Centre, Perth, WA, Australia, 6000
and the West Australian Institute for Medical
Research, Queen Elizabeth II Medical Centre,
Perth, WA, Australia, 6009

W. R. Smythe
Department of Surgery,
Texas A&M University,
2401 S31st St,
Temple TX 76508, USA

B. Souberbielle
Department of Molecular Medicine,
Kings College Hospital, London, UK

J. P. C. Steele
Mesothelioma Unit,
St Bartholomew's Hospital and
London Lung Cancer Group,
University of London,
London, UK

D. H. Sterman
Thoracic Oncology Research Laboratory,
Pulmonary, Allergy, and Critical Care
Division, Department of Medicine,
University of Pennsylvania Medical Center,
Philadelphia, PA 19104–4283, USA

C. W. Stevens
Division of Radiation Oncology,
H. Lee Moffitt Cancer Center & Research
Institute,
12902 Magnolia Drive,
Tampa, FL 33612–9497, USA

J. R. Testa
Human Genetics Program,
Fox Chase Cancer Center,
Philadelphia, PA 19111, USA

M. Tuncer
Director of National Cancer Control
Department, Ministry of Health,
Ankara, Turkey

E. A. Van Marck
Department of Pathology,
University Hospital Antwerp,
Wilrijkstraat 10, B-2650,
Edegem, Belgium

P. B. Vermeulen
Translational Cancer Research Group
(General Hospital Sint-Augustinus &
Antwerp University), Antwerp, Belgium

D. A. Vorobiof
Sandton Oncology Center,
Johannesburg, South Africa

D. A. Waller
Department of Thoracic Surgery,
Glenfield Hospital,
Groby Road,
Leicester LE3 9QP, UK

N. White
University of Cape Town,
Cape Town, South Africa

U. Zangemeister-Wittke
Department of Oncology,
Laboratory of Molecular Oncology,
University Hospital Zurich,
Halideliweg 4,
8044 Zurich, Switzerland

Chapter 1

The epidemiology and aetiology of malignant mesothelioma

J. E. King and P. S. Hasleton

Introduction

Malignant mesothelioma is a primary tumour of the serosal membranes (mesothelium) which line the thoracic and abdominal cavities. It is most commonly described in the pleura, which accounts for approximately 75 per cent of cases in most series, but can also arise in the peritoneum, pericardium, and tunica vaginalis.

The UK is currently in the midst of a 'mesothelioma epidemic' (Fig. 1.1). The incidence of malignant mesothelioma has been increasing for more than 30 years, and is predicted to continue rising for at least another decade [1–4]. The majority of cases of mesothelioma in Great Britain can be attributed to occupational or para-occupational exposure to amphibole asbestos. Although the industrial use of asbestos has been regulated since the late 1960s, the majority of new cases involve men who were exposed to asbestos before regulations were introduced or who worked in unregulated occupations [5]. The risk of mesothelioma induction in the pleura after

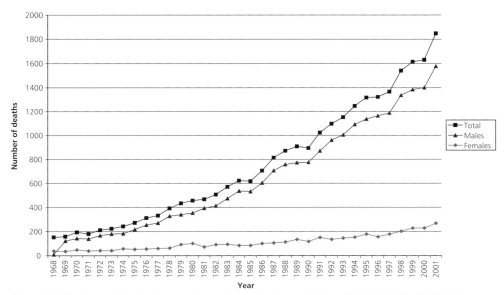

Figure 1.1 Number of deaths from malignant mesothelioma in Great Britain (1968–2001). (Data reproduced with permission from Health and Safety Executive, *Mesothelioma Mortality in Great Britain: Estimating the Future Burden*. London: Health and Safety Executive, 2003.)

amphibole asbestos exposure is not entirely dose dependent, and it is unlikely that there is a minimum safe threshold below which mesothelioma does not develop. Therefore it is possible that many thousands of men may have been exposed to pathologically significant amounts of asbestos during their working lives. In contrast, malignant peritoneal mesothelioma tends to be associated with higher levels of asbestos exposure and the presence of asbestosis [6].

Historical perspectives

Malignant pleural mesothelioma was previously a very uncommon tumour. Indeed, for many years it was disputed whether mesothelioma actually existed as a separate pathological entity. Sporadic reports of tumours involving the pleura had been described as long ago as the eighteenth century [7]. E. Wagner is credited as one of the first to publish a formal description of mesothelioma in 1870 [8]. In this paper he describes the gross and microscopic appearances of the lungs and pleura in 13 patients who had initially been diagnosed as having tuberculosis. He believed that they all showed evidence of a malignant tumour originating in the pleura.

The concept of a primary mesothelial tumour was not generally accepted for several years. Many influential pathologists thought that all pleural tumours were secondary tumours, invading the pleura from adjacent lung or metastasizing from elsewhere in the body [7, 9]. The subject remained contentious, despite increasing experimental evidence that mesothelioma was histologically distinct from primary pulmonary tumours [10]. By the 1950s opinion was changing. The pioneering work of Klemperer and Rabin [10], Stout and Murray [11], Campbell [12] and McCaughey [13] was reinforced by the publication of a landmark paper in 1960 by yet another Wagner!

In this paper Wagner *et al.* [14] described 33 cases of malignant tumours involving the pleura that had presented to the Pneumoconiosis Research Unit in Johannesburg, South Africa, during the period 1956–1960. All tumours were histologically consistent with mesothelioma. Twenty-eight of these patients had worked directly with crocidolite (blue asbestos) during mining work in the northwest Cape Province. A further four patients had lived close to asbestos mines. Eighty per cent of those patients who had lung tissue available also showed evidence of asbestos-related lung fibrosis (asbestosis). In contrast, during the same 5 year period no cases of mesothelioma had been reported in over 10 000 lungs from individuals not working or living near asbestos deposits examined by the Pneumoconiosis Bureau or similar institutes in South Africa.

The publication of this observational study triggered much research on the subject of mesothelioma and asbestos. It is now accepted that mesothelioma exists as a distinct pathological entity. Numerous epidemiological studies have confirmed a causal relationship between amphibole asbestos and mesothelioma, although the evidence that serpentine asbestos (chrysotile) induces mesothelioma is less convincing. The majority of series have found that approximately 85 per cent of cases of mesothelioma are asbestos related. Changes in mesothelioma incidence closely reflect previous amphibole asbestos usage in the UK, as demonstrated by Peto *et al.* [2] (Fig. 1.2).

The epidemiology of malignant mesothelioma

Amphibole asbestos has now been regulated or banned in most of Europe and the USA, although it continues to be used in some developing countries [5]. Chrysotile now accounts for more than 99 per cent of the total world asbestos production [15]. Because most asbestos exposure in Europe occurs via occupational exposure, mesothelioma rates are higher in those areas based around industries utilizing asbestos, such as shipbuilding and insulation work. Mesothelioma

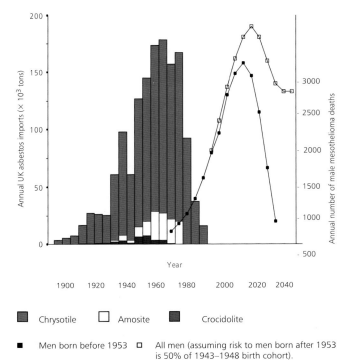

Figure 1.2 Predicted mesothelioma deaths in British men and UK asbestos imports. The bar chart indicates annual UK asbestos imports (1900–1995). The curves show the actual and predicted mesothelioma deaths as cited by Peto *et al.* [2]. (Reproduced with permission from Professor Peto.)

accounts for more than 10 per cent of deaths in workers in these industries [16]. As these occupations are markedly male dominated, the male-to-female ratio in malignant mesothelioma is high (>3:1), and the greatest increase in incidence attributed to asbestos usage has been seen in men. A notable exception is in women who were exposed to asbestos during war work (e.g. manufacture of gas masks) who have an incidence of mesothelioma similar to that in men [17, 18].

Some geographical areas are associated with higher mesothelioma rates. These include areas where asbestos occurs naturally and is mined (e.g. Russia, Quebec Province in Canada, Northern Italy, Wittenoom in Australia, Kazakhstan, and Cape Province in South Africa). Non-asbestiform fibrous minerals are also capable of causing mesothelioma. In Turkey, high mesothelioma rates are associated with the fibrous zeolite erionite [19] which is a crystalline aluminosilicate whose fibres have similar dimensions and carcinogenic potential to those of amphibole asbestos.

Ten to fifteen per cent of patients with malignant mesothelioma cases have had no apparent exposure to asbestos. A proportion of these may have been unwittingly exposed to asbestos at work or in the home. The ability of asbestos to cause mesothelioma is not dose dependent, and relatively minor asbestos exposure can probably induce malignant mesothelioma in predisposed individuals. This is classically demonstrated in women with mesothelioma whose only exposure is via their husband's work-clothes or from living, but not working, in the vicinity of asbestos mines or factories [14, 20, 21]. There have been reports of families with more than one member afflicted by mesothelioma [22]. In these cases it is often difficult to exclude common environmental or para-occupational factors. There is evidence that some of the cases of erionite-induced mesotheliomas in Turkey are in part due to familial genetic susceptibility [23]. Mesothelioma is extremely rare in children, and is far less likely to be related to asbestos exposure as it appears that a minimum lag phase of 10 years from exposure is required for tumour development [24, 25]. No other causal agents have yet been confirmed, although chronic pleural inflammation, simian virus 40 (SV40) and ionizing radiation have been suggested as candidates. These are discussed in more detail later in this chapter and elsewhere in this book.

Predictions of future mesothelioma incidence in the UK

The Health and Safety Executive (HSE) first compiled their mesothelioma register in 1967 to coincide with the introduction of updated asbestos regulations [5]. This register has recorded all known deaths from mesothelioma in the UK from that time. The Epidemiology and Medical Statistics Unit (EMSU) of the HSE has twice used this data to estimate the future incidence of malignant mesothelioma in the UK [2, 4]. In both cases projections were based on data for male deaths only.

In 1995 Peto *et al.* [2] published their first estimate of future mesothelioma incidence based on the register figures for the period 1968–1991. They employed a simple multiplicative birth cohort model which assumed that the incidence of mesothelioma was directly related to date of birth, which itself reflected asbestos usage at that time. Projections of mesothelioma incidence up to 1991 fitted this model well, and appeared to reflect a direct correlation between mesothelioma incidence and UK asbestos imports (Fig. 1.2). The model predicted that the incidence of mesothelioma would continue to rise for at least another 20 years, peaking at a level of 2700–3300 deaths per annum in 2020 before decreasing to a 'background level' of approximately 100–200 cases per annum.

More recently, the HSE has published an updated prediction using a different statistical model [4]. They had found that although their previous model appeared to predict mesothelioma deaths accurately up to 1991, more recent register data fitted less well. A second statistical model was devised, based on the assumption that the risk of mesothelioma to a population can be described by a single age-related figure and that the risk of mesothelioma development is proportional to exposure to the power of 2.6. This revised model predicts that the peak mesothelioma incidence in males in the UK will be in the period 2011–2015, with 1950–2450 deaths annually. The cohort of workers who had most asbestos exposure is likely to have been those aged 20–49 years in 1967, just before the introduction of the asbestos regulations, i.e. men born in the period 1918–1947.

The prediction of future mesothelioma incidence is complicated by the presence of several confounding factors that are themselves difficult to evaluate. Statistical models make assumptions regarding the amount of asbestos exposure and its inherent risk of mesothelioma induction. Since the introduction of asbestos regulations, heavy industrial asbestos exposure has been stopped and those who still work with asbestos do so under protected conditions. However, it is thought that many thousands of (predominantly) men have been exposed to biologically significant asbestos doses through work in less well-regulated industries such as the building trade. Therefore it is very difficult to evaluate the risk of mesothelioma in younger birth cohorts. The long lag phase of mesothelioma also poses epidemiological problems as it takes an average of 30–40 years for mesothelioma to develop after exposure to asbestos [26, 27]. Asbestos also causes bronchogenic carcinoma, and its carcinogenicity is synergistic with cigarette smoke. It is impossible to say how many smokers have died of lung cancer or cardiovascular disease before they had a chance to show evidence of their mesothelioma.

The relationship between asbestos and mesothelioma in women is less predictable, and 10–15 per cent of all cases of mesothelioma have no apparent asbestos exposure. Finally, the carcinogenetic potential of asbestos is in part related to fibre dimensions, rather than its chemical composition [28]. The potential risk of man-made fibres with similar dimensions that have been introduced to replace asbestos has not yet been fully appraised.

Asbestos mineralogy

Asbestos is the commercial collective name for a group of naturally occurring fibrous hydrated silicates that share similar chemical and physical properties. Named from the Greek for 'unquenchable', these minerals have been greatly valued for their thermal resistance, tensile strength, flexibility and durability, and in ancient times were imbued with almost magical properties. Asbestos deposits are widespread, although relatively few are commercially exploitable. Although asbestos has been utilized by humans for over 6000 years, widespread commercial mining and manufacturing only began in earnest in the second half of the nineteenth century [29, 30].

Asbestos minerals are subclassified into two groups, amphibole and serpentine, according to their fibre morphology. Both consist of a silicate core. The type and proportion of other metals within the core structure influences the physical and chemical properties of asbestos, and may explain differing carcinogenic potential between fibres [31].

Amphibole asbestos consists of sharp brittle javelin-shaped fibres with a high length-to-width ratio. This group includes crocidolite (blue asbestos), amosite (brown asbestos), tremolite, actinolite, and anthophyllite. The basic amphibole structure is a double chain of silica tetrahedra cross-linked by bridging cations. Although described by an idealized formula, cation substitutions occur freely. This results in significant chemical variations between asbestos mineral types from different geographical areas. All the amphiboles exhibit good stability in acid conditions and have decomposition temperatures above 400°C. Different asbestos types can be found together in the same area, and can contaminate other mineral deposits such as talc.

In contrast, serpentine asbestos, of which chrysotile (white asbestos) is the only commercial form, has long curved fibres that are less aerodynamically shaped and more friable than those of the amphiboles. Chrysotile is a sheet silicate of uniform composition. The silica tetrahedra are planar-linked with a layer of brucite (magnesium hydroxide). Differences in size and alignment between the two layers produce a structural mismatch. The resulting fibres resemble scrolls with a hollow central core. The fibres are held together by hydrogen bonds, producing bundles with splayed ends that are 1–20 mm long in their natural state. Chrysotile, in contrast with the amphiboles, is stable in alkaline solution but susceptible to acid attack.

It is recognized that fibrous minerals other that asbestos can cause mesothelioma. This implies that chemical composition alone is not the only determinant of carcinogenicity. Erionite is a fibrous zeolite (aluminosilicate) that differs substantially from asbestiform minerals in terms of its structure and chemical composition. It resembles the amphiboles in that it is durable, it has a very large active surface area, and the fibre dimensions are within the range deemed critical for mesothelioma induction [28]. Deposits of erionite are prominent in Turkey, and have resulted in endemic mesothelioma through the use of erionite-bearing rock for house construction [19]. Erionite is no longer commercially exploited, although non-fibrous zeolites are widely used as catalysts and adsorbents in industry. The chemical and physical properties of the asbestos minerals and erionite are summarized in Table 1.1.

Asbestos fibres and lung clearance mechanisms

An appreciation of the way that the body deals with inhaled fibres is essential to understanding the mechanism behind asbestos-related toxicity in the lung and pleura. Asbestos fibres occur naturally in the environment and may contaminate water supplies, however, there is no definitive evidence that they are carcinogenic unless inhaled.

Several mechanisms exist to prevent the passage of inhaled particles into the respiratory tract [32]. The proportion of an inhaled particle load that remains in the lung depends on the balance

Table 1.1 Chemical and physical properties of fibrous minerals implicated as causing malignant mesothelioma

Name	Fibre type	Colour	Decomposition temperature (°C)	Idealized chemical formula
Actinolite	Amphibole	Green	620–960	$Ca_2(Mg,Fe)_5(Si_8O_{22})(OH)_2$
Amosite	Amphibole	Pale grey/brown	600–800	$(Fe,Mg)_7(Si_8O_{22})(OH)_2$
Anthophyllite	Amphibole	White/grey/brown	600–850	$(Mg,Fe)_7(Si_8O_{22})(OH)_2$
Chrysotile	Serpentine	White	450–700	$Mg_3(Si_2O_5)(OH)_4$
Crocidolite	Amphibole	Blue	400–600	$Na_2Fe^{2+}{}_3Fe^{3+}{}_2(Si_8O_{22})(OH)_2$
Erionite	Fibrous zeolite	White	Not known	$(K_2Na_2Ca)MgA1_8Si_{28}O_{72} \bullet 28H_2O$
Tremolite	Amphibole	White/pale grey	950–1040	$Ca_2Mg_5(Si_8O_{22})(OH)_2$

between initial load size and subsequent clearance. Clearance is influenced by the physical properties (size, shape, density) and chemical properties of a particle. The overall process can be divided into five stages: inhalation, sedimentation, deposition, translocation, and dissolution.

Inhalation of particles is predominantly through the nose during normal respiration. The nasal passages trap all particles more than 15 mm in diameter. Mouth breathing bypasses this mechanism, and therefore is far less efficient at protecting the upper airways from particles inhaled during physical exertion. Exercise also alters the dynamics of breathing. Therefore the amount and character of an inhaled particle load is influenced by the circumstances in which it is inhaled.

Once in the upper airways, most particles will be deposited on the epithelial surface, particularly at bronchial airway bifurcations. Here they are trapped in mucus and removed via the mucociliary escalator and/or engulfed (phagocytosed) by alveolar macrophages. Mucociliary clearance and macrophage function are impaired in smokers, resulting in prolonged particle contact with the bronchial epithelium. This may partly explain the synergism between smoking and asbestos in lung cancer development.

The probability that a particle will be deposited increases with its size. Exceptions are straight fibres with high length-to-width ratios, such as those characteristically seen in amphibole asbestos. Some of these fibres will align with the long axis of the airways, allowing them to travel further than less aerodynamic particles of a similar size. In the distal airways particles are distributed by sedimentation and can impact on the epithelium or penetrate into the interstitium. From here they can only be removed by translocation into the lymphatic system, or by phagocytosis and dissolution by local macrophages.

Macrophages internalize particles and then attempt to destroy them through the production of lytic enzymes and an acid environment. In particular, highly reactive oxygen species (ROS) are formed. ROS production is catalysed at available surface redox (reduction–oxidation) sites via cation exchange, particularly in the presence of reduced iron. The most toxic ROS are superoxide and hydroxyl ions. These can react directly with individual DNA molecules, as well as causing damage indirectly by promoting lipid peroxidation. Under normal circumstances termination of free-radical activity occurs once the initiating particle is inactivated through spontaneous decay or the production of antioxidants (e.g. transferrin, glutathione, vitamin E). Experimental chromosomal damage from ROS is partly blocked by the addition of antioxidants and iron chelators such as desferrioxamine [33, 34]. The durable nature of amphibole asbestos fibres, and in partic-

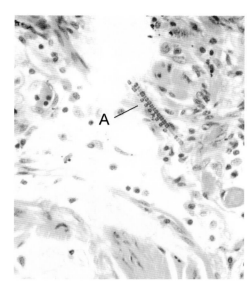

Figure 1.3 Asbestos body (A) within a section of lung tissue affected by asbestosis (haematoxylin–eosin stain).

ular their stability in acid solution, resists these effects. This 'frustrated phagocytosis' perpetuates ROS generation and enables further DNA damage.

If unsuccessful, macrophage cell death results in the release of these enzymes and other inflammatory mediators (e.g. cytokines) into the local environment. Macrophages will also attempt to ameliorate the toxic effects of persisting particles by coating them with an iron-rich protein and mucopolysaccharide layer to form ferruginous or asbestos bodies, depending on the core material. An asbestos fibre within a section of lung tissue is shown in Figure 1.3.

It was recognized that pathways between the pleural space and subpleural lymphatics existed long before they could be demonstrated morphologically. Water and small molecules can pass between mesothelial cells directly into lymphatics. Larger molecules, up to a size of approximately 1 mm, are phagocytosed and actively transported across mesothelial cell cytoplasm. Particles of size greater than 1 mm cannot be transported through cells, yet they can still leave the pleural space. Electron microscope studies have confirmed that pleural translocation pathways exist, with a net flow from the visceral to the parietal pleura [35]. A variable proportion of an inhaled asbestos fibre load will be translocated to the parietal pleura via these pathways. Fibres that are too large to pass into the subpleural lymphatics will accumulate in these areas and stimulate defence mechanisms within the pleura.

Macrophage recruitment and mesothelial cell proliferation in the pleura occur within days of asbestos inhalation in animal models, well before asbestos fibres can be demonstrated within the pleural space [36, 37]. It seems likely that these changes are induced by increasing levels of pulmonary-derived cytokines secreted in response to asbestos in the airways and lung parenchyma. Once asbestos fibres reach the pleural space, pleural macrophages and activated mesothelial cells will attempt phagocytosis within a matter of hours. This will further increase pleural concentrations of chemotactic and mitogenic factors, induce an inflammatory cascade, and contribute to the development of a stimulatory autocrine loop.

The prolonged production of the inflammatory cytokines transforming growth factor-β_1 (TGF-β_1) and platelet-derived growth factor (PDGF) has been implicated in the development and progression of mesothelioma. Mesothelial cells secrete these cytokines in response to an inflammatory stimulus, and their production has been shown to be increased in mesothelioma [38–40]. Increased local production of cytokines may also induce tumour angiogenesis and invasion through their effects on the extracellular matrix and fibroblasts.

The ability of macrophages to clear inhaled particles is finite. If mucociliary clearance mechanisms are impaired or a large particulate load is inhaled, not all fibres can be cleared. Asbestos fibres, particularly amphiboles, pose particular problems for lung-clearance mechanisms. The natural fibres are friable and easily fragment into smaller particles within the respirable range. Their aerodynamic shape enables them to pass deep into the airways where they are too large for efficient phagocytosis. This results in a relative accumulation of long fibres, with the short fibres being preferentially cleared. Finally, asbestos fibres are able to resist acid attack within macrophages, stimulating prolonged release of inflammatory cytokines and related factors. In summary, the physical properties of asbestos facilitate passage and its chemical properties resist removal.

Asbestos-induced carcinogenesis and the development of mesothelioma

Advances in molecular biology have identified some of the cellular processes that initiate and control malignant transformation. *In vitro* and *in vivo* systems have been developed to assess the carcinogenic potential of a wide range of substances. The cellular processes that control the cell cycle and DNA repair mechanisms, and the contribution of oncogenes and tumour suppressor genes to the development of cancer are being unravelled. Despite these advances, the exact mechanism by which malignant mesothelioma develops is uncertain.

The long latent period seen in asbestos-related cases of mesothelioma suggests that a multistep carcinogenic mechanism is involved. Unfortunately, there are discrepancies between cell culture and *in vivo* results, and between animal and human models. Different species, and different cell types from the same species, vary greatly in their susceptibility to the effects of carcinogens and promoter substances. The experimental method of fibre delivery can also influence subsequent carcinogenic potential.

A carcinogen is defined as a substance that induces neoplastic change in a cell [41]. A complete carcinogen can induce this change in a cell after a single exposure. There is experimental evidence that asbestos fibres are complete carcinogens for bronchial epithelial cells, as well as being fibrogenic in the lung and pleura. Whether asbestos is a complete carcinogen for the mesothelial cell remains the subject of some debate. Standard experimental studies of carcinogenicity are based on bacterial tests (Ames' test) or animal (usually rodent) models [41]. Bacterial tests have failed to confirm the carcinogenicity of asbestos. As bacterial cells do not ingest asbestos fibres, the potential for toxic effects is reduced compared with phagocytic mammalian cells. Extrapolation from animal studies assumes little or no interspecies variation in sensitivity to the effects of a carcinogen, which is not the case. It is recognized that the development of cancers in humans can be critically influenced by genetic, physiological, and environmental factors. Differences between species are likely to be greater than those within species. Within the rodent family, significant differences are seen in the sensitivity to the mutagenic effects of asbestos: hamsters are very sensitive, whilst guinea pigs are relatively resistant [42]. Therefore it is necessary to exercise caution when extrapolating animal experimental results to humans.

One problem relates to size. The length-to-width aspect of amphibole asbestos appears to be critical to mesothelioma induction [28]. Obviously, rodent airways are smaller than those of humans, which will limit the size of fibres that can pass beyond mucociliary clearance mechanisms. Rodent macrophages are also smaller than their human equivalents, which is an important consideration when assessing asbestos carcinogenicity according to fibre size [43].

Another problem with experimental models of mesothelioma induction relates to the method of asbestos delivery. In animal models, asbestos fibre delivery is often by non-physiological means (e.g. direct intratracheal or intrapleural installation). Therefore many of the physiological processes vital to asbestos clearance may be bypassed or overloaded. This markedly changes the amount and distribution of fibres within the lung and pleura compared with standard inhalation models, and makes evaluation of a threshold level difficult [42].

The lag phase seen in the development of mesothelioma in humans can also pose problems in the construction of experimental models. Most rodents have a lifespan of only 2–3 years. Conducting experiments over many years using cultured human cells is impractical. There is also some evidence that particulates, including asbestos, can facilitate transfection of foreign genes into mammalian cells [44]. This represents another potential oncogenic mechanism that may be relevant to the development of mesothelioma.

Three different mechanisms probably contribute to the genotoxicity of asbestos.

1. The chemical composition of asbestos promotes cation exchange.

2. The chemical and structural durability of asbestos induces and maintains ROS production, causing direct DNA damage.

3. Phagocytosed asbestos fibres physically interfere with cytoplasmic functions such as spindle formation during mitosis.

Asbestos is an insulator and therefore resists the free passage of electrons at physiological temperatures. Low-grade ion exchange from the active surface can occur within cells until the fibre is destroyed or its surface rendered passive. The most active part of the fibre surface is at the free end; interestingly, this is the part that shows most coating when asbestos bodies are formed. Chrysotile has a hollow central core, which can act as an ion reservoir and may explain why it appears more toxic than some amphiboles in cell culture studies [45]. Amphiboles have solid cores, but contain many surface sites that facilitate cation exchange. Erionite also has a very large surface area, most of which is internal and communicates with the fibre surface via tiny pores. One gram of erionite has an active surface area of over 200 m^2; crocidolite and chrysotile have surface areas of approximately 10 m^2/g and 24 m^2/g, respectively. These surface pores facilitate the passage of cations but are too small for larger antioxidant molecules, produced to counteract the toxic effects of ROS, to reach the most active parts of the fibre. Blocking surface pores with isopentane reduces erionite cytotoxicity by 50 per cent [46]. Redox reactions involving the fibre surface are perpetuated by a local supply of ions and enhanced by the presence of reduced iron (Fe^{3+}). Crocidolite is also capable of absorbing organic carcinogens, such as polyaromatic hydrocarbons, onto its surface. This may be another factor contributing to the synergistic effects of asbestos and smoking in the development of lung cancer [47, 48].

The length and width of an asbestos fibre, and particularly their ratio, is deemed critical for carcinogenesis. The definitive work of Stanton et al. [28] demonstrated that fibres more than 8 mm long and less than 0.25 mm wide were the most toxic. This fibre length is comparable to the diameter of a mesothelial cell. Intracytoplasmic asbestos fibres may therefore have a deleterious effect during mitosis. Spindle formation is vital to achieving the correct alignment and separation of sister chromatids, ensuring that each daughter cell receives an equal number of chromosomes. It has been shown experimentally that asbestos fibres collect in the perinuclear region following phagocytosis [49]. In this position they are well placed to affect spindle formation, thereby predisposing to chromosomal non-dysjunction and karyotypic abnormalities. The molecular biological changes associated with asbestos exposure will be discussed in detail in Chapter 6.

Chromosomal changes in malignant pleural mesothelioma

Chromosomal changes have been demonstrated in both animal and human models of mesothelioma. Some of these changes appear to be random, but others occur sufficiently frequently to imply that they may be critical to the development of mesothelioma. These include changes in regions containing proto-oncogenes and tumour suppressor genes already implicated in the development of other tumours

Some of the earliest *in vitro* work investigating asbestos-related chromosomal changes was that of Lechner *et al.* [50]. They initially studied the mutagenic effects of asbestos on human mesothelial cells derived from non-malignant pleural effusions. These were cultured with UICC standard amosite, chrysotile, and crocidolite fibres, and assessed for both cytotoxicity and carcinogenicity. Human mesothelial cells were 10 times more sensitive to the cytotoxic effects of asbestos than bronchial epithelial cells. Chrysotile was the most toxic, followed by amosite and crocidolite. In carcinogenicity testing, prolonged culture with amosite produced multiple karyotypic changes, particularly losses from chromosomes 11 and 21. The *in vitro* finding that chrysotile was the most genotoxic fibre conflicts with the currently held view that pure serpentine asbestos rarely, if ever, causes mesothelioma *in vivo*. This may relate to the type of fibres used. At the time of this study the UICC standard crocidolite was composed of relatively short fibres (<2.5 mm) which are now recognized as being less pathogenic than longer fibres [51]. Using crocidolite fibres within the Stanton range has confirmed that amphiboles are more genotoxic than serpentine asbestos [46]. An alternative interpretation of these data is that chrysotile can induce mesothelioma, but only if it is able to reach the pleura.

In 1989 Olofsson and Mark [52] investigated the effects of incubating human mesothelial cells with crocidolite, chrysotile, or amosite. All fibres caused numerical and structural chromosomal abnormalities, which were predominantly seen in chromosomes 1, 4, 6, 9, 13, and 17. The authors concluded that asbestos has a propensity to preferentially induce changes in specific chromosomes. Their failure to detect abnormalities seen more commonly in mesothelioma (e.g. monosomy 22) may indicate that such changes develop later, after initial asbestos-induced changes have occurred.

Several groups have investigated the type and number of karyotypic changes in human mesothelioma cells. In contrast with the previously mentioned *in vitro* experiments on non-malignant mesothelial cells exposed to asbestos, these experiments describe chromosomal changes that have persisted or accompanied mesothelioma development. Comparisons can then be made with non-asbestos-related tumours to determine whether different genetic mechanisms are implicated in tumour development. Karyotyping studies have demonstrated that most mesotheliomas have multiple chromosomal abnormalities, with the majority having 10 or more identifiable alterations [53–78]. Changes in association with oncogenes and tumour suppressor genes already implicated in the development of other tumours have been identified. These include p53, p15 and p16, NF2 (neurofibromatosis-2), WT1 (Wilms tumour product-1), SEN6, Rb1 (retinoblastoma-1), and the viral oncogene v-*cis*. The genetic changes seen in mesothelioma are discussed in more detail elsewhere in this book.

DNA flow cytometry has also been used to evaluate chromosomal changes in mesothelioma [53, 79–85]. Most mesotheliomas remain diploid or pseudodiploid. Aneuploid tumours appear to have a poorer prognosis [53, 85]. The genetic abnormalities associated with mesothelioma will be discussed in further detail in Chapter 11.

Other causes of malignant mesothelioma

Simian virus 40

The role of simian virus 40 (SV40) in the pathogenesis of malignant pleural mesothelioma is a contentious issue. The following section gives an overview of the data pertaining to SV40 in this disease which will be discussed further in Chapters 2 and 7.

There have been few indications as to whether any other aetiological factors are important in the development of mesothelioma. It remains a fact that a significant number of patients with mesothelioma irrefutably have had no personal exposure to asbestos above 'normal' environmental levels. These tumours appear to be histologically and clinically identical to their asbestos-related counterparts. This poses the question as to whether there are other patient-related factors or carcinogens yet to be identified. Two possible causal agents have been suggested: SV40 and ionizing radiation. The potential influence of other carcinogens and genetic factors on the development of mesothelioma has been reviewed by Heineman *et al.* [22] and Peterson *et al.* [86].

SV40 is a papovavirus that is endemic and non-pathogenic in rhesus and cynomolgus monkeys. There is experimental evidence that SV40 is oncogenic in rodents and in some human cells *in vitro*. The isolation of SV40-like DNA sequences from human tumours, including mesothelioma, has been suggested as evidence that it may also be oncogenic in humans. In the 1950s and 1960s millions of adults and children were inadvertently vaccinated with polio- and adenovirus vaccines contaminated with SV40, raising the possibility of a major public health scare if the oncogenic effects of SV40 were to be confirmed.

Vaccination programmes against poliomyelitis were introduced in the 1950s. These vaccines were initially produced in culture from monolayers of rhesus monkey kidney cells. When culture methods were changed and green monkey kidney cells were used, the presence of an infecting agent was noted. Sweet and Hilleman [87] first reported vacuolation in the kidney cell cultures in 1960. By 1962 it had been confirmed that live SV40 had contaminated several batches of both forms of poliovaccine, as well as some adenovirus vaccines [88]. It was still uncertain whether this should cause concern, as SV40 was thought to be non-pathogenic in humans. By 1964 it was confirmed that SV40 was oncogenic in rodents and was capable of transforming human cells *in vitro* [89, 90]. Despite more than three decades of research, the risk to humans from these contaminated vaccines remains unclear.

Mesothelioma is one of the human tumours in which SV40 has been implicated. Experimental studies of SV40 oncogenesis were first performed in hamsters, which are particularly sensitive to its transforming effects. Tumours developed following inoculation by several different routes, and were most frequent in young animals. Fibrosarcomas developed at the site of subcutaneous injection, and ependymomas after intracerebral injection [91]. Cicala *et al.* [92] injected SV40 directly into the pleura and peritoneum of young hamsters; mesothelioma rates were 100 per cent and 67 per cent, respectively, within 3–6 months. Mesotheliomas also developed in 60 per cent of young hamsters after intracardiac injection of SV40; the remaining animals developed osteosarcomas and lymphomas.

Although SV40 appears to be inactivated when administered by the oral route, it is excreted in stool for up to 5 weeks after ingestion [93]. Antibodies to SV40 are demonstrable for at least 3 years after inoculation, and are also seen in a small proportion of those who have never received contaminated vaccines [94]. Hence, although the parenteral forms of vaccine potentially pose the greater risk to humans, the possibility of other mechanisms of infection (e.g. faeco-oral spread) cannot be entirely dismissed.

The effects of SV40 on human cells *in vitro* have been investigated. SV40 can transform and immortalize some human cells, and this effect is enhanced by the presence of asbestos [95, 96]. The transformed cells are tumorigenic when injected into human volunteers [97]. As in the rodent model, it appears that SV40 predominantly affects ependyma, choroid plexus, bone, and mesothelium.

After SV40 was first identified there were sporadic reports of SV40-like DNA sequences isolated from tumours in humans [98]. The technology for DNA sequencing was still quite primitive at that time, and it was not certain whether some of these results were actually due to contamination of reagents with SV40, cross-reactions with related viruses, or differences in experimental technique and primers. In 1992 Bergsagel *et al.* [99] used a polymerase chain reaction (PCR) technique to demonstrate SV40-like sequences in human ependymomas and choroid plexus tumours. Subsequently, Carbone *et al.* [95] showed that 60 per cent of mesotheliomas tested were also positive for this sequence. Normal lung tissue in individuals with mesothelioma did not contain this viral sequence; neither did tumours originating from other tissues. Interestingly, Finnish researchers were unable to demonstrate SV40 sequences in pleural mesothelioma. Finland has a low incidence of mesothelioma, and Finnish poliovaccine was never demonstrably contaminated with SV40.

In order to investigate the relationship between SV40 and mesothelioma definitively, an international multi-institutional study was initiated by the International Mesothelioma Interest Group (IMIG) in 1997. Twelve samples of snap-frozen tumours provided by an independent source were sent to each of four separate laboratories and were analysed for SV40 sequences using a fixed protocol and standard primers. Nine of the 12 samples provided identical results in all four laboratories; the others were non-consistently positive. Two of the three negative samples were also negative for the presence of the SV40-related antigen Tag on immunohistochemistry [100].

Another approach to investigating the relationship between SV40 and human cancer is to see whether the incidence of the specific tumours produced by SV40 in animals has increased in humans since administration of contaminated vaccines. Three separate groups have reported the results of such studies [101–103]. Unfortunately, all the tumours that may relate to SV40 are rare, which makes the evaluation of changes in incidence difficult. In particular, mesothelioma in children has only been described in a handful of cases worldwide [24, 25].

The results of a 20-year follow-up study of 1073 children born between 1960 and 1962, who were potentially exposed to SV40 as neonates, were published in 1981 [101]. No cancer deaths were seen in the children in this group; however, only one childhood cancer death would be expected in a cohort of this size. Therefore this study could have missed a statistically significant increase in cancer deaths in those lost to follow-up, and was probably not large enough to evaluate absolute risk.

Another study investigating cancer rates in SV40-exposed children was published in 1998 [103]. This retrospective cohort study specifically addressed whether there was a demonstrable increase in incidence of those cancers most strongly associated with SV40: ependymomas, osteosarcomas, and mesotheliomas. Cancer rates were calculated from the Surveillance, Epidemiology and End Results (SEER) data (1973–1993), which covers almost 10 per cent of the population of the USA, the Connecticut Tumor Registry (1950–1969), and national mortality statistics (1947–1973). There was no discernible increase in any of these tumours in exposed individuals. The study methodology has been criticized, particularly regarding age comparisons, as the cancer registry data age stratification is not comparable to the age cohorts chosen in the study group. It has again been questioned whether this study was statistically powerful enough to identify a significant increase in tumours; it reported a threefold increase in risk for developing mesothelioma, yet this failed to reach statistical significance. It has also been claimed that although gross cancer rates have not increased, the age-specific rates for ependymomas and osteosarcomas have increased by 20 per cent since 1973 [104].

In conclusion, there is evidence of an association between SV40 and some human tumours, including mesothelioma. Whether this is a causal association is still not clear. Is SV40 a pathogen or a passenger?

Ionizing radiation

Ionizing radiation is recognized as causing direct DNA damage. Pleural mesothelioma has been experimentally produced in rodents following inhalation of plutonium, and peritoneal tumours have resulted from the intraperitoneal implantation of plutonium oxide ($^{239}PuO_2$) [105]. Therefore it is biologically plausible that some cases of mesothelioma may have resulted from previous radiotherapy treatment or other sources of radiation. There have also been a small number of case reports of development of mesothelioma following radiotherapy, particularly for Hodgkin's disease [106, 107].

Three retrospective studies have investigated a possible relationship between mesothelioma and radiation [106, 108, 109]. Cavazza et al. [109] undertook a retrospective study to evaluate the proportion of mesotheliomas that might be radiotherapy related. This was done in two ways. Initially they searched for mesothelioma patients with a history of previous cancers treated with radiotherapy. Eight patients were identified: six following treatment for Hodgkin's disease, and two following treatment for breast carcinoma. Secondly, a population-based study was performed using cancer statistics provided by the SEER registry. Out of a total of 1 489 643 registered cancer patients, 142 were recorded as having developed mesothelioma as a second cancer. Only 37 of these 142 had undergone prior radiotherapy treatment. Most of the mesotheliomas developed within 10 years of their first cancer, and not all tumours were within the original radiotherapy field. The investigators concluded that radiotherapy is a very uncommon cause of mesothelioma. In the same year, Weissmann et al. [106] investigated the possible relationship between radiotherapy and mesothelioma. They followed up a 12-year cohort (1982–1993) of patients with Hodgkin's disease. Four cases of subsequent mesothelioma were identified, two pleural and two peritoneal. The mean interval from treatment to mesothelioma development was 17 years.

One of the largest retrospective studies has been undertaken by Neugut et al. [108]. They followed up two large cohorts of patients with breast cancer ($n = 251 750$) and Hodgkin's disease ($n = 13 743$) registered by SEER in the period 1973–1993. Approximately a quarter ($n = 62 453$) of the breast cancer patients and half ($n = 6961$) of the Hodgkin's patients had received radiotherapy as part of their treatment. Cases diagnosed within 5 years of the first cancer were excluded, as were those with missing clinical information. Six cases of pleural mesothelioma were identified in the breast cancer group, four of whom had not received radiotherapy. There were no cases of mesothelioma in the Hodgkin's group. The estimated relative risk for the development of mesothelioma was calculated at 1.56 (95 per cent confidence interval, 0.18–5.63). With such a wide confidence interval it is difficult to make a firm conclusion regarding the influence of radiotherapy. It should also be remembered that both breast cancer and lymphoma commonly metastasize to the pleura, and may resemble mesothelioma histologically. Thoracic radiation can cause lung cancer within the radiotherapy field, and such tumours can also mimic mesothelioma clinically, radiologically, and pathologically. The authors did not state whether histological review was undertaken in the six cases of mesothelioma in the breast cancer group.

In conclusion, although it is biologically plausible that a small number of cases of mesothelioma may arise from radiotherapy treatment, the overall contribution of radiation to the development of mesothelioma is likely to be slight.

Conclusions

The biology of mesothelioma is complex and incompletely understood. Amphibole asbestos is accepted as the primary cause of most cases of mesothelioma in the UK, but the mechanisms by which asbestos induces malignant change in the mesothelium have not been entirely elucidated. Whether chrysotile causes mesothelioma remains a contentious issue.

Other causes of mesothelioma have not been confirmed with any certainty. Familial studies and chromosomal analysis of tumour specimens have suggested that genetic factors may be important, but no single specific gene or chromosome abnormality has yet been implicated. Concerns remain regarding the putative relationship between mesothelioma and SV40, but it is likely to be some time before an unequivocal conclusion as to the importance of SV40 can be made. Chronic pleural inflammation and thoracic radiation remain as potential causes of mesothelioma, but the overall number of cases likely to arise from them is small.

References

1. Office for National Statistics. *Cancer Statistics—Registrations (England and Wales 1992). Series MBI No. 25.* London: Stationery Office, 1992.
2. Peto J, Hodgson J, Matthews F, *et al.* Continuing increase in mesothelioma mortality in Britain. *Lancet* 1995; **345**: 535–9.
3. Peto J, Decarli A, La Vecchia C, *et al.* The European mesothelioma epidemic. *Br J Cancer* 1999; **79**: 666–72.
4. Health and Safety Executive. *Mesothelioma Mortality in Great Britain: Estimating the Future Burden.* London: Health and Safety Executive, 2003.
5. *Asbestos Regulations 1969 (SI 1969 No. 690).* London: HMSO, 1969.
6. Neumann V, Muller KM, Fischer M. [Peritoneal mesothelioma—incidence and etiology]. *Pathologe* 1999; **20**: 169–76 (in German).
7. Robertson H. Endothelioma of the pleura. *J Cancer Res* 1924; **8**: 317–75.
8. Wagner E. Das tuberkelähnliche Lymphadenom. *Archiv Heilk* 1870; **11**: 497–528.
9. Willis R. *Pathology of Tumours*, 2nd edn. London: Butterworths, 1953.
10. Klemperer P, Rabin C. Primary neoplasms of the pleura: a report of five cases. *Arch Pathol* 1931; **141**: 385–412.
11. Stout A, Murray M. Localised pleural mesothelioma. *Arch Pathol* 1941; **34**: 951–64.
12. Campbell W. Pleural mesothelioma. *Am J Pathol* 1950; **26**: 473–87.
13. McCaughey W. Primary tumours of the pleura. *J Pathol Bacteriol* 1958; **76**: 517–29.
14. Wagner J, Sleggs C, Marchand P. Diffuse pleural mesothelioma and asbestos exposure in the north western Cape Province. *Br J Ind Med* 1960; **17**: 260–71.
15. Asbestos Institute, 2002. Available online at: www.asbestos-institute.ca
16. Ribak J, Lilis R, Suzuki Y, *et al.* Malignant mesothelioma in a cohort of asbestos insulation workers: clinical presentation, diagnosis and causes of death. *Br J Ind Med* 1988; **45**: 182–7.
17. McDonald A, McDonald J. Mesothelioma after crocidolite exposure during gas mask manufacture. *Environ Res* 1978; **17**: 340–6.
18. Jones J, Smith P, Pooley F, *et al.* The consequences of exposure to asbestos dust in a wartime gas-mask factory. In: Wagner JC, ed. *The Biological Effects of Mineral Fibre.* Lyon: IARC Scientific Publications, 1980; 637–53.
19. Baris Y, Sahin A, Ozesmi M, *et al.* An outbreak of pleural mesotheliomas and chronic fibrosing pleurisy in the village of Karain/Urgup in Anatolia. *Thorax* 1978; **33**: 181–92.
20. Vianna N, Polan A. Non-occupational exposure to asbestos and malignant mesothelioma in females. *Lancet* 1978: 1061–3.

21. Newhouse M, Thompson H. Mesothelioma of the pleura and peritoneum following exposure to asbestos in the London area. *Br J Ind Med* 1965; **22**: 261–9.

22. Heineman E, Bernstein L, Stark A, *et al*. Mesothelioma, asbestos, and reported history of cancer in first-degree relatives. *Cancer* 1996; **77**: 549–54.

23. Roushdy-Hammady I, Siegel J, Emri S, *et al*. Genetic-susceptibility factor and malignant mesothelioma in the Cappadocian region of Turkey. *Lancet* 2001; **357**: 444–5.

24. Grundy G, Miller R. Malignant mesothelioma in childhood. *Cancer* 1972; **30**: 1216–18.

25. Wasserman M, Wasserman D, Steinitz R, *et al*. Mesothelioma in children. In: Wagner JC, ed. *The Biological Effects of Mineral Fibre*. Lyon: IARC Scientific Publications, 1980; 253.

26. Selikoff I, Hammond E, Seidman H. Latency of asbestos disease among insulation workers in the United States and Canada. *Cancer* 1980; **46**: 2736–40.

27. Bianchi C, Giarelli L, Grandi G, *et al*. Latency periods in asbestos-related mesothelioma of the pleura. *Eur J Cancer Prev* 1997; **6**: 162–6.

28. Stanton M, Layard M, Tegeris A, *et al*. Relation of particle dimension to carcinogenicity in amphibole asbestoses and other fibrous minerals. *J Natl Cancer Inst* 1981; **67**: 965–75.

29. Abratt RP, Vorobiof DA, White N. Asbestos and mesothelioma in South Africa. *Lung Cancer* 2004; **45** (Suppl 1): S3–6.

30. Nishimura S, Broaddus V. Asbestos-induced pleural disease. *Clin Chest Med* 1998; **19**: 311–29.

31. Guthrie Jr G. Mineral properties and their contributions to particle toxicity. *Environ Health Perspect* 1997; **105**: 1003–11.

32. Lippmann M, Yeates D, Albert R. Deposition, retention, and clearance of inhaled particles. *Br J Ind Med* 1980; **37**: 337–62.

33. Dong H, Buard A, Renier A, *et al*. Role of oxygen derivatives in the cytotoxicity and DNA damage produced by asbestos on rat pleural mesothelial cells *in vivo*. *Carcinogenesis* 1994; **15**: 1251–5.

34. Jaurand M-C. Mechanisms of fiber-induced genotoxicity. *Environ Health Perspect* 1997; **105**: 1073–84.

35. Wang N-S. Anatomy of the pleura. *Clin Chest Med* 1998; **19**: 229–39.

36. Adamson I. Early mesothelial cell proliferation after asbestos exposure: *in vivo* and *in vitro* studies. *Environ Health Perspect* 1997; **105**: 1205–8.

37. Choe N, Tanaka S, Xia W, *et al*. Pleural macrophage recruitment and activation in asbestos-induced pleural injury. *Environ Health Perspect* 1997; **105**: 1257–60.

38. Garlepp M, Leong C. Biological and immunological aspects of malignant mesothelioma. *Eur Respir J* 1995; **8**: 643–50.

39. Gerwin B, Lechner J, Reddel R, *et al*. Comparison of production of transforming growth factor-β and platelet derived growth factor by normal human mesothelial cells and mesothelioma cell lines. *Cancer Res* 1987; **47**: 6180–4.

40. Walker C, Bermudez E, Stewart W, *et al*. Growth factor and growth factor receptor expression in transformed rat mesothelial cells. In: Brown RC, Hoskins JA, Johnson NF, ed. *Mechanisms in Fibre Carcinogenesis*. New York: Plenum Press, 1991; 377–83.

41. Tennant R, Wigley C, Balmain A. Chemical carcinogenesis. In: Teich N, ed. *Introduction to the Cellular and Molecular Biology of Cancer*, 3rd edn. Oxford: Oxford University Press, 1998; 106–29.

42. Bignon J, Brochard P. Animal and cell models for understanding and predicting fibre-related mesothelioma in man. In: Brown RC, Hoskins JA, Johnson NF, ed. *Mechanisms in Fibre Carcinogenesis*. New York: Plenum Press, 1991; 515–30.

43. Krombach F, Münzing S, Allmeling A-M, *et al*. Cell size of alveolar macrophages: an interspecies comparison. *Environ Health Perspect* 1995; **105**: 1261–3.

44. Jaurand M-C. Mechanisms of fibre genotoxicity. In: Brown RC, Hoskins JA, Johnson NF, ed. *Mechanisms in Fibre Carcinogenesis*. New York: Plenum Press, 1991; 287–307.

45. Lechner J, Tesfaigzi J, Gerwin B. Oncogenes and tumor-suppressor genes in mesothelioma: a synopsis. *Environ Health Perspect* 1997; **105**: 1061–7.

46. Coffin D, Ghio A. Relative intrinsic potency of asbestos and erionite fibers: proposed mechanism of action. In: Brown RC, Hoskins JA, Johnson NF, ed. *Mechanisms in Fibre Carcinogenesis*. New York: Plenum Press, 1991; 71–80.

47. Fubini B. Surface reactivity in the pathogenic response to particulates. *Environ Health Perspect* 1997; **105**: 1013–20.

48. Meldrum M. *Review of Fibre Toxicity (OELS)*. London: Health and Safety Executive, 1996.

49. Barrett J. Mechanisms of action of known carcinogens. In: McMichael A, ed. *Mechanisms of Carcinogenesis in Risk Identification*. Lyon: IARC Scientific Publications, 1992; 115–34.

50. Lechner J, Tokiwa T, La Veck M, *et al.* Asbestos-associated chromosomal changes in human mesothelial cells. *Proc Natl Acad Sci USA* 1985; **82**: 3884–8.

51. Davis J. Experimental studies on mineral fibre carcinogenesis: an overview. In: Brown RC, Hoskins JA, Johnson NF, ed. *Mechanisms in Fibre Carcinogenesis*. New York: Plenum Press, 1991; 51–58.

52. Olofsson K, Mark J. Specificity of asbestos-induced chromosomal aberrations in short-term cultured human mesothelial cells. *Cancer Genet Cytogenet* 1989; **41**: 33–9.

53. Tiainen M, Rautonen J, Pyrhonen S, *et al.* Chromosome number correlates with survival in patients with malignant pleural mesothelioma. *Cancer Genet Cytogenet* 1992; **62**: 21–4.

54. Taguchi T, Jhanwar S, Siegfried J, *et al.* Recurrent deletions of specific chromosomal sites in 1p, 3p, 6q, and 9p in human malignant mesothelioma. *Cancer Res* 1993; **53**: 4349–55.

55. Mark J. Monosomy 14, monosomy 22 and 13q: three chromosomal abnormalities observed in cells of two malignant mesotheliomas studied by banding techniques. *Acta Cytol* 1978; **22**: 398–401.

56. Popescu N, Chahinian A, DiPaolo J. Non-random chromosome alterations in human malignant mesothelioma. *Cancer Res* 1988; **48**: 142–7.

57. Flejter W, Li F, Antman K, *et al.* Recurring loss involving chromosomes 1, 3, and 22 in malignant mesothelioma: possible sites of tumour supressor genes. *Genes Chromosomes Cancer* 1989; **1**: 148–54.

58. Tiainen M, Tammilehto L, Rautonen J, *et al.* Chromosomal abnormalities and their correlations with asbestos exposure and survival in patients with mesothelioma. *Br J Cancer* 1989; **60**: 618–26.

59. Hagemeijer A, Versnel M, Van Drunen E, *et al.* Cytogenetic analysis of malignant mesothelioma. *Cancer Genet Cytogenet* 1990; **47**: 1–28.

60. Pelin-Enlund K, Husgafvel-Pursiainen K, Tammilehto L, *et al.* Asbestos-related malignant mesothelioma: growth, cytology, tumorigenicity and consistant chromosome findings in cell lines from five patients. *Carcinogenesis* 1990; **11**: 673–81.

61. Tammilehto L, Tuomi T, Tiainen M, *et al.* Malignant mesothelioma; clinical characteristics, asbestos mineralogy and chromosomal abnormalities of 41 patients. *Eur J Cancer* 1992; **28A**: 1373–9.

62. Center R, Lukeis R, Deitzch E, *et al.* Molecular deletion of 9p sequences in non-small cell lung cancer and malignant mesothelioma. *Genes Chromosomes Cancer* 1993; **7**: 47–53.

63. Cheng J, Jhanwar S, Lu Y, *et al.* Homozygous deletions within 9p21-p22 identify a small critical region of chromosomal loss in human malignant mesothelioma. *Cancer Res* 1993; **53**: 4761–3.

64. Cheng J, Jhanwar S, Klein W, *et al.* p16 alterations and deletion mapping of 9p21-p22 in malignant mesothelioma. *Cancer Res* 1994; **54**: 5547–51.

65. Lu Y, Jhanwar S, Cheng J, *et al.* Deletion mapping of the short arm of chromosome 3 in human malignant mesothelioma. *Genes Chromosomes Cancer* 1994; **9**: 76–80.

66. Bianchi A, Mitsunaga S, Cheng J, *et al.* High frequency of inactivating mutations in the neurofibromatosis type 2 gene (NF2) in primary malignant mesotheliomas. *Proc Natl Acad Sci USA* 1995; **92**: 10854–8.

67. Sekido Y, Pass H, Bader S, *et al.* Neurofibromatosis type 2 (NF2) gene is somatically mutated in mesothelioma but not in lung cancer. *Cancer Res* 1995; **55**: 1227–31.

68. Shivapurkar N, Virmani A, Wistuba I, *et al.* Deletions of chromosome 4 at multiple sites are frequent in malignant mesothelioma and small cell lung carcinoma. *Clin Cancer Res* 1999; **5**: 17–23.

69. Xio S, Li D, Vijg J, *et al.* Codeletion of p15 and p16 in primary malignant mesothelioma. *Oncogene* 1995; **11**: 511–15.

70. Cheng J, Lee W, Klein M, *et al*. Frequent mutations of NF2 and allelic loss from chromosome 22q12 in malignant mesothelioma: evidence for a two-hit mechanism of NF2 inactivation. *Genes Chromosomes Cancer* 1999; **24**: 238–42.

71. Balsara B, Bell D, Sonoda G, *et al*. Comparative genomic hybridization and loss of heterozygosity analyses identify a common region of deletion at 15q11.1–15 in human malignant mesothelioma. *Cancer Res* 1999; **59**: 450–4.

72. Björkqvist A-M, Tammilehto L, Anttila S, *et al*. Recurrent DNA copy number changes in 1q, 4q, 6q, 9p, 13q, 14q, and 22q detected by comparative genomic hybridization in malignant mesothelioma. *Br J Cancer* 1997; **75**: 523–7.

73. Björkqvist A-M, Tammilehto L, Nordling S, *et al*. Comparison of DNA copy number changes in malignant mesothelioma, adenocarcinoma and large-cell anaplastic carcinoma of the lung. *Br J Cancer* 1998; **77**: 260–9.

74. Bell D, Jhanwar S, Testa J. Multiple regions of allelic loss from chromosome arm 6q in malignant mesothelioma. *Cancer Res* 1997; **57**: 4057–62.

75. Lee W, Balsara B, Liu Z, *et al*. Loss of heterozygosity analysis defines a critical region in chromosome 1p22 commonly deleted in human malignant mesothelioma. *Cancer Res* 1996; **56**: 4297–301.

76. Ribotta M, Roseo F, Salvio M, *et al*. Recurrent chromosome 6 abnormalities in malignant mesothelioma. *Monaldi Arch Chest Dis* 1998; **53**: 228–35.

77. Deguen B, Goutebroze L, Giovannini M, *et al*. Heterogeneity of mesothelioma cell lines as defined by altered genomic structure and expression of the NF2 gene. *Int J Cancer* 1998; **77**: 554–60.

78. Pass H, Stevens E, Oie H, *et al*. Characteristics of nine newly derived mesothelioma cell lines. *Ann Thorac Surg* 1995; **59**: 835–44.

79. Dressler L, Bartow S. DNA flow cytometry in solid tumours: practical aspects and clinical applications. *Semin Diagn Pathol* 1989; **6**: 55–82.

80. Croonen A, van der Valk P, Herman C, *et al*. Cytology, immunopathology and flow cytometry in the diagnosis of pleural and peritoneal mesothelioma. *Lab Invest* 1988; **58**: 725–32.

81. Burner G, Rabinovitch P, Kulander B, *et al*. Flow cytometric analysis of malignant pleural mesothelioma. *Hum Pathol* 1989; **20**: 777–83.

82. Pyrhonen S, Laasonen A, Tammilehto L, *et al*. Diploid predominance and prognostic significance of s-phase cells in malignant mesothelioma. *Eur J Cancer* 1991; **27**: 197–200.

83. Dazzi H, Thatcher N, Hasleton P, *et al*. DNA analysis by flow cytometry in malignant pleural mesothelioma: relationship to histology and survival. *J Pathol* 1990; **162**: 51–5.

84. Esteban J, Sheibani K. DNA ploidy analysis of pleural mesotheliomas: its usefulness for their distinction from lung adenocarcinomas. *Mod Pathol* 1992; **5**: 626–30.

85. Isobe H, Sridhar K, Doria R, *et al*. Prognostic significance of DNA aneuploidy in diffuse malignant mesothelioma. *Cytometry* 1995; **19**: 86–91.

86. Peterson J, Greenberg S, Buffler P. Non-asbestos-related malignant mesothelioma. *Cancer* 1984; **54**: 951–60.

87. Sweet B, Hilleman M. The vacuolating virus, SV_{40}. *Proc Soc Exp Biol Med* 1960; **105**: 420–7.

88. Eddy B. Identification of the oncogenic substance in rhesus monkey kidney cells as simian virus 40. *Virology* 1962; **17**: 65–75.

89. Eddy B. Simian virus 40: an oncogenic virus. *Prog Exp Tumour Res* 1964; **4**: 1–26.

90. Shein H, Enders J. Multiplication and cytopathogenicity of simian vacuolating virus 40 in cultures of human tissues. *Proc Soc Exp Biol Med* 1962; **109**: 495–500.

91. Kirschstein R, Gerber P. Ependymomas produced after intracerebral inoculation of SV40 into newborn hamsters. *Nature* 1962; **195**: 299–300.

92. Cicala C, Pompetti F, Carbone M. SV40 induces mesotheliomas in hamsters. *Am J Pathol* 1993; **142**: 1524–33.

93. Melnick J, Stinebaugh S. Excretion of vacuolating SV-40 virus (papova virus group) after ingestion as a contaminant of oral poliovaccine. *Proc Soc Exp Biol Med* 1962; **109**: 965–8.

94. Shah K, McCrumb F, Daniel R, *et al.* Serologic evidence for a simian-virus-40-like infection of man. *J Natl Cancer Inst* 1972; **48**: 557–61.

95. Carbone M, Pass H, Rizzo P, *et al.* Simian virus 40-like DNA sequences in human pleural mesothelioma. *Oncogene* 1994; **9**: 1781–90.

96. Mayall FG, Jacobson G, Wilkins R. Mutations of p53 gene and SV40 sequences in asbestos associated and non-asbestos-associated mesotheliomas. *J Clin Pathol* 1999; **52**: 291–3.

97. Jensen F, Koprowski H, Pagano J, *et al.* Autologous and homologous implantation of human cells transformed *in vitro* by SV40. *J Natl Cancer Inst* 1964; **32**: 917–25.

98. Carbone M, Rizzo P, Pass H. Association of simian virus 40 with rodent and human mesotheliomas. In: Friedman H, ed. *DNA Tumour Viruses: Oncogenic Mechanisms.* New York: Plenum Press, 1995; 75–90.

99. Bergsagel D, Finegold M, Butel J, *et al.* DNA sequences similar to those of simian virus 40 in ependymomas and choroid plexus tumours of childhood. *N Engl J Med* 1992; **36**: 988–93.

100. Testa J, Carbone M, Hirvonen A, *et al.* A multi-institutional study confirms the presence and expression of simian virus 40 in human malignant mesothelioma. *Cancer Res* 1998; **58**: 4505–9.

101. Mortimer E, Lepow M, Gold E, *et al.* Long-term follow-up of persons inadvertently inoculated with SV40 as neonates. *N Engl J Med* 1981; **305**: 1517–18.

102. Geissler E. SV40 and human brain tumours. *Prog Med Virol* 1990; **37**: 211–22.

103. Strickler H, Rosenberg P, Devesa S, *et al.* Contamination of poliovirus vaccines with simian virus 40 (1955–1963) and subsequent cancer rates. *JAMA* 1998; **279**: 292–5.

104. Carbone M, Rizzo P, Pass H. Simian virus 40, poliovaccines and human tumours: a review of recent developments. *Oncogene* 1997; **15**: 1877–88.

105. Sanders C. Pleural mesothelioma in the rat following exposure to ^{239}PuO$_2$. *Health Phys* 1992; **63**: 695–7.

106. Weissmann L, Corson J, Neugut A, *et al.* Malignant mesothelioma following treatment for Hodgkin's disease. *J Clin Oncol* 1996; **14**: 2098–2100.

107. Peto J, Seidman H, Selikoff I. Mesothelioma mortality in asbestos workers: implications for models of carcinogenesis and risk assessment. *Br J Cancer* 1982; **45**: 124–35.

108. Neugut A, Ahsan H, Antman K. Incidence of malignant pleural mesothelioma after thoracic radiotherapy. *Cancer* 1997; **80**: 948–50.

109. Cavazza A, Travis L, Travis W, *et al.* Post-irradiation malignant mesothelioma. *Cancer* 1996; **77**: 1379–85.

Chapter 2

Malignant mesothelioma: epidemiological snapshots from around the world

A brief history of asbestos use

R. P. Abratt

Asbestos has remarkable properties and has been used by humans for many centuries. The word 'asbestos' means inextinguishable or unquenchable. It is flexible and has great tensile strength. These properties make it an ideal compound for use in the construction industry and insulation.

Asbestos was initially used for wicks in lamps and candles as far back as 4000 BC. Between 2000 and 3000 BC the embalmed bodies of Egyptian pharaohs were wrapped in asbestos cloths to offset the ravages of time. In Finland, asbestos was used to strengthen clay pots in the period around 2500 BC. There is anecdotal evidence that Charlemagne (742–814 AD) had a tablecloth made from woven asbestos. The Mediterranean people used chrysotile from Cyprus and tremolite from upper Italy for the fabrication of cremation cloths, mats, and wicks for temple lamps from 1000 AD. Marco Polo visited an asbestos mine in China in the latter half of the thirteenth century. He concluded that asbestos was a stone and laid to rest the myth that it was the hair of a woolly lizard. Asbestos papers and boards were made in Italy from the early eighteenth century. Benjamin Franklin bought a purse made of asbestos which is now in the Natural History Museum, London.

In 1828 a US patent was issued for asbestos insulating material used in steam engines. By 1853 asbestos helmets and jackets were being worn by the Parisian Fire Brigade, and from 1866 moulded lagging materials were made from waterglass and asbestos. The first asbestos brake linings were made by Ferodo Ltd in England in 1896. In 1900 high-pressure asbestos gaskets were made by Klinger in Austria, and in 1913 the first asbestos pipes were developed in Italy. Standard corrugated sheets were introduced in Australia by Hardies in 1919. During the Second World War the use of asbestos included fireproof suits and parachute flares. Perhaps most appropriately, in the film *The Wizard of Oz*, released in 1939, the Wicked Witch of the West appeared on a broom made of asbestos.

The post-war years saw a rapid expansion in the use of asbestos as many construction projects relied heavily on it, and its use reached an all-time high in 1973. Indeed, in the 1990s the solid fuel boosters of the space shuttle were insulated with asbestos.

As a result of its widespread use, asbestos-related diseases, and particularly malignant mesothelioma, have become a worldwide problem (Fig. 2.1). These diseases will have a particular impact in the developing world in the future where fibres are still being sold for building and insulation purposes.

The following sections describe the epidemiology and aetiology of malignant mesothelioma from four countries and give a flavour of the problems faced by each.

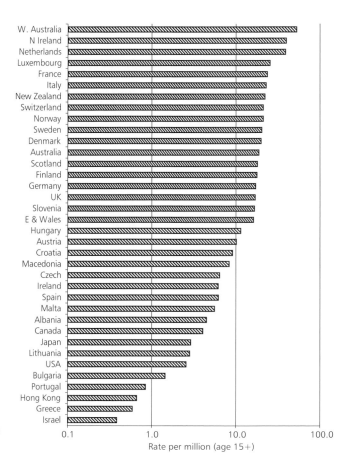

Figure 2.1 World mesothelioma mortality in males (1995).

Malignant mesothelioma in Australia

A. W. Musk and N. H. de Klerk

Introduction

Data describing the epidemic of malignant mesothelioma in Australia has been derived from mandatory death and cancer registrations in all states, a survey of incident cases dating back as far as records existed in which all pathologists from major hospitals and laboratories in Australia were contacted in collaboration with the Royal Australasian College of Pathologists [1], the Australian Mesothelioma Surveillance Program [2] which was established in January 1980, and follow-up of workers in the Wittenoom crocidolite industry [3] and residents of the township of Wittenoom, Western Australia [4].

In Australia more chrysotile than amphibole asbestos was mined until 1939 when production of crocidolite from Wittenoom, Western Australia, which commenced in 1937, exceeded local production of other forms [5]. Wittenoom production also exceeded imported amosite and approached levels of imported chrysotile during the 1950s. Locally produced chrysotile increased rapidly during the 1970s, but both production and importation diminished progressively during the early 1980s. Consumption of asbestos peaked in about 1975 at about 70 000 tons/year. In addition to production and importation of asbestos fibre, Australia also imported many manufactured asbestos products including asbestos cement articles, asbestos yarn, cord, fabric, joints, millboard, friction materials and gaskets mainly from the USA, the UK, Germany, and Japan. By 1954 Australia was fourth in the Western world in gross consumption of asbestos cement products (after the USA, the UK, and France) and therefore highest on a per capita basis. Ninety per cent of all consumption of asbestos fibre was for asbestos cement manufacture. Australia continued to import small amounts of chrysotile fibre and some asbestos products for friction material and gaskets until all asbestos production and importation was totally banned on 1 January 2004.

Crocidolite was mined at Wittenoom in Western Australia from 1937 to 1966 [6]. From 1943 the principal leases were mined by a single company, the Australian Blue Asbestos Company, a subsidiary of Colonial Sugar Refinery Ltd (CSR), which employed 6500 people mainly for short periods of time (the median duration of employment was 3 months). The employment records of the company have formed the basis for an ongoing cohort mortality study of the workforce. A cohort of 5000 persons who lived in the township but were not employed by the industry has also been assembled [3]. These cohorts, together with data on exposure from compliance monitoring by the Mines Department of the Government of Western Australia (a single survey of dustiness in the industry undertaken in 1966 shortly before the industry closed and periodic dust sampling in the township of Wittenoom up until the town itself was closed in 1990) have allowed detailed exposure–response relationships for mesothelioma (and other diseases) to be obtained. The crocidolite exposure estimates used have been validated with lung fibre content analyses [7] The workers' and residents' cohorts are unique, as few members ever worked in the asbestos industry elsewhere and were therefore exposed almost exclusively to crocidolite in estimable quantities. The Wittenoom crocidolite industry has had a profound effect on the occurrence of all asbestos-related diseases in the State of Western Australia.

Disease occurrence

As in other countries, the increasing incidence of mesothelioma in Australia has followed asbestos production and importation by 20–30 years [8] The first documented case of mesothelioma in Australia occurred in Victoria in 1947 [1], and the first case from Wittenoom occurred in 1960 [9]. The incidence (and mortality) rates have increased rapidly since the 1960s, although recently they appear to have been levelling out. In 1998 the age-standardized mortality rates for Western Australia were 4.8 per 100 000 for males and 0.3 per 100 000 for females, while the age-standardised incidence rates were 4.7 for males and 0.5 for females. The mortality rate for males in the state of Western Australia was higher than in any other industrialized country in 1995, the year for which the most recent WHO statistics are available (Fig. 2.1). Overall mortality rates for mesothelioma in males in Australia were ranked 11th in the world. In females in Western Australia the mesothelioma mortality was the third highest in the world, behind Italy and Slovenia, and, in Australia as a whole, 22nd in the world after Spain [8]. As with most cancers, the age-specific mortality rates are highest in the oldest age groups in both males and females. In 1988, 429/459 cases (93 per cent) were known to originate in the pleura, and only 20/459 (4 per cent) were known to originate in the peritoneum. The median age at diagnosis of cases in Western Australia was previously in the fifth decade, but is now in the sixth decade consistent with known relationships between risk and time since exposure for mesothelioma and asbestos exposure.

In Western Australia the percentage of cases attributed to work at Wittenoom has decreased from 45 per cent in 1960–1979 to 21 per cent in 1980–1994 [10, 11]. The percentage of cases in patients with other occupational exposures increased from 26 to 48 per cent for the same peri-

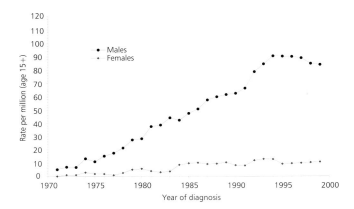

Figure 2.2 Mesothelioma (all types) n Western Australia: 3 year moving average.

ods. The numbers of cases with no identifiable asbestos exposure has remained steady (7 and 8 per cent) and the numbers with unknown exposure status in the Western Australia Mesothelioma Registry has increased slightly from 5 to 9 per cent. Rates of mesothelioma incidence for cases with unknown or no known exposure have been stable over the past 20 years, while rates in those with known exposure have been increasing, although overall rates appear to have levelled off (Fig. 2.2). Apart from Wittenoom cases the major occupational groups experiencing high rates of mesothelioma in Western Australia and Australia have been railway workshop workers, asbestos cement manufacturing workers, wharf workers (particularly at Point Sampson where Wittenoom crocidolite was loaded onto ships and at Fremantle where it was unloaded from ships from Point Sampson and overseas), other transport workers, insulation workers, boilermakers, cleaners and welders, building construction and supply workers, automotive repair workers, and workers in the armed forces, particularly the Navy. The incidence of malignant mesothelioma is also particularly high in the Aboriginal inhabitants of the Pilbara region of Western Australia, which includes Wittenoom. Aborigines worked at the mine and mill at Wittenoom but were not formally employed by the Australian Blue Asbestos Company [12], just as Aborigines were not entitled to vote until 1962 (after being disenfranchised in 1902) and were not granted citizenship until 1967.

Fibre clearance and future predictions

In the Wittenoom people, studies of the fibre content of lungs obtained from post-mortem and resected lung tissue have shown that clearance of crocidolite from the lungs takes place at a rate of up to 10 per cent of the load per year [7, 13]. Statistical modelling of mesothelioma incidence rates suggests that the peak in the number of cases in the Wittenoom cohort is occurring at present [3], although individual risks continue to increase at an exponential rate (although the magnitude of the exponent on years since first exposure has decreased from a peak of 3.4 to 3.2, probably as a result of fibre clearance) as the ageing cohort size is diminishing. The peak for the whole country is expected to occur in about the year 2020 because of later exposures. These estimates based on exposure information and asbestos production and utilization may be incorrect as a result of increased longevity of the population with reduced deaths from other causes, as well as clearance of particles from the lungs and, in Western Australia, a cancer prevention programme using vitamin A for people with past asbestos exposure [14, 15].

Exposure to asbestos and derived products in Poland

J. Niklinski

The overall incidence of mesothelioma in Poland is low with 120 cases reported per annum. The incidence is comparable to that observed in Hungary (78 cases per annum) and Romania (133 cases per annum), significantly less than that reported in Western Countries [16]. Nonetheless a number of important studies have evaluated the effects of asbestos exposure in Poland. Although asbestos is not mined in Poland many of the observed mesothelioma cases resulted from industrial exposure from the 4 asbestos cement plants in Poland which are now closed. In one case the local community, particularly the workers in the plant, was permitted to make use of the production waste for surfacing roads, paths and farmyards or for construction materials. As a result the asbestos exposure of factory workers and the general population living in the vicinity of the plant was prolonged. The principal types of asbestos used in the plants were chrysotile, which accounted for 85 per cent, and crocidolite.

Two major studies have been performed that demonstrated an increased mortality from mesothelioma in the exposed plant worker population compared to the general population (Tables 2.1 and 2.2) [17,18]. The first study included a cohort of 1526 workers from one plant, including 1356 men and 170 women. These subjects had been exposed to asbestos for a minimum period of 3 months between 1959 and 1985 and were observed until 1996. Of these 306 had died. Of interest is the fact that, despite the increased mortality from mesothelioma, the overall standard mortality rates for the population were similar to those of the general population in Poland although a twofold excess in cancer mortality was observed in women. No excess in lung cancer deaths was seen in men, unusual given that asbestos is a co-carcinogen with cigarette smoking for the disease [17].

The second study evaluated 3116 employees from other plants, including 2525 men and 591 women. The most pertinent observation was that mesothelioma mortality increased with increased duration of exposure to asbestos. Interestingly, despite the increase in mesothelioma, the overall standard mortality rates were lower than the general population suggesting a 'healthy worker' effect. Again the low incidence of lung cancer in this population is remarkable. A higher incidence of colon cancer was seen as has been observed in other series [18].

As elsewhere in the world these studies demonstrate the robust link between asbestos exposure and the incidence of mesothelioma.

Table 2.1 Mortality from cancer of Polish subjects exposed to asbestos in plant I [17]

Cause of death	Standard mortality rate (95% CI)	
	Males	**Females**
All cancer	99 (79–123)	216 (112–377)
Trachea, bronchus, lung	99 (66-142)	671 (138-1961)
Pleura Mesothelioma	8135 (3532–12 738)	20 292 (2435–73 254)
Colon	301 (121–620)	–
Pancreas	59 (7–213)	989 (120–3573)

Table 2.2 Mortality from cancer of Polish subjects exposed to asbestos in plants II and III [18]

Cause of death	Males			Females
	Duration <9 years	Duration 10–19 years	Duration >20 years	
All cancer	90 (67–119)	75 (49–111)	109 (54–195)	89 (43–164)
Trachea, bronchus, lung	79 (44–130)	94 (47–168)	77 (16–225)	382 (79–1116)
Pleura Mesothelioma	0	3606 (437–13 206)	16 646 (34 209–48 606)	11 275 (1368–40 714)
Colon	261 (71–668)	229 (28–827)	412	NA
Pancreas	128 (26–374)	0	0	NA

NA, not available.

Asbestos and mesothelioma in South Africa

R. P. Abratt, D. A. Vorobiof, and N. White

Asbestos and mesothelioma

The link between asbestos and mesothelioma was established in the Kimberley area in the Northern Cape region in South Africa [19]. In 1956, Wagner performed a necropsy on a black male shower attendant at a gold mine. He was surprised to find a tumour filling the right chest with collapsed lung in the centre. Tuberculosis had been endemic in the area, but antituberculous treatment, which was introduced in 1952, had a dramatic effect, except for cases from the area west of Kimberley. In 1956, C. A. Sleggs, the Chief Medical Officer of Kimberley Tuberculosis Hospital, collected the radiographs of 14 patients with a similar history. These were biopsied and showed mesothelioma. Most cases lived in the vicinity of asbestos mines. A long latent period with up to 44 years between exposure and mesothelioma was noted. Wagner reported the link between asbestos and mesothelioma in 1960.

In 1960, the South African Pneumoconiosis Research Unit undertook a survey of every 10th house in areas at risk. They found an alarming incidence of mesothelioma both within and outside the industry. In addition, 4.8 per cent of the general population had asbestos fibres in their sputum. The fibre concentration in the ambient atmosphere was measured at 0.09 fibres/ml. The mining houses were informed, but the report was denigrated. Funding for further research was discontinued, except for the final report on condition that it was not published externally. As a result of the withdrawal of support, studies were only restarted in the 1970s. In addition, the residents of areas which were at risk, such as Prieska, were not informed of the hazards and there was no control of atmospheric pollution.

There have been three sequential reports of the incidence of mesothelioma in South Africa (Fig. 2.3). Webster [20] reported the first series of 232 cases up to 1976 based on pathology reports sent to the National Centre of Occupational Health. Zwi et al. [21] reported on 1347 cases diagnosed between 1976 and 1984. They actively sought out cases in addition to those reported to a central asbestos tumour board. Only 59 per cent of their biopsy-proven cases were known to the tumour board. The South African National Cancer Registry (SANCR) has reported cases since 1986 and has relied on a passive reporting system based on the forwarding of pathology

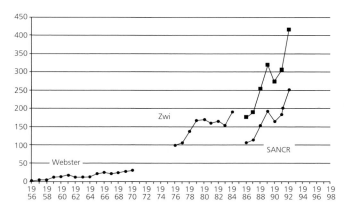

Figure 2.3 Annual number of cases of mesothelioma in South Africa (see text). The broken curve for the period 1986–1992 is an extrapolation of data based on pathological reports only.

reports [22]. This resulted in under-reporting of proven cases as shown by Zwi and colleagues. During the 9-year study by Zvi *et al.* [21] the age-standardized incidence rate (ASIR) in white males rose from 23.6 per million in 1976 to 40.5 per million in 1984. The comparable figure from the SANCR is 54 per million, giving an indication of a steady increase in mesothelioma incidence over the years.

The incidence of mesothelioma in South Africa is amongst the highest in the world. It is six times higher than that in England and at least as high as in Western Australia. The male-to-female ratio is 2.5:1. The available data are probably a serious underestimate of the true incidence. The low incidence documented in black South Africans is particularly suggestive of of underdiagnosis of mesothelioma. Zwi and colleagues speculated that this was due to the reluctance of physicians to undertake invasive procedures for untreatable conditions, the shorter life expectancy of blacks, and the migrant labour system whereby blacks would return to rural areas of South Africa or to other countries where they were not followed up or medical care was rudimentary. Mesothelioma usually develops 20 or more years after the first exposure, and the peak incidence is 35–45 years after exposure. The cumulative lifetime risk of developing mesothelioma rises as a constant multiplied by the third or fourth power of years since first exposure.

Asbestos mining in South Africa

The major types of asbestos encountered in South Africa are crocidolite, chrysotile, and amosite. Hausman, a German geologist, coined the name crocidolite in 1831 from the Greek *krokis* (woolly) and *lithos* (rock). Also known as blue asbestos, crocidolite was first discovered in South Africa in 1805 and was originally named 'woolstone'. All commercial asbestos fibres were mined in South Africa. South African mining of crocidolite began in the mid-nineteenth century. Initially, the mining took place with many small digging operations, 'outcrop mining'. The mining and milling processes are highly labour intensive, with the fibre cobbed from the rock by hand-held hammers, sieved by hand, sorted by a combination of manual and mechanized methods, and transported in hessian sacks (Fig. 2.4). Crocidolite is less heat resistant than other forms of asbestos, but very acid resistant as well as very elastic. It is used mainly as a reinforcing agent for binding with cement, rubber, and plastics, friction materials (brake linings), packing, and jointing products. The last crocidolite mine closed in 1994.

Chrysotile is also called white asbestos, although the fibres are pale green. In South Africa the area near Barberton was mined since the beginning of the twentieth century. In 1937 the Msauli mine in South Africa started mining operations in the largest deposit of chrysotile in the world. Operations closed in 2001. Chrysotile fibres have less tensile strength and less resistance to corro-

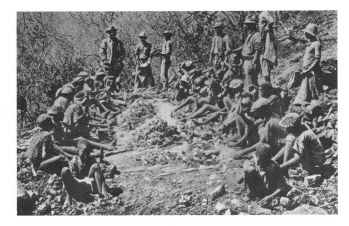

Figure 2.4 A group of workers sit and cobb blue asbestos ore by hand in the early twentieth century. Child labour for ore processing was a common practice at that time.

sion by acid. They are more suitable for spinning and weaving and more heat resistant than other asbestos fibres, and so chrysotile is used mainly in fire-resistant and insulator materials.

Amosite is a pale silvery fibrous mineral which is also called brown asbestos. Asbestos Mines of South Africa Ltd (Amosa) first mined the fibre at the turn of the twentieth century. It occurs mainly in the area of Penge and has been mined there for the past 80 years, mainly with small operations and crude technologies, causing extensive environmental pollution and exposing the labour force to high levels of dust. The Penge deposit is the largest in the world, and stretches for 40 km (25 miles)

Asbestos mining reached its peak in South Africa in 1977, when more than 380 000 tons was exported and 20 000 miners were employed. Asbestos is no longer mined in South Africa. However, given the latency period for mesothelioma, all those exposed during the 1970s and 1980s will be approaching the peak for their risk of this disease. Therefore it can be expected that the mesothelioma epidemic in South Africa will continue at least for the lifetime of those large numbers of people exposed to amphibole asbestos in mining, in industry, and environmentally.

Asbestos exposure and mesothelioma in South Africa

Four case series detailing the source of exposure in more than 500 cases of histologically proven malignant mesothelioma have been reported in South Africa [20, 23–25].

Mining industry If we remove the cases with unknown exposure and no exposure, mining-related exposure represents 40 per cent of those mesotheliomas for which exposure is known. The majority are related to exposure to crocidolite, which appears to be more mesotheliomagenic than the other fibres.

Secondary industry The majority of the reported mesothelioma cases result from exposure to asbestos in its many and varied uses in secondary industry. The major occupations at risk are the maintenance of steam locomotive and other rail-related procedures, the asbestos cement industry, and boilermakers and other artisans who use asbestos for insulation applications.

Environmental origin A high proportion (26 per cent) of mesothelioma in patients in South Africa can be attributed to environmental origin, particularly in the Northern Cape area. Of all environmental cases in South Africa, 93 per cent originate from exposure to crocidolite in that area. An interesting observation is the high incidence of women and children affected, accounting for more than 70 per cent of all reported environmental cases. In this area extensive use was made of asbestos waste as a cheap construction material for houses and public buildings.

Windborne pollution from mills and dumps was extensive, given the arid climate, and presumably asbestos was brought home in the hair and clothes of the miners. Therefore the closure of the last mine is not the end of the problem. There are 82 asbestos mine dumps in the Northern Cape alone, many still requiring rehabilitation.

Summary

Until recently, the story of mesothelioma within South Africa has been dismal. More than 2700 South Africans are documented as having died of mesothelioma. Government officials failed to prevent the disease and protect citizens. Mine owners focused excessively on profit. The legal system has offered no practical means of redress for patients with mesothelioma resulting from environmental exposure, and the medical community has had minimal impact on policy and/or practice.

Some recent developments are more encouraging. There has been a concerted focus by the South African legislature on asbestos-related matters. New and more stringent asbestos control regulations exist under the Occupational Health and Safety Act. Asbestos is no longer mined in South Africa and the government has an active programme of rehabilitating mine dumps. Cape plc, a UK asbestos mining company that left South Africa in 1976, is being sued by more than 5000 former South African employees suffering from asbestos-related diseases in a court case in London. Hopefully, future prospects in mesothelioma prevention and treatment will offer hope to those who are still at risk

Malignant pleural mesothelioma in Turkey

S. Emri, M. Tuncer, and Y. I. Baris

Background

Turkey has one of the highest prevalence rates for endemic asbestos-related pulmonary disease in the world [26]. This can be attributed to the large population of the country and to the geology, which includes numerous asbestos outcrops (Fig. 2.5). Historically, asbestos deposits have been

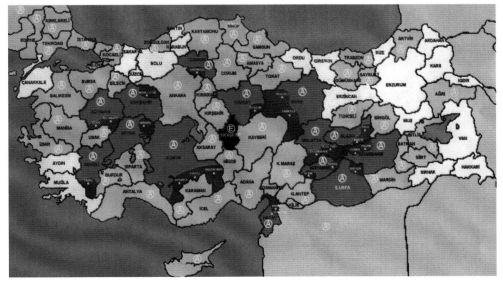

Figure 2.5 Map of Turkey showing areas of asbetos and erionite deposits: black, intense exposure to mineral fibres; red, moderate exposure; pink, least exposure.

Types of Asbestos Exposure.

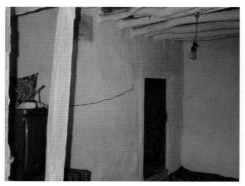

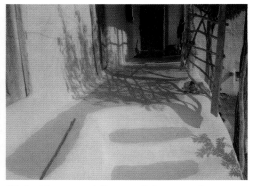

(a) **Interior of house plastered with asbestos-containing 'white soil'**

(b) **Outdoors and floors of the same house plastered with asbestos-containing 'white soil'**

Asbestos exposure starts at birth and can be considered lifelong

Figure 2.6 (a) Interior of a house plastered with asbestos-containing 'white soil'. (b) Outside walls and terrace of the same house also plastered with 'white soil'.

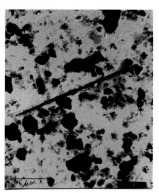

TEM view of a TREMOLITE fibre

GLOBAL CHEMICAL ANALYSIS BY ELECTRON MICROSCOPY

Visual estimation of particle concentration : high

Element	Weight %
Na_2O	1.7
MgO	4.5
Al_2O_3	18.2
SiO_2	56.8
K_2O	4.3
CaO	0.9
TiO_2	1.9
FeO	11.1
others	0.7

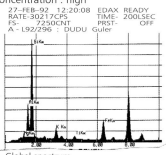

Global spectrum

Figure 2.7 Mineralogical analysis revealed that, in addition to tremolite, which is the most prominent asbestos type found as a contaminant of white stucco in Turkey, chrysotile asbestos and in certain districts (Mihallic[,]c[,]ık and Edige) anthophyllite asbestos also contaminate white stucco.

used in rural areas to make a whitewash or stucco which is applied to the walls, floors, and roofs of houses (Fig. 2.6) and is also used as a substitute for baby powder and gripewater. Mineralogical analysis has revealed that tremolite is the most prominent type of asbestos found as a contaminant of white stucco. In addition, chrysotile asbestos and in some districts, including Mihallic[,]c[,]ık and Edige, anthophyllite asbestos have also been found as contaminants of white stucco [27] (Fig. 2.7).

Erionite

A different non-asbestos mineral fibre has also been found, particularly in three villages (Karain, Tuzköy, and Sarihidir) located in the Cappadocian region of Central Anatolia [28] (Fig. 2.8),

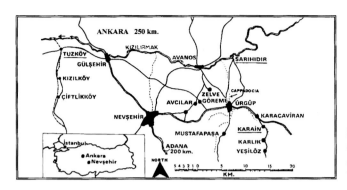

Figure 2.8 Map of the Cappadocia region showing the erionite villages of Karain, Tuzköy, and Sarihidir.

which has been identified as the fibrous zeolite erionite. Erionite fibres, formed by bundles of individual fibrils with a diameter of approximately 0.5 μm, are 5–6 μm in diameter and 30–40 μm long. There are three principal types of erionite, erionite sodium, erionite potassium, and erionite calcium, all of which are considered to be carcinogens. This fibre is present in the volcanic tuffs from which blocks have been cut to build houses in these villages (Fig. 2.9). Where used for construction, erionite is not only present in the houses, outhouses, and village streets but can also be detected in air samples, resulting in continuous exposure of the population. Experimental studies have shown that erionite is 300–800 times more carcinogenic than chrysotile, and 100–500 times more potent than crocidolite when given to hamsters by the intrapleural route [29].

Both asbestos and erionite can cause a variety of benign and malignant chest diseases. Among the latter, pleural mesothelioma is the most serious public health problem in central and eastern Anatolia. It has been estimated that about 16 million people living in rural Anatolia have been environmentally exposed to mineral fibres. In a study in 65 Turkish subjects from asbestos areas bronchoalveolar lavage revealed the asbestos fibre burden to be in the same range as that of

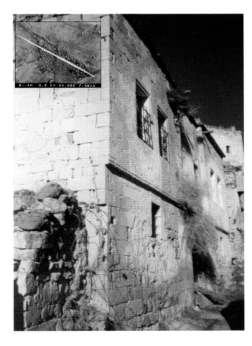

Figure 2.9 Houses constructed from blocks containing erionite fibres.

Belgian subjects occupationally exposed to commercial amphiboles [30]. This indicates that environmental exposure in Turkey is a much more serious health hazard than in other Western countries where it does not pose a health risk [31].

Asbestos, erionite, and malignant mesothelioma

The estimated incidence of mesothelioma has been reported to be 43 per million in southeastern Turkey [32] and 996 per 100 000 in the 'erionite villages' of Cappadocia [28], where more than 50 per cent of deaths are caused by malignant mesothelioma [33]. In a pivotal study in Sweden, Metintas *et al.* reported 14 deaths (78 per cent) due to mesothelioma among the 18 deaths occurring between 1965 and 1997 in a cohort of 162 Turkish immigrants from Karain, one of the erionite villages [34]. Compared with the incidence in the general population in Sweden, that of the Turkish study population was 135 times higher in males and 1336 times higher in females. The risk was also shown to correlate with the duration of residence in the village. A recent survey of the incidence and distribution of malignant mesothelioma in Turkey revealed a total of 506 new cases (464 pleural, 42 peritoneal) for the year 2000 [35]. The female-to-male incidence ratio was 213:293. The mean age at diagnosis was 56 years (range 24–88 years) and was similar for both men and women. No history of occupational exposure to either asbestos or erionite was obtained in any these cases. Six per cent of the cases (30/506) were reported from the erionite villages.

Recent mortality data from villages near the three known erionite villages in Cappadocia (Tuzköy, Karain, and Sarihidir) for the period 1994–1997 suggest that malignant mesothelioma might also occur in some of them [36]. These villages include Karacaören, Boyali, Cökek, Karlik, and Yesilöz. Out of the total 64 reported deaths due to mesothelioma, 53 were from the three erionite villages, six were from Karacaören, and five from the other four villages. No mesotheliomas were found in Karlik despite the fact that the village is only 1.5 km from Karain and built from the same stones used in Karain. Thus mesothelioma cases are more prevalent in the erionite villages than in the neighbouring villages [37]. This could be due to differences in genetic suscep-

Like many other places in Cappodocia, these villages are characterised by ancient rock dwelling and caves dug in soft volcanic tuff.

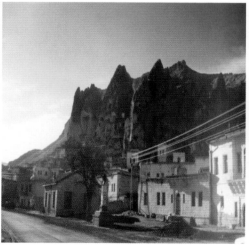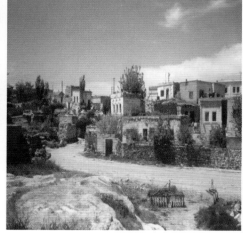

(a) **Karain village (population ~ 600)**   (b) **Tuzköy village (population ~ 1,400)**

Photographs of the well known erionite villages.

Figure 2.10 Two of the erionite villages: (a) Karain; (b) Tuzköy.

tibility to mesothelioma [38]. The type of erionite did not differ between houses in Karain and Tuzköy (Fig. 2.10).

Genetic predisposition to mesothelioma

Individuals in adjacent houses in the same village seem to have a very different incidence of mesothelioma, despite similar erionite exposure. The first indications for a genetic predisposition to mesothelioma arose from a case–control study of 31 patients with mesothelioma undertaken in 1998 by Karakoca *et al.* [39]. HLA-B41, HLA-B58, and HLA-DR16 antigens were significantly higher in the mesothelioma patients than in two control groups, including 118 healthy renal donors and 119 inhabitants of Tuzköy. However, HLA-B27 antigen appeared to be protective against mesothelioma [39]. A recent genetic–epidemiological study addressing this issue investigated the possibility that susceptibility to erionite carcinogenicity was determined by a genetic factor. Analysis of a six-generation extended pedigree of 526 individuals showed that malignant pleural mesothelioma was genetically transmitted and suggested that the transmission occurs in an autosomal dominant fashion [38]. Further studies are in progress to identify the gene(s) that predispose individuals to malignant mesothelioma (see also Chapter 11).

Lack of evidence for viral factors in the aetiology of mesothelioma in Turkey

It has been shown that simian virus 40 (SV40), a DNA tumour virus that contaminated poliovaccines distributed worldwide in the late 1950s and early 1960s, is a cofactor in the development of human mesotheliomas in the USA [40]. However, a recent study showed that SV40 was not a cofactor in the pathogenesis of environmentally related malignant mesothelioma in Turkey [41]. This appears to be related to the fact that SV40-contaminated vaccines were never administered in Turkey.

The potential role of human herpesvirus 8 (HHV-8) in the pathogenesis of malignant mesothelioma has also been studied in the Turkish population. This recently described virus has been shown to be associated with Kaposi's sarcoma and 'body-cavity-based' B-cell lymphomas. It is known that HHV-8 upregulates the level of interleukin 6 (IL-6) which is also secreted by mesothelioma cells. However, the pleura and the peritoneum are not targets for HHV-8 and environmentally induced mesothelioma in Turkey does not appear to be related to HHV-8 [42].

The role of viral factors in the aetiology of mesothelioma is discussed in detail in Chapter 7.

Summary

Turkey has one of the highest incidences of malignant mesothelioma in the world because of the geology of the country with numerous outcrops of asbestos and its traditional widespread use, particularly by the rural population. Turkey also has a population in Cappadocia relatively uniquely exposed to the zeolite erionite, commonly used for building materials. Evidence from studies in Turkey indicates the presence of susceptibility genes for the development of malignant mesothelioma which should prove an exciting area for research in the future.

Conclusions

The epidemiology of asbestos and, in Turkey, erionite seen in these four countries provide an insight into the diversity of patterns of exposure experienced by different populations. In all countries the exposure is contributed to by local, national, and international industry. The studies support the continued international effort to ban the use of asbestos globally and for continued vigilance to prevent potential exposure in those countries where asbestos was widely used in the past.

References

1. Musk AW, Dolin PJ, Armstrong BK, Ford JM, de Klerk NH, Hobbs MST. The incidence of malignant mesothelioma in Australia, 1947–1980. *Med J Aust* 1989; **150**: 242–6.

2. National Occupational Health and Safety Commission. *The Incidence of Mesothelioma in Australia 1996–1998*. Australian Mesothelioma Register Report, 2001.

3. Berry G, de Klerk NH, Reid A, *et al.* Malignant pleural and peritoneal mesotheliomas in former miners and millers of crocidolite at Wittenoom, Western Australia. *Occup Environ Med* 2004 ;**61**: E14.

4. Hansen J, de Klerk NH, Musk AW, Hobbs MST. Environmental exposure to crocidolite and mesothelioma. exposure–response relationships. *Am J Respir Crit Care Med* 1998; **157**: 69–75.

5. Zhong X, Armstrong BK, Blunsdon B, Rogers JM, Musk AW, Shilkin KB. Trends in mortality from malignant mesothelioma of the pleura and production and use of asbestos in Australia, 1968 to 1981. *Med J Aust* 1985; **143**: 185–7.

6. Musk AW, de Klerk NH, Eccles JL, *et al.* Wittenoom, Western Australia: a modern industrial disaster. *Am J Ind Med* 1992; **21**: 735–47.

7. de Klerk NH, Musk AW, Williams V, Filion PR, Whitaker D, Shilkin KB. Comparison of measures of exposure to asbestos in former crocidolite workers from Wittenoom Gorge, Western Australia. *Am J Ind Med* 1996; **30**: 579–87.

8. de Klerk NH, Musk AW. Epidemiology of mesothelioma. In: Robinson BWS, Chahinian P, eds. *Mesothelioma*. London: Martin Dunitz, 2002; 339–49.

9. McNulty JC. Malignant pleural mesothelioma in an asbestos worker. *Med J Aust* 1962; **2**: 953–4.

10. Threlfall TJ, Morgan A. *Malignant Mesothelioma in Western Australia, 1960–1994. Data from the WA Mesothelioma Register*. Statistical Series no. 46. Perth: Health Department of Western Australia, 1996.

11. Western Australian Cancer Registry. *Cancer Incidence and Mortality in Western Australia*. Statistical Series no. 61. Perth: Health Department of Western Australia, 2000.

12. Musk AW, Eccles JL, Shilkin KB, de Klerk NH. Malignant mesothelioma in Pilbara Aboriginals. *Aust J Public Health* 1995;**19**: 520–2

13. Williams VM, Shilkin KB, Filion P, de Klerk NH, Musk AW, Whitaker D. Assay of pulmonary asbestos body and asbestos fibre burden in subjects with malignant mesothelioma and other conditions related to exposure to asbestos in Western Australia. *Aust J Med Sci* 1996; **17**: 75–8.

14. Musk AW, de Klerk NH, Ambrosini GL, *et al.* Vitamin A and cancer prevention. I: Observations in workers previously exposed to asbestos in Wittenoom, Western Australia. *Int J Cancer* 1998; **75**: 355–61.

15. de Klerk NH, Musk AW, Ambrosini GL, *et al.* Vitamin A and cancer prevention. II: Comparison of the effects of retinol and β-carotene. *Int J Cancer* 1998; **75**: 362–7.

16. Bianchi C, Brollo A, Ramani L, Bianchi T. Malignant mesothelioma in Central and Eastern Europe. *Acta Med Croatica* 2000; **54**: 161–4.

17. Szeszenia-Dabrowska N, Wilczynska U, Szymczak W. Environmental exposure to asbestos in asbestos-cement workers: a case of additional exposure from indiscriminate use of industrial wastes. *Int J Occup Med Environ Health* 1998; **11**: 171–7.

18. Szeszenia-Dabrowska N, Strzelecka A, Wilczynska U, Szymczak W. Mortality of workers at two asbestos-cement plants in Poland. *Int J Occup Med Envir Health* 2000; **13**: 121–30.

19. Wagner JC, Sleggs CA, Marchand P. Diffuse pleural mesotheliomas and asbestos exposure in the Northwestern Cape Province. *Br J Ind Med* 1960; **17**: 260–71.

20. Webster I. Asbestosis and Malignancy. *S Afr Med J* 1973; **47**: 165–71.

21. Zwi AB, Reid G, London SP, Kiek-Kowski D, Sitas F, Becklake MR. Mesothelioma in South Africa <1976–84: incidence and case characteristics. *Int J Epidemiol* 1989; **18**: 320–9.

22. *Cancer in South Africa. Annual Reports of the National Cancer Registry (NCR) of South Africa*. Johannesburg: SAIMR, 1986–1992.

23. Cochrane JC, Webster I. Mesothelioma in relation to asbestos fibre exposure. *S Afr Med J* 1978; **54**: 279–81.

24. Solomons K. Malignant mesothelioma—clinical and epidemiological features: a report of 80 cases. *S Afr Med J* 1984; **866**: 407–12.

25. Rees D, Goodman K, Fourie E, *et al. Asbestos Exposure and Mesothelioma in South Africa*, 1998 (unpublished).

26. Karakoca Y, Emri S, Cangır AK, Barıs YI. Environmental pleural plaques due to asbestos and fibrous zeolite exposure in Turkey. *Indoor Built Environ* 1997; **6**: 100–05.

27. Dogan M, Emri S. Environmental health problems related to mineral dusts in Ankara and Eskisehir, Turkey. *Yerbilimleri* 2000; **22**: 149–61.

28. Baris YI, Simanato l, Artvinli M, *et al.* Epidemiological and environmental evidence of health effect of exposure to erionite fibers: a four-year study in the Cappadocian region of Turkey. *Int J Cancer* 1987; **39**: 10–17.

29. Carthew P, Hill RJ, Edwards RE, Lee PN. Intrapleural admistration of fibers induces mesothelioma in rats in the same relative order of hazards as occurs in man after exposure. *Hum Exp Toxicol* 1992; **11**: 530–4.

30. Dumortier P, Çoplü L, de Maertelaer V, Emri S, Baris I, De Vuyst P. Assessment of environmental asbestos exposure in Turkey by bronchoalveolar lavage. *Am J Respir Crit Care Med* 1998; **158**: 1815–24.

31. Dumortier P, Çoplü L, Broucke I, *et al.* Erionite bodies and fibres in bronchoalveolar lavage fluid (BALF) of residents from Tuzköy, Cappadocia, Turkey. *Occup Environ Med* 2001; **58**: 261–6.

32. Senyi_it A, Babyi_it C, Gökirmak M, *et al.* Incidence of malignant pleural mesothelioma due to environmental asbestos fiber exposure in the southeast of Turkey. *Respiration* 2000; **67**: 610–14.

33. Baris B, Demir AU, Shehu V, Karakoca Y, Kısacık G, Baris YI. Environmental fibrous zeolite/erionite exposure and malignant tumors other than mesothelioma. *J Environ Pathol Toxicol Oncol* 1996; **15**: 183–9.

34. Metintas M, Hillerdal H, Metintas S. Malignant mesothelioma due to environmental exposure to erionite: follow of a Turkish cohort. *Eur Respir J* 1999; **13**: 523–6.

35. Emri S, Demir AU. Malignant pleural mesothelioma in Turkey, 2000–2002. *Lung Cancer* 2004; **45** (Suppl 1): S17–20.

36. Emri S, Demir A, Dogan M, *et al.* Lung diseases due to environmental exposures to erionite and asbestos in Turkey. *Toxicol Lett* 2002; **127**: 251–7.

37. Dogan AU. Cappadocian mesothelioma villages. Presented at: Symposium on Nutrition, Environment, and Cancer, Ankara, 2002.

38. Hammady I-Roushdy, Siegel J, Emri S, Testa JR, Carbone M. Genetic-susceptibility factor and malignant mesothelioma in the Cappadocian region of Turkey. *Lancet* 2001; **357**: 444–5.

39. Karakoca Y, Emri S, Bagci T, Erdem Y, Baris E, Sahin AA. Environmentally induced malignant pleural mesothelioma and HLA distribution in Turkey. *Int J Tuberc Lung Dis* 1998; **2**: 1017–22.

40. Carbone M, Fisher S, Powers A, Pass HI, Rizzo P. New molecular and epidemiological issues in mesothelioma: role of SV40. *J Cell Physiol* 1999; **180**: 167–72.

41. Emri S, Kocagoz T, Olut A, Güngen Y, Mutti L, Baris YI. Simian virus 40 is not a cofactor in the pathogenesis of environmentally induced malignant pleural mesothelioma in Turkey. *Anticancer Res* 2000; **20**: 891–4.

42. Olut A, Ertugrul D, Kocagoz T, Er M, Emri S. HHV-8 is not a cofactor in the pathogenesis of environmentally induced malignant pleural mesothelioma. *Monaldi Arch Chest Dis* 2000; **55**: 110–13.

Chapter 3

Malignant pleural mesothelioma: clinical presentation, radiological evaluation and diagnosis

M. D. Peake, J. Entwisle, and S. G. Gray

Introduction

It is difficult to appreciate now, when mesothelioma is increasing in frequency and has a relatively high profile, that it is only comparatively recently that it was unequivocally recognized as a distinct clinical entity. The first cases were probably reported by Joseph Lieutand as early as 1767 [1] and the pathology was described in 1870 [2], although 16 years earlier Von Rokitanski [3] had reported on a primary peritoneal 'colloid tumour' which was probably mesothelioma. The name 'mesothelioma' (i.e. from the mesothelium) was suggested by Klemperer and Rabin [4], who reported the unique features of these diffuse tumours of the pleura. Later, diagnostic criteria were proposed for malignant pleural mesothelioma (MPM) by Godwin [5] and for the peritoneal variety by Winslow and Taylor [6]. Over the 20 years or so following these reports, MPM gradually became accepted as a tumour separate from bronchial carcinoma and metastatic disease [7, 8].

The first 'large' series of 33 cases of MPM was reported in the Northwestern Cape province of South Africa in 1960 [9], and virtually all of them had a history of significant occupational or environmental exposure to asbestos. Five years later Wagner [10] went on to report a total of 89 cases of which two originated in the peritoneum and all except another two had a clear history of asbestos exposure. Since then many reports from a variety of countries have confirmed the relationship between asbestos exposure and the development of mesothelioma. In many reports such exposure has been of occupational origin [11, 12], but in a significant number environmental exposure has been of equal or even greater significance [13–16].

The approach to diagnosis

It is worth stating at the outset that mesothelioma is not an easy disease to diagnose. Its early symptomatology and, to a lesser extent, its radiological features are often non-specific, and in addition obtaining sufficient pathological material to establish firmly what is, in turn, a difficult histological diagnosis [17] is not always straightforward. Clinical vigilance and maintaining a high index of suspicion combined with a careful structured approach to the diagnosis is required. Early referral to a clinical team widely experienced in the diagnosis and assessment of disease is essential for the consistent achievement of the best outcomes for these unfortunate individuals.

Site of disease

Malignant mesothelioma can present as a tumour in either the pleura or the peritoneum. The proportion of cases in which the tumour appears to originate in one or other of these two sites in an asbestos-exposed population varies widely between published reports. In a North American

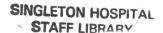

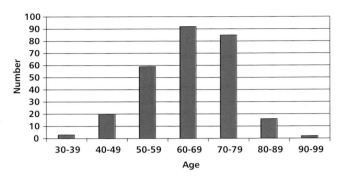

Figure 3.1 Distribution of age at presentation. (Reproduced from D. H. Yates *et al.* Malignant mesothelioma in south east England: clinicopathological experience of 272 cases. *Thorax* 1997; 5 2: 507–12.)

series Ribak *et al.* [11] found that 62 per cent of their 356 histologically confirmed cases were of peritoneal origin. However, this is highly atypical compared with other series. For example, in Australia only 4 per cent of cases reported originate in the peritoneum [18], and in a UK series of 327 cases only 11 per cent were peritoneal, with a further 7.6 per cent of cases where it was not possible to define the primary site [19]. In the pleura, a slight preponderance for the right side (60:40) of the thorax has been shown in some series [20, 21], and it has been suggested that this may be related to the slightly higher surface area of the pleura on that side. Very occasionally tumours appear to arise in other sites such as the pericardium and tunica vaginalis [20].

Age and sex distribution

The average latent interval between first asbestos exposure and onset of disease is very long. One careful UK study estimated a mean interval of 41 years with a range of 15–67 years [20]. As a result of this, the average age at onset is about 60 years (Fig. 3.1), varying from 48 to 65 years in published series [11, 19–22], which is about 10 years younger than the average age at diagnosis of lung cancer patients in the UK. Since the median survival from the time of diagnosis is about 7–12 months [20, 23], the mean age at death is only marginally greater, being 59.4 years (range 29–88 years) in Elmes' series from the 1960s and 1970s [19] and 65.2 years in Yates's series of patients diagnosed in the late 1980s and 1990s [20].

There is a strong male preponderance in most series, although this varies a great deal depending on the relative contribution of environmental and occupational sources of exposure in the population studied. In pleural mesothelioma the reported male-to-female ratio varies from 1.4:1 in Turkey [24[, 1.9:1 in Italy [25], and 2.5:1 in South Africa [16] at the low end to 12.6:1 in a UK series [20]. The average ratio is about 6:1. This gender difference may be larger for pleural than for peritoneal tumours; a male-to-female ratio as low as 1.5:1 was quoted for peritoneal tumours in one large study [21].

Occupational groups at risk

The range of occupational groups exposed to asbestos and at current risk of developing mesothelioma is huge, especially in international terms, and is more fully covered in Chapter 1. The most common occupations of those seen with the condition in the UK are shown in Table 3.1, although the proportions will vary widely between different regions of the country depending on the industrial geography. It is of particular importance to recognize that many people who worked in the industries listed were not aware of their exposure at the time and may not give an unequivocal history of exposure. This is particularly true of those who have worked in the building industry.

Table 3.1 Occupational exposure to asbestos in cases of mesothelioma from the South East of England (modified from Yates *et al.*, 1997–ref 20)

Industry	Percentage of cases
Shipbuilding and repair	15.4
Boiler, pipe, and heating	14.7
Carpenters	11
Electricians	9.9
Construction and demolition	8.5
Asbestos manufacturing and sales	5.1
Insulation work, laggers	4.8
Electricity generation	4.0
Laboratory and research	2.6
Stevedores and dockers	2.2
Railway coach construction	2.2
Navy seamen	1.1
Other	5.9

Other aetiological factors

In every reported series of mesothelioma there is no history of asbestos exposure in a proportion of cases. This proportion is usually considered to be about 10 per cent [20], although it has been reported to be as high as 60 per cent in some series [26]. In some instances this can be explained by unknown casual exposure such as is seen in the wives of men working with asbestos or workers unknowingly exposed (e.g. electricians and carpenters in the building trade). However, it is clear that there is a relatively constant 'background' incidence (see Chapter 1) and thus consideration has to be given to the possibility of involvement of other aetiological agents. Conversely, there has to be some element of variability in genetic susceptibility, since not everyone exposed to asbestos, even in high-exposure areas such as some Turkish villages [27], develops the disease. The occurrence of the disease in children not exposed to asbestos [28] also argues in favour of other causes in a minority of cases. Simian virus 40 (SV40) has been suggested as a possible aetiological agent [29, 30], although the consensus view is that the evidence for this is controversial [31].

Other causative agents that have been proposed include organic fibres in sugar cane workers [32] and other mineral fibres, particularly erionite, found locally in some villages in Turkey [24]. There is no good evidence that exposure to man-made mineral fibres is associated with an increased incidence of mesothelioma, although there is evidence of some excess mortality from lung cancer in exposed individuals [33]. A relatively high prevalence of smoking among patients with mesothelioma has been reported in several studies [11]. However, there is no evidence that cigarette smoking itself is a risk factor for the development of mesothelioma [34–36].

Clinical features

Symptoms: pleural mesothelioma

In the vast majority of patients the onset of symptoms is insidious, with chest pain and breathlessness being the most common features. Both these symptoms are commonly mild at the outset and are often attributed to other causes, delaying referral to specialist care. Indeed, patients themselves often find it difficult to define the date of onset to within a month [19]. Since the disease occurs in a demographic group that has a high incidence of other respiratory diseases such as chronic obstructive pulmonary disease (COPD), the breathlessness can be manifested as either the new onset of dyspnoea or the deterioration of the existing symptom. In one series the presenting complaint was the recent onset of new breathlessness in 25 per cent of patients, and in a further 22 per cent the increase of existing dyspnoea led to them seeking medical advice [11]. The chest pain is frequently described as being like a 'heaviness' or 'coldness' in one side of the chest/abdomen. Referral of this rather vague chest pain to the shoulder or upper abdomen (probably because of involvement of the diaphragmatic pleura) may lead to inappropriate investigation and further diagnostic delays. Of course pain and breathlessness can coexist in the same patient, but in about a third the mode of symptomatic onset is breathlessness related to pleural effusion without pain [20]. Rarely, the presentation is relatively acute, with dyspnoea and pain leading to emergency admission [19]. A 'dry' cough is a common feature during the course of the disease but is rarely troublesome in the early stages, being seen in about 10 per cent of patients at presentation [37].

Other relatively common features include fatigue and lassitude, weight loss, and intermittent low-grade fever [38]. Occasionally the tumour is found incidentally during the radiological investigation of some other problem. This was the mode of presentation in about 4 per cent of cases in one series from the UK [20]. Pneumothorax is another rare mode of presentation [20, 39]. The relative incidence of these symptoms is summarized in Table 3.2.

By the time of referral to secondary care the picture has often changed. Because of the insidious onset, the interval between first symptom and referral is often long, 3–39 months in one

Table 3.2 Reported Frequency of presenting symptoms of malignant mesothelioma

Pleural mesothelioma	
Chest pain [11, 19, 20, 84]	22%–56%
Breathlessness [11, 19, 20, 84]	36%–41.5%
Recent *onset* only	24%
Recent *deterioration* only [84]	22%
Due to pleural effusion without pain [20]	33%
Non-specific symptoms (lassitude ± weight loss) [19]	6.4%
Weight loss alone [84]	44%
Cough [37]	10%
Asymptomatic (incidental finding) [11, 19, 20, 84]	2.2%–7.7%
Chest wall mass [20]	4%
Peritoneal mesothelioma	
Abdominal pain [11]	40%
Abdominal distension [11]	37%
Weight loss ± fatigue [11, 19]	5%–6.4%
Intestinal obstruction [11]	3.6%
Abdominal mass [11]	2%
Ascites [11]	1%

study [19]. Even when chest pain was the main factor, a mean period of 3 months elapsed before referral. Other complaints have usually been added to the 'list' by the time of referral, so that pain appears in patients where breathlessness was the initial feature and vice versa. Over time, typically dry cough, weight loss, and general malaise appear [37]. The initial 'heaviness' changes to more definite and continuous pain, often described as 'like a toothache', but not usually pleuritic in nature. Paraesthesiae are sometimes experienced in the chest wall. Occasionally patients are perceived as having no organic basis for their symptoms for significant periods of time.

Clinical features of local invasion

Local invasion is the most common form of spread of malignant mesothelioma and, in addition to the worsening of the presenting symptoms, a whole host of other symptoms and syndromes have been described. These include:

- dysphagia related to oesophageal compression [19]
- neurological syndromes such as Horner's syndrome [40]
- sympathetic nerve involvement of the arm [41]
- recurrent laryngeal nerve palsy [42]
- invasion of spinal canal with paraplegia [43]
- chest wall mass
- severe chest wall pain as a result of invasion and nerve root involvement
- malignant pericardial effusion/pericardial invasion
- superior venal caval obstruction [44]
- tracking along the route of previous surgical intervention in up to 50 per cent [45]
- intermittent hypoglycaemia (probably more common with rare localized fibrous mesothelioma—see below).

Relationship with pleural plaques and asbestosis

Clearly, people with pleural plaques have been exposed to asbestos and one would expect them to be at higher risk of developing malignant mesothelioma. Some studies have reported an increased risk in patients with plaques [46, 47], and mesothelioma is much more common in those areas of the world where plaques are more or less endemic [8]. Up to 15 per cent of patients with asbestosis will develop malignant mesothelioma [48, 49].

Physical signs: pleural and peritoneal

About a third of patients have signs of a significant pleural effusion at the time of presentation, and more obvious reduction of chest wall movement, dullness, and reduced breath sounds often appear as the disease progresses. Mediastinal displacement towards the side of the lesion usually occurs at some stage as the pleural tumour becomes a severe restriction on the expansion of underlying lung. Spinal curvature can occur in long-standing cases. Chest wall masses are occasionally detected at presentation but are more usually associated with 'seeding' of the disease along the track of pleural tap or biopsy or surgical interventions. Basal crackles are occasionally heard, although it is unclear whether this is related to undiagnosed asbestosis [19].

Clubbing of the fingers occurs in a minority (9.5 per cent in Elmes' series [19]) and hypertrophic pulmonary osteoarthropathy (HPOA) is extremely rare. Both of these manifestations appear more common when there is associated asbestosis [40]. Evidence of more distant spread such as palpable supraclavicular lymphadenopathy and hepatomegaly are rarely seen at presentation, although it was reported in as many as 11 per cent of patients in one series [50].

Solitary fibrous mesothelioma

There is a rare form of the disease, taking the form of a localized pleural tumour, which accounts for up to 5 per cent of cases and for which there appears to be no clear relationship to asbestos exposure. It is often almost symptom free and pleural effusions are uncommonly seen. Finger clubbing and HPOA are much more common than in the more usual diffuse manifestation of the disease, and the rare syndrome of intermittent hypoglycaemia has been reported as being associated with it [51].

Pattern of metastasis

Spread to the mediastinal lymph nodes is common and probably occurs in about half of cases; a level of 44 per cent was detected in one post-mortem study [52]. Spread outside the thorax is detected in 54–82 per cent of cases during the course of the disease, although this includes the peritoneum. Metastases have been reported to the liver, the adrenal glands (10 per cent in a small series compared with 37 per cent in a parallel series of bronchial carcinoma [7]), and occasionally the brain. Distant metastases appear more common in sarcomatous mesothelioma [52]. Death resulting directly from distant metastases is uncommon [53]. Metastatic disease is being experienced more commonly in patients living longer as a result of radical therapies such as extrapleural pneumonectomy.

Laboratory investigations

At the time of diagnosis routine blood tests including full blood count, inflammatory markers, and biochemical screen are often normal and there is, as yet, no blood test that is specific to the diagnosis of mesothelioma. However, non-specific haematological abnormalities such as normochromic normocytic anaemia, low-grade leucocytosis, and/or thrombocytosis are relatively common. In one series mild anaemia (<14g/dl) was found in 32 per cent of patients, leucocytosis (>8.3×10^9/litre) in 57 per cent, and thrombocytosis (>400×10^9/litre) in 35 per cent [54]. The presence of each of these abnormalities was associated with a poorer prognosis (see also Chapter 5). An elevated erythrocyte sedimentation rate is common, sometimes to high levels [19], and hypergammaglobulinaemia of a polyclonal type is not infrequent [55]. Mild elevation of liver enzymes and hypoalbuminaemia are also sometimes present, especially as the disease progresses.

The syndrome of inappropriate ADH secretion resulting in hyponatraemia has been described occasionally [56], as has intermittent hypoglycaemia although, as mentioned above, this may be more frequent in localized fibrous tumours [51].

Tumour markers

Carcinoembryonic antigen and tissue polypeptide antigen

Serum levels of carcinoembryonic antigen (CEA) have not been found to be elevated in mesothelioma [57]; if they were elevated in a particular patient, this would argue in favour of adenocarcinoma of the pleura, possibly metastatic from a gastrointestinal source, in the absence of clear-cut histological confirmation. Tissue polypeptide antigen (TPA) is a cytoskeleton marker characteristic of mesothelial cells corresponding to cytokeratins 8, 18, and 19. It is expressed differently in mesothelioma than in lung cancer, and it has been suggested that combining the measurements of serum levels of TPA and CEA could help in the differential diagnosis of malignant pleural disease [58].

Mesothelin

Clearly, a serum marker that could assist in the diagnosis, early detection, and monitoring of progress in mesothelioma would be of enormous value. One such candidate currently under evaluation is mesothelin [59]. Mesothelin is a glycoprotein attached to the cell surface and thought to have a role in cell adhesion and possibly cell-to-cell signalling. It exists in a variety of forms which can be detected in serum using monocolonal antibody techniques in the form of soluble mesothelin related proteins (SMR). Elevated levels of SMR have been found in patients with ovarian carcinoma [60]. Robinson *et al.* [59] have demonstrated that 37/44 patients with malignant mesothelioma in their Australian series had elevated levels of SMR compared with only 10/228 of a mixed group of appropriate controls. Seven of these 10 patients were apparently healthy asbestos-exposed individuals, three of whom subsequently went on to develop mesothelioma. SMR levels appeared higher in epithelioid tumours and were directly related to tumour mass. In this study the test had a sensitivity of 84 per cent and a specificity of 100 per cent when compared with other pleural diseases being investigated in their centre, 95 per cent when compared with other lung tumours, and 83 per cent when compared with other healthy asbestos-exposed individuals. Such results need confirmation, but the approach looks very promising.

Osteopontin

Another potential tumour marker recently identified as part of a systematic search for tools for the early diagnosis of mesothelioma is osteopontin [61]. A glycoprotein, osteopontin is overexpressed in a variety of solid tumours including lung, breast, colo-rectal, gastric and ovarian cancers. It acts as a mediator of cell matrix interactions and inter-cell signalling through its binding with integrin and CD44 receptors. It is, in turn, regulated by cell signalling proteins that are known to be active in asbestos-induced carcinogenesis. Pass and his co-workers [61] have demonstrated elevated serum levels of osteopontin in individuals with mesothelioma compared with control subjects. They found no significant differences in serum levels between the asbestos-exposed controls and those with no history of asbestos exposure, although modest elevations were found in subjects with a combination of established asbestos-related pulmonary fibrosis and pulmonary plaques. They were also able to demonstrate positive immunohistochemical staining for osteopontin in the vast majority of resected tissue samples of patients with mesothelioma. There was no correlation of serum osteopontin levels and the stage of disease in patients with mesothelioma but elevated levels were seen in stage 1 disease, tempting speculation that it could be used in screening for early disease in high-risk subjects. Clearly further work needs to be done to establish the place of this promising marker in the diagnostic armamentarium.

Radiology in the diagnostic evaluation of mesothelioma

Chest radiography

It is important emphasize the central role of the plain chest radiograph in the early diagnosis of mesothelioma. It is a simple, cheap, and easily available tool that should be employed at the first hint of suspicious symptoms in at-risk individuals. Between 75 and 90 per cent of patients will have a unilateral pleural effusion of variable size detectable on chest radiograph at the time of diagnosis and may be associated with the presence of pleural plaques [62]. Figure 3.2 shows a

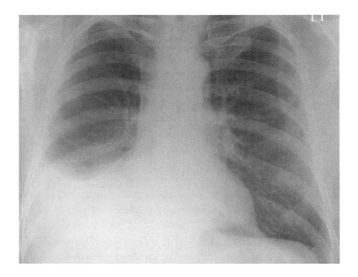

Figure 3.2 Typical appearance of mesothelioma chest radiograph. There is a right pleural effusion and the mediastinum is central.

typical radiological appearance at presentation. Some authors have stated that the chest radiograph is invariably abnormal at the time of presentation [19] but occasionally patients who present with chest pain and normal radiology go on to develop abnormalities as the disease progresses. Pleural effusions may or may not be accompanied by obvious pleural thickening and this, in turn, can be present without obvious effusion. Such thickening may have a lobulated appearance and characteristically spreads to the mediastinal surface of the pleura. A minority of cases of

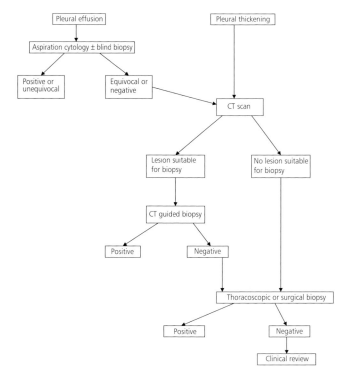

Figure 3.3 Diagnostic strategy for suspected pleural mesothelioma. (Reproduced with permission from British Thoracic Society. Statement on malignant mesothelioma in the United Kingdom. *Thorax* 2001; 5 6: 250–65.)

pleural mesotheliomas, probably less than 5 per cent, occur without serous effusion at any stage [19, 21]. Occasionally the mass can appear to be intrapulmonary rather than pleural on the chest radiograph [62]. Contrast-enhanced CT scanning is an essential next step in establishing both a diagnosis and assessing the stage of disease [63, 64] (Fig. 3.3).

Computed tomography

CT is the primary imaging modality used for the radiological evaluation of malignant mesothelioma. Enhanced CT with iodinated contrast is normally used. Malignant or inflammatory pleural disease enhances strongly, and the contrast allows differentiation between any thickness pleura, effusion, and underlying aerated or collapsed lung. Modern multidetector CT (MDCT) allows a scan of the entire chest to be performed in less than 10 seconds. The use of a narrow scan slice (<1 mm thick) allows the final images to be visualized in any plane.

The anatomy of the pleura is complex and is not always appreciated. The inferior margins of the pleura in the posterior costodiaphragmatic recesses of the hemithorax extend considerably lower than the corresponding border of the lung at the level of the 12th dorsal vertebra. The diaphragm extends more inferiorly and the right crus arises from the anterolateral surfaces of the bodies and the intravertebral discs of the upper three lumbar vertebra. In patients with established MPM being considered for surgery, the entire pleural and diaphragmatic surfaces need to be scanned contiguously from the thoracic inlet to the level of the third lumbar vertebra. This allows coronal and sagital images to be reconstructed to interrogate for subdiaphragmatic extension which is deemed unresectable.

The lymphatic drainage of the pleura is equally complex. Although the visceral pleural lymphatics follow the same pattern of drainage as the lung, the lymphatic drainage of the parietal pleura is very different. The anterior parietal pleura drains to internal mammary nodes. The posterior parietal pleura drains to the extrapleural lymph nodes which lie in the paraspinal fat adjacent to the heads of the ribs. The diaphragm is commonly involved by MPM. The anterior and lateral diaphragmatic lymphatics drain to internal mammary and anterior peridiaphragnmatic nodes. The posterior diaphragm drains to para-aortic and posterior mediastinal nodes. There are free anastamoses between lymphatics on both surfaces of the diaphragm, and coeliac axis or gastrohepatic nodal enlargement may be seen (Fig. 3.4). In practice the lymphatic drainage can be thought of as a circle of nodes in the extrapleural space. Any nodes visualized here should be viewed with suspicion. In addition to inspection of the thorax, a thorough search for enlarged nodes should be made in the retrocrural region and upper abdomen.

CT allows evaluation of the detailed morphology of pleural disease allowing differentiation of malignant disease from benign pleural or other pleural malignant disease (Figs 3.4–3.6 and Table 3.3). Leung et al. [65] studied 74 consecutive patients with diffuse pleural disease. CT features used to distinguish malignant from benign pleural disease were circumferential pleural thickening, nodular pleural thickening, parietal pleural thickening greater than 1 cm, and mediastinal pleural involvement. The specificities of these findings were 100 per cent, 94 per cent, 94 per cent, and 88 per cent, respectively. The sensitivities were 41 per cent, 51 per cent, 36 per cent, and 56 per cent, respectively. Using these criteria, Traill et al. [66] studied 40 consecutive patients. Contrast-enhanced CT correctly identified 28 of 32 patients with malignant disease and all eight patients with benign disease, giving a sensitivity of 84 per cent and a specificity of 100 per cent for the technique. This study found circumferential thickening a less reliable indicator for malignancy, and this was seen in equal numbers in the benign and malignant groups.

It is important in patients with suspected pleural malignancy to differentiate between MPM and other pleural malignancy. Metintas et al. [66] looked at this issue and reviewed the CT

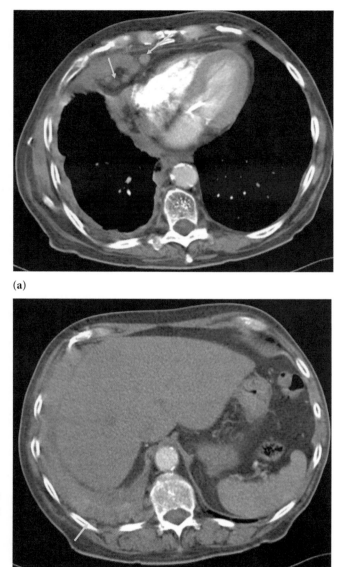

(a)

(b)

Figure 3.4 The lymphatic drainage of the parietal pleura is complex and drains to a 'ring' of nodes surrounding the pleura. This is demonstrated on these two axial CT images in the same patient with a right-sided tumour with several extrapleural nodes (yellow arrows).

findings of 215 patients, 99 with MPM, 39 with metastatic pleural disease, and 77 with benign pleural disease. The most common CT features in patients with MPM were circumferential nodular lung encasement, pleural thickening with irregular pleuropulmonary margins, and pleural thickening with superimposed nodules. In the 70 per cent of cases of MPM, there was rind-like extension of tumour on the pleural surfaces. In multivariate analysis, the CT findings of 'rind-like pleural involvement', 'mediastinal pleural involvement', and 'pleural thickness more than 1 cm' were independent findings in differentiating mesothelioma from other malignant pleural disease.

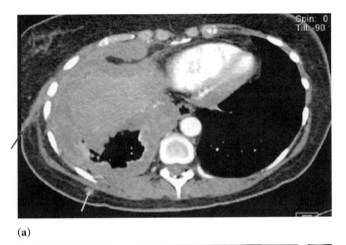

(a)

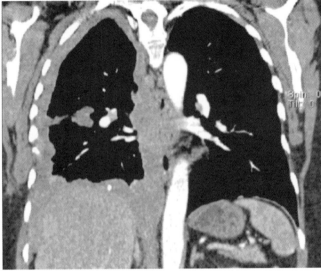

(b)

Figure 3.5 Axial and coronal contrast-enhanced CT showing an advanced right-sided malignant pleural mesothelioma. There is irregular circumferential involvement of the right hemithorax. Two foci of chest wall involvement are seen posteriorly (yellow arrow) and laterally (red arrow).

Other features found at CT include the presence of calcified plaques in approximately 20 per cent of patients with mesothelioma. There may also be contraction of the affected hemithorax with associated ipsilateral mediastinal shift, narrowed intercostal spaces, and elevation of the ipsilateral hemidiaphragm. This is a tumour that is locally aggressive with frequent invasion of the chest wall, mediastinum, and diaphragm. As stated above, chest wall involvement is common at sites of previous intervention including biopsy, drain, and surgical sites [45]. There should be careful evaluation of these areas which can be marked with a suitable radio-opaque marker to aid this. Chest wall involvement may manifest as obliteration of extrapleural fat planes, invasion of intercostal muscles, displacement of ribs, or bone destruction. Direct extension of the tumour into the major vessels and mediastinum may occur. Mesothelioma may invade the pericardium and can be seen at CT as nodular pericardial thickening or pericardial effusion [63, 64].

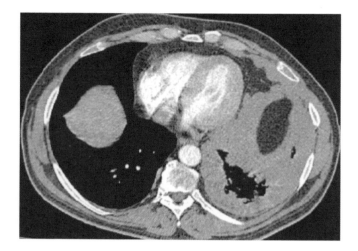

Figure 3.6 Axial contrast-enhanced CT. There is pericardial invasion by a left MPM. The pericardium is thickened and there are contralateral pleural plaques.

Table 3.3 CT features of malignant pleural mesothelioma

Common features

Pleural thickening

Irregular/nodular

Rind like

Pleural effusion

Mediastinal pleural thickening

Interlobar fissural involvement

Volume contraction

Chest wall invasion

Uncommon features

Discrete pleural nodules or masses

Rib destruction

Vertebral body erosion

Mediastinal invasion

Diaphragmatic invasion

Features discriminating MPM from other pleural malignancies

Rind-like pleural involvement

Mediastinal pleural involvement

Pleural thickness >1 cm

Pleural plaques

Magnetic resonance imaging

MRI can play an important role in defining the extent of malignant disease in patients with MPM. Through the use of different pulse sequences and gadolinium-based contrast material, MRI can help differentiate between tumour and normal tissue. Relative to adjacent chest wall muscle, malignant mesothelioma is typically iso- or slightly hyper-intense on T_1-weighted images and moderately hyper-intense on T_2-weighted images. The tumour enhances with use of gadolinium-based contrast material. The excellent contrast resolution of MRI can allow improved detection of tumour extension, especially to the chest wall and diaphragm, and better prediction of overall likelihood of resectability. Anatomical and morphological MRI features similar to those seen at CT are used to establish local invasion of mesothelioma. Loss of normal fat planes, extension into the mediastinal fat, and tumour encasement of more than 50 per cent of the circumference of mediastinal structures are some of the MRI features that suggest tumour extension. MRI is the most useful tool for evaluating patients with questionable areas of local tumour extension at CT or in whom intravenous administration of iodinated contrast material is contraindicated [68, 69] (Fig. 3.7). It has historically had an advantage in view of its multiplanar capability, but this is likely to be overcome with the advent of multi detector CT scans.

The use of MRI contrast agents has been shown to be of value in the prediction of malignancy in patients with asbestos exposure. Benign plaques typically show low signal intensity on unenhanced and enhanced T_1- and T_2-weighted images. Malignant mesothelioma typically shows hyper-intensity on T_2-weighted imaging and enhances following intravenous gadolinium contrast on T_1-weighted images. Boraschi et al. [70] described 30 patients with asbestos-related pleural disease. The sensitivity, specificity, and diagnostic accuracy of MRI in classifying a lesion as suggestive of malignancy were 100 per cent, 95 per cent, and 97 per cent respectively. These appearances are not specific and are similar for other malignant pleural disease, and contrast enhancement may be seen in benign asbestos-related pleural disease if there is an inflammatory component to this. Enhancement may be seen following pleurodesis of a benign effusion [68].

Hierholzer et al. [71] retrospectively studied 42 patients and compared CT with MRI Mediastinal pleural involvement, circumferential pleural thickening, nodularity, irregularity of pleural contour, and infiltration of the chest wall and/or diaphragm were found to be most suggestive of a malignant cause on both CT and MRI. Pleural calcification on CT was suggestive of a benign cause. High signal intensity in relation to intercostal muscles on T_2-weighted and/or

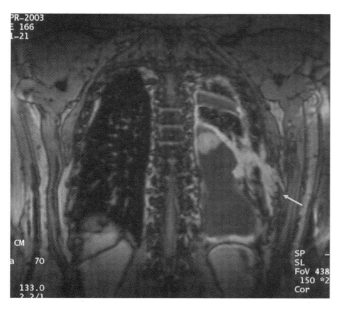

Figure 3.7 Coronal contrast-enhanced MRI of a left MPM with enhancement in the left lateral chest wall due to tumour involvement, (yellow arrow).

contrast-enhanced T_1-weighted images was significantly suggestive of malignant disease. Using these morphological features in combination with the signal intensity features, MRI had a sensitivity of 100 per cent and a specificity of 93 per cent in the detection of pleural malignancy and was thought to be superior to CT. In a comparative study of MRI and CT Knuuttila *et al.* [72] found that contrast-enhanced MRI was superior in demonstrating focal thickening and enhancement of interlobar fissures, a useful sign in detecting early malignant pleural disease.

Ultrasound

Where examination of a normal lung is of limited value, ultrasound can be very useful in identifying pathology of the pleura. The presence of a pleural effusion can substantially enhance the usefulness of ultrasound investigations; the liquid acts as an acoustic window and can enable the detection of intrapleural and intrapulmonary processes. Pleural effusions and thickening can be readily appreciated by ultrasound and discrete malignant nodules may be seen [73].

Positron emission tomography

Positron emission tomography (PET) scanning uses the positron-emitting radionuclides of several biologically fundamental elements to obtain quantitative tomographic images. 2-[^{18}F]fluoro-2-deoxy-D-glucose (FDG) PET is the most commonly used technique. The standardized uptake value (SUV) of FDG is used as a semiquantitative measure of the metabolic activity of a lesion. The SUV is significantly higher in MPM than in benign pleural diseases such as inflammatory pleuritis and asbestos-related pleural plaques, however, some mesotheliomas are relatively low-grade tumours and may not be intensely hypermetabolic on FDG-PET [74].

PET can play a role in differentiating benign from malignant disease. Duysinx *et al.* [75] prospectively studied 98 patients presenting with either pleural thickening or an exudate pleural effusion. FDG-PET was performed on each subject prior to sampling. Sixty-one of 63 patients with histologically confirmed malignant disease showed FDG uptake within the area of pleural thickening. FDG-PET imaging showed an absence of FDG uptake, and correctly classified 31 and 35 benign lesions. In the remaining four lesions, intense FDG uptake was seen in one case of parapneumonic effusion, while moderate and localized uptake was observed in one parapneumonic, one tuberculous, and one uraemic pleurisy. The sensitivity of the method to identify malignancy was 96.8 per cent with a negative predictive value of 93.9 per cent, while its specificity was 88.5 per cent and its positive predictive value was 93.8 per cent. In a prospective study, Kramer *et al.* [76] studied 32 patients, 19 with malignant and 13 with benign disease. PET was true positive in 18 patients and true negative in 12 patients, with an accuracy and negative predictive value of 94 per cent and 92 per cent, respectively. PET was false positive in a patient with infectious pleuritis and false negative for a slowly growing malignant solitary fibrous tumour.

There is dispute as to whether the SUV correlates with the T stage [77], but it appears to be higher in those with nodal and metastatic disease, and is associated with an unfavourable prognosis [74, 77, 78]. SUV does not appear to be related to histological grade. Care should be taken with patients who have previously undergone talc pleurodesis, as the inflammatory process caused by this procedure can cause a false-positive result. Correlation with CT is needed to demonstrate the high-attenuation pleural thickening due to talc administration [79].

Areas of pleural thickening may not necessarily correspond to areas of high metabolic activity, and the most appropriate biopsy site may not be apparent from CT findings. Because FDG-PET can provide information about metabolically active areas when findings are correlated with anatomical imaging information, it can be used to help determine the most appropriate biopsy site for obtaining positive results. This is particularly useful in a patient with a suspected false-negative result.

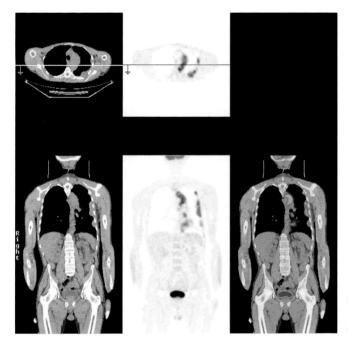

Figure 3.8 CT–PET images of a left-sided MPM in the axial and coronal planes.

Although FDG-PET gives valuable functional information, its spatial resolution is inferior to CT and MRI and it may be difficult to localize metabolic activity to PET. This is particularly difficult in differentiating malignant lymphadenopathy from closely adjacent mediastinal pleural involvement. Co-registration techniques that involve the fusion of CT and PET scans can provide more accurate identification of abnormalities seen with the two modalities separately, and the same is true for CT–PET imaging (Fig. 3.8).

Staging

The staging of mesothelioma is not easy and a number of criteria have been proposed. Staging is particularly important in patients being considered for radical surgery and included amongst the elements of this process is the requirement for mediastinal node biopsy prior to extrapleural pneumonectomy. This topic is fully covered in Chapter 13. The prognostic importance of staging is discussed in Chapter 5.

Establishing a histological or cytological diagnosis

Clearly, tissue confirmation of the diagnosis is very important since the differential diagnosis of pleural effusion and thickening encompasses a wide range of disease entities. Comprehensive discussion of the differential diagnosis of pleural effusions is beyond the scope of this chapter, but has recently been systematically reviewed and guidelines have been published in the UK [80].

Pleural fluid

The first step in the diagnosis of a unilateral pleural effusion will usually be a needle aspiration. Unfortunately, in malignant mesothelioma this does not provide more than supportive evidence of the diagnosis in the majority of patients. However, simple aspiration is minimally invasive and if it is to be carried out, it is best done with a simple 21G needle with aspiration of the fluid into a 50 ml syringe with samples being sent for cytology, bacteriology (including AAFBs), and biochemical analysis. This should include its protein content and lactate dehydrogenase level, and the pH and glucose level should also be requested if infection is suspected. A 20 ml sample is usually sufficient for cytological analysis. More reliable results are obtained when the specimen is fresh [80], although storage for up to 4 days at 4°C is acceptable [81]. In the presence of a large effusion this procedure can be safely carried out in an outpatient or ward setting, but if the effusion is small it is best performed under ultrasound or CT guidance to reduce the risk of pneumothorax. The appearance of the pleural fluid is serous in about 50 per cent of patients and blood-stained to a varying extent in the remainder [82]. Bleeding into the effusion is very heavy in some patients [83].

The fluid is invariably an exudate, usually with protein content higher than 35g/l, although it can be lower in the presence of a low serum albumin. Elevated levels of hyaluronate can occasionally make the fluid very viscous, and some authors have proposed that an elevated level of hyaluronate in the pleural fluid is a finding specific to mesothelioma [84]. Cytological examination of the pleural fluid will give a diagnosis of malignancy in 50–60 per cent of malignant pleural effusions, but even with modern immunocytochemical techniques its specificity for the diagnosis of mesothelioma is only 32 per cent [85] and pleural biopsy of some description is required in the majority of cases.

Closed pleural biopsy

Figure 3.3 shows one algorithm proposed for the diagnosis of pleural effusion [31]. Pleural biopsy can be carried out in several ways: closed, blind biopsy with Abrams, Cope, or Ramel reverse cutting needles, CT (or ultrasound) guided-needle biopsy, and open biopsy by either thoracoscopy or surgical incision. Abrams needle is the most widely used, yielding somewhat larger tissue samples than the Cope needle, and is relatively free of complications in the presence of an effusion of significant size. Complications include pneumothorax, vasovagal syncope, haemothorax, haematoma at the biopsy site, and ipsilateral shoulder pain [86, 87].

Ideally a contrast-enhanced CT scan should be carried out before biopsy, but this is not always practicable and it is reasonable to have a single attempt at blind pleural biopsy, ideally at the same time as pleural aspiration, before a scan is available. At least four biopsy samples need to be taken during this procedure [80, 88]. Since 'seeding' of the tumour is common with mesothelioma after

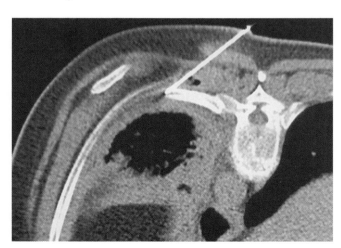

Figure 3.9 A CT-guided pleural biopsy of a left-sided MPM with the patient prone.

such procedures, the number of invasive investigations should be kept to a minimum and there is no place for repeated closed biopsy. The addition of Abrams biopsy to simple cytology improves the diagnostic rate of mesothelioma from about 33 per cent to nearer 50 per cent [89].

The best of the non-surgical techniques now appears to be image-guided cutting-needle biopsy of suitable pleural masses which can be performed using either ultrasound [90] or CT scanning [91, 92] (Fig. 3.9). Direct visualization of the pleura using these techniques allows biopsy of the most thickened areas of pleura and can be performed safely in the absence of a pleural effusion. Using ultrasound-guided core-needle biopsy, Heilo *et al.* [90] biopsied 70 patients with a tentative diagnosis of mesothelioma. Fifty-two of these (74 per cent) had a final diagnosis of malignant pleural mesothelioma. Twelve of 14 inadequate biopsy specimens were false negative for mesothelioma and there were no false-positive biopsy results. They calculated that ultrasound-guided core-needle biopsy had a sensitivity of 77 per cent in the detection of mesothelioma. Metintas *et al.* [67] described CT-guided closed pleural biopsy (using Cope, Ramel, or Abrams needles) in 30 patients with a final diagnosis of mesothelioma with a sensitivity of 83 per cent and a specificity of 100 per cent in diagnosing mesothelioma.

Maskell *et al.* [92] directly compared Abrams and CT cutting-needle biopsy. Fifty consecutive patients with cytologically negative suspected malignant pleural effusions were randomly allocated to either Abrams pleural biopsy or CT-guided cutting-needle biopsy. Abrams biopsy correctly diagnosed malignancy in eight of 17 patients (sensitivity, 47 per cent; specificity, 100 per cent). CT-guided biopsy correctly diagnosed malignancy in 13 of 15 (sensitivity, 87 per cent; specificity, 100 per cent). The difference of 40 per cent in sensitivity between Abrams and CT-guided biopsy was significant (95 per cent confidence interval 10–69; $P = 0.02$). The diagnostic advantage was similar in patients proving to have mesothelioma and other forms of malignancy.

Thoracoscopy and open surgical biopsy

The most assured method of obtaining sufficient pathological material to make the histological diagnosis of pleural mesothelioma is surgical biopsy. Some authors have proposed a routine open surgical approach [93], but in many centres thoracoscopy is now the preferred method of surgical biopsy. The procedure can be carried out under local or general anaesthesia, and there is an increasing trend, in Europe at least, towards 'medical' thoracoscopy being carried out by suitably trained and experienced respiratory physicians [94]. The diagnostic sensitivity for malignant pleural effusions has been reported to be 95 per cent or more [95–97]. Apart from allowing for the removal of relatively large amounts of tissue from macroscopically abnormal areas of pleura, it can assist in the staging process and allow for therapeutic interventions such as talc pleurodesis. Ideally, this technique should probably be the biopsy method of first choice in a suspected malignant pleural effusion, an approach that would be likely to save many repeated and unsuccessful theoretically less invasive procedures.

Microarray gene expression profiles

The advent of microarray technology has enabled researchers to examine many genes simultaneously under the same conditions [98]. The wealth of data generated enables reclassification of tumours [99–101], identification of prognostic characteristics [102], characterization of disease-related genes [103], detection of regulatory motifs [104], and examination of the kinetics of promoter occupancy of transcriptional coactivators [105]. Other uses for microarray technology include the development of microarray-based comparative genomic hybridization (array-CGH) to identify chromosomal losses and gains within tumours [106] and epigenomic analysis [107–109]. Within the clinical setting an exciting use of microarrays is their potential to predict clinical outcome [110–114], resistance to chemotherapy [115], and the pharmacogenomics of drug response [116].

In the adjuvant setting, in order to avoid missing the few patients who may benefit from such treatment, most cancer patients are currently overtreated. Microarray-based technologies may allow personalized therapies geared towards the individual based on the molecular profiles of the tumour [117]; however, a caveat to the current potential of microarray-based personalized therapies is that many studies utilize samples with contaminating admixtures of stromal and other cell types. This can not only lead to complications not only in the precise delineation of gene profiling between non-tumours and tumours [118], but issues of reproducibility and accuracy can also cause problems with regulatory agencies [119, 120].

Altered gene expression in mesothelioma

Several gene expression profiling studies have been carried out on normal mesothelial tissue, mesothelioma-derived cell lines, and primary tumours. In the following sections we shall give a brief overview of the results obtained.

Rihn *et al.* [121] used both a cDNA microarray comprising 6969 probes and a high-density filter array to identify gene expression changes between a control simian virus 40 (SV40) transformed mesothelial cell line (Met-5A) and a mesothelioma derived cell line (MSTO-211H) [121]. From this analysis they identified genes involved with macromolecule stability and metabolism (upregulation of *GADD45A* and *PCNA*), adhesion (upregulation of *integrins a3, a4, a6* and *b-like 1*), and invasion [downregulation of *fibronectin 1* and upregulation of plasminogen activator inhibitor-2 (*PAI-2*) and tissue inhibitor of matrix metalloproteinase-3 (*TIMP-3*)] in the malignant line. Other genes which were altered involved cell cycle regulation and growth (upregulation of *cyclin H, cdk-7*, Ki-*ras*, c-*myc*, and basic fibroblast growth factor *bFGF/FGF2*), and oxidative stress response genes [superoxide dismutase Cu/Zn (*SOD1*)]. In a study examining gene expression changes during asbestos-induced carcinogenesis in rats several genes were found to be upregulated including c-*myc*, c-*jun*, integrin-linked kinase (*ilk*), epidermal growth factor receptor (*EGFR*) and Fos-related antigen-1 (*Fra-1*) [122]. Confirmation that the genes *Fra-1*, *GADD45*, and c-*myc* were significantly upregulated in mesothelioma came from additional studies using both rat and human mesothelioma cells [123, 124]. Two studies examining gene expression in mesothelioma cell lines have demonstrated upregulation of Jun-B [123, 125]. A subsequent study found that the upregulation of Jun-B was discriminatory for the epithelial subtype of mesothelioma [126].

Additional fibroblast growth factors have also been shown to have altered expression in mesothelioma including upregulation of *FGF3* and *FGF12* and downregulation of *FGF-1* and *FGF-7* [125]. A follow-up analysis of histological subgroups of malignant mesothelioma found that *bFGF/FGF2* was upregulated in epithelial and sarcomatoid forms but not in biphasic tumours [126]. This same study also identified the FGF receptor activating protein (*FRAG1*) as an upregulated gene within mesotheliomas with an epithelial histopathological classification [126].

Genes whose function involves apoptotic pathways have frequently been shown to be altered in array studies of mesothelioma [123, 127, 128]. It is interesting to note that overexpression of the antiapoptotic genes Bcl-2 and survivin was observed in one study, and targeting survivin led to the induction of apoptosis in these cells [128]. In a similar study where the authors were comparing changes in gene expression of mesothelioma cells under conditions of oxidative stress downregulation of Bcl-2 was observed [123].

One emerging subset of genes which has been shown to be altered in mesothelioma concerns the insulin-like growth factor axis. This axis has previously been shown to be altered in mesothelioma [129], and has frequently been reported as a cause of tumour-induced hypoglycaemia [130–132]. Microarray analysis has shown that several members of this axis have also been altered, confirming the importance of this pathway in mesothelioma. Two commonly downregulated genes from the IGF axis in mesothelioma are *IGFBP-4* and *IGFBP-5* [125, 133–135]. Commonly overexpressed genes include *IGFBP-3*, *IGFBP-7/MAC25*, and an exon-specific isoform of IGF-I (IGF-I, exon 1A) [126, 136, 137]. Increased *IGFBP-5* exression was linked to the long term (more than 12 months after operation) [135]. However, in a separate study downregulation of IGFBP-5 was observed to be a common feature in mesothelioma, but no survival data are available for these samples [126]. IGFBP-3 is another gene whose overexpression has been linked to poor outcome tumours [136].

Kratzke's group noted the dysregulation of the IGF axis in an early microarray study [126] and reanalysed their microarray data specifically for members of this axis. They subsequently identified additional genes which were overexpressed in mesotheliomas (*IGF1R*, *IRS-2*, *IGFBP-3*, and *IGFBP-6*) [138]. Albelda's group also identified *IGF1R* as a gene with altered expression in mesothelioma [127]. The analysis by Hoang *et al.* [138] led to the discovery that there is selective activation of the insulin receptor substrates 1 and 2 (*IRS-1*, *IRS-2*) associated with a distinct subset of malignant pleural mesotheliomas. This study highlights one of the advantages of microarray data, as all experiments can be reanalysed as new information becomes available.

An additional subset of genes whose expression is frequently observed to be altered in mesotheliomas are those associated with cytoskeletal reorganization [121, 122, 125, 127, 133–136]. Altered expression of various keratins [121, 125–127, 139] integrins [121, 125, 127, 133–135, 139], annexins [127, 140], and cadherins [133, 139], and type-specific upregulation of integrin beta 4 (*ITG-4*) and P-cadherin, have also been observed for epithelioid mesotheliomas [133].

Oxidative stress genes have also been identified in gene expression arrays as having altered expression in mesotheliomas. Two genes have frequently been observed to be altered in several studies. These are *SOD1* [121, 127, 137] and thioredoxin [121, 137, 139].

Gene profiling in the diagnosis of MPM

Despite the fact that MPM has relatively unique biological features and the development of more robust diagnostic immunohistochemistry tests, the differentiation of the disease from other metastatic and benign pleural disease can be difficult. In a recent collaborative study between Leicester University and Oxford University, the gene array profiles of MPM (14 cases) were compared with those of adenocarcinoma (three cases) and benign pleura (five cases) using good-quality RNA as assessed by the Agilent 2100 bioanalyser and Affymetrix HU133A chip technology analysed using GeneSpring version 6.2.1. A significant number of genes, including the cytokeratins (*CK7* and *CK19*), E- and P-cadherin, growth factors (c-*met*), and proteinase inhibitors (anti-leucoproteinase), were elevated more than fourfold in MPM compared with benign tissue. Calretinin, uroplakin, *FGF-9* and annexins 3 and 9 were significantly elevated in MPM compared with adenocarcinoma [140]. In contrast a number of genes, including CD24, tight junction proteins such as claudins 3, 4 and 7, and mucin proteins, were elevated in adenocarcinomas compared with MPM (Fig. 3.10). This work is ongoing and remains to be validated with larger patient numbers and a testing cohort. An earlier study by Gordon *et al.* [141] used microarray gene expression clustering to separate MPM from adenocarcinomas of the lung with 95 per cent accuracy for MPM.

Mesotheliomas are classified histologically into three subtypes, designated as epithelioid, biphasic, and sarcomatoid according to the WHO–IASLC classification scheme. Gene expession profiling has been shown to have the ability to identify tumour subtypes accurately [99–101].

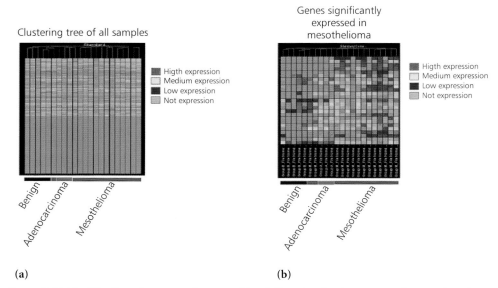

Figure 3.10 Identification of a gene subset capable of discrminating between malignant pleural mesothelioma (MPM), metastatic adenocarcinoma, and benign pleura.[139] (a) A tree cluster showing all samples separated on the basis of expression levels from highest to no-expression. (b) A tree cluster showing the subset of genes which have a high expression in MPM compared with adenocarcinoma and benign pleura.

While several gene expression profiling studies have been carried out on mesothelioma, classifying mesotheliomas into subtype by gene expression changes has been limited. In the study by Albelda's group, no distinct subclassifications were identified following clustering of gene expression profiles [127].

More recently, two groups have successfully used microarray gene expression profiling to cluster mesotheliomas on the basis of their histological subtype. Knuutila's group, using microarray analysis, identified 10 genes which can potentially distinguish between the three histological subtypes of MPM [133]. Kratzke's group identified a 180-gene subset which could discriminate differentially between histological subtype. Using this gene subset, the authors subsequently classified two unknown MPM cell lines into the epithelial subtype on the basis of their gene expression profiles [126].

Conclusions

The principal techniques for diagnosing MPM include clinical suspicion, a careful review focusing on social history and presenting symptoms, radiological investigations and obtaining adequate biopsy material for histological assessment. The use of serum mesothelin and osteopontin levels to screen patients at high risk of developing MPM, and as tools to monitor response to and subsequent relapse following therapy require evaluation in prospective randomised studies. The role of genomics as a diagnostic, prognostic and predictive tool is an area of ongoing research that holds promise not only for directing patient management but also for the discovery of future novel therapeutic targets.

References

1. Robertson HE. Endothelia of the pleura. *J Cancer Res* 1924; **8**: 317.

2. Wagner E. Das tuberkelahnliche Lymphadenom. *Arch Heilk* 1870; **11**: 497.

3. Von Rokitanski C. *Manual of Pathological Anatomy*. London: Sydenham Society Transactions 1854, 265.

4. Klemperer P, Rabin CB. Primary neoplasms of the pleura (a report of five cases). *Archives of Pathology* 1931; **141**: 385–412.

5. Godwin MC. Diffuse mesothelioma with comment on their relation to localized fibrous mesotheliomas. *Cancer* 1957; **10**: 298–319.

6. Winslow DJ, Taylor HB. Malignant pleural mesothelioma. *Cancer* 1960; **13**: 127–36.

7. Roberts GH. Diffuse pleural mesothelioma, a clinical and pathological study. *Br J Dis Chest* 1970; **64**: 201–11.

8. Hillerdal G. Asbestos-related pleural disease including diffuse malignant mesothelioma. *Eur Respir Mon* 2002; **22**: 189–203.

9. Wagner JC, Slegges CA, Marchand P. Diffuse pleural mesothelioma and asbestos exposure in the North Western Cape Province. *Br J Ind Med* 1960; **17**: 260–71.

10. Wagner JC. Epidemiology of diffuse mesothelial tumours: evidence of an association from studies in South Africa and United Kingdom. *Ann NY Acad Sci* 1965; **132**: 575–8.

11. Ribak J, Lilis R, Suzuki Y, Penner L, Selikoff IJ. Malignant mesothelioma in a cohort of asbestos insulation workers: clinical presentation, diagnosis and causes of death. *Br J Ind Med* 1988; **45**: 182–7.

12. Bittersohl G, Ose H. Epidemiology of mesothelioma. *Z Gesamte Hyg* 1971; **17**, 861–4.

13. Newhouse ML, Thompson H. Mesothelioma of the pleura and peritoneum following exposure to asbestos in the London area. *Br J Ind Med* 1965; **22**: 261–9.

14. Meurman LO, Kiviluoto R, Hakama M. Mortality and morbidity among the working population of anthophyllite asbestos miners in Finland. *Br J Ind Med* 1974; **31**: 105–12.

15. Magnani C, Terracini B, Ivaldi C, Botta M, Mancini A, Andrion A. Pleural malignant mesothelioma and non-occupational exposure to asbestos in Casale Monferrate, Italy. *Occup Environ Med* 1995; **52**, 362–7.

16. Abratt RP, Vorobiof DA, White N. Asbestos and mesothelioma in South Africa. *Lung Cancer* 2004; **45** (Suppl): S3–6.

17. Henderson DW, Shilkin KB, Whitaker D. Reactive mesothelial hyperplasia vs mesothelioma, including mesothelioma *in situ*: a brief review. *Am J Clin Pathol* 1998; **110**: 397–404.

18. Musk AW, de Klerk NH. Epidemiology of malignant mesothelioma in Australia. *Lung Cancer* 2004; **45** (Suppl): S21–3.

19. Elmes PC, Simpson MJC. The clinical aspects of mesothelioma. *Q J Med* 1976; **45**: 427–9.

20. Yates DH, Corrin B, Stidolph PN, Browne K. Malignant mesothelioma in south east England: clinicopathological experience of 272 cases. *Thorax* 1997; **52**: 507–12.

21. Hillerdal G. Malignant mesothelioma 1982: review of 4710 published cases. *Br J Dis Chest* 1983; **77**: 321–43.

22. Selcuk ZT, Çöplü L, Emri S, Kalyoncu AF, Sarin AA, BarisYI. Malignant pleural mesothelioma due to environmental mineral fiber exposure in Turkey. Analysis of 135 cases. *Chest* 1992; **102**: 790–6.

23. McLean AN, Patel KR. Clinical features and epidemiology of malignant mesothelioma in west Glasgow 1987–1992. *Scot Med J* 1997; **42**: 37–9.

24. Emri S, Demir AU. Malignant pleural mesothelioma in Turkey. *Lung Cancer* 2004; **45** (Suppl): S17–20.

25. Filiberti R, Montanaro F. Epidemiology of pleural mesothelioma in Italy. *Lung Cancer* ; **45** (Suppl): S25–7.

26. Shepherd KE, Oliver LC, Kazemi H. Diffuse malignant pleural mesothelioma in an urban hospital: clinical spectrum and trend in incidence over time. *Am J Ind Med* 1989; **16**: 373–83.

27. Baris B, Demir AU, Shehu V, Karakoca Y, Kisacik G, Baris YI. Environmental fibrous (zeolite/erionite) exposure and malignant tumours other than mesothelioma. *J Environ Pathol Toxicol Oncol* 1996; **15**: 183–9.

28. Fraire AE, Cooper S, Greenberg SD, Buffler P, Langston C. Mesothelioma of childhood. *Cancer* 1988; **62**: 838–47.

29. Carbone M, Pass HI, Rizzo P, *et al.* Simian virus 40-like DNA sequences in human pleural mesothelioma. *Oncogene* 1994; **9**: 1781–90.

30. Gibbs AR, Jasani B, Pepper C, Navabi H, Wynford-Thomas D. SV40 DNA sequences in mesotheliomas. *Dev Biol Stand* 1998; **94**: 41–5.

31. British Thoracic Society. Statement on malignant mesothelioma in the United Kingdom. *Thorax* 2001; **56**: 250–265

32. Rothschild H, Mulvey JJ. An increased risk for lung cancer mortality associated with sugar cane farming. *J Natl Cancer Inst* 1982; **68**: 755–60.

33. Niklinski J, Nicklinska W, Chyczewska E, *et al.* The epidemiology of asbestos-related diseases. *Lung Cancer* 2004; **45** (Suppl): S7–S15.

34. McDonald AD, McDonald JC. Malignant mesothelioma in North America. *Cancer* 1980; **46**: 1650–6.

35. Muscat JE, Wynder EL. Cigarette smoking, asbestos and malignant mesothelioma. *Cancer Res* 1991; **51**: 2263–7.

36. Pisani RJ, Colby TV, Williams DE. Malignant mesothelioma of the pleura. *Mayo Clin Proc* 1988; **63**: 1234–44.

37. Rusch VW. Diagnosis and treatment of pleural mesothelioma. *Semin Surg Oncol* 1990; **6**: 279–84.

38. Suziki Y. Pathology of human malignant mesothelioma. *Semin Oncol* 1981; **8**: 268–82.

39. Ehrenhaft JL, Sensenig DM, Lawrence MS. Mesotheliomas of the pleura. *J Thorac Cardiovasc Surg* 1960; **40**, 393–409.

40. Baris YI, Artvinli M, Sahin AA. Environmental mesothelioma in Turkey. *Ann NY Acad Sci* 1980; **330**: 423–32.

41. Stanford F. Sympathetic nerve involvement with mesothelioma of the pleura. *Br J Dis Chest* 1976; **70**: 134–7.

42. Porter JM, Cheek JM. Pleural mesothelioma. Review of histogenesis and report of 12 cases. *J Thorac Cardiovasc Surg* 1968; **55**: 882–90.

43. Cooper D. Malignant mesothelioma invading the spinal canal. *Postgrad Med J* 1974; **50**: 718–23.

44. Chandurkar SN, Khandekar AL, Shirde AV, Kher AV. Primary pleural mesothelioma. *India J Chest Dis* 1975; **17**: 139.

45. Boutin C, Rey F, Viallat JK. Prevention of malignant seeding after invasive diagnostic procedures in patients with pleural mesothelioma. *Chest* 1995; **108**: 754–8.

46. Hillerdal G. Pleural plaques and risk for bronchial carcinoma and mesothelioma: a prospective study. *Chest* 1994; **105**: 144–50 .

47. Edge JR. Asbestos-related disease in Barrow-in-Furness. *Environ Res* 1976; **11**: 244–7.

48. Selikoff IJ, Hammond EC, Seidman H. Mortality experience of insulation workers in the United States and Canada, 1943–1976. *Ann NY Acad Sci* 1979; **330**: 91–116.

49. Berry G. The prognosis following certification with asbestosis in the United Kingdom. In: Wagner JC, ed. *Biological Effects of Mineral Fibre.* Lyon: IARC Scientific Publications, 1980; 603–8.

50. Chailleux E, Dabouir G, Pioche D. Prognostic factors in diffuse malignant mesothelioma. *Chest* 1988; **93**: 159–62.

51. Briselli M, Mark EJ, Dickersin GR. Solitary fibrous tumours of the pleura: 8 new cases and review of 360 cases in the literature. *Cancer* 1981; **47**: 2678–89.

52. Kim SB, Varkey B, Choi H. Diagnosis of malignant pleural mesothelioma by axillary lymph node biopsy. *Chest* 1987; **91**: 279–82.

53. Pass HI, Pogrebniak HW. Malignant pleural mesothelioma. *Curr Prob Surg* 1993; **30**: 921–1012.

54. Edwards JG, Abrams KR, Leverment JN, Spyt TJ, Waller DA, O'Byrne KJ. Prognostic factors for malignant mesothelioma in 142 patients: validation of CALGB and EORTC prognostic scoring systems. *Thorax* 2000; **55**: 731–5.

55. Onodera S, Inaba R, Nikawa K, Oikawa K, Yoshinaga K. Peritoneal mesothelioma associated with polyclonal hyperimmunoglobulinaemia. *Tohuku J Exp Med* 1974; **114**: 195–203.

56. Perks WH, Stanhope R, Green M. Hyponatraemia and mesothelioma. *Br J Dis Chest* 1979; **73**: 89–91.

57. Albin M, Jakobsen K, Attenell R, Johansson L, Welinder H. Mortality and cancer morbidity in cohorts of asbestos cement workers and referents. *Br J Ind Med* 1990; **47**: 602–10.

58. Pluygers E, Baldewyns P, Minette P, Beauduin M, Robinet P. Biomarker assessments in asbestos-exposed workers as indicators for selective prevention of mesothelioma or bronchogenic carcinoma: rationale and practical implementation Part I. *Eur J Cancer Prev* 1991; **1**: 57–68. Part II. *Eur J Cancer Prev* 1992; **1**: 129–38.

59. Robinson BWS, Creaney J, Lake R, *et al.* Mesothelin-family proteins and diagnosis of mesothelioma. *Lancet* 2004; **362**: 1612–16.

60. Scholler N, Fu N, Yang Y, *et al.* Soluble member(s) of the mesothelin/megakaryocyte potentiating factor family are detectable in sera from patients with ovarian carcinoma. *Proc Natl Acad Sci USA* 1999; **96**: 11531–6.

61. Pass HI, Cott D, Lonardo F, *et al.* Asbestos Exposure, Pleural mesothelioma and Serum Osteopontin Levels. *N Eng J Med* 2005; **353**: 1564–73.

62. Heller RM, Janower ML, Weber AL. The radiological manifestations of malignant pleural mesothelioma. *Am J Roentgenol* 1970; **108**: 53–9.

63. Kreel L. Computed tomography in mesothelioma. *Semin Oncol* 1981; **8**: 302–12.

64. Kawashima A, Libschitz HI. Malignant pleural mesothelioma: CT manifestations in 50 cases. *Am J Roentgenol* 1990; **155**: 965–9.

65. Leung AN, Muller NL, Miller RR. CT in differential diagnosis of diffuse pleural disease. *Am J Roentgenol* 1990; **154**: 487–92.

66. Traill ZC, Davies RJ, Gleeson FV. Thoracic computed tomography in patients with suspected malignant pleural effusions. *Clin Radiol* 2001; **56**: 193–6.

67. Metintas M, Ozdemir N, Isiksoy S, *et al.* CT-guided pleural needle biopsy in the diagnosis of malignant mesothelioma. *J Comput Assist Tomogr* 1995; **19**, 370–4.

68. Entwisle J. The use of magnetic resonance imaging in malignant mesothelioma. *Lung Cancer* 2004; **45** (Suppl 1): S69–71.

69. Stewart D, Waller D, Edwards J, Jeyapalan K, Entwisle J. Is there a role for pre-operative contrast-enhanced magnetic resonance imaging for radical surgery in malignant pleural mesothelioma? *Eur J Cardiothorac Surg* 2003; **24**: 1019–24.

70. Boraschi P, Neri S, Braccini G, Gigoni R, Leoncini B, Perri G. Magnetic resonance appearance of asbestos-related benign and malignant pleural diseases. *Scand J Work Environ Health* 1999; **25**: 18–23.

71. Hierholzer J, Luo L, Bittner RC, *et al.* MRI and CT in the differential diagnosis of pleural disease. *Chest* 2000; **118**: 604–9.

72. Knuuttila A, Kivisaari L, Kivisaari A, Palomaki M, Tervahartiala P, Mattson K. Evaluation of pleural disease using MR and CT with special reference to malignant pleural mesothelioma. *Acta Radiologica* 2001; **42**: 502–7.

73. Herth F. Diagnosis and staging of mesothelioma with transthoracic ultrasound. *Lung Cancer* 2004: **45** (Suppl 1); S63–7.

74. Benard F, Sterman D, Smith RJ, Kaiser LR, Albelda SM, Alavi A. Metabolic imaging of malignant pleural mesothelioma with fluorodoexyglucose positron emission tomography. *Chest* 1998; **114**: 713–22.

75. Duysinx B, Nguyen D, Louis R, *et al.* Evaluation of pleural disease with 18-fluorodeoxyglucose positron emission tomography imaging. *Chest* 2004; **125**: 489–93.

76. Kramer H, Pieterman RM, Slebos DJ, *et al.* PET for the evaluation of pleural thickening observed on CT. *J Nucl Med* 2004; **45**: 995–8.

77. Flores RM, Akhurst T, Gonen M, Larson SM, Rusch VW. Positron emission tomography defines metastatic disease but not locoregional disease in patients with malignant pleural mesothelioma. *J Thorac Cardiovasc Surg* 2003; **126**: 11–16.

78. Gerbaudo VH, Britz-Cunningham S, Sugarbaker DJ, Treves ST. Metabolic significance of the pattern, intensity and kinetics of 18F-FDG uptake in malignant pleural mesothelioma. *Thorax* 2003; **58**: 1077–82.

79. Kwek BH, Aquino SL, Fischman AJ. Fluorodeoxyglucose positron emission tomography and CT after talc pleurodesis. *Chest* 2004; **125**: 2356–60.

80. Maskell NA, Butland RJA. BTS guidelines for the investigation of unilateral pleural effusion in adults. *Thorax* 2003; **58** (Suppl II): ii8–17.

81. Boddington M. Serous effusions. In: Coleman DV, ed. *Clinical Cytotechnology.* London: Butterworths, 1989; 271–5.

82. Light RW. *Pleural Diseases*, 4th edn. Philadelphia, PA: Lippincott–Williams & Wilkins, 2001; 139

83. Kattan YB. Pleural mesothelioma with intrathoracic haemorrhage. *Br J Dis Chest* 1970; **64**: 179.

84. Nurminen M, Dejmek A, Martensson G, Thylen A, Hjerpe A. Clinical utility of liquid-chromatographic analysis of effusions for hyaluronate content. *Clin Chem* 1994; **40**: 777–80.

85. Renshaw AA, Dean BR, Antman KH, Sugarbaker DJ, Cibas DS. The role of cytological evaluation of pleural fluid in the diagnosis of malignant mesothelioma. *Chest* 1997; **111**: 106–9.

86. Levine H, Cugell DW. Blunt-end needle biopsy of pleura and rib. *Arch Int Med* 1971; **109**: 516–25.

87. Morrone N, Algranti E, Barreto E. Pleural biopsy with Cope and Abrams needles. *Chest* 1987; **92**, 1050–2.

88. Jiménez D, Pérez-Rodriguez E, Diaz G, *et al.* Determining the optimal number of specimens to obtain with needle biopsy of the pleura. *Respir Med* 2001; **96**: 14–17.

89. Whittaker D, Shilkin KB. Diagnosis of malignant pleural mesothelioma in life: a practical approach. *J Pathol* 1984; **143**: 147–75.

90. Heilo A, Steinwig AE, Solheim OP. Malignant pleural mesothelioma: US-guided histologic core-needle biopsy. *Radiology* 1999; **211**: 657–9.

91. Adams RF, Gray W, Davies RJO, Gleeson FV. Percutaneous image-guided cutting needle biopsy of the pleura in the diagnosis of malignant mesothelioma. *Chest* 2001; **120**: 1798–1802.

92. Maskell NA, Gleeson FV, Davies RJO. Standard pleural biopsy versus CT-guided cutting-needle biopsy for diagnosis of malignant disease in pleural effusion: a randomised controlled trial. *Lancet* 2003; **361**: 1326–30.

93. Herbert A, Gallagher PJ. Pleural biopsy in the diagnosis of malignant mesothelioma. *Thorax* 1982; **37**: 816–21.

94. Enk B, Viskum K. Diagnostic thoracoscopy. *Eur J Respir Dis* 1981; **62**: 344–51.

95. Harris RJ, Kavuru MS, Rice TW, Kirby TJ. The diagnostic and therapeutic utility of thoracosopy. A review. *Chest* 1995; **108**: 828–41.

96. Page RD. Thoracoscopy: a review of 121 consecutive surgical procedures. *Ann Thorac Surg* 1989; **48**: 66–8.

97. Astoul P, Boutin C. Pleuroscopy in the management of malignant pleural mesothelioma. In: Robinson WS, Chahinian AP, eds. *Mesothelioma.* London: Martin Dunitz, 2002; 127–42.

98. Meltzer PS. Spotting the target: microarrays for disease gene discovery. *Curr Opin Genet Dev* 2001; **11**: 258–63.

99. Alizadeh AA, Eisen MB, Davis RE, *et al.* Distinct types of diffuse large B-cell lymphoma identified by gene expression profiling. *Nature* 2000; **403**: 503–11.

100. Hedenfalk I, Duggan D, Chen Y, *et al.* Gene-expression profiles in hereditary breast cancer. *N Engl J Med* 2001; **344**: 539–48.

101. Takahashi M, Yang XJ, Sugimura J, *et al.* Molecular subclassification of kidney tumors and the discovery of new diagnostic markers. *Oncogene* 2003; **22**: 6810–18.

102. Takahashi M, Rhodes DR, Furge KA, *et al.* Gene expression profiling of clear cell renal cell carcinoma: gene identification and prognostic classification. *Proc Natl Acad Sci USA* 2001; **98**: 9754–9.

103. Lawn RM, Wade DP, Garvin MR, *et al.* The Tangier disease gene product ABC1 controls the cellular apolipoprotein-mediated lipid removal pathway. *J Clin Invest* 1999; **104**: R25–31.

104. Mukherjee S, Berger MF, Jona G, *et al.* Rapid analysis of the DNA-binding specificities of transcription factors with DNA microarrays. *Nat Genet* 2004; **36**: 1331–9.

105. Smith JL, Freebern WJ, Collins I, *et al.* Kinetic profiles of p300 occupancy *in vivo* predict common features of promoter structure and coactivator recruitment. *Proc Natl Acad Sci USA* 2004; **101**: 11554–9.

106. Mantripragada KK, Buckley PG, de Stahl TD, Dumanski JP. Genomic microarrays in the spotlight. *Trends Genet* 2004; **20**: 87–94.

107. Kondo Y, Shen L, Yan PS, Huang TH, Issa JP. Chromatin immunoprecipitation microarrays for identification of genes silenced by histone H3 lysine 9 methylation. *Proc Natl Acad Sci USA* 2004; **101**: 7398–403.

108. Chiba T, Yokosuka O, Arai M, *et al.* Identification of genes up-regulated by histone deacetylase inhibition with cDNA microarray and exploration of epigenetic alterations on hepatoma cells. *J Hepatol* 2004; **41**: 436–45.

109. Ballestar E, Paz MF, Valle L, *et al.* Methyl-CpG binding proteins identify novel sites of epigenetic inactivation in human cancer. *EMBO J* 2003; **22**: 6335–45.

110. van de Vijver MJ, He YD, van't Veer LJ, *et al.* A gene-expression signature as a predictor of survival in breast cancer. *N Engl J Med* 2002; **347**: 1999–2009.

111. van 't Veer LJ, Dai H, van de Vijver MJ, *et al.* Gene expression profiling predicts clinical outcome of breast cancer. *Nature* 2002; **415**: 530–6.

112. Onda M, Emi M, Nagai H, *et al.* Gene expression patterns as marker for 5-year postoperative prognosis of primary breast cancers. *J Cancer Res Clin Oncol* 2004; **130**: 537–45.

113. Nagahata T, Onda M, Emi M, *et al.* Expression profiling to predict postoperative prognosis for estrogen receptor-negative breast cancers by analysis of 25 344 genes on a cDNA microarray. *Cancer Sci* 2004; **95**: 218–25.

114. Robison JE, Perreard L, Bernard PS. State of the science: molecular classifications of breast cancer for clinical diagnostics. *Clin Biochem* 2004; **37**: 572–8.

115. Lee CH, Macgregor PF. Using microarrays to predict resistance to chemotherapy in cancer patients. *Pharmacogenomics* 2004; **5**: 611–25.

116. Villeneuve DJ, Parissenti AM. The use of DNA microarrays to investigate the pharmacogenomics of drug response in living systems. *Curr Top Med Chem* 2004; **4**: 1329–45.

117. Wulfkuhle J, Espina V, Liotta L, Petricoin E. Genomic and proteomic technologies for individualisation and improvement of cancer treatment. *Eur J Cancer* 2004; **40**: 2623–32.

118. Player A, Barrett JC, Kawasaki ES. Laser capture microdissection, microarrays and the precise definition of a cancer cell. *Expert Rev Mol Diagn* 2004; **4**: 831–40.

119. Shi L, Tong W, Goodsaid F, *et al.* QA/QC: challenges and pitfalls facing the microarray community and regulatory agencies. *Expert Rev Mol Diagn* 2004; **4**: 761–77.

120. Olson JA Jr. Application of microarray profiling to clinical trials in cancer. *Surgery* 2004; **136**: 519–23.

121. Rihn BH, Mohr S, McDowell SA, *et al.* (2000) Differential gene expression in mesothelioma. *FEBS Lett* 2000; **480**: 95–100.

122. Sandhu H, Dehnen W, Roller M, Abel J, Unfried K. mRNA expression patterns in different stages of asbestos-induced carcinogenesis in rats. *Carcinogenesis* 2000; **21**: 1023–9.

123. Kepler TB, Crosby L, Morgan KT. Normalization and analysis of DNA microarray data by self-consistency and local regression. *Genome Biol* 2002; **3**: RESEARCH0037.

124. Ramos-Nino ME, Scapoli L, Martinelli M, Land S, Mossman BT. Microarray analysis and RNA silencing link *Fra-1* to *Cd44* and c-*met* expression in mesothelioma. *Cancer Res* 2003; **63**: 3539–45.

125. Kettunen E, Nissen AM, Ollikainen T, *et al.* Gene expression profiling of malignant mesothelioma cell lines: cDNA array study. *Int J Cancer* 2001; **91**: 492–6.

126. Hoang CD, D'Cunha J, Kratzke MG, *et al.* Gene expression profiling identifies matriptase overexpression in malignant mesothelioma. *Chest* 2004; **125**: 1843–52.

127. Singhal S, Wiewrodt R, Malden LD, *et al.* Gene expression profiling of malignant mesothelioma. *Clin Cancer Res* 2003; **9**: 3080–97.

128. Xia C, Xu Z, Yuan X, *et al.* Induction of apoptosis in mesothelioma cells by antisurvivin oligonucleotides. *Mol Cancer Ther* 2002; **1**: 687–94.

129. Lee TC, Zhang Y, Aston C, *et al.* Normal human mesothelial cells and mesothelioma cell lines express insulin-like growth factor I and associated molecules. *Cancer Res* 1993; **53**: 2858–64.

130. Sakamoto T, Kaneshige H, Takeshi A, Tsushima T, Hasegawa S. Localized pleural mesothelioma with elevation of high molecular weight insulin-like growth factor II and hypoglycemia. *Chest* 1994; **106**: 965–7.

131. Baxter RC, Daughaday WH. Impaired formation of the ternary insulin-like growth factor-binding protein complex in patients with hypoglycemia due to nonislet cell tumors. *J Clin Endocrinol Metab* 1991; **73**: 696–702.

132. Hodzic D, Delacroix L, Willemsen P, *et al.* Characterization of the IGF system and analysis of the possible molecular mechanisms leading to IGF-II overexpression in a mesothelioma. *Horm Metab Res* 1997; **29**: 549–55.

133. Kettunen E, Nicholson AG, Nagy B, *et al.* L1CAM, INP10, P-cadherin, tPA and ITGB4 over-expression in malignant pleural mesotheliomas revealed by combined use of cDNA and tissue microarray. *Carcinogenesis* 2005; **26**: 17–25.

134. Kettunen E, Vivo C, Gattacceca F, Knuutila S, Jaurand MC. Gene expression profiles in human mesothelioma cell lines in response to interferon-gamma treatment. *Cancer Genet Cytogenet* 2004; **152**: 42–51.

135. Pass HI, Liu Z, Wali A, *et al.* Gene expression profiles predict survival and progression of pleural mesothelioma. *Clin Cancer Res* 2004; **10**: 849–59.

136. Gordon GJ, Jensen RV, Hsiao LL, *et al.* Using gene expression ratios to predict outcome among patients with mesothelioma. *J Natl Cancer Inst* 2003; **95**: 598–605.

137. Mohr S, Bottin MC, Lannes B, *et al.* Microdissection, mRNA amplification and microarray: a study of pleural mesothelial and malignant mesothelioma cells. *Biochimie* 2004; **86**: 13–19.

138. Hoang CD, Zhang X, Scott PD, *et al.* Selective activation of insulin receptor substrate-1 and -2 in pleural mesothelioma cells: association with distinct malignant phenotypes. *Cancer Res* 2004; **64**: 7479–85.

139. Mohr S, Keith G, Galateau-Salle F, Icard P, Rihn BH. Cell protection, resistance and invasiveness of two malignant mesotheliomas as assessed by 10K-microarray. *Biochim Biophys Acta* 2004; **1688**: 43–60.

140. Lee GYC, Street T, O'Byrne KJ, *et al.* Global gene expression profiling of malignant pleural mesothelioma. *Am J Respir Crit Care Med* 2005; in press.

141. Gordon GJ, Jensen RV, Hsiao LL, *et al.* Translation of microarray data into clinically relevant cancer diagnostic tests using gene expression ratios in lung cancer and mesothelioma. *Cancer Res* 2002; **62**: 4963–7.

Chapter 4

Histopathology of malignant pleural mesothelioma

J. E. King, F. Galateau-Sallé, and P. S. Hasleton

Introduction

It is well recognized that malignant mesothelioma can be a difficult tumour to diagnose histologically. Malignant pleural mesothelioma may be difficult to distinguish from malignant primary and metastatic pleural carcinomas or sarcomas, and also from benign mesothelial disease.
Although there have been great advances in diagnostic histopathology in the last three decades,
there is still no single test that can reliably identify malignant mesothelial cells. The correct
classification of pleural malignancy is important to ensure that appropriate treatment is given
and, in the case of patients with occupational asbestos exposure, to support claims for industrial compensation.

Anatomical sites

Malignant mesothelioma is a primary tumour of the serosal membranes. Therefore it can arise in
the pleura, peritoneum, tunica vaginalis and other related anatomical sites. The majority of reported cases in the UK involve the pleura, and a history of exposure to amphibole asbestos is evident in
more than three-quarters of cases [1]. The risk of developing mesothelioma is proportional to the
degree of asbestos exposure, but there is no apparent minimum threshold. In contrast, peritoneal
mesothelioma is associated with higher levels of asbestos exposure and asbestosis [2–4].

Primary pericardial mesothelioma is uncommon and needs to be distinguished from pleural
tumours extending to involve the pericardium. It is unclear whether primary pericardial
mesothelioma is related to asbestos exposure [5–7]. This tumour is seen in a wide age range of
12–77 years (mean 47 years) with a male-to-female ratio of 2:1 [8]. Patients most commonly
present with dyspnoea, arrhythmias, and the signs and symptoms of cardiac tamponade [8, 9].
The prognosis is understandably poor. A single case of mesothelioma of the atrioventricular
node has been documented at a national reference centre over a 46-year period [10]. It is possible
that this tumour may actually be endodermal or ectodermal in origin, rather than mesothelial,
and it is most probably not associated with asbestos exposure [11]. Malignant mesothelioma of
the tunica vaginalis or ovary is very uncommon, accounting for only 0.3 per cent of all mesotheliomas in one large Japanese series, and 0.09 per cent in a British study [12–14]. They have also
been associated with asbestos exposure [15].

The anatomy and histology of normal pleura

All the serosal membranes are derived from the intracoelomic mesoderm, which is itself derived
from cells of the epiblast (future endoderm) in the third week of embryological development [16].

Other mesodermal derivatives include connective tissues, muscle, heart, and blood vessels, kidneys, gonads, adrenal cortex, and spleen.

The pleura consists of two layers, parietal and visceral, which are continuous at the pulmonary hilum. The parietal pleura covers the internal surface of the thoracic cage. The visceral pleura covers the surface of the lung and extends deep into each interlobar fissure. The visceral and parietal pleura meet at the hilum as the pulmonary ligament.

Both parietal and visceral pleura are composed of five distinct layers [17]. The surface consists of a single layer of mesothelial cells, the mesothelium. The mesothelial cells sit on a thin layer of submesothelial connective tissue, which includes the basal lamina. The third layer, the superficial elastic layer, is separated from the deep elastic layer by an intervening layer of loose connective tissue. The deep elastic layer is adherent to underlying lung, diaphragm, or chest wall.

The submesothelium consists primarily of fibroblasts within a stroma rich in collagen, laminin and acid mucoproteins. Stromal constituents are produced by both mesothelial and submesothelial cell populations [17]. Submesothelial cells resemble fibroblasts in the resting state, acquiring a more epithelioid morphology when stimulated. Immunohistochemical studies have confirmed the different embryological origins of mesothelial and submesothelial cells.

Mesothelial cell morphology reflects the level of cellular activity. In the normal resting state they are flattened, with bulging nuclei. The cell diameter is normally in the range 16–40 mm [17]. Cell margins are well defined, except at the apical surface, where the presence of microvilli produces a 'frilly' indistinct appearance. Microvilli are a striking feature of mesothelial cells. They are most prominent on the visceral pleura, particularly caudally. Mesothelial cells are also characterized by the dual presence of the cytoplasmic filaments vimentin and cytokeratin [18].

Pleural lymphatic pathways and asbestos fibre clearance

An appreciation of the way that the body deals with inhaled fibres is essential to understanding the mechanism behind asbestos-related toxicity in the lung and pleura.

Several mechanisms exist to prevent the passage of inhaled particles into the respiratory tract [19]. As discussed in Chapter 1, the proportion of an inhaled particle load that remains in the lung depends on the balance between initial load size and subsequent clearance. Clearance is influenced by the physical (size, shape, density) and chemical properties of a particle. The probability of a particle being deposited increases with its size. The exceptions are straight fibres with high length-to-width ratios, such as is characteristically seen in amphibole asbestos. Some of these fibres will align with the long axis of the airways, allowing them to travel further down the airway than less aerodynamic particles of a similar size. In the distal airways particles are distributed by sedimentation and can impact on the epithelium or penetrate into the interstitium. From here they can only be removed by translocation into the lymphatic system, or by phagocytosis and dissolution by local alveolar macrophages.

Asbestos fibres, particularly amphiboles, pose particular problems for lung clearance mechanisms. The natural fibres are friable and easily fragment into smaller particles within the respirable range. Their aerodynamic shape enables them to pass deep into the airways where they are too large to be efficiently phagocytosed. This results in a relative accumulation of long fibres, which in turn induces the production of local inflammatory mediators.

That asbestos fibres reach the pleural space is undisputed; they have been demonstrated within pleural tissue and parietal pleural plaques in humans [20]. This may reflect passive accumulation of fibres beyond the reach of clearance mechanisms. Alternatively, it could represent active transportation (translocation) of fibre-carrying alveolar macrophages via peribronchovascular spaces and lymphatic channels to the pleura in an attempt to clear fibres.

The histopathology of pleural disease

It is important to understand the processes involved in mesothelial inflammation and healing, as these can influence the histopathological changes seen in both benign and malignant pleural disease. Infection, radiation, malignant invasion, acute and chronic inflammatory conditions, collagen vascular disease, and intracavity treatments (chemical pleurodesis) can all induce these changes [21]. Mesothelial cell proliferation and submesothelial stromal activity increases pleural thickness to a variable extent. Morphological changes in the mesothelium include a marked increase in cell size and a reduction in cell border definition. Microvillus proliferation emphasizes the frilly cell margins and may produce small intercellular gaps. These 'windows' can be identified in cytological preparations derived from pleural effusions, and may aid the distinction between reactive mesothelial cells and metastatic carcinoma [22]. Mesothelial cell nuclei become larger, hypochromatic, and vesicular, but exhibit little pleomorphism. Nucleoli are prominent. An inflammatory cell infiltrate is often seen.

The pattern of mesothelial proliferation can also be important: complex papillary proliferation is a worrying feature, particularly if groups of cells are budding away from the pleural surface and have established fibrous cores [23, 24]. Such changes are uncommon in benign disease. Mesothelial necrosis in the absence of inflammation is uncommon in benign disease, but may be seen in up to 20 per cent of early mesotheliomas [24]. Cellular or nuclear pleomorphism is rarely prominent in malignant mesothelioma.

Another important diagnostic feature that distinguishes between benign and malignant mesothelial disease is that of invasion. The basement membrane is poorly defined in the pleura, making invasion difficult to assess. Extension of abnormal cells to involve chest wall structures such as fat or muscle is very suggestive of malignancy. It is important to differentiate between invasion, pseudo-invasion, and mesothelial sequestration. Pseudo-invasion is an artefact resulting from tangential sectioning of biopsy material. Surface mesothelium can also become sequestered deep within the pleura, secondary to inflammation and granulation tissue formation at the pleural surface. In these cases the mesothelial cells and associated capillaries usually lie parallel to the pleural surface, and may be accompanied by an inflammatory infiltrate. Sequestered cells normally elicit little in the way of a stromal reaction themselves. A final consideration when assessing invasion is the knowledge that desquamated surface mesothelial cells can pass into pleural lymphatics via stomata, which increase in size in response to pleural injury. This can resemble lymphatic invasion [25].

Electron microscopy

Electron microscopy has identified several cellular features that are characteristic of mesothelial tissue. These include apical microvilli, giant desmosomes, and perinuclear cytoplasmic intermediate filaments [18]. These features are retained despite malignant transformation, and therefore may aid differentiation between mesothelioma and other pleural tumours. Unfortunately, electron microscopy is expensive, time consuming, and generally found only in research institutions, which limits its usefulness in everyday diagnostic histopathology.

Apical microvilli

Microvilli are a striking feature of mesothelial cells, reflecting their integral role in the secretion and absorption of fluid from the pleural cavity. Not only do they increase the apical surface area available for these functions, but they also entrap glycoproteins on the cell surface. The resulting glycocalyx increases lubrication between the pleural surfaces. Microvilli are usually 1–3 mm long, and are often complex, with secondary and tertiary branching [17]. The length-to-diameter ratio (LDR) of mesothelial microvilli is high, often of the order of 12–15. Adenocarcinoma cells may possess microvilli, but their LDR is usually less than 10 [26]. As well as being shorter, adenocarcinoma microvilli are simple and club like, with occasional glycocalyceal bodies and visible rootlets on electron microscopy [27]. Differences in microvillus appearance can potentially aid the distinction between epithelioid mesothelioma and adenocarcinoma. There is significant degree of overlap in LDR between the two cell types, which limits its usefulness as a diagnostic test.

Desmosomes

Desmosomes are structures that anchor adjacent cell membranes. Microscopically they can be identified as areas of densely thickened membrane associated with filaments radiating from them into the cytoplasm. The intercellular gap is widened or unchanged, and may be filled with dense material [18]. Desmosomes are predominantly features of epithelial cells, but are also seen in some endothelia and the mesothelium. Giant desmosomes (>1 mm) are typical of mesothelial cells [28].

Intermediate filaments

Intracytoplasmic protein filaments are found in many cells, particularly those with motile ability. Actin (diameter 4–7 nm) and myosin (11–16 nm) are characteristic of mesenchymal-derived cells. Mesothelial cells are characterized by the additional presence of two types of intermediate size (6–12 nm diameter) filaments, vimentin and cytokeratin (CK) [18]. Vimentin filaments are found in all tissues of mesenchymal origin. Mesothelial cells also have numerous low molecular weight CK-positive filaments. These are arranged in wavy bundles in the perinuclear region and can readily be identified on electron microscopy and by immunohistochemistry.

Pleural biopsy techniques

Cytology and needle biopsy

The majority of patients with pleural malignancy have demonstrable pleural effusion or pleural thickening at presentation. Aspiration of pleural fluid, with or without a percutaneous needle biopsy, is commonly performed for both therapeutic and diagnostic reasons. Unfortunately, the diagnostic sensitivity and specificity of aspiration cytology and blind needle biopsy are not high for mesothelioma.

The diagnostic sensitivity of pleural fluid cytology has been reported to be as high as 90 per cent in expert hands [29]. Few published series have been able to reproduce such impressive results, even with the use of immunohistochemistry. Tomlinson and Sahn [30] have published a review of 14 papers that had assessed the diagnostic accuracy of cytology and needle pleural biopsies during the period 1958–1985. This review included a total of almost 3000 pleural biopsy samples, and concluded that diagnostic accuracy approached 60 per cent in effusions caused by carcinoma. The ability of pleural biopsy to diagnose mesothelioma confidently is nearer to 30 per cent [31–35]. Abrams needle biopsy with multiple samples is very sensitive for the diagnosis of tuberculous pleuritis when combined with microbiological analysis [36].

There are two reasons why cytology and needle biopsy are of limited diagnostic value in mesothelioma. The first relates to the nature of the cytology specimen; not all malignant pleural disease results in an effusion that contains exfoliated cells. In those that do, the effusion contains two separate cell populations: neoplastic cells and reactive mesothelial cells. Therefore it is necessary to distinguish between these different cells and confirm which population is malignant.

Immunocytochemistry is of limited value in effusions caused by malignant mesothelioma, as there are no reliable markers that differentiate between benign and malignant mesothelial cells.

The second problem is technical. It can be difficult to accurately target abnormal pleural tissue with a blind technique as used with an Abrams needle [37]. Therefore percutaneous pleural biopsy samples may not be representative of the rest of the pleura, or may only contain muscle and fibrous tissue. Crush artefact may also be present. Four or more biopsies at a single site may improve the diagnostic yield [38]. The use of radiological techniques to target abnormal pleura in combination with needle biopsies appears to improve diagnostic accuracy significantly. A recent trial comparing CT-guided cutting-needle biopsy with a standard Abrams needle technique has been reported [39]. Fifty consecutive patients with pleural effusion were randomized to one of these diagnostic techniques. The CT-guided biopsies had almost double the diagnostic sensitivity of the Abrams needle technique for malignancy (87 vs. 47 per cent).

Thoracoscopy

Thoracoscopy involves the direct visualization of the pleural surface, and therefore enables better targeting of abnormal areas when biopsies are taken. 'Medical' thoracoscopy can be performed under local anaesthesia or intravenous sedation in an endoscopy suite. Thus it is considerably cheaper and does not subject the patient to the risks of a general anaesthetic. However, it may not be possible to enter the pleural cavity because of adhesions or pleural thickening.

Surgical thoracoscopy [video-assisted thoracic surgery (VATS)] is performed under a general anaesthetic and requires single-lung anaesthesia. There may be better visualization of the pleura, and the port-site incisions can be readily converted to a limited thoracotomy if the pleural cavity has been obliterated. Therapeutic manoeuvres, such as pleurectomy or chemical pleurodesis, are also possible. It is unusual to find facilities and equipment for VATS outside cardiothoracic or specialist thoracic surgical units.

The diagnostic accuracy of biopsies obtained at thoracoscopy is far superior to that of needle biopsies. Boutin and Rey [40] have compared the diagnostic value of medical thoracoscopic biopsy, fluid cytology, and Abrams needle biopsy in an 18-year cohort of patients with mesothelioma. In most patients, thoracoscopy allowed complete visualization of the pleural cavity and provided good-quality biopsy samples, with 10–20 biopsies taken from multiple sites. In 51 patients, inspection was limited by adhesions that were divided to obtain biopsy. Diagnosis was achieved by thoracoscopy in 98 per cent of patients, by fluid cytology in 26 per cent, and by needle biopsy in 21 per cent.

The pathology of malignant pleural mesothelioma: macroscopic features

Pleural mesotheliomas are more commonly right-sided (right-to-left ratio 3:2) [41]. This difference may be explained by the greater size of the right pleural cavity. Alhough usually unilateral at presentation, it is not infrequent to find histological evidence of mesothelioma in the contralateral pleura. Macroscopic evidence of synchronous bilateral pleural tumours is rare. Pleural plaques are often identified in the pleural cavity but their absence does not negate a diagnosis of mesothelioma. It is not infrequent to see plaque histologically amidst mesotheliomatous tissue.

In the early stages of disease mesothelioma is seen as nodules on the parietal or, less commonly, the visceral pleura. The distribution of both tumour nodules and benign pleural plaques tends to follow the distribution of pleural lymphatic pathways. There may an associated pleural effusion, which is most commonly seen in association with epithelioid mesotheliomas (see below).

Transmission electron microscopy analysis of the pleura from asbestos-exposed subjects has confirmed that amphibole asbestos fibres outnumber chrysotile fibres and are located close to aggregates of parietal pleura lymphatic tissue [42].

As mesothelioma progresses the tumour nodules coalesce, commonly fusing the two layers of the pleura and thereby obliterating the pleural cavity. A thick rind of malignant tissue is produced that encases, compresses, and eventually invades the underlying lung, often extending into and through the diaphragm, and along the lobar fissures. Rarely, mesothelioma may present as a localized pleural or apparent pulmonary mass [43–45]. In such cases it is important to exclude primary pulmonary tumours and malignant variants of localized pleural tumours.

At post-mortem mesothelioma is seen as a dense pleural thickening by firm grey–white or even yellow tissue, which may show cystic areas containing glary 'mucoid-like' material. Epithelioid mesotheliomas commonly produce large amounts of hyaluronic acid. Sarcomatoid tumours may contain large amounts of dense collagenous tissue. Mesothelioma is highly invasive, and chest wall, pericardial, and mediastinal invasion may be identified. Tumour can encircle the oesophagus, aorta, and other great vessels. It has a tendency to track along the site of surgical incisions or chest drains. In some cases there is replacement of a lobe or an entire lung by tumour, often making it impossible to exclude a primary bronchial carcinoma macroscopically.

It is becoming rarer in the UK and North America to find asbestosis (asbestos-induced pulmonary fibrosis) in association with mesothelioma. This reflects the effects that health and safety regulations have had on overall exposure, as the development of asbestosis directly relates to the magnitude of asbestos exposure [46]. It can be difficult to quantify asbestos exposure reproducibly. One study found that 50 per cent of cases had asbestos fibre counts that would be incompatible with identification of fibres using light microscopy [47].

Metastatic spread

Malignant mesothelioma is capable of extensive local and distant metastatic spread. The pattern of spread reflects histological subtype; epithelioid tumours behave as carcinomas and sarcomatoid variants like sarcomas. Epithelioid tumours primarily spread to the adjacent lymph nodes and from there into the lymphatic system. Therefore secondary deposits are found in the hilar, the mediastinal, and then the supraclavicular or axillary nodes. It permeates lymphatics, as well as thin-walled pulmonary veins (Fig. 4.1) and arteries. Lymphatic involvement may also con-

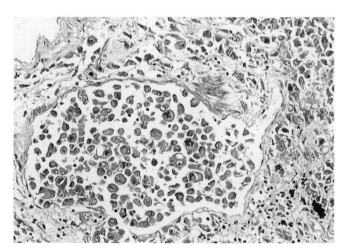

Figure 4.1 Mesothelioma surrounding and present in the lumen of thin-walled vein.

tribute to the development of pleural effusions. Tumour may grow along the interstitium and alveolar walls as well as into their lumina, simulating bronchioloalveolar carcinoma.

Trans-diaphragmatic extension to the liver and peritoneum is also more common in epithelioid mesotheliomas. Distant metastases can be seen in the brain, vertebral column, liver, pancreas, adrenals, kidney, and contralateral lung. A search of all pulmonary and abdominal viscera should be made to exclude a non-pleural primary tumour at post-mortem examination of those dying of suspected mesothelioma.

Sarcomatoid tumours often grow quickly, producing bulky lobulated tumours, and are less commonly associated with large pleural effusions. They metastasize through vascular rather than lymphatic invasion. Therefore distant metastases are more common in sarcomatoid mesotheliomas [48]. Biphasic tumours are intermediate in their biological behaviour.

The pathology of malignant pleural mesothelioma: microscopic features

Histopathology is the mainstay of diagnosis since macroscopically and radiologically mesotheliomas can be confused with many other tumours that can involve the lung and pleura. Mesothelioma is capable of showing a variety of histological patterns; this diversity of cell types is one of the causes of diagnostic difficulty.

The World Health Organization has classified mesothelioma into epithelioid, biphasic, and sarcomatoid subtypes [49]. The epithelioid subtype comprises approximately 50 per cent of cases in most reported series, with biphasic accounting for 30 per cent and sarcomatoid the remaining 20 per cent. There can be significant differences in the reported incidence of the different subtypes of mesothelioma, which in part may reflect sampling error. A tumour that comprises more than 10 per cent of both epithelioid and sarcomatoid areas should be classified as biphasic. It has been shown that the incidence of biphasic mesothelioma increases as a larger number of blocks are taken from any one tumour [50].

Malignant pleural mesotheliomas frequently contain areas of non-malignant connective tissue (stroma). This stroma is variable in both amount and appearance. It may consist of moderately cellular fibrous tissue with some myxoid change, which should not be confused with malignant sarcomatoid foci. In some cases it may be difficult to differentiate the biphasic pattern from the epithelioid because of stromal cellularity. Desmoplasia (dense paucicellular collagenous areas) may be seen in any subtype of tumour but is most common in sarcomatoid forms. If this comprises more than 50 per cent of the total, the tumour is subclassified as the desmoplastic variant [49].

Epithelioid mesothelioma

Epithelioid mesotheliomas most typically exhibit a tubulo-papillary pattern of differentiation consisting of cuboidal or polyhedral tumour cells. There may be simple papillary (Fig 4.2), tubular, or in some cases solid sheets of polygonal cells (Fig 4.3).

The papillae have fibrous cores, a feature less commonly seen in benign mesothelial proliferations [24]. Some tubules form complex branching patterns. In rare cases a squamoid pattern of differentiation is seen. Microcystic differentiation, in which a network of flattened mesothelial cells produces a lace-like pattern similar to that seen in adenomatoid tumours, has been described. Rare cases may show an adenoid cystic or deciduoid pattern. Up to 10 per cent of cases have psammoma bodies within the cores of proliferating cells. A summary of recognized histological patterns in epithelioid mesotheliomas is shown in Table 4.1.

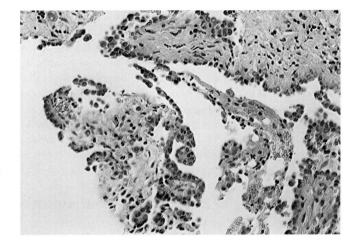

Figure 4.2 Epithelioid mesothelioma with a papillary pattern. Even though this is a low magnification there is a hint of the regular nature of the nuclei.

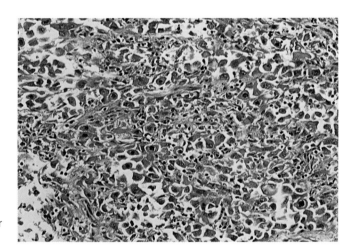

Figure 4.3 Mesothelioma composed of polygonal cells with focal nuclear hyperchromatism. No acinar or papillary pattern is seen.

The nuclei in epithelioid mesothelioma are usually regular, open, and vesicular, with prominent nucleoli. In keeping with the nuclear features there is a constant nuclear-to-cytoplasmic ratio [51]. These features, although non-specific, are useful as an initial guide in differentiating mesothelioma from adenocarcinoma. The latter tumour usually consists of larger cells with hyperchromatic irregular nuclei (Fig. 4.4).

Mitoses, nuclear pleomorphism, tumour giant cells, and atypical mitoses are unusual in most mesotheliomas, but can be seen after chemotherapy or radiotherapy. In such cases immunohisto-chemistry (see below) is also often of little help in distinguishing mesothelioma from carcinoma, and other diagnostic techniques (e.g. electron microscopy) may be required.

The cytoplasm of mesotheliomas is often eosinophilic and cell borders are well defined. There may be cytoplasmic vacuolation, producing a signet-ring appearance (Fig. 4.5). These vacuoles may contain hyaluronic acid, which can resemble the mucin found in some adenocarcinomas. Mucin histochemistry (see below) should help to distinguish between these. Mesotheliomas have rarely been shown to demonstrate true mucin positivity, and when present this is usually focal and involves less than 30 per cent of the cells [27, 52, 53].

Table 4.1 Histological patterns identified in epithelioid malignant pleural mesothelioma

In situ

Tubulo-papillary

Acinar and complex acinar

Microcystic ('adenomatoid')

Deciduoid

Poorly differentiated

Pleomorphic

Mesothelioma with psammoma bodies

Signet ring

Clear cell

Small-cell

Lymphohistiocytoid

Mesothelioma with small amounts of mucin

Biphasic

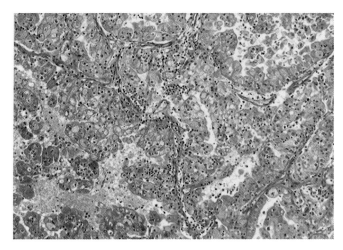

Figure 4.4 Adenocarcinoma of lung growing along the alveolar basement membrane. The cells are large and vacuolated but do not have marked nuclear hyperchromatism.

Variants of epithelioid mesothelioma

The classification of histological patterns seen in epithelioid mesothelioma is probably of little clinical significance as there is no convincing evidence that these patterns influence subsequent biological behaviour. However, the presence of several different patterns of differentiation within the same tumour is more characteristic of mesothelioma than other epithelioid tumours. They are documented here for completeness.

Deciduoid mesothelioma

This subtype is characterized by the presence of large round cells with abundant eosinophilic cytoplasm. Originally described in the peritoneal cavity in young women, this subtype has recently also been described in the pleural cavity in older male patients [54, 55]. Therefore it

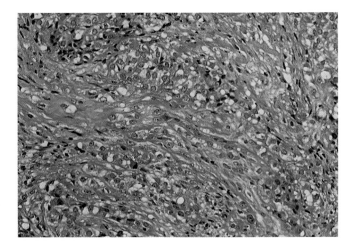

Figure 4.5 Epithelioid mesothelioma with many cells showing cytoplasmic vacuolation.

should probably be regarded as part of the histological spectrum of epithelioid mesothelioma rather than a separate pathological entity.

Well-differentiated papillary mesothelioma (WDPM)

This is a rare variant which was first described by Foyle in 1981 [56]. It is important to differentiate it from malignant mesothelioma as it may have a lower malignant potential. It is most common in the peritoneal cavities of younger women, but has rarely been described in the pleura or in men. A causal link with asbestos has not been established. Microscopically, WDPM is characterized by the presence of a surface papillary proliferation with associated myxoid stroma, but it is cytologically bland with no evidence of invasion into deep structures. The morphological features that help to distinguish WDPM from reactive pleuritis and mesothelioma have been summarized by Daya and McCaughey [57]. It usually follows a relatively benign course, but may produce ascites in advanced cases [15, 58].

Multicystic mesothelioma

This uncommon variant may affect the pleura in a similar way to the peritoneal cavity [59]. It is characterized by the presence of macroscopically thin-walled cysts separated by connective tissue and lined by a single layer of flattened cuboidal epithelium. These lesions are continuous with the parietal pleura and also adherent to the visceral pleura. Small buds or clumps of mesothelial cells are sometimes seen within the cystic spaces. Occasionally an adenomatoid pattern is identified. The tumour may be indistinguishable from a conventional epithelioid mesothelioma.

Small-cell mesothelioma

This tumour may superficially resemble a small-cell carcinoma or lymphoma, both of which are uncommon in the pleura. A small-cell pattern is seen in less than 6 per cent of mesotheliomas [60–62]. The French Mesopath Group have not seen a single case in over 3000 validated mesotheliomas. If multiple blocks are examined, this subtype usually contains areas of more typical mesothelioma. The immunophenotype is that of a mesothelioma.

Lymphohistiocytoid mesothelioma

This is considered a subtype of sarcomatoid mesotheliomas, but is mentioned here because of its resemblance to the small-cell variant. It is discussed in more detail below.

Giant-cell mesothelioma

A rare variant of malignant mesothelioma is the pleomorphic or giant-cell type. This tumour may be confused with giant-cell carcinoma of lung. A mucin stain may help to exclude an adeno-carcinoma or a large-cell carcinoma. Immunohistochemistry is often unhelpful in differentiating this tumour from a pleomorphic carcinoma of the lung [63]. Electron microscopy has been recommended in such cases.

In situ mesothelioma

There is a degree of controversy as to whether *in situ* mesothelioma exists as a pathological entity. The concept of a pre-invasive (*in situ*) stage, in which cytologically malignant cells are identifiable but have not yet crossed the basement membrane, is recognized in other epithelial tumours. In mesothelioma the basement membrane is poorly defined and the cytological distinction between benign and malignant cells is more difficult.

Henderson *et al.* [24] have defined *in situ* mesothelioma as 'the replacement of benign surface mesothelium by mesothelial cells that have cytoarchitectural features of malignancy' without defining any level of invasion. The main differentials of *in situ* mesothelioma include benign (reactive) processes as well as other tumours. Immunohistochemistry is of limited value in this area, but the use of mesothelial cell markers may help to emphasize the pattern and extent of sequestrated or invasive surface cells within the submesothelium (Fig. 4.6). In practical terms it is unusual to diagnose *in situ* mesothelioma except in the presence of invasive mesothelioma elsewhere in a surgical specimen or in association with definite mesothelioma in the contralateral pleura.

Biphasic mesothelioma

Biphasic mesothelioma exhibits both epithelioid and sarcomatoid patterns of differentiation within the same tumour (each greater than 10 per cent of total) [49]. The diagnosis of biphasic mesothelioma requires unequivocal malignancy in both components. There are often large areas where only one histological pattern predominates, but after extensive sampling the biphasic nature of the tumour becomes evident. Different patterns are characteristically adjacent to each other with little separation. Although epithelioid mesothelioma is the most common pattern of differentiation, biphasic mesothelioma is considered the 'classical' pattern. Other tumours that

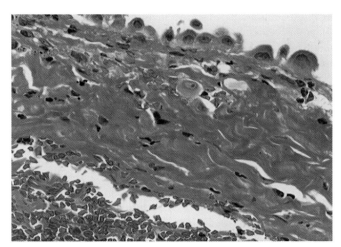

Figure 4.6 Mesothelioma *in situ*. There is nuclear pleomorphism of the surface cells. The presence of scanty cells in the underlying layers would require examination of extra levels to exclude an invasive tumour.

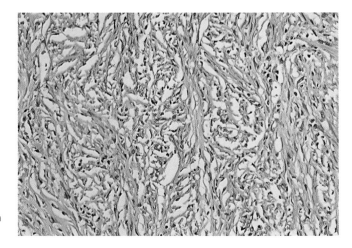

Figure 4.7 Sarcomatoid mesothelioma with a storiform pattern.

exhibit a biphasic pattern of differentiation are relatively uncommon in the pleura. The differential diagnosis includes pleomorphic carcinoma, carcinosarcoma of the lung, biphasic synovial sarcoma, sarcoma with areas of epithelioid differentiation, and pulmonary blastoma.

Sarcomatoid mesothelioma

Sarcomatoid mesothelioma is composed of relatively featureless spindle-shaped cells (Fig 4.7). Although small foci of epithelioid cells may be seen, by definition these should comprise less than 10 per cent of the tumour overall. Transitional forms, in which the fibroblastic cells retain some features of epithelioid cells, such as microvilli, may be seen on electron microscopy. Sarcomatoid mesothelioma is frequently seen in association with desmoplasia—dense collagenous paucicellular stroma that may resemble chronic fibrous pleurisy and pleural plaque. Rarely, this desmoplasia may account for most of the tumour. Sarcomatoid mesothelioma can exhibit areas of subdifferentiation which can make it difficult to distinguish from soft tissue tumours on small biopsies. Conversely, some of the tumours that have already been discussed in the differential diagnosis of epithelioid and biphasic mesothelioma contain prominent areas of sarcomatoid differentiation; sampling errors can obscure the predominant pattern. Osseous and/or cartilaginous differentiation may be identified [64, 65]. Liposarcomatous differentiation in a sarcomatoid mesothelioma, which is very rare, must be differentiated from a mesothelioma growing around existing fat spaces or a primary pleural liposarcoma. The differential diagnosis of sarcomatoid mesothelioma includes sarcomas, solitary (localized) fibrous tumours of the pleura, malignant fibrous histiocytomas, and peripheral nerve sheath tumours.

Desmoplastic mesothelioma

An uncommon but important variant of sarcomatoid mesothelioma is desmoplastic malignant mesothelioma [66–68]. This subtype accounts for approximately 5 per cent of all mesotheliomas. The desmoplastic area should comprise at least 50 per cent of the tumour. In most cases the tumour cell type is sarcomatoid, but it can also be identified as a component of biphasic tumours. Cellular and desmoplastic areas often merge imperceptibly (Fig. 4.8). A useful diagnostic feature is collagen necrosis, which is seen in 70 per cent of cases. This is bland and often, but not always, without associated inflammation. This variant of mesothelioma is very difficult to diagnose and may be confused with a healing reactive pleurisy. The demonstration of stromal

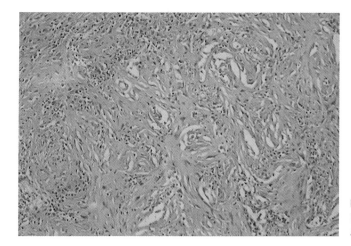

Figure 4.8 A small focus of bland fibrosis (desmoplasia) in a sarcomatoid mesothelioma.

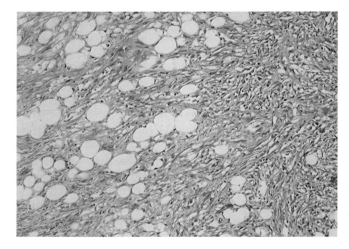

Figure 4.9 Infiltration of fat by a sarcomatoid mesothelioma. This is a valuable indicator of malignancy.

invasion is the most helpful diagnostic feature, i.e. tumour growth around the fat spaces (Fig. 4.9) and muscle in the parietal pleura. The US–Canadian Mesothelioma Reference Panel has stressed the diagnostic importance of focal invasion of the pulmonary parenchyma, as well as extension along interlobar fissures and intralobular septa in desmoplastic mesothelioma. This is virtually never seen in a reactive pleurisy.

In reactive processes mesothelial cells can be entrapped within areas of fibrosis, which can create diagnostic problems. In addition, the reactive mesothelial cells may show cellular atypia. Reactive lesions also show surface hypercellularity which decreases deeper in the lesion. No zonation is seen in desmoplastic mesothelioma. There is a lack of inflammation in desmoplastic mesotheliomas, unlike the superficial portions of a reactive pleurisy. Necrosis is not identified in reactive lesions; hence its presence is helpful in the confirmation of malignancy. Cytokeratin stains are useful to emphasize stromal invasion, and the authors have seen cases misdiagnosed because of mesothelial cells entrapped in reactive fibrosis. Rarely, an empyema may be superimposed on a desmoplastic mesothelioma.

Lymphohistiocytoid mesothelioma

This very rare variant accounts for less than 1 per cent of mesotheliomas. It may be misdiagnosed as lymphoma or small-cell carcinoma [69, 70]. The tumour tissue shows populations of large histiocytic cells which vary from round to spindle-shaped. The nuclei vary from round to ovoid and contain finely divided chromatin with small prominent nucleoli. A diffuse but variable lymphoplasmacytoid infiltrate is also present. Eosinophils may occasionally be prominent, giving an initial resemblance to Hodgkin's disease, but no Reed–Sternberg cells are identified. The lymphocytes show T-cell predominance in 50 per cent of cases, T and B cells are equal in number in 25 per cent, and B cells predominate in the remainder [69]. Electron microscopy of the lymphohistiocytoid variant shows predominantly mesenchymal cells with a mixed population of fibroblasts, fibrohistiocytic cells, histiocytes, myofibroblasts, rare xanthoma cells, and undifferentiated mesenchymal cells resembling those seen in malignant fibrous histiocytoma.

Rhabdomyoblastic differentiation

Rare cases with rhabdomyoblastic differentiation have been described [71].

Differential diagnosis of malignant mesothelioma

A wide range of primary and secondary tumours can present in the thorax. Therefore it is unsurprising that diagnostic difficulties occur [72]. This problem is compounded by the fact that expert mesothelioma reference panels disagree in up to 30 per cent of referred cases [53]. Since the Pneumoconiosis Medical Panel was disbanded in the UK, general pathologists are now left to make diagnostic decisions and attend inquests in suspected mesothelioma cases. The problem has been compounded by the reluctance in recent years of some coroners to sanction the retention of organs or tissue for post-mortem examination following the Alder Hey and Bristol Reports (http://www.rlcinquiry.org.uk/ and http://www.bristol-inquiry.org.uk/). These reports concentrated on the retention of tissue from paediatric and adult post-mortems without consent. The impact on the apparent incidence of mesothelioma of changes in attitude to organ retention following these reports is uncertain.

The differential diagnosis of pleural tumours according to histological subtype is summarized in Figure 4.10. The rational use of immunohistochemistry (IHC) and other techniques relies on the correct identification of the initial growth pattern of the tumour. There are broadly four main categories of histological pattern that a pathologist should consider. These are reactive lesions, epithelioid tumours, which include carcinomas, lymphomas, and some epithelioid sarcomas, biphasic tumours, including pleomorphic carcinomas and sarcomatoid tumours.

It is impossible to consider all the lesions referred to in the differential diagnosis within the scope of this chapter. The reader is referred to standard pathology texts such as *Spencer's Pathology of the Lung* [73]. Any such text rapidly becomes outdated with the development of new monoclonal antibodies and the description of different histological patterns. The latter problem is not decreasing, since a recent report from France, which has a well-developed certification and verification system, indicates that the diagnosis of rare variants of mesothelioma has increased in incidence (from 6 per cent in 1998 to 15 per cent in 2002) [74].

Malignant mesothelioma can appear in many different histological guises. This variability of appearance, and the wide range of tumours that can metastasize to the pleura, means that the diagnosis of mesothelioma has now come to rely heavily on adjuvant diagnostic techniques. The diagnostic process can be considered as a hierarchy: simple microscopy of sections stained with haematoxylin and eosin (H&E), the routine initial stain employed by all pathologists, is the first level, followed by tissue histochemistry, then IHC, and finally electron microscopy [75].

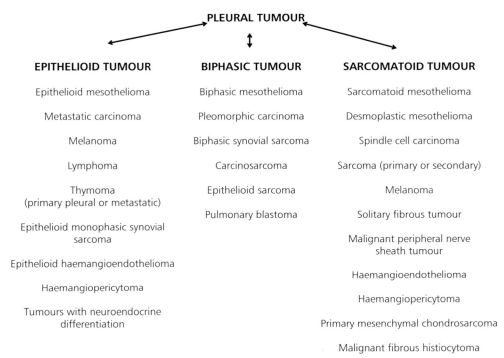

Figure 4.10 Differential diagnosis of pleural mesothelioma. (Reproduced by permission of the editor of *Histopathology.*)

Although the first three of these techniques are readily available in most pathology departments, electron microscopy is often limited to research facilities. Therefore IHC tends to be the highest diagnostic arbiter in routine practice.

Clinical, radiological, H&E, and IHC findings must all be taken into account before reaching a final diagnosis. The presence of pleural plaques or interstitial fibrosis is suggestive of previous asbestos exposure. As both these conditions also predispose to the development of carcinoma of the lung, definitive histology is required to differentiate between pulmonary tumours involving the pleura and primary pleural tumours. A relevant drug history may also be important. For example, bromocriptine, a drug used in Parkinson's disease, may cause pleural fibrosis in patients previously exposed to asbestos [76, 77]. This reaction can be confused with mesothelioma. Therefore it is essential that sufficient clinical data is given to the pathologist. The physician or surgeon must discuss any discrepant pathology report with the histopathologist when mesothelioma is a possible diagnosis.

The experiences of the Joint US–Canadian Mesothelioma Registry serve as a good illustration of the most common problems that a pathologist has to face when correctly classifying pleural tumours [53]. In a review of the first 200 referred cases, of which three-quarters were pleural, areas causing difficulty were as follows. The most common problem was differentiating epithelioid mesothelioma from pleural-based carcinoma. The next largest group was where the diagnosis of mesothelioma was made by the referring pathologist, but panel confirmation was requested. This accounted for less than 20 per cent of cases. The differentiation between mesothelial hyperplasia and mesothelioma and between reactive pleuritis and desmoplastic mesothelioma both accounted for approximately 13 per cent of cases. The problem of sarcoma vs. sarcomatoid mesothelioma was seen in 9 per cent of cases, and the remaining 13 per cent of referrals comprised a mixture of other diagnostic problems such as unusual variants of mesothelioma. This pattern of referrals is similar to that reported by other reference panels [78]. The extent of agreement within the panel for any given case was variable. A consensus opinion (>75 per cent) was achieved in 70 per cent of all cases. An even split was seen in less than 5 per cent. The categories affording the least disagreement were those involving simple confirmation of mesothelioma, and the distinction between epithelioid mesothelioma and carcinoma. Consensus was achieved in 70–83 per cent of these cases. Least agreement was seen in the sarcomatoid mesothelioma vs. sarcoma (46 per cent) and benign vs. malignant pleural disease categories (59 per cent).

Immunohistochemistry

IHC utilizes antibodies raised against specific cellular epitopes. Ideally, these epitopes should be exclusive to one particular cell type and therefore can be used to identify the tissue of origin of a tumour. Initial hopes that IHC could solve most diagnostic dilemmas in histopathology have been tempered with the realization that, whilst useful, its value is limited in many areas. Although IHC has made a significant contribution to the distinction between mesothelioma and other pleural tumours, the hope that a specific mesothelioma marker would be identified has not yet been realized [79–87].

Numerous factors influence the results of IHC staining. Differences in tissue preparation, fixation, and processing can critically affect epitope sites, as can the degree of tumour differentiation [88]. Sampling errors may be introduced by the inclusion of non-representative areas, especially in small specimens, or in the presence of necrosis [78]. The pattern of IHC staining may vary between the initial biopsy and subsequent post-mortem material in the same patient, especially if tumour growth is associated with histological dedifferentiation [89, 90]. Antibody specificity and sensitivity varies according to the manufacturer batch, and some antibodies require antibody retrieval techniques to ensure reproducible results [91]. Interpretation of the pattern and intensity of staining is subject to both inter- and intra-observer variation, and may be overly influenced by clinical factors such as a history of asbestos exposure [92].

The ideal diagnostic antibody would be 100 per cent sensitive (no false negatives) and 100 per cent specific (no false positives) for any given epitope. Over the past two decades many antibodies have been heralded as highly specific and sensitive mesothelial markers, only to be discredited when applied to larger numbers of pleuropulmonary tumours. It should be remembered that the discriminative value of a diagnostic test can only be truly evaluated if a pathologist is confident of the diagnosis in each test group. This is one of the greatest problems when evaluating IHC in mesothelioma. Because there is no gold standard for pathological identification of mesothelioma, there is always the possibility that results could be skewed by the inclusion of even a small number of other tumours.

As previously mentioned, the most common diagnostic problem for a pathologist faced with a biopsy of a pleural tumour is usually the distinction between epithelioid mesothelioma and pulmonary adenocarcinoma. Therefore many of the antibodies utilized in suspected mesothelioma cases are selected for their ability to differentiate between mesothelial and epithelial cells, and can be divided into two broad groups. Those that identify cells of epithelial origin include mucins, carcinoembryonic antigen (CEA), the glycoprotein markers Ber-EP4 and B72.3, Leu-M1, and thyroid transcription factor-1 (TTF-1) among others. These are often referred to as 'carcinoma markers'. This is a useful generic term to distinguish them from antibodies that are usually positive in cells of mesothelial origin ('mesothelioma markers'), but it is important to realize that they may also be positive in cells of non-epithelial origin [93]. These antibodies do not distin-

Table 4.2 Immunohistochemical diagnostic antibodies commonly used to distinguish between carcinoma and mesothelioma

Carcinoma markers	Mesothelioma markers
Epithelial mucins	Calretinin
Carcinoembryonic antigen (CEA)	CK 5/6
Ber-EP4	HBME-1
B72.3	Thrombomodulin
Leu-M1	N-cadherin
MOC-31	Wilms tumour product 1
E-cadherin	
Thyroid transcription factor-1 (TTF-1)	
Lewis^y	

guish between benign and malignant proliferations of a given cell type, in which case basic principles of tumour diagnosis, such as pattern of spread, the presence of necrosis, and cellular and nuclear morphology are employed. Commonly used carcinoma and mesothelioma markers are listed in Table 4.2.

There are other IHC antibodies employed to confirm the diagnosis of mesothelioma that cannot be exclusively classified into one or other of these groups. For example, low-molecular-weight cytokeratins (LMWCK) and some glycoprotein antigens [e.g. epithelial membrane antigen (EMA)] are present in both pulmonary adenocarcinoma and mesothelioma, but the pattern of distribution of the IHC marker may have discriminatory value. The vascular markers CD31 and CD34 help to distinguish epithelioid mesothelioma from vascular tumours, and desmoplastic mesothelioma from solitary fibrous pleural tumour. The use of IHC stains may also contribute to the diagnosis of mesothelioma by emphasizing areas of invasion not apparent on simple H&E sections.

Meta-analysis of published studies of immunohistochemistry in the diagnosis of malignant pleural mesothelioma

In an attempt to confirm which IHC antibodies are of most use in everyday practice, we have analysed the results of 115 studies devoted to the role of IHC in the diagnosis of mesothelioma. Individual papers were analysed to determine the diagnostic criteria used, and wherever possible individual results were extracted for each case of mesothelioma. These results were then compared with the IHC results of the tumours that are their main differential in normal practice. For example the results for epithelioid mesothelioma were compared with those for pulmonary adenocarcinoma. Those for sarcomatoid and desmoplastic mesothelioma were contrasted with sarcomas and benign pleural disease respectively.

In comparing the ability of an antibody to identify a particular tissue or tumour type correctly, results are best expressed in terms of diagnostic sensitivity and specificity. Sensitivity is defined as the ability of a diagnostic test to identify positive cases correctly, implying a low false-negative rate. Specificity is defined as the ability of a test to identify a negative result correctly, i.e. it has a low false-positive rate [94]. Both sensitivity and specificity are expressed as percentages, and convention dictates that results are expressed with reference to the positive test result. Studies that compared staining in epithelioid or biphasic mesothelioma with pulmonary adenocarcinoma

Table 4.3 Summary of the results of published studies that have evaluated the sensitivity and specificity of immunohistochemical markers in distinguishing between pulmonary adenocarcinoma (PACA) and epithelioid mesothelioma (EM): carcinoma markers

IHC marker	No. of studies analysed	No. of PACA cases included	No. of EM cases included	Sensitivity of antibody for PACA (%)	Specificity of antibody for PACA (%)
All cases CEA	51	1524	1818	83	95
Monoclonal CEA	24	949	1007	81	97
Ber-EP4	17	702	899	80	90
B72.3	16	769	700	80	93
Leu-M1	26	1473	1204	72	93
E-cadherin	7	183	218	86	82
MOC-31	7	213	276	93	93
TTF-1	5	366	240	72	100
Lewis^y (BG8)	4	231	197	93	93

were combined to calculate the overall sensitivity and specificity for each antibody. Not all published studies of the IHC of mesothelioma have compared their results with other tumours: Therefore they cannot be used to calculate sensitivity and specificity. Those studies that have reported IHC staining only in mesothelioma were combined to calculate the overall incidence of positive staining for each antibody. The results of this analysis are summarized in Tables 4.3 and 4.4.

There are significant problems inherent in performing this sort of meta-analysis. When analysing published papers, case selection criteria are often unapparent. Some authors state that the diagnosis of mesothelioma was made 'according to standard texts'. This leads to the suspicion that only easily diagnosable well-differentiated tumours are included in the study. Difficult or undifferentiated tumours are perhaps excluded. Inclusion of too many post-mortem or needle biopsy cases may also skew data. These cases cause most diagnostic difficulty.

There are also problems when comparing IHC results from different institutions. There may be differences in processing tissue that may influence the sensitivity or specificity of an antibody.

Table 4.4 Summary of the results of published studies that have evaluated the sensitivity and specificity of immunohistochemical markers in distinguishing between pulmonary adenocarcinoma (PACA) and epithelioid mesothelioma (EM): mesothelioma markers

IHC marker	No. of studies analysed	No. of PACA cases included	No. of EM cases included	Sensitivity of antibody for EM (%)	Specificity of antibody for EM (%)
CK 5/6	8	284	402	83	85
Vimentin	17	815	773	62	75
Calretinin	17	912	885	82	85
HBME-1	14	676	769	85	43
Thrombomodulin	17	964	831	61	80
N-cadherin	5	121	151	78	84
WT1	6	213	264	77	96

Staining methodologies vary between manufacturers, particularly in terms of optimum antibody concentration. Antigen retrieval techniques, such as microwave or pressure cooker heat treatments, may also have been used. Poorly preserved or autolysed tissue may loose characteristic epitope sites and fail to stain with an antibody that is expected to be positive. Conversely, necrotic tissue with an inflammatory infiltrate may produce a false-positive reaction with some IHC markers such as Leu-M1. Pooling of antibody complexes at the periphery of a tissue section can be misinterpreted as a positive reaction, and the pattern of distribution can be critical in the interpretation of IHC results. Many papers do not provide enough methodological detail to ascertain whether any of these factors could be relevant. Finally, few papers give indications of the percentage of cells stained positively and the intensity of staining. In the future medical editors could do worse than to agree a protocol for these issues and reject papers, which do not conform.

Tissue histochemistry

Mucins

Histochemistry was one of the first diagnostic tests used to distinguish between pulmonary carcinomas and epithelioid mesothelioma. Both epithelium and mesothelium can produce intracellular mucins. These are polyanionic compounds composed of a protein core associated with variable chains of glycosaminoglycans. The predominant type of glycosaminoglycan varies between different tissues of origin; in mesothelium it is almost exclusively hyaluronic acid. Positive mucin reactions in mesothelioma are frequently due to hyaluronic acid, and are usually abolished by hyaluronidase pretreatment. Staining for hyaluronic acid directly is often unhelpful, as it is leached from tissues when water-based fixatives such as formalin are used [53]. Approximately 60–70 per cent of pulmonary adenocarcinomas are mucin positive [52, 95, 96]. The incidence of mucin-positive mesotheliomas in series utilizing hyaluronidase pretreatment is 5 per cent or less [27, 52, 53]. Mesotheliomas uncommonly exhibit positive mucin staining, when combined diastase and periodic acid–Schiff (D-PAS) is used [97, 98].

Mucin histochemistry is relatively cheap and quick to perform, and still has a diagnostic role despite the introduction of IHC [99]. A diffuse strongly positive D-PAS in an epithelioid pleural tumour is strongly suggestive of adenocarcinoma, whilst weak and/or focal staining is of less diagnostic value.

Carcinoma markers

Carcinoembryonic antigen (CEA)

CEA is an oncofetal glycoprotein identified by Gold and Freeman [100]. It is seen in adenocarcinomas arising from different tissues, particularly those from the colon and lung. Mesothelial cells characteristically do not possess CEA epitopes. Therefore the CEA antibody was recognized nearly 25 years ago as a potential discriminator between these two tumours, and remains one of the most useful diagnostic antibodies for distinguishing between pulmonary adenocarcinoma and epithelioid mesothelioma [101].

Initial studies with CEA used a polyclonal antibody. This also reacted with CEA-related sites [non-specific cross-reacting antigen (NCA)]. These NCA sites can be demonstrated in mesothelioma cells, resulting in false-positive CEA staining. Studies evaluating polyclonal CEA in mesothelioma have reported positive results in up to 45 per cent of cases [102–114]. Preabsorption with spleen powder or NCA can reduce the false-positive rate, but the value of polyclonal CEA is still limited. The introduction of monoclonal (Mo) CEA antibodies has improved its diagnostic specificity, with far fewer mesotheliomas reported as CEA positive (0–8 per cent). Interestingly, CEA-positive mesotheliomas often also give positive reactions for mucin. Both Robb [115] and Hammar *et al.* [52] have demonstrated that CEA reactivity in mesotheliomas is abolished or diminished by predigestion with hyaluronidase. Therefore it appears likely that other cross-reacting antigens exist and may influence results with both polyclonal and monoclonal antibodies.

Papers reporting significant levels of CEA-positive reactions in mesothelioma usually describe them as weak and focal. Thus the criteria for cut-off levels of staining should be indicated in papers. The level at which staining is deemed to be negative can vary from zero to over 10 per cent, and could be responsible for a false impression of the incidence of CEA positivity in mesothelioma.

We have identified a total of 58 studies that have evaluated CEA expression in mesothelioma [27, 81, 87, 91, 95, 96, 98, 99, 101–114, 116–151]. A total of 1524 cases of pulmonary adenocarcinoma and 2077 cases of epithelioid (or biphasic) mesothelioma were examined. The incidence of positive CEA staining was 83 per cent in adenocarcinomas and 4.4 per cent in mesotheliomas. When only those studies that had compared pulmonary adenocarcinomas with mesotheliomas were considered, the sensitivity and specificity of CEA were 83 per cent and 95 per cent, respectively. In the 24 studies that utilized monoclonal CEA, sensitivity was reduced to 81 per cent but specificity improved to 97 per cent [27, 91, 95, 99, 104, 106, 116, 119–121, 123, 124, 126, 128, 129, 131, 134, 135, 142, 144, 146, 147, 149, 151].

Glycoproteins Ber-EP4 and B72.3

Ber-EP4 is a formalin-resistant antibody raised against a 34–49 kDa glycoprotein expressed on most epithelial cells, except those with squamous differentiation. Early studies suggested that it had a high sensitivity and specificity for adenocarcinoma [81, 103, 147], whilst positive reactions were reported in less than 1 per cent of mesotheliomas by others [91, 93, 152].

Seventeen studies have compared Ber-EP4 staining in PACA ($n = 702$) and EM ($n = 899$) [81, 87, 91, 93, 103, 104, 106, 120, 123, 124, 128, 134, 147, 149, 150, 152, 153]. The proportion of mesotheliomas exhibiting positive reactions with Ber-EP4 ranged from zero to 20 per cent. The overall sensitivity and specificity of Ber-EP4 for distinguishing between pulmonary adenocarcinomas and epithelioid mesotheliomas were 80 per cent and 90 per cent, respectively.

B72.3 is a monoclonal antibody raised in mice against a tumour-associated glycoprotein complex expressed in breast carcinoma cell lines [154]. As with Ber-EP4, initial studies suggested that B72.3 could be an important tool for differentiating between pulmonary adenocarcinomas and mesotheliomas [155]. Further investigation led to a dampening of enthusiasm, with some authors reporting positive reactions in up to 47 per cent of mesotheliomas [108]. Analysis of 16 studies that include 769 cases of pulmonary adenocarcinomas and 700 cases of mesotheliomas show it to have an 80 per cent sensitivity and 93 per cent specificity for adenocarcinoma, figures that compare favourably with more established IHC antibodies [75, 81, 91, 95, 106, 108, 117, 120, 124, 126, 127, 131, 134, 149, 155, 229].

MOC-31

MOC-31 is a monoclonal antibody that reacts with a 38 kDa epithelium-associated transmembranous glycoprotein raised from a small-cell lung cancer cell line. MOC-31 has been investigated in a small number of studies ($n = 7$) as a means of distinguishing pulmonary adenocarcinomas ($n = 213$) from mesotheliomas ($n = 276$) in tissue block preparations [84, 85, 87, 147, 150, 151,

156]. These studies have confirmed that MOC-31 has a high sensitivity and specificity for pulmonary adenocarcinoma (93 per cent for both). However, there is a single study of MOC-31 in mesothelioma and metastatic pleural carcinoma that reports a positive staining incidence of MOC-31 in mesothelioma of 17 per cent [157]. This was not incorporated into our meta-analysis as the primary source of the metastatic carcinomas was not reported. MOC-31 positivity in cytological preparations has also been studied by three groups who report slightly less impressive results, with a sensitivity of 88 per cent and a specificity of 93 per cent overall [158–160].

E-cadherins

The cadherins are a group of heterodimeric calcium-dependent membrane-associated glycoproteins in the cell adhesion molecule (CAM) family [161]. The type of cadherin expressed by a cell reflects its embryological origin. E-cadherin is typically expressed in epithelia. In contrast, N-cadherin is expressed by cells originating from mesodermal and neural crest tissue, such as mesothelium.

Seven studies have evaluated E-cadherin as a discriminator between mesotheliomas ($n = 218$) and pulmonary adenocarcinoma ($n = 183$) [86, 87, 134, 148, 162–164]. E-cadherin appears to have reasonable diagnostic value with an overall sensitivity and specificity for adenocarcinoma of 86 per cent and 82 per cent, respectively.

Thyroid transcription factor-1 (TTF-1)

This factor is exclusively expressed in thyroid and lung epithelium [165, 166]. The TTF-1 gene is highly conserved and its expression is retained despite malignant transformation. Five papers have investigated the differential expression of this antibody in a total of 366 pulmonary adenocarcinomas and 240 mesotheliomas [86, 87, 148, 167, 168]. None of the mesotheliomas were positive for TTF-1, and 85 carcinomas were negative (28 per cent) (Fig. 4.11). The sensitivity and specificity of TTF-1 for distinguishing between PACA and EM are 72 per cent and 100 per cent, respectively.

Blood group antigens (Lewis[y])

Several blood group antigens have been examined as potential discriminators between adenocarcinomas and mesotheliomas. These include Lewis[y], ABO blood group related antigen (BGRA-g)

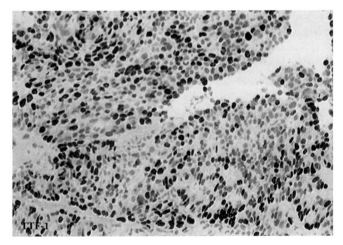

Figure 4.11 Diffuse TTF-1 nuclear positivity in a primary pulmonary carcinoma.

[144] and *Helix pomotia* agglutinin (HPAgg) [140]. Lewis^y is the only one of these that has consistently proved its worth. Four studies have evaluated Lewis^y, using the BG8 antibody, in a total of 231 cases of pulmonary adenocarcinomas and 197 mesotheliomas [86, 87, 91, 169]. Combined sensitivity and specificity were both 93 per cent.

Intermediate filaments and cytokeratins

The type of cytokeratin (CK) expressed by a cell is influenced by embryological origin and differentiation, and is usually retained despite malignant transformation. Low-molecular-weight cytokeratins (LMWCKs) are preferentially expressed in glandular tissue, with heavier CKs seen in tissues with transitional or squamous differentiation. Studying the distribution of specific CK types within a tumour cell can help identify its tissue of origin.

Two of the more commonly used CK antibodies are AE1/AE3 and CAM5.2. AE1/AE3 is a cocktail of two monoclonal antibodies which between them identify most cytokeratins found in human epithelium (AE1 is CK19, AE3 is CK8). They have little cross-reactivity with members of the other intermediate filament groups [170]. CAM5.2 is a monoclonal antibody which preferentially recognizes the CK8/18 pair [171]. The majority of mesotheliomas (87 per cent, $n = 963$) and adenocarcinomas (90 per cent, $n = 768$) express LMWCK [81, 91, 98, 105, 108–114, 116–118, 120–122, 126, 127, 130, 133, 135, 136, 140–142, 144, 146, 151, 172–174]. Thus the use of broad-spectrum LMWCK is limited when distinguishing between these tumours, as both produce positive results with a similar pattern of distribution. However, the demonstration of LMWCK positivity in an epithelioid tumour that is negative for other common carcinoma markers (CEA, Ber-EP4 or Leu-M1) supports a diagnosis of mesothelioma. Cytokeratins are also very valuable in distinguishing between sarcomatoid mesothelioma and its differentials, as is the co-expression of cytokeratin and vimentin [120].

Mesothelioma markers

The other group of antibodies that have been extensively investigated are 'mesothelioma markers'. These preferentially stain cells of mesenchymal or mesothelial origin. The most commonly used markers were listed earlier in Table 4.2. There are significant advantages to including mesothelium-specific antibodies in a mesothelioma diagnostic panel. First, the antibody can usually be used to evaluate all three histological subtypes of mesothelioma. Secondly, assuming that a negative 'carcinoma marker' result confirms the diagnosis of mesothelioma does not take account of the possibility of false-negative results. A negative result could reflect poor staining technique or inadequate antigen retrieval. The appropriate use of positive and negative controls reduces misinterpretation of results. A laboratory should routinely use whichever two of these antibodies it finds most reliable and reproducible.

Cytokeratin 5/6

As previously mentioned, because both mesothelial cells and carcinomas express cytokeratin, the use of broad spectrum LMWCK is of limited diagnostic value in distinguishing between these two groups. However, expression of specific cytokeratin subtypes has a diagnostic role. Mesothelial cells express both LMWCK (pairs CK5/14, 8/18, 7 and 19) and vimentin (intermediate filament group III member). Pulmonary adenocarcinoma ACA expresses CK7, 8/18 and 19 [175]. Thus the presence of CK5 and/or CK14 is an important discriminator between pulmonary adenocarcinoma and mesothelioma.

Initial reports of the diagnostic value of CK5/6 suggested close to 100 per cent sensitivity and specificity [176, 177]. More recent papers have reported less impressive results. There have also been reports of CK5/6 positivity in other epithelioid tumours capable of metastasizing to the pleura. For example, in a study by Chu and Weiss [178], although most tumours showed less prominent CK5/6 positivity than mesotheliomas, focal staining was seen in 25 per cent of ovarian carcinomas, 40 per cent of ductal breast carcinomas, and 38 per cent of pancreatic carcinomas. Eight thymomas were also CK5/6 positive. All these tumours enter the differential diagnosis of mesothelioma, particularly in the peritoneum, which may limit the value of CK5/6 at this site.

Eight groups have studied CK5/6 expression in pleural tumours [87, 99, 148, 150, 176–179]. The combined results of these studies include a total of 284 cases of pulmonary adenocarcinomas and 402 mesotheliomas. The overall sensitivity and specificity of CK5/6 for mesothelioma were 83 per cent and 85 per cent, respectively.

Calretinin

Calretinin is a 29 kDa calcium-binding molecule which is a member of the EF-hand protein group. It is probably involved in the calcium-dependent intracellular signalling mechanisms that control the cell cycle. Although characteristically expressed in central and peripheral nervous system tissue, it can also be demonstrated in the mesothelium [180].

Initial studies of calretinin reported high sensitivity and specificity, with almost all epithelioid mesotheliomas and the majority of sarcomatoid mesotheliomas demonstrating calretinin positivity [103, 181]. As more tumours have been studied it has become apparent that a small but significant number of pulmonary adenocarcinomas demonstrate calretinin positivity, albeit weak and focal. There has been debate as to whether any of the commercially available calretinin antibodies is superior, but there is no convincing evidence for this above and beyond the sort of interlaboratory discrepancies that could be expected.

To date a total of 17 studies have assessed the value of calretinin in distinguishing between mesothelioma and pulmonary adenocarcinoma [85, 87, 91, 99, 103, 104, 128, 134, 147–150, 179–183]. These comprise a combined total of 912 cases of PACA and 885 cases of EM. Overall calretinin sensitivity was 82 per cent, whilst specificity was 85 per cent.

The pattern of calretinin staining is important, with nuclear rather than cytoplasmic staining probably being of greater diagnostic value (Fig. 4.12). The majority of those groups that studied calretinin in mesothelioma found it was primarily expressed in cytoplasm, although four groups also reported nuclear staining [85, 103, 128, 182]. Nuclear staining may be less evident in post-

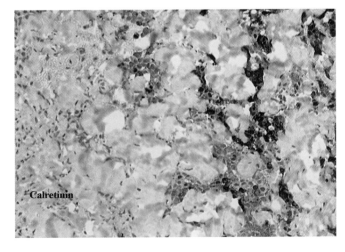

Figure 4.12 Epithelioid mesothelioma demonstrating both nuclear and cytoplasmic calretinin positivity.

mortem samples compared with pre-mortem samples from the same patients [89]. As many studies use post-mortem samples of mesothelioma, this may be of relevance.

The disappointing sensitivity and specificity results for calretinin may have a biological explanation beyond that of IHC technique. In the original paper by Gotzos *et al.* [180] calretinin was described as only being expressed in activated (cuboidal) mesothelial cells with an epithelioid appearance. Quiescent endothelial-like cells were negative, as were areas of sarcomatoid differentiation. Other studies have confirmed that between 10–30 per cent of mesothelial cells are consistently negative for calretinin. Calretinin expression may therefore be cyclical, and is most common during the G_1 phase of the cell cycle [180].

N-cadherin

The diagnostic value of cell adhesion molecules, in particular the cadherins, has been mentioned previously. Mesothelium expresses N-cadherin. An initial study by Peralta-Soler *et al.* [163], using frozen-section material, confirmed that N-cadherin was expressed in mesothelioma with maximum sensitivity and specificity (100 per cent) compared with pulmonary adenocarcinoma. The introduction of an antibody suitable for use with paraffin-embedded tissue has enabled further study of N-cadherin. Han *et al.* [162] reported that N-cadherin had a high sensitivity and specificity for mesothelioma (100 per cent and 94 per cent, respectively). Thirkettle *et al.* [164] reported slightly less impressive results for N-cadherin, at 90 per cent sensitivity and 83 per cent specificity for epithelioid mesothelioma in a small study, with 29 mesotheliomas but only six pulmonary adenocarcinomas. More recently Abutaily *et al.* [148] reported that N-cadherin sensitivity and specificity was only 74 per cent. Ordonez [87] has also reported more disappointing results, with a sensitivity of 63 per cent and a specificity of 82 per cent. The combined result of these five studies implies an overall sensitivity of 78 per cent and specificity of 84 per cent.

Wilms tumour gene product (WT1)

The Wilms tumour gene product has also been investigated as a potential diagnostic marker for mesothelioma. WT1 is expressed in fetal spleen, mesothelium, and mesonephric ridge derivatives such as the kidney. In the adult, WT1 continues to be expressed by mesothelium, spleen, the glomerular cells of the kidney, testicular Sertoli cells, uterine decidual cells, granulosa cells of the ovary and myoepithelial cells in the breast [184]. WT1 positivity can also be seen in stromal cells and blood vessels.

The value of WT1as a diagnostic marker for mesothelioma in tissue samples has been investigated by eight groups [85–87, 182, 184–187]. Overall, WT1 has a sensitivity of 77 per cent and specificity of 96 per cent in distinguishing between epithelioid mesothelioma ($n = 264$) and pulmonary adenocarcinoma ($n = 213$) in tissue sections.

There are potential problems with using WT1 in the diagnostic panel for mesothelioma. In a comparative study primarily examining differences in IHC staining between biopsy and post-mortem tissue samples, Oates *et al.* [85] found that only 43 per cent of mesotheliomas showed WT1 positivity. None of the post-mortem samples stained with WT1, and biopsy sample results were highly dependent on fixation technique. Problems can also arise if renal or ovarian tumours are included in the differential diagnosis. Renal cell carcinoma can metastasize to the pleura, and conversely mesothelioma and pulmonary adenocarcinoma can metastasize to the kidney and adrenal glands. Renal cell carcinoma shares a similar IHC profile (CEA/Ber-EP4 negative, CK positive, vimentin positive) with mesothelioma. Renal cell carcinomas may also contain areas of sarcomatoid differentiation resembling sarcomatoid mesothelioma. Clear cell variants of epithelioid mesothelioma have been reported, and clear cell change has also been described in chondro- and osteosarcomas [188–190].

Although WT1 expression has been extensively investigated in paediatric renal tumours, expression in renal cell carcinoma in adults has been less commonly studied [86, 185, 191]. The ability of IHC to distinguish between mesothelioma and renal carcinomas has not been investigated by many groups. In 1995 Attanoos *et al.* [192] studied the ability of Ber-EP4, Leu-M1, thrombomodulin, and Tamm–Horsfall protein to distinguish between mesothelioma and renal cell carcinoma. They concluded that Leu-M1 was the best discriminator with a sensitivity and specificity of 70 per cent and 95 per cent, respectively, for renal cell carcinoma. In their original description of calretinin immunolocalization, Doglioni *et al.* [103] reported that all four renal cell carcinomas studied were calretinin negative. More recently Osborn *et al.* [193] studied the IHC profile of 37 cases of mesothelioma with epithelioid differentiation and 40 cases of renal cell carcinomas with five antibodies commonly used in mesothelioma panels (CEA, Ber-EP4, CK5/6, thrombomodulin and calretinin). They concluded that calretinin was the most useful antibody, staining 97 per cent of mesotheliomas and only 10 per cent of renal tumours. CK5/6 positivity was seen in 78 per cent of mesotheliomas and only 5 per cent of renal cell carcinomas. None of the other antibodies had significant discriminatory value. The value of CK5/6 has been independently confirmed by Chu and Weiss [178], who found no positive CK5/6 staining in a series of 19 renal cell carcinomas, and Ordóñez [176] who reported negative staining in 10 cases of renal tumours.

Therefore it would seem prudent to avoid the use of WT1 if renal or ovarian tumours are considered in the differential, and they should be excluded by appropriate radiology, such as renal ultrasound or abdominal CT, if clinically suspected.

Thrombomodulin and HBME-1

Thrombomodulin and HBME-1 are two previously widely used mesothelioma markers that now compare less favourably with newer antibodies such as calretinin, N-cadherin, and WT1. HBME-1 is a monoclonal antibody raised from the mesothelioma cell line SPC111 [194]. The exact nature of the target antigen is unknown but it is predominantly located on microvilli. An early study by Bateman *et al.* [195] compared HBME-1 staining in 17 mesotheliomas and 14 adenocarcinomas. They reported 100 per cent HBME-1 positivity in the mesotheliomas, but 10 of the adenocarcinomas were also positive. Three of the adenocarcinomas were of pulmonary origin, and their results were not stratified according to tissue of origin; hence their results were not included in our meta-analysis. Since then a total of 14 other studies have reported their experiences using HBME-1 to distinguish between epithelioid mesothelioma and pulmonary adenocarcinoma [81–83, 85, 87, 91, 99, 104, 128, 147, 149, 151, 196, 197]. The overall sensitivity and specificity of HBME-1 for mesothelioma are 85 per cent and 43 per cent, respectively, when the results of these studies are combined. These are based on a total of 769 mesotheliomas and 676 pulmonary adenocarcinomas.

Thrombomodulin is a 75 kDa glycoprotein that is expressed by endothelium, mesothelium, synovium, and placental syncytiotrophoblasts [119]. It was first described in 1982 [198] and its value in the recognition of vascular tumours was soon recognized [199]. Collins and colleagues [119, 200] were the first to investigate the expression of thrombomodulin in mesothelioma. They found it to have excellent sensitivity (100 per cent) and specificity (92 per cent) for epithelioid mesothelioma compared with adenocarcinoma. Thrombomodulin has subsequently been evaluated in a further 15 studies, but with less impressive results [81, 83, 87, 91, 95, 103, 104, 128, 147–150, 179, 182, 183, 196]. Combining the results of these 17 studies indicates that the sensitivity and specificity of thrombomodulin for mesothelioma are poor, at 61 per cent and 80 per cent, respectively. This is based on a total of 964 cases of pulmonary adenocarcinoma and 831 cases of epithelioid mesothelioma.

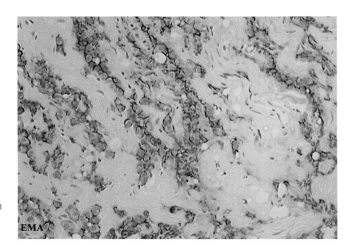

Figure 4.13 Mesothelioma with membranous EMA antibody staining.

Miscellaneous IHC markers

Several other IHC antibodies have been investigated for their potential to differentiate between mesothelioma and adenocarcinoma. Epithelial membrane antigen (EMA) is positive in both tumours, but the distribution of the staining differs between the two. In mesothelial cells, EMA is located predominantly on the cell surface (Fig. 4.13) in association with microvilli. In contrast, EMA is exclusively intracytoplasmic in adenocarcinoma [201, 202].

Human milk fat globulins, particularly HMFG-2, share a similar pattern of staining distribution to EMA. Both EMA and HMFG stain PAS-positive material, implying a common antigenic moiety. Almost 50 per cent of anaplastic (CD30+) large-cell lymphomas are positive for EMA, and EMA positivity has also been described in the epithelioid areas of synovial sarcomas and epithelioid sarcomas [203]. Therefore these antibodies are less commonly favoured when trying to distinguish between mesothelioma and adenocarcinoma.

An immunohistochemical algorithm for differentiating between mesothelioma and adenocarcinoma

Novel antibodies that aid the distinction between mesothelioma and adenocarcinoma have expanded the pathology diagnostic panel. Although these may improve diagnostic accuracy, they have the disadvantages of being expensive and time consuming. Not infrequently, results for different antibodies are contradictory. Studies that have assessed the contribution of IHC to the diagnosis of mesothelioma have reported conflicting results. Moch *et al.* [204] found that only 25 per cent of suspected cases of mesothelioma were confidently diagnosed using clinical factors, H&E and D-PAS stains. The additional use of a panel of IHC antibodies increased the proportion confidently diagnosed to almost 80 per cent. Conversely, Betta *et al.* [205] considered that 63–81 per cent of prospective mesotheliomas could be diagnosed without the use of IHC. Using IHC improved the diagnostic rate to between 67 and 92 per cent.

An ideal panel would consist of a small number of complementary antibodies, some with high sensitivity and others with high specificity. This panel would at best identify all cases of mesothelioma, or at least act as a useful screening panel to prompt further analyses. Several groups have attempted to extrapolate from their own IHC results to produce a small but robust antibody panel and/or associated algorithm to address this problem [95, 134, 148, 149, 204, 205].

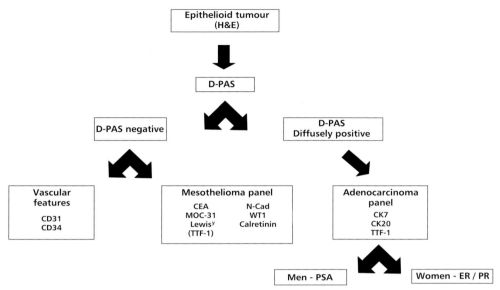

Figure 4.14 Diagnostic algorithm to guide the choice of immunohistochemical antibodies to distinguish between epithelioid mesothelioma and pulmonary adenocarcinoma.

Extrapolating from our own literature search and analysis, we suggest the following diagnostic algorithm, illustrated in Fig. 4.14. After identification of the presence of an epithelioid pleural tumour on H&E sections, a D-PAS stain should be performed. A diffusely positive D-PAS is highly suggestive of adenocarcinoma and should direct further investigations towards identifying the tissue of origin. These might include the use of TTF-1, and appropriate anticytokeratins (e.g. CK 7 and CK 20), hormone [oestrogen or progesterone receptors (ER/PR)], or tumour-specific markers [prostate-specific antigen (PSA)] chosen after consideration of the mostly likely diagnosis according to patient sex, age, and clinical details. A negative D-PAS result would prompt the use of the 'mesothelioma panel'. This should comprise two antibodies with the best sensitivity and specificity for adenocarcinoma and mesothelioma, respectively. Each laboratory should use the antibodies that provide the most consistent and reliable results in their hands.

Monoclonal CEA (97 per cent specific, 81 per cent sensitive) has repeatedly shown itself to be of great value in a large number of cases. This should be combined with another antibody with better sensitivity, such as E-cadherin or MOC-31. TTF-1 is an alternative, but is of less value when considering a carcinoma of non-pulmonary or thyroid origin.

The panel should also contain two antibodies that specifically identify mesothelioma. The best two antibodies for this appear to be calretinin and WT-1. It will be necessary to adapt this panel if ovarian or renal tumours are differentials.

The presence of histological or clinical factors atypical for mesothelioma or adenocarcinoma should alert the pathologist to the possibility of other rarer differentials, such as vascular tumours, melanoma, or thymoma. Epithelioid haemangioendotheliomas are sometimes positive for CAM 5.2 or AE1/3.

The role of immunohistochemistry in the diagnosis of biphasic and sarcomatoid mesothelioma

Less attention has been paid to the role of IHC in characterizing pleural tumours containing areas of sarcomatoid differentiation. This is partly due to the fact that biphasic and sarcomatoid mesotheliomas are less common than their epithelioid counterparts, and therefore constitute less of a diagnostic problem. A biphasic pleural tumour has a smaller number of differential diagnoses, which include mesothelioma, carcinosarcoma, biphasic synovial sarcoma, and pleomorphic carcinoma of the lung (Fig. 4.10). A staining profile consistent with mesothelioma in epithelioid areas or demonstration of cytokeratin positivity within sarcomatoid areas is generally considered diagnostic of mesothelioma. There is the important caveat that some sarcomas (e.g. epithelioid haemangioendotheliomas, synovial sarcomas, peripheral nerve sheath tumours, pleomorphic carcinomas and rarely leiomyosarcomas) may be cytokeratin positive.

Pure sarcomatoid pleural tumours are rare. The main differentials of sarcomatoid mesothelioma (Fig 4.10) include primary and secondary sarcomas, vascular tumours, spindle cell carcinoma, melanoma, and solitary fibrous tumours. Important differentials of desmoplastic mesothelioma include benign reactive pleural fibrosis and the rare pleural fibromatosis. The use of IHC to identify cells of mesothelial origin is of less diagnostic value in these cases.

There have been far fewer published papers that have specifically examined the differences in IHC expression of sarcomatoid mesothelioma and its differentials. In our IHC meta-analysis we identified a total of 29 studies that reported specific IHC results for biphasic and sarcomatoid mesotheliomas [70, 82, 83, 85, 99, 102, 103, 105, 106, 116, 128, 132, 134, 147, 148, 157, 162–164, 173, 177, 178, 180, 182, 185, 186, 206–208]. Many of these studies did not compare the IHC profile of mesothelioma with that of other tumours; therefore these results cannot be used to calculate diagnostic sensitivity and specificity. However, the results can act as a crude surrogate marker for IHC expression in sarcomatoid mesothelioma for comparison with other pleural tumours.

Cytokeratins

Cytokeratin expression is a useful diagnostic feature when trying to identify sarcomatoid pleural tumours correctly. Cytokeratin expression in sarcomas can be either of two types. Some sarcomas are characterized by areas of true epithelial differentiation, i.e. their epithelioid areas express epithelial markers. The classical examples of this are epithelioid sarcomas and synovial sarcomas [203]. The other pattern of cytokeratin expression involves the production of anomalous cytokeratins. In these cases CK is expressed in areas that are not epithelioid in appearance. These are usually non-specific LMWCKs, such as CK8/18, and are seen in dot-like aggregations in a perinuclear distribution, usually in a small proportion of the tumour overall. Anomalous cytokeratin expression has been described in smooth muscle tumours, melanomas, and vascular tumours. It may be enhanced by the use of heat-induced epitope retrieval techniques.

The expression of broad-spectrum LMWCK in biphasic and sarcomatoid mesothelioma has been reported in 11 papers [70, 105, 106, 116, 120, 128, 157, 173, 206–208]. Four of these studied CAM 5.2 expression, with a combined total of 106 tumours [106, 120, 128, 173]. The range of positive staining was similar in each group (90–94 per cent). Overall, CAM 5.2 was expressed in 99 tumours, corresponding to an overall incidence of 93 per cent. Four other studies used the AE1/AE3 antibody in a total of 72 tumours, with positivity reported in 64 cases (89 per cent) [105, 157, 206, 207]. Lucas *et al.* [208] studied the expression of a pan-cytokeratin antibody cocktail (CAM 5.2, AE1/AE3 and CK-904) in sarcomatoid mesotheliomas and other sarcomatoid tumours. The majority of sarcomatoid areas in biphasic ($n = 9$, 90 per cent) and sarcomatoid mesotheliomas ($n = 7$, 70 per cent) demonstrated positive staining, albeit less strong than in epithelioid mesothelioma. A further two studies have reported cytokeratin expression using a pan-cytokeratin cocktail of antibodies which included AE1/AE3, CAM5.2, and CK7 [70, 116]. The incidence of pan- cytokeratin expression was 83 per cent.

The intermediate filament that has most extensively been studied in sarcomatoid mesothelioma is vimentin. There have been 11 published studies, which have included a total of 207 tumours [70, 99, 102, 105, 106, 116, 128, 132, 147, 157, 173]. Vimentin positivity was reported to range from 55 to 100 per cent, with an average of 81 per cent overall.

CK5/6

The expression of the CK5/6 antibody in sarcomatoid mesothelioma has been evaluated in seven studies that include a total of 94 tumours [99, 148, 177, 178, 186, 206, 208]. CK5/6 positivity ranged from zero to 86 per cent for individual studies. The highest incidence was reported by Kayser et al. [99] with six of seven tumours CK5/6 positive. In contrast, four other groups have reported CK5/6 incidence of less than 20 per cent in sarcomatoid mesothelioma [148, 177, 186, 208]. The overall incidence of CK5/6 positive staining is 22 per cent when the results of all of these studies are combined.

Calretinin

Thirteen groups have studied calretinin expression in mesotheliomas showing sarcomatoid differentiation [70, 85, 99, 103, 128, 134, 147, 148, 180, 182, 186, 206, 208]. They include a combined total of 141 mesotheliomas. Four of these have reported 100 per cent calretinin expression in sarcomatoid mesotheliomas, albeit in small numbers of cases [103, 134, 147, 186]. Conversely, four other studies report calretinin positivity in less than a third of tumours [128, 148, 180, 182]. The mean incidence of calretinin positivity when all these studies were combined was 46 per cent.

Three groups also evaluated calretinin expression in other sarcomatoid pleural tumours [186, 206, 208]. In the first of these studies calretinin expression was assessed in 103 synovial sarcomas, 30 mesotheliomas, and a small number of other sarcomas [186]. Calretinin positivity was seen in all mesotheliomas. Sarcomatoid areas within biphasic and sarcomatoid synovial sarcomas demonstrated focal calretinin positivity in a little over half of all cases (55 per cent), with much less positivity in any epithelioid areas (14 per cent). Two peripheral nerve sheath tumours demonstrated focal calretinin positivity, but all other sarcomas were negative.

Attanoos et al. [206] reported conflicting results. In their comparative study of 31 sarcomatoid mesotheliomas and a similar number of other spindle cell tumours, calretinin positivity was demonstrable in less than half of the mesotheliomas ($n = 12$, 39 per cent). However, none of the other spindle cell tumours were positive for calretinin, suggesting low sensitivity but 100 per cent specificity for mesothelioma. Lucas et al. [208] have also evaluated calretinin expression in sarcomatoid mesothelioma and its differentials. Four sarcomas (17 per cent of all cases studied) and six sarcomatoid carcinomas (60 per cent) were calretinin positive. In the sarcomas calretinin positivity was less than 5 per cent in three tumours. Only two of the six sarcomatoid carcinomas exhibited strong and diffuse calretinin positivity. Therefore it appears that, although calretinin is a useful to differentiate between mesothelioma and other epithelioid pleural tumours, a positive result in biphasic or sarcomatoid tumours is not necessarily diagnostic of mesothelioma. However, strong calretinin positivity is uncommon in other sarcomatoid pleural tumours. Biphasic synovial sarcoma should always be considered as a differential diagnosis.

HBME-1, thrombomodulin, N-cadherin, and WT-1

Nine groups have studied HBME-1 expression in sarcomatoid mesothelioma [82, 83, 85, 99, 128, 147, 157, 186]. These include a total of 81 cases of mesothelioma with a positive staining incidence of only 25 per cent. Thrombomodulin expression in sarcomatoid mesothelioma has been studied by seven groups [70, 128, 148, 182, 186, 206, 208]. Thrombomodulin positivity was noted in 34 out of a total of 92 cases of sarcomatoid mesothelioma (37 per cent).

Although studied by only three groups, and in a very small number of cases ($n = 22$), N-cadherin expression has been reported in all but one sarcomatoid mesothelioma studied (95 per cent expression) [148, 162, 163]. More recently Laskin *et al.* [209] have studied cadherin expression in a series of sarcomatoid tumours with epithelioid features that included cases of mesothelioma and synovial sarcoma. They reported 100 per cent expression of E-cadherin in the epithelioid areas of biphasic synovial sarcoma, with more than 50 per cent E-cadherin expression in cases of melanoma and monophasic sarcomatoid synovial sarcoma. In contrast, only 20 per cent of mesotheliomas were positive. When N-cadherin was considered, high levels of expression were seen in biphasic synovial sarcoma (86 per cent), malignant melanoma (56 per cent), and mesothelioma (70 per cent). Therefore it would appear likely that, although N-cadherin is of great diagnostic value in differentiating mesothelioma from other epithelioid tumours, it may be less useful when synovial sarcoma is a differential. Synovial sarcomas are associated with a specific genetic abnormality: a balanced translocation between Ch 18 and the X chromosome, t(X;18)(p11.2; q11.2) [210, 211]. The demonstration of the SYT/SSX gene product is now the gold standard for the diagnosis of synovial sarcoma [186].

WT-1 has also been evaluated in only a small number of studies ($n = 5$) and tumours ($n = 43$).[85, 182, 185, 186, 208]. Overall incidence of WT-1 expression was 37 per cent. Only one study reported no WT-1 positivity in any case of sarcomatoid mesothelioma [186]. Therefore WT-1 is of limited value in the distinction of sarcomatoid mesothelioma from other sarcomatoid tumours.

The role of immunohistochemistry in differentiating between benign and malignant mesothelial proliferations

The final diagnostic consideration when studying pleural pathology is the differentiation between benign and malignant mesothelial proliferations. This can be particularly challenging in the presence of infection (empyema) or when dealing with desmoplastic tumours, in which a bland appearance belies their aggressive invasive behaviour and poorer prognosis. The distinction between benign and malignant pleural disease is one of the most important to make, as the repercussions of an incorrect diagnosis can be far more devastating for a patient.

IHC is of limited value in this area as both benign and malignant mesothelial proliferations have similar IHC profiles. Staining with LMWCK can emphasize the distribution of mesothelial cells within stroma and highlight areas of invasion with are critical in confirming the diagnosis of malignancy [24]. Similarly, the use of macrophage markers (CD68) may help to better define cellular areas associated with an inflammatory infiltrate [212].

Several IHC antibodies have been evaluated for their ability to distinguish between benign and malignant mesothelial proliferations. The most extensively investigated include p53 and EMA. Other potential diagnostic markers include p-170, desmin, Bcl-2, and the gene products c-*fos* and c-*myc* [24]. The diagnostic sensitivity and specificity of the most widely examined of these markers are summarized in Table 4.5. Another diagnostic technique that has been studied is the quantitative distribution of argyrophil nucleolar organizer regions (AgNOR) [24].

Table 4.5 Summary of the results of published studies that have evaluated the diagnostic value of immunohistochemical markers in distinguishing between benign and malignant mesothelial proliferations

IHC marker	No. of studies analysed	No. of mesothelioma cases	No. of reactive pleuritis cases	Sensitivity of antibody for MPM (%)	Specificity of antibody for MPM (%)
p53	10	416	193	58	90
EMA	5	353	170	74	88
Desmin	3	114	60	83	83
Bcl-2	3	108	93	5	100
p-170	3	154	61	45	97

p53

Changes in the tumour suppressor gene p53 have been implicated in the origin in many human cancers including malignant mesothelioma. The normal (wild-type) form of p53 has a very short half-life and therefore is difficult to demonstrate with IHC techniques unless degradation mechanisms have been altered or subjected to high levels of cellular stress. Mutated forms of p53 are resistant to normal degradation, and therefore accumulate in the nucleus in quantities that are proportional to cell proliferation rate. Thus the immunohistochemical demonstration of p53 is suggestive, but not diagnostic, of malignant proliferation. Anti-p53 antibodies are sensitive to differences in fixation techniques, and are most reliably demonstrated in small tissue sections or cytological preparations.

p53 has been investigated as a marker for malignancy in mesothelioma by 13 groups, of which 10 have also assessed its incidence in benign mesothelial proliferations.[117, 128, 185, 213–222]. Combining their results suggests that the incidence of p53 staining in mesothelioma is 57 per cent (range 25–100 per cent). The sensitivity of p53 is 58 per cent and the specificity is 90 per cent when used to distinguish between mesothelioma ($n = 416$) and benign mesothelial proliferations ($n = 193$).

Epithelial membrane antigen

EMA has been discussed regarding its ability to distinguish between epithelioid mesothelioma and adenocarcinoma. It has also been evaluated as a discriminator between benign and malignant mesothelial processes [24, 128, 215, 221, 222]. Although EMA can be demonstrated on the microvilli of normal mesothelial cells, the intensity of staining is much less than that seen in mesothelioma. Overall EMA has a sensitivity of 74 per cent and a specificity of 88 per cent when compared in reactive pleuritis ($n = 170$) and mesothelioma ($n = 353$).

Desmin

Desmin is an intracellular intermediate filament that can be characteristically demonstrated in smooth and skeletal muscle. It has also been described in non-myogenous tumours, including primitive neuroectodermal tumour, Wilms tumour, and mesothelioma [223, 224]. Three groups have specifically evaluated desmin in terms of its ability to distinguish between mesothelioma and reactive pleuritis [222, 223, 225]. These studies included a total of 114 mesotheliomas and 60 cases of reactive pleuritis. The sensitivity and specificity of desmin for mesothelioma were equal at 83 per cent.

Bcl-2 and p-170

Bcl-2 is a protein that has anti-apoptotic activity, and its overexpression in carcinomas is associated with a poorer prognosis. Three groups have studied the expression of Bcl-2 in mesothelioma ($n = 108$) and reactive pleuritis ($n = 93$) [215, 222, 226]. Bcl-2 positivity was seen in 5 per cent of mesotheliomas and no cases of reactive pleuritis. p-170 is the glycoprotein product of the *mdr 1* gene [222]. It has been studied in mesothelioma and reactive pleuritis by three groups and found to have a sensitivity of only 45 per cent, although specificity is better at 97 per cent [128, 213, 222].

Argyrophil nucleolar organizer regions

Nucleolar organizer regions are argyrophil acidic proteins associated with areas within chromosomes 13, 14, 15, 21, and 22 that code for ribosomal RNA [129]. Therefore an increase in the number of NORs may reflect an increase in transcriptional or proliferative activity. The use of silver labelling facilitates the recognition and counting of NORs within the nucleus. An increase in AgNOR numbers has been shown to be of value in distinguishing between benign and malignant lymphoid and breast tissue, and has also been studied in mesothelial tissue [24, 129, 227, 228]. Although the incidence of AGNORs is increased in malignant mesothelioma compared with reactive disease, the degree of overlap between the values for benign and malignant tissue reduces its discriminatory value overall. Henderson *et al.* [24] have reported a diagnostic sensitivity of 95 per cent for distinguishing between reactive and malignant mesothelium when AgNOR (expressed as the proportion of the nucleus that was occupied by AgNOR-positive material) and EMA were combined.

Conclusions

The diagnosis of all subtypes of mesothelioma can be difficult. A pathologist should not be content to diagnose a mesothelial malignancy just because the patient has a history of asbestos exposure [92]. As asbestos also predisposes to the development of carcinoma of the lung, this factor has limited discriminatory value. A great deal of input from other clinicians (e.g. physician, radiologist, and surgeon) may be necessary before a final diagnosis can be made.

Diagnostic histochemistry and IHC have been embraced wholeheartedly in the search for a gold standard for the diagnosis of mesothelioma, and this subject has resulted in the publication of dozens of papers over the last 20 years. Unfortunately, although much has been learned from these studies, we are still left without any IHC antibody that is reproducibly 100 per cent sensitive and specific for mesothelioma compared with other pleural tumours. Therefore it is essential that IHC is used to complement rather than override both clinical and histopathological factors.

The tendency to use an ever-expanding panel of diagnostic antibodies should not be encouraged. This is time consuming and expensive, and the greater the number of antibodies, the greater the difficulty in interpretation if conflicting results are found. It is essential that the limitations of immunohistochemical stains are recognized. A pathologist should not be overly influenced by the results of novel antibodies, unless they have been shown to be repeatable in different laboratories and in large numbers of cases.

Other factors must be remembered when attempting a critical analysis of the contribution of IHC to mesothelioma diagnosis. Studies often state that the diagnosis of mesothelioma was made using 'standard diagnostic criteria' without definition. It may well be that authors are only including well-differentiated tumours, and therefore ignoring pleomorphic mesothelioma which causes most diagnostic problems. Most diagnostic adjuncts, even electron microscopy, are not

100 per cent accurate. Many studies of mesothelioma have included small numbers of cases. The inclusion of even one or two carcinomas in a group of mesotheliomas can give a false impression of the value of a diagnostic antibody.

References

1. Health and Safety Executive. *Mesothelioma mortality in Great Britain: Estimating the Future Burden.* London: Health and Safety Executive, 2003.
2. Neumann V, Muller KM, Fischer M. [Peritoneal mesothelioma—incidence and etiology.] *Pathologe* 1999; **20**: 169–76 (in German).
3. Hodgson JT, Darnton A. The quantitative risks of mesothelioma and lung cancer in relation to asbestos exposure. *Ann Occup Hyg* 2000; **44**: 565–01.
4. British Thoracic Society. Statement on malignant mesothelioma in the United Kingdom. *Thorax* 2001; **56**: 250–65.
5. Kahn EI, Rohl A, Barrett EW, *et al.* Primary pericardial mesothelioma following exposure to asbestos. *Environ Res* 1980; **23**: 270–81.
6. Maltoni C, Pinto C, Carnuccio R, *et al.* Mesotheliomas following exposure to asbestos used in railroads: 130 Italian cases. *Med Lav* 1995; **86**: 461–77.
7. Churg A, Warnock ML, Bensch KG. Malignant mesothelioma arising after direct application of asbestos and fiber glass to the pericardium. *Am Rev Respir Dis* 1978; **118**: 419–24.
8. Thomason R, Schlegel W, Lucca M, *et al.* Primary malignant mesothelioma of the pericardium. Case report and literature review. *Tex Heart Inst J* 1994; **21**: 170–4.
9. Chung CM, Chu PH, Chen JS, *et al.* Primary pericardial mesothelioma with cardiac tamponade and distant metastasis: case report. *Changgeng Yi Xue Za Zhi* 1998; **21**: 498–502.
10. Veinot JP, Burns BF, Commons AS, *et al.* Cardiac neoplasms at the Canadian reference centre for cancer pathology. *Can J Cardiol* 1999; **15**: 311–19.
11. Kawano H, Okada R, Kawano Y, *et al.* Mesothelioma in the atrioventricular node. Case report. *Jpn Heart J* 1994; **35**: 255–61.
12. Clement PB, Young RH, Scully RE. Malignant mesotheliomas presenting as ovarian masses. A report of nine cases, including two primary ovarian mesotheliomas. *Am J Surg Pathol* 1996; **20**: 1067–80.
13. Murai Y. Malignant mesothelioma in Japan: analysis of registered autopsy cases. *Arch Environ Health* 2001; **56**: 84–8.
14. Attanoos RL, Gibbs AR. Primary malignant gonadal mesotheliomas and asbestos. *Histopathology* 2000; **37**: 150–9.
15. Butnor KJ, Sporn TA, Hammar SP, *et al.* Well-differentiated papillary mesothelioma. *Am J Surg Pathol* 2001; **25**: 1304–9.
16. Sadler T, ed. *Langman's Medical Embryology,* 7th edn. Baltimore, MD: Williams & Wilkins, 1995.
17. Carter D, True L, Otis C. Serous membranes. In: Sternberg S, ed. *Histology for Pathologists.* New York: Raven Press, 1992; 499–514.
18. Ghadially F. *Ultrastructural Pathology of the Cell and Matrix,* 2nd edn. London: Butterworths, 1982.
19. Lippmann M, Yeates D, Albert R. Deposition, retention, and clearance of inhaled particles. *Br J Ind Med* 1980; **37**: 337–62.
20. Bignon J, Brochard P. Animal and cell models for understanding and predicting fibre-related mesothelioma in man. In: Brown R, Hoskins J, Johnson N, eds. *Mechanisms in Fibre Carcinogenesis.* New York: Plenum Press, 1991; 515–30.
21. Hasleton P, ed. *Spencers Pathology of the Lung.* New York: McGraw-Hill, 1995.
22. McKee G. *Cytopathology.* London: Mosby–Wolfe, 1997.
23. Attanoos R, Gibbs A. Pathology of malignant mesothelioma. *Histopathology* 1997; **30**: 403–18.

24. Henderson D, Shilkin K, Whitaker D. Reactive mesothelial hyperplasia vs. mesothelioma, including mesothelioma *in situ*. *Am J Clin Pathol* 1998; **110**: 397–404.

25. Suárez Vilela D, Izquierdo Garcia F. Embolization of mesothelial cells in lymphatics: the route to mesothelial inclusions in lymph nodes? *Histopathology* 1998; **33**: 570–5.

26. Warhol M, Corson J. An ultrastructural comparison of mesotheliomas with adenocarcinomas of the lung and breast. *Hum Pathol* 1985; **16**: 50–5.

27. Dewar A, Valente M, Ring N, *et al*. Pleural mesothelioma of epithelial type and pulmonary adenocarcinoma: An ultrastructural and cytochemical comparison. *J Pathol* 1987; **152**: 309–16.

28. Burns T, Johnson E, Cartwright J, *et al*. Desmosomes of epithelial malignant mesothelioma. *Ultrastruct Pathol* 1988; **12**: 385–8.

29. Grunze H. The comparative diagnostic accuracy, efficiency and specificity of cytologic technics used in the diagnosis of malignant neoplasm in serous effusions of the pleural and pericardial cavities. *Acta Cytol* 1964; **40**: 150–63.

30. Tomlinson J, Sahn S. Invasive procedures in the diagnosis of pleural disease. *Semin Respir Med* 1987; **9**: 30–6.

31. Prakash UB, Reiman HM. Comparison of needle biopsy with cytologic analysis for the evaluation of pleural effusion: analysis of 414 cases. *Mayo Clin Proc* 1985; **60**: 158–64.

32. Nance KV, Shermer RW, Askin FB. Diagnostic efficacy of pleural biopsy as compared with that of pleural fluid examination. *Mod Pathol* 1991; **4**: 320–4.

33. Escudero Bueno C, Garcia Clemente M, Cuesta Castro B, *et al*. Cytologic and bacteriologic analysis of fluid and pleural biopsy specimens with Cope's needle. Study of 414 patients. *Arch Intern Med* 1990; **150**: 1190–4.

34. Frist B, Kahan AV, Koss LG. Comparison of the diagnostic values of biopsies of the pleura and cytologic evaluation of pleural fluids. *Am J Clin Pathol* 1979; **72**: 48–51.

35. Renshaw A, Dean B, Antman K, *et al*. The role of cytologic evaluation of pleural fluid in the diagnosis of maligant mesothelioma. *Chest* 1997; **111**: 106–9.

36. Kirsch CM, Kroe DM, Azzi RL, *et al*. The optimal number of pleural biopsy specimens for a diagnosis of tuberculous pleurisy. *Chest* 1997; **112**: 702–6.

37. Abrams L. A pleural biopsy punch. *Lancet* 1958; i: 30.

38. Mungall IP, Cowen PN, Cooke NT, *et al*. Multiple pleural biopsy with the Abrams needle. *Thorax* 1980; **35**: 600–2.

39. Maskell NA, Gleeson FV, Davies RJ. Standard pleural biopsy versus CT-guided cutting-needle biopsy for diagnosis of malignant disease in pleural effusions: a randomised controlled trial. *Lancet* 2003; **361**: 1326–30.

40. Boutin C, Rey F. Thoracoscopy in pleural malignant mesothelioma: a prospective study of 188 consecutive patients. Part 1: Diagnosis. *Cancer* 1993; **72**: 389–93.

41. Hillerdal G. Malignant mesothelioma 1982: review of 4710 published cases. *Br J Dis Chest* 1983; **77**: 321–43.

42. Boutin C, Dumortier P, Rey F, *et al*. Black spots concentrate oncogenic asbestos fibers in the parietal pleura. Thoracoscopic and mineralogic study. *Am J Respir Crit Care Med* 1996; **153**: 444–9.

43. Roy GC, Saha DK, Chandra A. Localised malignant mesothelioma of visceral pleura. *J Indian Med Assoc* 1994; **92**: 339–44.

44. Erkilic S, Sari I, Tuncozgur B. Localized pleural malignant mesothelioma. *Pathol Int* 2001; **51**: 812–15.

45. Okuma S, Kashara M, Kuroda M, *et al*. [Sarcomatous malignant mesothelioma diagnosed after death.] *Nihon Kyobu Shikkan Gakkai Zasshi* 1996; **34**: 312–16 (in Japanese).

46. Mossman BT, Churg A. Mechanisms in the pathogenesis of asbestosis and silicosis. *Am J Respir Crit Care Med* 1998; **157**: 1666–80.

47. Hasleton P, Hammar S. Malignant mesothelioma. *Curr Diagn Pathol* 1996; **3**: 153–164.

48. Law M, Hodson M, Heard B. Malignant mesothelioma of the pleura: relation between histological type and clinical behaviour. *Thorax* 1982; **37**: 810–15.

49. Travis W, Colby T, Corrin B, *et al. WHO International Histological Classification of Tumours: Histological Typing of Lung and Pleural Tumours*, 3rd edn. Berlin: Springer-Verlag; 1999.

50. Van Gelder T, Hoogsteden H, Vandenbroucke J, *et al.* The influence of the diagnostic technique on the histopathological diagnosis in malignant mesothelioma. *Virchows Arch A Pathol Anat Histopathol* 1991; **418**: 315–17.

51. Adams V, Unni K. Diffuse malignant mesothelioma of pleura: diagnostic criteria based on an autopsy study. *Am J Clin Pathol* 1984; **82**: 15–23.

52. Hammar S, Bockus D, Remington F, *et al.* Mucin-positive mesotheliomas: a histochemical, immunohistochemical and ultrastructural comparison with mucin-producing pulmonary adenocarcinomas. *Ultrastruct Pathol* 1996; **20**: 293–325.

53. McCaughey W, Colby T, Battifora H, *et al.* Diagnosis of diffuse malignant mesothelioma: experience of a US/Canadian mesothelioma panel. *Mod Pathol* 1991; **4**: 342–53.

54. Shanks J, Harris M, Banerjee S, *et al.* Mesotheliomas with deciduoid morphology. *Am J Surg Pathol* 2000; **24**: 285–94.

55. Nascimento AG, Keeney GL, Fletcher CD. Deciduoid peritoneal mesothelioma. An unusual phenotype affecting young females. *Am J Surg Pathol* 1994; **18**: 439–45.

56. Foyle A, Al-Jabi M, McCaughey WT. Papillary peritoneal tumors in women. *Am J Surg Pathol* 1981; **5**: 241–9.

57. Daya D, McCaughey WT. Pathology of the peritoneum: a review of selected topics. *Semin Diagn Pathol* 1991; **8**: 277–289.

58. Mark EJ, Shin DH. Diffuse malignant mesothelioma of the pleura: a clinicopathological study of six patients with a prolonged symptom-free interval or extended survival after biopsy and a review of the literature of long-term survival. *Virchows Arch A Pathol Anat Histopathol* 1993; **422**: 445–51.

59. Ball NJ, Urbanski SJ, Green FH, *et al.* Pleural multicystic mesothelial proliferation. The so-called multicystic mesothelioma. *Am J Surg Pathol* 1990; **14**: 375–8.

60. Mayall F, Gibbs A. The histology and immunohistochemistry of small cell mesothelioma. *Histopathology* 1992; **20**: 47–51.

61. Cook HC. Small cell mesothelioma. *Histopathology* 1993; **22**: 294–5.

62. Attanoos RL, Webb R, Dojcinov SD, *et al.* Malignant epithelioid mesothelioma: anti-mesothelial marker expression correlates with histological pattern. *Histopathology* 2001; **39**: 584–8.

63. Rossi G, Cavazza A, Sturm N, *et al.* Pulmonary carcinomas with pleomorphic, sarcomatoid, or sarcomatous elements: A clinicopathologic and immunohistochemical study of 75 cases. *Am J Surg Pathol* 2003; **27**: 311–24.

64. Yousem SA, Hochholzer L. Malignant mesotheliomas with osseous and cartilaginous differentiation. *Arch Pathol Lab Med* 1987; **111**: 62–6.

65. Goldstein B. Two malignant pleural mesotheliomas with unusual histological features. *Thorax* 1979; **34**: 375–9.

66. Kannerstein M, Churg J. Desmoplastic diffuse malignant mesothelioma. *Prog Surg Pathol* 1980; **2**: 19–29.

67. Cantin R, Al-Jabi M, McCaughey W. Desmoplastic diffuse mesothelioma. *Am J Surg Pathol* 1982; **6**: 215–22.

68. Wilson G, Hasleton P, Chatterjee A. Desmoplastic malignant mesothelioma: a review of 17 cases. *J Clin Pathol* 1992; **45**: 295–8.

69. Henderson D, Attwood H, Constance T, *et al.* Lymphohistiocytoid mesothelioma: A rare lymphomatoid variant of predominantly sarcomatoid mesothelioma. *Ultrastruct Pathol* 1988; **12**: 367–84.

70. Khalidi HS, Medeiros LJ, Battifora H. Lymphohistiocytoid mesothelioma. An often misdiagnosed variant of sarcomatoid malignant mesothelioma. *Am J Clin Pathol* 2000; **113**: 649–54.

71. Roggli VL, Kolbeck J, Sanfilippo F, *et al.* Pathology of human mesothelioma. Etiologic and diagnostic considerations. *Pathol Annu* 1987; **22**: 91–131.

72. Sahn S. Malignancy metastatic to the pleura. *Clin Chest Med* 1998; **19**: 351–61.

73. Hasleton P. Pleural disease. In: Hasleton P, ed. *Spencer's Pathology of the Lung*, 5th edn. New York: McGraw-Hill, 1996: 1131–1210.

74. Galateau-Sallé F. *Mod Pathol* 2002; **15**: 319A.

75. Wick M. Immunophenotyping of malignant mesothelioma. *Am J Surg Pathol* 1997; **21**: 1395–8.

76. Hillerdal G, Lee J, Blomkvist A, *et al.* Pleural disease during treatment with bromocriptine in patients previously exposed to asbestos. *Eur Respir J* 1997; **10**: 2711–15.

77. Knoop C, Mairesse M, Lenclud C, *et al.* Pleural effusion during bromocriptine exposure in two patients with pre-existing asbestos pleural plaques: a relationship? *Eur Respir J* 1997; **10**: 2898–901.

78. Andrion A, Magnani C, Betta P, *et al.* Malignant mesothelioma of the pleura: interobserver variability. *J Clin Pathol* 1995; **48**: 856–60.

79. Anderson T, Holmes E, Kosaka C, *et al.* Monoclonal antibodies to human malignant mesothelioma. *J Clin Immunol* 1987; 7: 254–61.

80. Sheibani K, Esteban J, Bailey A, *et al.* Immunopathologic and molecular studies as an aid to the diagnosis of malignant mesothelioma. *Hum Pathol* 1992; **23**: 107–16.

81. Ordóñez N. The value of antibodies 44-3A6, SM3, HBME-1, and thrombomodulin in differentiating epithelial pleural mesothelioma from lung adenocarcinoma. A comparative study with other commonly used antibodies. *Am J Surg Pathol* 1997; **21**: 1399–1408.

82. Donna A, Betta P-G, Chiodera P, *et al.* Newly marketed tissue markers for malignant mesothelioma: Immunoreactivity of rabbit AMAD-2 antiserum compared with monoclonal antibody HBME-1 and a review of the literature of so-called antimesothelioma antibodies. *Hum Pathol* 1997; **28**: 929–37.

83. Kennedy A, King G, Kerr K. HBME-1 and antithrombomodulin in the differential diagnosis of malignant mesothelioma of pleura. *J Clin Pathol* 1997; **50**: 859–62.

84. Ordóñez N. Value of the MOC-31 monoclonal antibody in differentiating epithelial pleural mesothelioma from lung adenocarcinoma. *Hum Pathol* 1998; **29**: 166–9.

85. Oates J, Edwards C. HBME-1, MOC-31, WT-1 and calretinin: an assessment of recently described markers for mesothelioma and adenocarcinoma. *Histopathology* 2000; **36**: 341–7.

86. Ordóñez N. Value of thyroid transcription factor-1, E-cadherin, BG8, WT1, and CD44S immunostaining in distinguishing epithelial pleural mesothelioma from pulmonary and non-pulmonary adenocarcinoma. *Am J Surg Pathol* 2000; **24**: 598–606.

87. Ordonez NG. The immunohistochemical diagnosis of mesothelioma: a comparative study of epithelioid mesothelioma and lung adenocarcinoma. *Am J Surg Pathol* 2003; **27**: 1031–51.

88. Legier J, Maddox J. Immunohistochemical diagnosis of mesothelioma. In: Jaurand M, Bignon J, eds. *The Mesothelial Cell and Mesothelioma*. New York: Marcel Dekker, 1994. 103–19.

89. Roberts F, McCall A, Burnett R. Malignant mesothelioma: a comparison of biopsy and postmortem material by light microscopy and immunohistochemistry. *J Clin Pathol* 2001; **54**: 766–70.

90. Attanoos R, Webb R, Dojcinov S, *et al.* Malignant epithelioid mesothelioma: Anti-mesothelial marker expression correlates with histological pattern. *Histopathology* 2001; **39**: 584–8.

91. Riera J, Astengo-Osuna C, Longmate J, *et al.* The immunohistochemical diagnostic panel for epithelial mesothelioma. A reevaluation after heat-induced epitope retrieval. *Am J Surg Pathol* 1997; **21**: 1409–19.

92. Skov B, Brændstrup O, Hirsch F, *et al.* Are pathologists biased by clinical information? A blinded cross-over study of the histopathological diagnosis of mesothelial tumours versus pulmonary adenocarcinoma. *Lung Cancer* 1994; **11**: 365–72.

93. Latza U, Niedobitek G, Schwarting R, *et al.* Ber-EP4: New monoclonal antibody which distinguishes epithelia from mesothelia. *J Clin Pathol* 1990; **43**: 213–19.

94. Daly L, Bourke G. *Interpretation and Uses of Medical Statistics*, 5th edn. Oxford: Blackwell Science, 2000.

95. Brown R, Clark G, Tandon A, *et al.* Multiple-marker immunohistochemical phenotypes distinguishing malignant pleural mesothelioma from pulmonary adenocarcinoma. *Hum Pathol* 1993; **24**: 347–54.

96. Whitaker D, Sterrett G, Shilkin K. Detection of tissue CEA-like substance as an aid in the differential diagnosis of malignant mesothelioma. *Pathology* 1982; **14**: 255–8.

97. Benjamin CJ, Ritchie AC. Histological staining for the diagnosis of mesothelioma. *Am J Med Technol* 1982; **48**: 905–8.

98. Walz R, Koch H. Malignant pleural mesothelioma: some aspects of epidemiology, differential diagnosis and prognosis. *Pathol Res Pract* 1990; **186**: 124–34.

99. Kayser K, Bohm G, Blum S, *et al.* Glyco- and immunohistochemical refinement of the differential diagnosis between mesothelioma and metastatic carcinoma and survival analysis of patients. *J Pathol* 2001; **193**: 175–80.

100. Gold P, Freeman S. Specific carcinoembryonic antigens of the human digestive system. *J Exp Med* 1965; **122**: 467–81.

101. Wang N, Huang S, Gold P. Absence of carcinoembryonic antigen-like material in mesothelioma: an immunohistochemical differentiation from other lung cancers. *Cancer* 1979; **44**: 937–43.

102. Dejmek A, Hjerpe A. Carcinoembryonic antigen-like reactivity in malignant mesothelioma. A comparison between different commercially available antibodies. *Cancer* 1994; **73**: 464–9.

103. Doglioni C, Dei Tos A, Laurino L, *et al.* Calretinin: a novel immunocytochemical marker for mesothelioma. *Am J Surg Pathol* 1996; **20**: 1037–46.

104. Brockstedt U, Gulyas M, Dobra K, *et al.* Optimized battery of eight antibodies that can distinguish most cases of epithelial mesothelioma from carcinoma. *Am J Clin Pathol* 2000; **114**: 203–9.

105. Cagle P, Truong L, Roggli V, *et al.* Immunohistochemical differentiation of sarcomatoid mesotheliomas from other spindle cell neoplasms. *Am J Clin Pathol* 1989; **92**: 566–71.

106. Garcia-Prats M, Ballestin C, Sotelo T, *et al.* A comparative evaluation of immunohistochemical markers for the differential diagnosis of malignant pleural tumours. *Histopathology* 1998; **32**: 462–72.

107. Lee I, Radosevich J, Chejfec G, *et al.* Malignant mesotheliomas. Improved differential diagnosis from lung adenocarcinomas using monoclonal antibodies 44–3A6 and 624A12. *Am J Pathol* 1986; **123**: 497–507.

108. Szpak C, Johnston W, Roggli V, *et al.* The diagnostic distinction between malignant mesothelioma of the pleura and adenocarcinoma of the lung as defined by a monoclonal antibody (B72.3). *Am J Pathol* 1986; **122**: 252–60.

109. Corson J, Pinkus G. Mesothelioma: Profile of keratin proteins and carcinoembryonic antigen: An immunoperoxidase study of 20 cases and comparison with pulmonary adenocarcinomas. *Am J Pathol* 1982; **108**: 80–7.

110. Holden J, Churg A. Immunohistochemical staining for keratin and carcinoembryonic antigen in the diagnosis of mesothelioma. *Am J Surg Pathol* 1984; **8**: 277–9.

111. Loosli H, Hurlimann J. Immunohistological study of malignant diffuse mesotheliomas of the pleura. *Histopathology* 1984; **8**: 793–803.

112. Tron V, Wright J, Churg A. Carcinoembryonic antigen and milk-fat globule protein staining of malignant mesothelioma and adenocarcinoma of the lung. *Arch Pathol Lab Med* 1987; **111**: 291–3.

113. Said J, Nash G, Banks-Schlegel S, *et al.* Keratin in human lung tumors. Patterns of localisation of different-molecular-weight keratin proteins. *Am J Pathol* 1983; **113**: 27–32.

114. Pfaltz M, Odermatt B, Christen B, *et al.* Immunohistochemistry in the diagnosis of malignant mesothelioma. *Virchows Arch A Pathol Anat Histopathol* 1987; **411**: 387–393.

115. Robb J. Mesothelioma versus adenocarcinoma: False positive CEA and Leu-M1 staining due to hyaluronic acid. *Hum Pathol* 1989; **20**: 400.

116. Al-Saffar N, Hasleton P. Vimentin, carcinoembryonic antigen and keratin in the diagnosis of mesothelioma, adenocarcinoma and reactive pleural lesions. *Eur Resp J* 1990; 3: 997–1001.

117. Cagle P, Brown R, Lebovitz R. p53 immunostaining in the differentiation of reactive processes from malignancy in pleural biopsy specimens. *Hum Pathol* 1994; 25: 443–448.

118. Chenard-Neu M, Bellocq J, Maier A, *et al.* Malignant mesothelioma of the pleura. Analysis of its immunohistochemical aspects. *Ann Pathol* 1990; 10: 20–27.

119. Collins C, Ordóñez N, Schaefer R, *et al.* Thrombomodulin expression in malignant pleural mesothelioma and pulmonary adenocarcinoma. *Am J Pathol* 1992; 141: 827–833.

120. Dejmek A, Hjerpe A. Immunohistochemical reactivity in mesothelioma and adenocarcinoma: A stepwise logistic regression analysis. *APMIS* 1994; 102: 255–264.

121. Ghosh A, Gatter K, Dunnill M, *et al.* Immunohistological staining of reactive mesothelium, mesothelioma, and lung carcinoma with a panel of monoclonal antibodies. *J Clin Pathol* 1987; 40: 19–25.

122. Gibbs A, Harach R, Wagner J, *et al.* Comparison of tumour markers in malignant mesothelioma and pulmonary adenocarcinoma. *Thorax* 1985; 40: 91–95.

123. Grove A, Paulsen S, Gregersen M. The value of immunohistohemistry of pleural biopsy specimens in the differential diagnosis between malignant mesothelioma and metastatic carcinoma. *Path Res Pract* 1994; 190: 1044–1055.

124. Moch H, Oberholzer M, Dalquen P, *et al.* Diagnostic tools for differentiating between pleural mesothelioma and lung adenocarcinoma in paraffin embedded tissue. Part I: Immunohistochemical findings. *Virchows Arch A Pathol Anat Histopathol* 1993; **423**: 19–27.

125. O'Hara C, Corson J, Pinkus G, *et al.* Me1: a monoclonal antibody that distinguishes epithelial-type malignant mesothelioma from pulmonary adenocarcinoma and extrapulmonary malignancies. *Am J Pathol* 1990; **136**: 421–8.

126. Ordóñez N. The immunohistochemical diagnosis of mesothelioma. *Am J Surg Pathol* 1989; **13**: 276–91.

127. Otis C, Carter D, Cole S, *et al.* Immunohistochemical evaluation of pleural mesothelioma and pulmonary adenocarcinoma. A bi-institutional study of 47 cases. *Am J Surg Pathol* 1987; **11**: 445–56.

128. Roberts F, Harper C, Downie I, *et al.* Immunohistochemical analysis still has a limited role in the diagnosis of malignant mesothelioma. A study of thirteen antibodies. *Am J Clin Pathol* 2001; **116**: 253–62.

129. Soosay G, Griffiths M, Papadaki L, *et al.* The differential diagnosis of epithelial-type mesothelioma from adenocarcinoma and reactive mesothelial proliferation. *J Pathol* 1991; **163**: 299–305.

130. Strickler J, Herndier B, Rouse R. Immunohistochemical staining in malignant mesotheliomas. *Am J Clin Pathol* 1987; **88**: 610–14.

131. Tuttle S, Lucas J, Bucci D, *et al.* Distinguishing malignant mesothelioma from pulmonary adenocarcinoma: an immuno-histochemical approach using a panel of monoclonal antibodies. *J Surg Oncol* 1990; **45**: 72–8.

132. Vortmeyer A, Preuss J, Padberg B, *et al.* Immunocytochemical differential diagnosis of diffuse malignant pleural mesotheliomas—a clinicomorphological study of 158 cases. *Anticancer Res* 1991; **11**: 889–94.

133. Bolen J, Hammar S, McNutt M. Reactive and neoplastic serosal tissue. A light-microscope, ultrastructural, and immunocytochemical study. *Am J Surg Pathol* 1986; **10**: 34–47.

134. Leers M, Aarts M, Theunissen P. E-cadherin and calretinin: a useful combination of immunochemical markers for differentiation between mesothelioma and metastatic adenocarcinoma. *Histopathology* 1998; **32**: 209–16.

135. Wirth P, Legier J, Wright G. Immunohistochemical evaluation of seven monoclonal antibodies for differentiation of pleural mesothelioma from lung adenocarcinoma. *Cancer* 1991; **67**: 655–62.

136. Battifora H, Kopinski M. Distinction of mesothelioma from adenocarcinoma. An immunohistochemical approach. *Cancer* 1985; **55**: 1679–85.

137. Friemann J, Otto H, Muller K. [Immunohistochemical studies for the differential diagnosis of primary and secondary pleural tumors.] *Verh Dtsch Ges Pathol* 1986; **70**: 311–16 (in German).

138. Jasani B, Edwards R, Thomas N, *et al.* The use of vimentin antibodies in the diagnosis of malignant mesothelioma. *Virchows Arch A Pathol Anat Histopathol* 1985; **406**: 441–8.

139. Kwee WS, Veldhuizen RW, Golding RP, *et al.* Histologic distinction between malignant mesothelioma, benign pleural lesion and carcinoma metastasis. Evaluation of the application of morphometry combined with histochemistry and immunostaining. *Virchows Arch A Pathol Anat Histol* 1982; **397**: 287–99.

140. Kawai T, Greenberg SD, Titus JL. Lectin histochemistry of normal lung and pulmonary adenocarcinoma. *Mod Pathol* 1988; **1**: 485–92.

141. Lucas J, Tuttle S. Diagnostic histochemical and immunohistochemical studies in malignant mesothelioma. *J Surg Oncol* 1987; **35**: 30–4.

142. Noguchi M, Nakajima T, Hirohashi S, *et al.* Immunohistochemical distinction of malignant mesothelioma from pulmonary adenocarcinoma with anti-surfactant apoprotein, anti-Lewis[a], and anti-Tn antibodies. *Hum Pathol* 1989; **20**: 53–57.

143. Pileri S, Rivano MT, Mancini AM. Immunohistochemical characterization of mesotheliomas. *Appl Pathol* 1983; **1**: 348–50.

144. Wick M, Loy T, Mills S, *et al.* Malignant epithelioid pleural mesothelioma versus peripheral pulmonary adenocarcinoma: a histochemical, ultrastructural, and immunohistologic study of 103 cases. *Hum Pathol* 1990; **21**: 759–66.

145. Marshall RJ, Herbert A, Braye SG, *et al.* Use of antibodies to carcinoembryonic antigen and human milk fat globule to distinguish carcinoma, mesothelioma, and reactive mesothelium. *J Clin Pathol* 1984; **37**: 1215–21.

146. Sheibani K, Battifora H, Burke J, *et al.* Leu-M1 antigen in human neoplasms: An immunohistologic study of 400 cases. *Am J Surg Pathol* 1986; **10**: 227–36.

147. Chenard-Neu M-P, Kabou A, Mechine A, *et al.* L'immunohistochimie dans le diagnostic différentiel entre mésothéliome et adénocarcinome. *Ann Pathol* 1998; **18**: 460–5.

148. Abutaily AS, Addis BJ, Roche WR. Immunohistochemistry in the distinction between malignant mesothelioma and pulmonary adenocarcinoma: a critical evaluation of new antibodies. *J Clin Pathol* 2002; **55**: 662–8.

149. Comin CE, Novelli L, Boddi V, *et al.* Calretinin, thrombomodulin, CEA, and CD15: a useful combination of immunohistochemical markers for differentiating pleural epithelial mesothelioma from peripheral pulmonary adenocarcinoma. *Hum Pathol* 2001; **32**: 529–36.

150. Carella R, Deleonardi G, D'Errico A, *et al.* Immunohistochemical panels for differentiating epithelial malignant mesothelioma from lung adenocarcinoma: a study with logistic regression analysis. *Am J Surg Pathol* 2001; **25**: 43–50.

151. Gumurdulu D, Zeren EH, Cagle PT, *et al.* Specificity of MOC-31 and HBME-1 immunohistochemistry in the differential diagnosis of adenocarcinoma and malignant mesothelioma: a study on environmental malignant mesothelioma cases from Turkish villages. *Pathol Oncol Res* 2002; **8**: 188–3.

152. Sheibani K, Shin S, Kezirian J, *et al.* Ber-EP4 antibody as a discriminant in the differential diagnosis of malignant mesothelioma vs. adenocarcinoma. *Am J Surg Pathol* 1991; **15**: 779–84.

153. Gaffey MJ, Mills SE, Swanson PE, *et al.* Immunoreactivity for Ber-EP4 in adenocarcinomas, adenomatoid tumors, and malignant mesotheliomas. *Am J Surg Pathol* 1992; **16**: 593–9.

154. Nuti M, Teramoto YA, Mariani-Costantini R, *et al.* A monoclonal antibody (B72.3) defines patterns of distribution of a novel tumor-associated antigen in human mammary carcinoma cell populations. *Int J Cancer* 1982; **29**: 539–45.

155. Warnock M, Stoloff A, Thor A. Differentiation of adenocarcinoma from mesothelioma: periodic acid–Schiff, monoclonal antibodies B72.3 and Leu-M1. *Am J Pathol* 1988; **133**: 30–8.

156. Sosolik RC, McGaughy VR, De Young BR. Anti-MOC-31: a potential addition to the pulmonary adenocarcinoma versus mesothelioma immunohistochemistry panel. *Mod Pathol* 1997; **10**: 716–19.

157. Gonzalez-Lois C, Ballestin C, Sotelo MT, *et al.* Combined use of novel epithelial (MOC-31) and mesothelial (HBME-1) immunohistochemical markers for optimal first line diagnostic distinction between mesothelioma and metastatic carcinoma in pleura. *Histopathology* 2001; **38**: 528–34.

158. Delahaye M, van der Ham F, van der Kwast T. Complementary value of five carcinoma markers for the diagnosis of malignant mesothelioma, adenocarcinoma metastasis, and reactive mesothelium in serous effusions. *Diagn Cytopathol* 1997; **17**: 115–20.

159. Edwards C, Oates J. OV 632 and MOC-31 in the diagnosis of mesothelioma and adenocarcinoma: an assessment of their use in formalin fixed paraffin embedded material. *J Clin Pathol* 1995; **48**: 626–30.

160. Ruitenbeek T, Gouw A, Poppema S. Immunocytology of body cavity fluids: MOC-31, a monoclonal antibody discriminating between mesothelioma and epithelial cells. *Arch Pathol Lab Med* 1994; **118**: 265–9.

161. Takeichi M. Cadherin cell adhesion receptors as a morphogenetic regulator. *Science* 1991; **251**: 1451–5.

162. Han A, Peralta-Soler A, Knudsen K, *et al.* Differential expression of N-cadherin in pleural mesotheliomas and E-cadherin in lung adenocarcinomas in formalin-fixed, paraffin-embedded tissues. *Hum Pathol* 1997; **28**: 641–5.

163. Peralta-Soler A, Knudsen K, Jaurand M. The differential expression of N-cadherin and E-cadherin distinguishes pleural mesotheliomas from lung adenocarcinomas. *Hum Pathol* 1995; **26**: 1363–9.

164. Thirkettle I, Harvey P, Hasleton P, *et al.* Immunoreactivity for cadherins, HGF/SF, met, and erbB-2 in pleural malignant mesotheliomas. *Histopathology* 2000; **36**: 522–8.

165. Civitareale D, Lonigro R, Sinclair A, *et al.* A thyroid-specific nuclear protein essential for tissue-specific expression of the thyroglobulin promoter. *EMBO J* 1989; **8**: 2537–542.

166. Guazzi S, Price M, De Felice M, *et al.* Thyroid nuclear factor 1 (TTF-1) contains a homeodomain and displays a novel DNA binding specificity. *EMBO J* 1990; **9**: 3631–9.

167. Khoor A, Whitsett J, Stahlman M, *et al.* Utility of surfactant protein b precursor and thyroid transcription factor 1 in differentiating adenocarcinoma of the lung from mesothelioma. *Hum Pathol* 1999; **30**: 695–700.

168. Di Loreto C, Puglisi F, Di Lauro V, *et al.* TTF-1 protein expression in pleural malignant mesotheliomas and adenocarcinomas of the lung. *Cancer Lett* 1998; **124**: 73–8.

169. Jordon D, Jagirdar J, Kaneko M. Blood group antigens Lewis[x] and Lewis[y] in the diagnostic discrimination of malignant mesothelioma versus adenocarcinoma. *Am J Pathol* 1989; **135**: 931–7.

170. Woodcock-Mitchell J, Eichner R, Nelson W, *et al.* Immunolocalisation of keratin polypeptides in human epidermis using monoclonal antibodies. *J Cell Biol* 1982; **95**: 580–8.

171. Makin C, Bobrow L, Bodmer W. Monoclonal antibody to cytokeratin for use in routine histopathology. *J Clin Pathol* 1984; **37**: 975–83.

172. Churg A. Immunohistochemical staining for vimentin and keratin in malignant mesothelioma. *Am J Surg Pathol* 1985; **9**: 360–5.

173. Al-Izzi M, Thurlow N, Corrin B. Pleural mesothelioma of connective tissue type, localized fibrous tumour of the pleura, and reactive submesothelial hyperplasia. An immunohistochemical comparison. *J Pathol* 1989; **158**: 41–4.

174. Blobel G, Moll R, Franke W, *et al.* The intermediate filament cytoskeleton of malignant mesotheliomas and its diagnostic significance. *Am J Pathol* 1985; **121**: 235–47.

175. Miettinen M. Keratin immunohistochemistry: update of applications and pitfalls. In: Rosen P, Fechner R, eds. *Pathology Annual.* New York: Appleton and Lange, 1993; 113–43.

176. Ordóñez N. Value of cytokeratin 5/6 in distinguishing epithelial mesothelioma of the pleura from lung adenocarcinoma. *Am J Surg Pathol* 1998; **22**: 1215–21.

177. Clover J, Oates J, Edwards C. Anticytokeratin 5/6: a positive marker for epithelioid mesothelioma. *Histopathology* 1997; **31**: 140–3.

178. Chu PG, Weiss LM. Expression of cytokeratin 5/6 in epithelial neoplasms: an immunohistochemical study of 509 cases. *Mod Pathol* 2002; **15**: 6–10.

179. Cury PM, Butcher DN, Fisher C, *et al.* Value of the mesothelium-associated antibodies thrombomodulin, cytokeratin 5/6, calretinin, and CD44H in distinguishing epithelioid pleural mesothelioma from adenocarcinoma metastatic to the pleura. *Mod Pathol* 2000; **13**: 107–12.

180. Gotzos V, Vogt P, Celio M. The calcium binding protein calretinin is a selective marker for malignant pleural mesotheliomas of the epithelial type. *Pathol Res Pract* 1996; **192**: 137–47.

181. Ordóñez N. Value of calretinin immunostaining in differentiating epithelial mesothelioma from lung adenocarcinoma. *Mod Pathol* 1998; **11**: 929–33.

182. Foster MR, Johnson JE, Olson SJ, *et al.* Immunohistochemical analysis of nuclear versus cytoplasmic staining of WT1 in malignant mesotheliomas and primary pulmonary adenocarcinomas. *Arch Pathol Lab Med* 2001; **125**: 1316–20.

183. Miettinen M, Sarlomo-Rikala M. Expression of calretinin, thrombomodulin, keratin 5, and mesothelin in lung carcinomas of different types: an immunohistochemical analysis of 596 tumors in comparison with epithelioid mesotheliomas of the pleura. *Am J Surg Pathol* 2003; **27**: 150–58.

184. Amin K, Litzky L, Smythe W, *et al.* Wilms' tumor 1 susceptibility (WT1) gene products are selectively expressed in malignant mesothelioma. *Am J Pathol* 1995; **146**: 344–56.

185. Kumar-Singh S, Segers K, Rodeck U, *et al.* WT1 mutation in malignant mesothelioma and WT1 immunoreactivity in relation to p53 and growth factor receptor expression, cell-type transition, and prognosis. *J Pathol* 1997; **181**: 67–74.

186. Miettinen M, Limon J, Niezabitowski A, *et al.* Calretinin and other mesothelioma markers in synovial sarcoma: analysis of antigenic similarities and differences with malignant mesothelioma. *Am J Surg Pathol* 2001; **25**: 610–17.

187. Hecht JL, Lee BH, Pinkus JL, *et al.* The value of Wilms tumor susceptibility gene-1 in cytologic preparations as a marker for malignant mesothelioma. *Cancer* 2002; **96**: 105–9.

188. Ordóñez N, Myhre M, Mackay B. Clear cell mesothelioma. *Ultrastruct Pathol* 1996; **20**: 331–6.

189. Nappi O, Mills SE, Swanson PE, *et al.* Clear cell tumors of unknown nature and origin: a systematic approach to diagnosis. *Semin Diagn Pathol* 1997; **14**: 164–74.

190. Dessy E, Falleni M, Braidotti P, *et al.* Unusual clear cell variant of epithelioid mesothelioma. *Arch Pathol Lab Med* 2001; **125**: 1588–90.

191. Campbell CE, Kuriyan NP, Rackley RR, *et al.* Constitutive expression of the Wilms tumor suppressor gene (WT1) in renal cell carcinoma. *Int J Cancer* 1998; **78**: 182–8.

192. Attanoos RL, Goddard H, Thomas ND, *et al.* A comparative immunohistochemical study of malignant mesothelioma and renal cell carcinoma: the diagnostic utility of Leu-M1, Ber-EP4, Tamm-Horsfall protein and thrombomodulin. *Histopathology* 1995; **27**: 361–6.

193. Osborn M, Pelling N, Walker MM, *et al.* The value of 'mesothelium-associated' antibodies in distinguishing between metastatic renal cell carcinomas and mesotheliomas. *Histopathology* 2002; **41**: 301–7.

194. Stahel R, O'Hara C, Waibel R, *et al.* Monoclonal antibodies against mesothelial membrane antigen discriminate between malignant mesothelioma and lung adenocarcinoma. *Int J Cancer* 1988; **41**: 218–23.

195. Bateman AC, al-Talib RK, Newman T, *et al.* Immunohistochemical phenotype of malignant mesothelioma: predictive value of CA125 and HBME-1 expression. *Histopathology* 1997; **30**: 49–56.

196. Attanoos RL, Goddard H, Gibbs AR. Mesothelioma-binding antibodies: thrombomodulin, OV 632 and HBME-1 and their use in the diagnosis of malignant mesothelioma. *Histopathology* 1996; **29**: 209–15.

197. Dahlstrom J, Maxwell L, Brodie N, *et al.* Distinctive microvillous brush border staining with HBME-1 distinguishes pleural mesotheliomas from pulmonary adenocarcinomas. *Pathology* 2001; **33**: 287–91.

198. Esmon NL, Owen WG, Esmon CT. Isolation of a membrane-bound cofactor for thrombin-catalyzed activation of protein C. *J Biol Chem* 1982; **257**: 859–64.

199. Yonezawa S, Maruyama I, Sakae K, *et al.* Thrombomodulin as a marker for vascular tumors. Comparative study with factor VIII and *Ulex europaeus* I lectin. *Am J Clin Pathol* 1987; **88**: 405–11.

200. Fink L, Collins C, Schaefer R. Thrombomodulin expression can be used to differentiate between mesotheliomas and adenocarcinomas. *Lab Invest* 1992; **66**: 113A.

201. Leong AS, Parkinson R, Milios J. 'Thick' cell membranes revealed by immunocytochemical staining: a clue to the diagnosis of mesothelioma. *Diagn Cytopathol* 1990; **6**: 9–13.

202. Leong AS, Vernon-Roberts E. The immunohistochemistry of malignant mesothelioma. *Pathol Annu* 1994; **29**: 157–79.

203. Folpe A, Gown A. Immunohistochemistry for analysis of soft tissue tumors. In: Weiss S, Goldblum J, eds. *Soft Tissue Tumors*, 4th edn. St Louis, MO: Mosby, 2001; 199–245.

204. Moch H, Oberholzer M, Christen H, *et al.* Diagnostic tools for differentiating between pleural mesothelioma and lung adenocarcinoma in paraffin embedded tissue. Part II: Design of an expert system and its application to the diagnosis of mesothelioma. *Virchows Arch A Pathol Anat Histopathol* 1993; **423**: 493–96.

205. Betta P, Andrion A, Donna A, *et al.* Malignant mesothelioma of the pleura. The reproducibility of the immunohistological diagnosis. *Pathol Res Pract* 1997; **193**: 759–765.

206. Attanoos R, Dojcinov S, Webb R, *et al.* Antimesothelial markers in sarcomatoid mesothelioma and other spindle cell neoplasms. *Histopathology* 2000; **37**: 224–31.

207. Montag A, Pinkus G, Corson J. Keratin protein immunoreactivity of sarcomatoid and mixed types of diffuse malignant mesothelioma: an immunoperoxidase study of 30 cases. *Hum Pathol* 1988; **19**: 336–42.

208. Lucas DR, Pass HI, Madan SK, *et al.* Sarcomatoid mesothelioma and its histological mimics: a comparative immunohistochemical study. *Histopathology* 2003; **42**: 270–9.

209. Laskin WB, Miettinen M. Epithelial-type and neural-type cadherin expression in malignant noncarcinomatous neoplasms with epithelioid features that involve the soft tissues. *Arch Pathol Lab Med* 2002; **126**: 425–31.

210. Enzinger F, Weiss S. *Soft Tissue Tumours*, 3rd edn. St Louis, MO: Mosby–Year Book, 1995.

211. Aubry MC, Bridge JA, Wickert R, *et al.* Primary monophasic synovial sarcoma of the pleura: five cases confirmed by the presence of SYT-SSX fusion transcript. *Am J Surg Pathol* 2001; **25**: 776–81.

212. Ordóñez N, Ro J, Ayala A. Lesions described as nodular mesothelial hyperplasia are composed of histiocytes. *Am J Surg Pathol* 1998; **22**: 285–92.

213. Ramael M, Lemmens G, Eerdekens C, *et al.* Immunoreactivity for p53 protein in malignant mesothelioma and non-neoplastic mesothelium. *J Pathol* 1992; **168**: 371–5.

214. Mayall FG, Goddard H, Gibbs AR. p53 immunostaining in the distinction between benign and malignant mesothelial proliferations using formalin-fixed paraffin sections. *J Pathol* 1992; **168**: 377–81.

215. Cury P, Butcher D, Corrin B, *et al.* The use of histological and immunohistochemical markers to distinguish pleural malignant mesothelioma and *in situ* mesothelioma from reactive mesothelial hyperplasia and reactive pleural fibrosis. *J Pathol* 1999; **189**: 251–7.

216. Kafiri G, Thomas DM, Shepherd NA, *et al.* p53 expression is common in malignant mesothelioma. *Histopathology* 1992; **21**: 331–4.

217. Mangano WE, Cagle PT, Churg A, *et al.* The diagnosis of desmoplastic malignant mesothelioma and its distinction from fibrous pleurisy: a histologic and immunohistochemical analysis of 31 cases including p53 immunostaining. *Am J Clin Pathol* 1998; **110**: 191–9.

218. Esposito V, Baldi A, De Luca A, *et al.* p53 immunostaining in differential diagnosis of pleural mesothelial proliferations. *Anticancer Res* 1997; **17**: 733–6.

219. Isik R, Metintas M, Gibbs AR, *et al.* p53, p21 and metallothionein immunoreactivities in patients with malignant pleural mesothelioma: correlations with the epidemiological features and prognosis of mesotheliomas with environmental asbestos exposure. *Respir Med* 2001; **95**: 588–93.

220. Cappello F, Barnes L. Synovial sarcoma and malignant mesothelioma of the pleura: review, differential diagnosis and possible role of apoptosis. *Pathology* 2001; **33**: 142–8.

221. Casalots J, Tarroch X, Forcada P. Utility of epithelial membrane antigen and p53 in the differential diagnosis of benign reactive processes from malignancy in pleural biopsy specimens. *Virchows Arch A Pathol Anat Histopathol* 1999; **435**: 286.

222. Attanoos RL, Griffin A, Gibbs AR. The use of immunohistochemistry in distinguishing reactive from neoplastic mesothelium. A novel use for desmin and comparative evaluation with epithelial membrane antigen, p53, platelet-derived growth factor-receptor, p-glycoprotein and Bcl-2. *Histopathology* 2003; **43**: 231–8.

223. Hurlimann J. Desmin and neural marker expression in mesothelial cells and mesothelioma. *Hum Pathol* 1994; **25**: 753–7.

224. Mayall F, Goddard H, Gibbs A. Intermediate filament expression in mesotheliomas: leiomyoid mesotheliomas are not uncommon. *Histopathology* 1992; **21**: 453–7.

225. Scoones D, Richman P. Expression of desmin and smooth muscle actin in mesothelial hyperplasia and mesothelioma. *J Pathol* 1993; **169s**: 188A.

226. Segers K, Backhovens H, Singh SK, *et al.* Immunoreactivity for p53 and mdm2 and the detection of p53 mutations in human malignant mesothelioma. *Virchows Arch A Pathol Anat Histopathol* 1995; **427**: 431–6.

227. Derenzini M, Nardi F, Farabegoli F, *et al.* Distribution of silver-stained interphase nucleolar organizer regions as a parameter to distinguish neoplastic from nonneoplastic reactive cells in human effusions. *Acta Cytol* 1989; **33**: 491–8.

228. Ayres JG, Crocker JG, Skilbeck NQ. Differentiation of malignant from normal and reactive mesothelial cells by the argyrophil technique for nucleolar organiser region associated proteins. *Thorax* 1988; **43**: 366–70.

229. Ordóñez NG. The immunohistochemical diagnosis of mesthelioma: A comparative study of epithelioid mesothelioma and lung adenocarcinoma. *Am J Surg Pathol* 2003; **27**: 1031–51.

Chapter 5

Clinicopathological prognostic factors and scoring systems in malignant pleural mesothelioma

J. A. Burgers and J. P. Hegmans

Introduction

Prediction of the future, whether it concerns economic welfare, the weather forecast, or health issues, has always fascinated mankind. In ancient Greece and Rome, major events in life were forecast by priests from the position of chicken bones that had been thrown in the air or the appearance of the liver of a goose that had been sacrificed, methods that we nowadays consider a 'wild guess'. In our modern era the wild guess is replaced by a 'calculated risk', introduced by statisticians. Focusing on statistical studies on cancer, we can identify prognostic factors which provide a forecast or statement of probability on a certain clinical outcome [1]. This statement predominantly applies to a group of patients, but can also be used in daily practice to make predictions and clinical decisions on individual patients.

Malignant pleural mesothelioma (MPM) is a disease with a heterogeneous clinical outcome. Although the prognosis is extremely poor in general, individual patients might live for an unexpectedly long time [2]. Similarly, although mesothelioma is known to be resistant to most tumour-directed therapies, individual patients might benefit from chemotherapy, radiotherapy, photodynamic therapy, immunotherapy, radical surgery, or multimodal treatment.

In this chapter some key issues on the science of prognosis will be highlighted before the individual prognostic factors that have been identified in MPM are described.

Prognostic factors

Prognostic factors are variables that can account for some of the heterogeneity that is associated with the expected course and outcome of a disease. They guide clinicians in clinical decision-making. The use of prognostic factors is hampered by the fact that the clinical outcome for the individual patient remains hard to predict, even when valid prognostic factors are available. Only groups of patients with mainly good or poor prognostic factors can be discriminated, and the median survival of a given group will be better or worse, respectively.

Not all prognostic factors have a clinically relevant impact on the prognosis. Since prognostic factors are not studied in a structured fashion, their relation and impact on prognosis is not evident in every situation [3].

A prognostic factor should be a significant and independent variable and should predict clinically important issues. Significant is meant to be statistically significant, and many, mostly univariate, tests are used for this purpose. An independent factor adds new and additional prognostic value to the already known prognostic factors. To show the additional value a multivariate analysis is required, which should preferentially be performed on prospectively collected data with adequate power to detect a small but significant prognostic value [1]. The number of events (e.g. death) should be at least 10 times the number of potential prognostic variables that are included in the model [4]. Therefore the ideal study of prognostic factors has a prospective design with a large study population in which the prognostic factor is evaluated by multivariate analysis.

Although the incidence of MPM is rising worldwide, it remains a relatively rare disease, and prospective evaluation of a novel prognostic factor would take a long period of time. Therefore the majority of studies on prognostic factors in MPM are retrospective analyses of clinical or pathological databases. A major flaw of these retrospective analyses is that data on 'confirmed' or already known prognostic factors are not always available and cannot be incorporated in the multivariate analysis to prove the 'additional' prognostic value of a new factor.

Most studies have an 'exploratory' nature, focusing on the prognostic potential of a factor, rather than 'confirmatory', applying known factors to other patient populations and thereby confirming their prognostic value [4]. Before being applied in clinical practice, a new prognostic factor should be validated in at least one confirmatory study.

Furthermore, prognostic factors not only predict issues relevant to daily clinical practice, but can also contribute to clinical and basic science. Currently, prognostic factors in malignant mesothelioma are most frequently used to select a particular patient population for a particular therapy or study protocol. Patients who participate in trials can be stratified according to their prognostic factors and, conversely, a description of the prognostic factors helps to identify the patients to whom the results can be applied. Proper description of the prognostic variables of all study groups that participate in randomized or other trials adds to the quality of the study reports [5, 6].

Progress in molecular and cellular biology might provide us with new prognostic markers. These markers have an additional benefit, since they reflect a specific feature of the biology of the tumour cell and lead to improved understanding of molecular pathogenesis [7, 8]. In the future, they might guide scientists in the development of new therapeutics, predict the sensitivity of the tumour for a particular treatment, and lead clinicians in their choice of the appropriate therapy.

Prognostic factor studies in malignant mesothelioma

Many papers have been published on prognostic factors in MPM, all of which focus on survival. These papers describe the prognostic value of more than 50 different factors. The majority of the studies are retrospective analyses of a particular patient population from a clinic or registry, or of patients who have participated in clinical trials, or concern reports on data obtained from pathology archives. Four studies which prospectively evaluate data from consecutive patients entering a hospital or receiving a particular treatment have been published [9–12].

One confirmatory study on prognostic factors in MPM has been published. Edwards *et al.* [13] applied the prognostic factors that had been identified by evaluation of the data from mesothelioma studies by the Cancer and Leukemia Group B (CALGB) [14] and the European Organization for Research and Treatment of Cancer (EORTC) [15] to their own population. By retrospective evaluation they showed that prognostic factors that had been determined in MPM patients involved in clinical trials also had a predictive value in a general hospital population [13].

Another landmark study on prognostic factors in mesothelioma is the study on the database of the Surveillance, Epidemiology and End Results (SEER) Program from 1988 [16]. It is the largest study of its kind, involving 1475 histologically confirmed cases of mesothelioma, and shows that age, sex, tumour stage, treatment, and geographical area of residence are important predictors of patient survival.

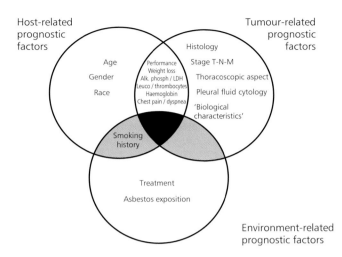

Host-related
prognostic
factors

Tumour-related
prognostic
factors

Histology

Age
Gender
Race

Performance
Weight loss
Alk. phosph / LDH
Leuco / thrombocytes
Haemoglobin
Chest pain / dyspnea

Stage T-N-M
Thoracoscopic aspect
Pleural fluid cytology
'Biological
characteristics'

Smoking
history

Treatment
Asbestos exposition

Environment-related
prognostic factors

Figure 5.1 Prognostic factors may be incorporated in more than one category, as illustrated in this diagram.

As MPM is generally seen as a disease with a rapid fatal outcome, quality of life is one of the most important issues for a patient. Although the quality of life might be reflected by the performance status, no data are available on the correlation between prognostic factors and quality of life, or on the role of quality of life as a prognostic factor. In this regard the clinical needs do not parallel the academic search for prognostic factors. All prognostic factors in mesothelioma studies, apart from one, focus on survival in an attempt to discriminate patient populations with a relatively good or relatively poor prognosis. Only one study focuses on recurrence-free survival [17], but no factors have been described that predict other clinical issues.

Prognostic factors can be separated into host-related prognostic factors, tumour-related factors, and environment-related factors [18]. The host-related factors typify the patient, the tumour-related factors characterize the disease, and the environment-related factors are external factors not directly related to either the disease or the patient. The prognostic factors that have been described for mesothelioma studies according to this classification are categorized in Figure 5.1. As illustrated, the prognostic factors may be included in more than one group. For instance, performance status is influenced by both comorbidity and tumour load, and therefore might be considered as both a host-related and a tumour-related factor. A remarkably large number of different factors have been evaluated for their prognostic significance, with a large number of biological parameters appearing to have an impact on prognosis. We will focus on the prognostic factors and describe their value as predictors of survival.

Host-related prognostic factors

Host-related prognostic factors include parameters that are unrelated or only indirectly related to the tumour, but have a major impact on the outcome of the disease. Factors of this type have been studied extensively in MPM. Although almost all studies concern retrospective analyses of hospital or study databases, they agree on the most important factors. These studies have been listed in a number of publications [7, 13–15, 19, 20].

Performance status

All MPM studies that included performance status data in their analysis showed a significant effect on the survival, with a better performance correlating with a better survival [10, 11, 13–15,

19, 21–25]. Only one study, which included only patients with WHO-performance status 0 and 1, did not confirm this result [26]. Since, until recently, the natural course of the disease could only be influenced minimally by treatment, the large impact of performance on survival was to be expected [27].

Since the first description of performance status by Karnofsky [28], its use has been widely accepted in clinical oncology [29]. It is considered to be a major parameter of the fitness of a patient and an important prognostic factor for many malignancies. The major drawback of performance status is the fact that it is not systematically documented in the records of all patients and therefore cannot be taken into account in all retrospective analyses [27, 30]. Moreover, oncologists tend to give the healthiest assessment, nurses an intermediate assessment, and patients themselves the poorest assessment of their performance status [31]. Despite these disadvantages, the performance of a patient remains one of the most important prognostic factors, and therefore a systematic and accurate documentation of the performance score should be in the charts of all MPM patients.

Weight loss

Weight loss is a poor prognostic factor in MPM [12–14, 22, 26, 32]. Patients without weight loss appeared to derive most symptomatic benefit from palliative surgery [26]. MPM patients with weight loss undergoing chemotherapy have fewer symptomatic and radiological responses and a shorter overall survival [33]. However, in all these studies weight loss lost its statistical significance as a prognostic factor when evaluated in a multivariate analysis.

Although weight loss has no independent prognostic significance in MPM, it is generally seen as a sign of a poor condition for patients with a malignancy. Clinical trials studying chemotherapeutic agents tend to focus on patients with the best prognosis and often exclude patients with a considerable weight loss. It is easy and reproducible to determine and is a helpful criterion for the selection of patients for chemotherapy or other treatments [34].

Leucocytes, platelets, and haemoglobin

Recently attention has been paid to the prognostic significance of these parameters by evaluation of the CALBG and EORTC databases [14, 15]. Appraisal of the EORTC database revealed that a high leucocyte count ($>8.3 \times 10^9$/litre) had a significant poor prognostic value [15], whereas a leucocyte count $>8.7 \times 10^9$/litre was predictive of a poor prognosis in univariate analysis of the CALBG data [14]. The confirmatory study by Edwards et al. [13] found an additive poor prognostic effect of a high leucocyte count in their population. Further but weaker support for this observation is provided by two other studies [19, 22]. One study did not detect a significant contribution of the leucocyte count to the survival [26].

Data concerning the prognostic significance of high platelet counts are variable. Three studies confirm a poor prognostic impact of a platelet count either $>400\,000$/µl [14, 32] or $>314\,000$/µl [17]. One study describes a univariate effect [13], and five studies do not verify any prognostic value of the platelet count [9, 15, 19, 25, 26]. Nevertheless, platelet count remains an interesting parameter theoretically. Platelets may affect the tumour by promoting proliferation of tumour cells by the secretion of agents such as vascular endothelial growth factor (VEGF) [35]. The effect of platelets on angiogenesis and the tumour vasculature via VEGF and other pro- and anti-angiogenic factors has recently been recognized [36]. Additionally, platelets act as a source of several inflammatory mediators [35]. The tumour may affect the number and activation state of platelets. Mesothelioma cells from a patient with a thrombocytosis produced large amounts of interleukin 6 (IL-6), an important promoter of thrombocytosis [37]. Thrombocytosis occurs rather frequently in mesothelioma patients, although thromboembolic complications such as severe thromboses and concurrent pulmonary emboli are only infrequently reported [11, 32, 38].

The haemoglobin level was one of the most significant prognostic factors in the study by Edwards *et al.* [13]. In two other studies the haemoglobin level had a significant prognostic value in univariate, but not multivariate, analyses [14, 15]. These latter studies concerned patients who had participated in chemotherapy trials and therefore had to have adequate cell counts. It is not known whether any or how many patients had received a blood transfusion before being entered in the trials, which might have biased the haemoglobin analysis. Two papers concentrating on haemoglobin as a prognostic factor did not confirm these data [19, 26]. Both studies used rather low median haemoglobin values for their patient population with cut-off levels of 12.6 g/dl and 13.2 g/dl, respectively. More data are needed to appreciate better the value of blood cell counts as prognostic indices in MPM.

Gender

Females with MPM tend to have a better prognosis than men in multivariate analysis [9, 10, 13, 15–17, 39]. The female gender is a good prognostic factor in univariate analysis in three other studies [23, 24, 40]. Although 12 studies could not confirm the good prognostic value of the female sex, they did not show the converse.

MPM preferentially affects males, probably because men are more likely to have an occupational exposure [32]. Therefore most studies only involve a small number of female patients, limiting the power to detect the prognostic importance of gender. Nevertheless, most data seem to point to a better prognosis for female patients with MPM. So far, the explanation for this observation remains to be elucidated.

Age

Most studies agree that older age is a poor prognostic factor, although this statement is not undisputed. Some studies state that an age higher than 50 or 60 years is associated with a worse survival [23, 41]. Other studies mention a worse survival at an age above 65 or 75 years [11, 14, 19, 25, 32, 42]. Only one study on 100 patients identifies older age as a good prognostic factor, when analysing age as a continuous variable in a multivariate analysis, but it does not provide an explanation for this contradictory result [30]. Eleven papers have been published that did not detect any significance for age as a prognostic factor. Older patients are likely to have more comorbidity, which again may have an impact on survival, especially since co-morbidity is usually poorly documented. This might upset the interpretation of data on the prognostic significance of age in MPM.

Chest pain and dyspnoea

Chest pain and dyspnoea are common symptoms at presentation of MPM. Chest pain might be a non-specific symptom but can also be caused by infiltration of the structures of the thoracic wall by tumour, and as such can be correlated with locally more advanced tumours. Therefore it might even be considered as a tumour-related prognostic factor. Several studies have shown an additional poor prognostic impact of the presence of chest pain [14, 32], whereas others showed this prognostic effect by univariate analysis only [13, 22]. However, the majority of studies did not detect any impact of the presence of chest pain on the survival of MPM patients [10, 19, 24, 25, 27, 40, 43].

A similar number of studies have analysed the prognostic effect of dyspnoea, but these unanimously conclude that dyspnoea does not have any impact on survival [10, 19, 23–25, 27, 40, 43].

Apparently, the presence and amount of pleural fluid, which is the major cause of dyspnoea in MPM, is not correlated with the extent of the tumour nor does it predict its natural course.

Race and ethnicity

One study including 19 per cent black and 81 per cent white patients demonstrated a significant survival advantage for white patients [24]. This effect was independent of other prognostic factors such as performance status, therapy, and tumour stage. No explanation was given for this phenomenon. A similar ethnic distribution was described in the SEER study but a better outcome for white MPM patients was not detected [16]. Race and ethnicity are only scantily reported in treatment and prevention trials in solid tumours including MPM [44] . Although the limited size of the patient population in most MPM studies does not allow subgroup analyses, information on the diversity of the participants substantially adds to the validity and applicability of the results [44].

Tumour-related prognostic factors

Tumour-related prognostic factors involve the anatomical tumour stage and histological and biological characteristics of the tumour.

Anatomical staging

Anatomical staging is a major prognostic factor in MPM. Almost all prognostic factor studies that include staging in their analysis reveal a significant impact on survival and show that this effect adds to the other prognostic factors. Twelve studies support this statement whilst only two cannot confirm it, as is summarized in Table 5.1. Despite this, staging is not generally accepted as a good prognostic factor for several reasons. Firstly, several different staging systems are in use, which makes direct comparison of the papers focusing on this subject difficult [40, 45–47]. Indeed, the radical multimodality therapy series of Sugarbaker *et al.* [40] describes a highly significant impact of one staging system on survival, while two other staging systems do not seem to have a predictive value in the same patient population. Secondly, proper staging of MPM requires a surgical procedure, which is a major disadvantage. Thorough staging is currently only indicated in patients eligible for major surgical procedures, and most patients tend to be inoperable at presentation. This implies that surgical staging is not routinely performed in all patients, and data on tumour stage are not available for every patient [27, 41]. Thirdly, the tools used for non-surgical staging differ considerably even within the populations from single hospitals [27, 30].

Some studies highlight specific aspects of the staging of MPM. In early stage MPM in particular, invasion of the visceral pleura was found to be a negative prognostic factor [12], and this feature was subsequently incorporated in staging systems [46]. In fact, a normal or purely inflammatory macroscopic appearance of the visceral pleura was associated with better survival than pleura with small nodules, which again had a better prognosis than completely involved visceral pleura (24months, 10.5 month, and. 6.9 months, respectively) [12]. A single observation points to the potential significance of the absence of neoplastic cells in the pleural fluid [25]. Negative microscopic resection margins positively influenced the survival of patients who had extrapleural pneumonectomy as part of trimodality treatment [40]. The statement 'negative resection margins' requires histological examination of at least 20 sections of the extrapleural pneumonectomy specimen, and therefore is difficult to reproduce since it is only valid for the minority of the patients who were candidates for this extensive therapy.

Although radiological techniques like CT and MRI scanning have their limitations in predicting local tumour spread and presence of mediastinal lymph node metastases, most centres rely

Table 5.1 Tumour stage as a prognostic factor in malignant pleural mesothelioma: different studies focusing on tumour stage as a prognostic factor in malignant mesothelioma

Reference	n	Patient selection	Staging system	Significance[a]	Staging method
Rusch and Venkatraman [9]	231	Prospective registry	TNM [46]	+	Thoracotomy
			T1 and 2 vs. T3 and 4	+	
			N0 vs. N2	+	
Tammilehto [10]	98	Prospective database	Mattson [111] stage I and IIA vs. higher stages	+	Clinical and surgical
Boutin et al. [12]	125	Prospective series	Butchart et al. [45]	+	Thoracoscopy
			Stage Ia vs. Ib	+	
Ohta et al. [39]	54	Random samples	Stage III and IV vs. I and II	+	Clinical
Metintas et al. [19]	100	Consecutive patients	Stage I vs. higher stage	+	CT
Van Gelder et al. [42]	167	'New cases'	Butchart	+	Clinical
Spirtas et al. [16]	1475	SEER Registry	Localized vs. regional vs. distant vs. unknown	+	
Ruffie et al. [32]	332	Pathological diagnosis	Butchart	+	From charts
Alberts et al. [24]	262	Histologically confirmed	Butchart	+	CT and thoracotomy
De Pangher Manzini et al. [25]	80	Consecutive patients	Butchart I and II vs. III and IV	Univariate[b]	Clinical
Sugarbaker et al. [40]	183	EPP and chemoradiotherapy	Sugarbaker et al. [47]	+	Extrapleural pneumonectomy
			Revised system [40]	+	
			TNM	−	
			Butchart	−	
Tammilehto et al. [21]	88	'With adequate CT'	TNM	+	CT
			T	+	
			N	−	
			M	−	

Direct comparison between the studies is severely hampered by the major differences in patient selection, staging systems, and methods used to stage the patients.

a+ The stage was a significant variable in a multivariate analysis of this series; − the stage was not significant.

[b]This study was not significant in multivariate analysis, possibly because 20 patients with an unknown stage and only four patients with stage II or IV were included.

on these tools for staging MPM. Estimation of the TNM stage from 88 preoperative CT scans revealed significant differences in prognosis correlated with the T categories and the TNM stages, but not with the N or M categories [21], although some centres feel that retrospective TNM staging is not sufficiently accurate [13]. Another CT parameter, tumour volume estimated by three-dimensional CT scan reconstruction, did predict the survival of patients who underwent resection of MPM [17]. The median survival for patients with a preoperative tumour volume less than 100 cm³ was 22 months compared with 11 months if the volume was more than 100 cm³.

MPM with a high metabolic activity, as assessed by fluorodeoxyglucose positron emission tomography (FDG PET), may have a worse prognosis [48]. A study of 17 patients with predominantly epithelioid and biphasic MPM showed a significantly worse survival for patients with a standardized uptake value (SUV) greater than 4 compared with the group with lower uptake of deoxyglucose and a lower metabolic activity. No information was available on other prognostic factors, which implies that this interesting finding needs to be confirmed by further studies.

Histology

The histological subtype is the best studied and most important prognostic factor of malignant mesothelioma (Fig. 5.2). Patients with an epithelioid type MPM have a significantly better prognosis than those with a sarcomatoid subtype [9, 40, 43, 49]. Differences in median survival may be as great as 200 days [27, 50]. Some patients have a mixed histology, with both epithelioid and sarcomatoid features. When larger pleura samples are taken for diagnosis, the mixed subtype of MPM is diagnosed more frequently [51, 52]. In survival analyses, mixed and sarcomatoid histology are often combined in one group since their incidence compared with the epithelioid subtype is rather low [9].

Almost all prognostic factor studies reveal data on the histological subtyping of the tumour. More than 50 per cent of the studies, including all prospective analyses, confirm its prognostic significance. Only six studies do not identify histological subtype as a significant factor [17, 19,

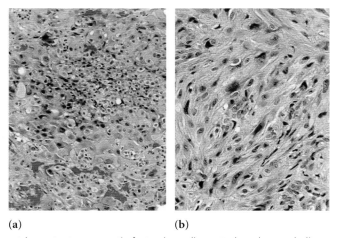

(a)   (b)

Figure 5.2 The most important prognostic factor in malignant pleural mesothelioma. (a) A mesothelioma with predominantly epitheloid cells in solid sheets; (b) a mesothelioma characterized by spindled cells with a fascicular pattern. The former epitheliod tumour has a far better prognosis than the latter sarcomatoid mesothelioma. In this particular situation both micrographs were obtained from the same patient, who consequently has an intermediate prognosis. (Courtesy of Dr M. den Bakker, Erasmus MC, Rotterdam, The Netherlands.)

24, 39, 41], among which is the largest study on prognostic factors in mesothelioma [16], but this paper listed the histological subtype for only 291 of the 1475 cases described. Other negative studies were also hampered by missing data [19], inter-observer error, leading to a lack of clarity regarding the histological subtype [24], or a long period of time over which the cases were gathered [27].

One study suggests that patients with a definite diagnosis of MPM survive longer than those with a possible or probable diagnosis [15]. Explanations given for this feature were a shorter time to obtain the diagnosis in the 'definite' group and/or the presence of more undifferentiated tumours in the 'probable or possible' group. The only other paper including this factor in its analysis could not confirm the prognostic significance of the certainty of histological diagnosis [13].

Origin

The influence of the site of origin on the survival of malignant mesothelioma is not clear. A malignant mesothelioma can originate from many serosal tissues, as is illustrated by the large SEER database which included pleural mesothelioma (81 per cent), peritoneal mesothelioma (15 per cent), and mesothelioma from the ovary, tunica vaginalis, heart, and lung [16]. Mesothelioma from the heart probably reflects pericardial mesothelioma, and that from the lung most likely reflects MPM. A survival difference between the different primary tissues was not described.

One series, including 136 pleural and 37 peritoneal mesotheliomas, revealed a poorer survival of patients with a pleural origin [23]. Otherwise, analysis of data from 57 patients with the pleura and 12 patients with the peritoneum as initial site of the tumour revealed a better survival for patients with pleural disease [11]. A further study with relatively few patients with peritoneal mesothelioma did not detect any survival difference [10]. Differentiation between peritoneal mesothelioma and female genital cancer can be difficult, and it is not clear to what extent the misdiagnosis of peritoneal mesothelioma confounds the results described earlier [10, 16].

Tumours from the testicular serosa are generally detected at a relatively early stage with a small tumour load and this might be reflected in the good survival observed. This probably also accounts for two patients with a mesothelioma originating from this site who had better survival than patients with primary pleural disease, despite the fact that their disease was metastasized [23].

Left- or right-sided pleural mesothelioma

Only one suggestion has been published so far on the favourable effect of left-sided tumours [41]. This study describes the prognosis of 167 MPM patients who were selected from the files of a pathology laboratory. No explanation is given for this observation, but it does not seem to be secondary to a higher complication or mortality rate for patients who had surgery for right-sided tumours. Other studies report similar survival rates for patients with right- and left-sided tumours [19, 25, 40].

Tumour markers

Recently, new markers have been explored by molecular and cellular biological techniques. Some markers seem to predict a better outcome of the disease in selected MPM patients, but confirmation by larger independent series is still lacking. More importantly, these markers give insight into the (extra)cellular processes associated with the development of MPM and shift the approach to MPM from anatomical, focusing on surgical staging and local (radiotherapeutic) treatment, towards systemic, focusing on the selection of patients for systemic therapy.

In general, tumour markers might be used for screening purposes, as a diagnostic, staging, or monitoring tool, or as a tool to predict the response to treatment or to foresee tumour recurrences [53]. Guidelines for the use of tumour markers in the management of various solid tumours such as breast, colorectal and prostate cancer have been published [53, 54]. Our knowledge of tumour markers in MPM is still too scanty to allow the implementation of the use of the markers in daily clinical practice, but they might be of help in the development of new diagnostic or therapeutic strategies.

Chromosomal changes

Chromosomal abnormalities associated with MPM are complex, involving both numerical and structural changes. Controversial results have been reported regarding the prognostic significance of, for example, DNA ploidy and lower S-phase fractions [55–58]. The number of copies of the short arm of chromosome 7 and hyperdiploid mean chromosomal number seem to correlate with shorter survival rates [59]. The proliferation index determined by flow cytometry and the expression of the cell-cycle-related proteins p27^{kip1}, PCNA and MIB1 (Ki-67 nuclear antigen) has been described as an independent prognostic factor [55, 60–63]. A low mitotic count and a low apoptotic index defined by *in situ* end-labelling is associated with a significant survival advantage [64]. Low expression of the p27 antigen in tissue sections of MPM is associated with a significantly worse prognosis [65].

Recent research has demonstrated that mice that developed pleural tumours induced by conditional knockout of different individual genes differed dramatically in overall survival time [66]. Whether this has its human counterpart in the expression-ratio-based microarray analysis that was able to predict treatment-related outcomes in selected MPM samples is not yet clear [67].

Tumour suppressor genes

Analogous to the frequent chromosomal aberrations, numerous mutations and deletions of tumour suppressor genes have been described in malignant mesothelioma [68–70]. An analysis of the significance of the expression of the tumour suppressor genes p53, Kristen ras (K-*ras*) and *rhoA* did not reveal a prognostic value of these markers [71, 72].

Aberrant methylation of the tumour suppressor gene RASSF1A has been associated with a poor prognosis in lung cancer patients [73]. Although a significant relationship with prognosis was not demonstrated, aberrant methylation was notably absent in four cases with survival that exceeded 36 months [74]. Expression of the cell cycle inhibitor p21$^{WAF1/CIP1}$ (p21), a downstream target of p53, bears a prognostic significance in patients in whom the SV40 sequence is found in the tumour tissue [75].

Simian virus 40

One study has shown a trend for increased survival in SV40-negative MPM patients [76]. Simian virus 40 (SV40), a DNA virus with potential transforming and carcinogenic effects, has been mainly studied as a possible aetiological, rather than prognostic, factor of mesothelioma [77]. DNA encoding SV40 Tag or SV40 Tag protein expression is primarily found in biphasic and sarcomatoid mesotheliomas [76], but it is still not clear whether SV40-positive MPM tumours behave more aggressively than SV40-negative tumours.

Angiogenesis

Angiogenesis, the process of generating new blood vessels, is essential for tumour growth beyond a few millimetres in diameter [78]. Increased microvascular density present mainly at the periphery of the tumour correlates with a shorter survival [22, 79]. Also, the spatial arrangement of the vessels, in addition to vessel density, correlated with survival, a feature that also applies to patients with cervical and colorectal cancers [80]. A number of factors are involved in the regulation of tumour angiogenesis. Although high levels of vascular endothelial growth factor (VEGF), acidic fibroblast growth factor (FGF-1), and transforming growth factor β (TGF-β) can be detected in serum and effusions, only FGF-2 and its binder syndecan-1 is significantly correlated with tumour aggressiveness and the prognosis of MPM [81, 82]. This study also showed that syndecan-1 is modulated by the Wilms tumour 1 transcriptional suppressor gene (WT1) product, which correlates with the histological type but did not correlate with prognosis.

The role of thrombospondin 1 (TSP-1) is still unclear. It was originally reported as an inhibitor of angiogenesis [83], but studies now suggest that it also may function as stimulator of angiogenesis [84]. The utility of TSP-1 overexpression as a prognostic factor in MPM had little value [85].

Cyclo-oxygenase-2 (COX-2) is overexpressed in MPM [86] and correlates with a worse survival in both univariate and multivariate analyses [87, 88]. COX-2 catalyses the initial rate-limiting steps of prostaglandin E_2 (PGE$_2$) synthesis from arachidonic acid in cell membranes. PGE$_2$ activates specific epithelioid receptors that increase cyclic AMP production, which in turn stimulates synthesis of VEGF, a trigger of angiogenesis.

Serum and pleural fluid markers

Hyaluronan is an extracellular polysaccharide present in pleural exudate from MPM patients. A retrospective analysis of 100 MPM patients by Thylen et al. [30] showed the prognostic significance of hyaluronan levels in the pleural fluid, with elevated levels indicating a longer survival.

High serum lactate dehydrogenase (LDH) levels (>500 IU/l) are associated with a worse prognosis, and since LDH is commonly measured in daily clinical practice it might be a useful marker for patient selection for specific treatments [14, 19]. More recently, Robinson et al. [89] assayed serum concentrations of soluble mesothelin-related proteins (SMRP) using a double-determinant ELISA and found that it correlated with the size of the tumour and increased during tumour progression. Although not tested widely, SMRP in serum could be a useful marker for monitoring MPM progression [89]. Finally, serum osteopontin levels could discriminate between subjects without malignancy who were exposed to asbestos and patients with pleural mesothelioma with a sensitivity of 78% and a specificity of 86% at an osteopontin cutoff value of 48.3 ng/ml [90].

Matrix metalloproteinases

Matrix metalloproteinases (MMPs) and their endogenous inhibitors (TIMPs) may have prognostic significance in MPM [91]. These proteins are involved in extracellular degradation of matrix proteins, such as collagen, laminin, and fibronectin, during normal tissue remodelling processes and implicated in the pathogenesis of diverse invasive processes including local cancer spread and metastasis. MMP-1 is overexpressed in MPM, but there is no significant variation in MMP and TIMP expression in patients with a better or worse prognosis [91]. Also, MMP-2 is abundantly present in MPM specimens [92]. High MMP-2 expression and activity seemed to be correlated with a poorer survival outcome.

Tissue polypeptide antigen and Cyfra 21–1

Tissue polypeptide antigen (TPA) assay measures a specific epitope structure of human cytokeratin 8, 18, and 19 fragments. The Cyfra 21–1 assay is specific for the cytokeratin 19 fragment. In contrast with cytokeratins themselves, cytokeratin fragments are soluble and thus detectable in serum and pleural effusions of MPM patients. In a retrospective study in 52 patients Schouwink et al. [93] showed that high serum TPS and Cyfra 21–1 levels were predictive for poorer survival in multivariate analysis. TPA and Cyfra 21–1 could not discriminate MPM from other malignant pleural diseases.

Antioxidant enzymes

Catalase is a hydrogen peroxidase scavenging enzyme which decomposes hydrogen peroxide to water and oxygen. Together with manganese superoxide dismutase, a superoxide scavenging enzyme, these antioxidant enzymes are more highly expressed in MPM than in healthy mesothelium or metastatic adenocarcinoma of the pleura [94–96]. High catalase, particularly high coordinated expression of catalase and manganese superoxide dismutase, in mesothelioma is associated with a better prognosis [97]. High prevalence of other detoxification enzymes such as glutathione S-transferases (GSTs) are in good agreement with the low responsiveness of mesothelioma to chemotherapy but their prognostic value is debatable [98, 99].

Proteomics and genomics

New powerful cellular, molecular, and proteomic-based technologies will undoubtedly lead to the identification of novel tumour markers. The application of new or improved techniques for immunohistochemistry [100], tissue immunoblotting, differential display, laser capture microdissection, phage antibody display technology [101], and flow cytometry [55] together with proteomic-based approaches, such as two-dimensional gel electrophoresis, mass spectrometry (MALDI–TOF/QTOF/SELDI–TOF) and protein (chip-based) expression array technology will enable this process to develop over the coming years and will undoubtedly affect clinical management of MPM in the future.

The advent of microarray gene expression profiling represents one such area. Early studies using microarray technology, which have been able to stratify mesothelioma according to outcome, have now been completed. The first prognostic set of genes, consisting of eight discriminatory genes, was identified by Bueno and colleagues, and a six-gene model based on these could significantly predict patient outcome after treatment [102]. Building on this, Bueno's group carried out a study to identify markers which had prognostic value for patients with widely divergent survival times. From this analysis 46 putative markers were identified. The authors identified four genes [*KIAA097*, GDP-dissociation inhibitor 1 (*GDIA1*), cytosolic thyroid hormone binding protein (*CTHBP*), and an EST similar to the L6 tumour antigen] which could correctly classify (100 per cent) a training sample. These genes were subsequently tested on 29 samples not previously subjected to microarray analysis, and were found to significantly predict outcome in these samples [103]. A later study compared two different microarray analysis methods to identify a common subset of 27 genes which could be used to predict both survival and progression of malignant pleural mesothelioma [104].

In summary, many molecular markers have been studied in MPM. The detection of these markers has led to the evaluation of a range of new targeted therapeutic agents, including inhibitors of angiogenesis and cell signalling, and survival pathways and immunomodulatory agents in the management of this disease [105]. In the future the powerful new technologies of proteomics and genomics will allow us not only to predict outcome for the individual patient and identify novel targets for therapy but also to individualize patient treatments based on likely outcomes from the various therapeutic options available.

Environment-related prognostic factors

Environment-related factors are external to the patient and his or her disease. They include treatment, exposure to asbestos, the availability of clinical care and social support, and the level of education and socio-economic status of the patient. Papers focusing on environment-related prognostic factors generally include patients with different malignancies. It is likely that the poor prognostic factors from these surveys, such as lower socio-economic status, poor education, and greater distance from medical centres and experience of medical professionals, also apply to mesothelioma patients and may account for regional survival differences [106–109]. Therefore a description of the clinical setting in which a study has been performed is potentially important when reporting on clinical trials. In this regard multicentre and multinational trials should consider stratification of the patients by centre of referral when analysing outcomes.

Exposure to asbestos

One paper describes a negative association between asbestos exposure and survival in 332 patients from the area around Ontario and Quebec [32]. Other studies, which investigated the correlation between asbestos exposure and survival, could not confirm this result. A history of exposure to asbestos *per se* is not an ideal prognostic factor since it is rather poorly reproducible. Many patients do not recall whether they have been exposed to asbestos, and when exposure to asbestos has occurred it is difficult to quantify. A more objective measure might be the amount of asbestos fibres in pleural biopsies or resection specimens after a surgical procedure. Correlation of asbestos fibre count with survival in 28 patients revealed that a lung tissue fibre count below 1×10^6 fibres/g tissue seemed to predict a relatively good prognosis, but its prognostic value was no longer apparent in a multivariate analysis [10].

The analysis of the SEER data for 1475 patients revealed poorer survival of patients from registries in areas that had shipbuilding as major industry [16]. A possible explanation for this phenomenon was higher asbestos exposure in these areas, but since individual data on exposure to asbestos were not available, the evidence for this statement was rather thin.

Smoking

The absence or presence of a smoking history does not have any prognostic significance for patients with MPM [10, 19, 23, 24, 32, 40].

Treatment

The data from the first phase III randomized trial in MPM have recently become available, and for the first time a particular chemotherapy schedule was proved to offer a survival benefit [110]. Until then only less conclusive data were available, including that from the studies focusing on therapy as a prognostic factor (Table 5.2).

Several papers show a beneficial effect on survival of tumour-directed therapy. However, three papers describing prospectively obtained data showed only a statistically weak or no treatment effect [9, 10, 12]. Three other papers which used a multivariate analysis and included the performance status as a prognostic factor did show a treatment effect. Pleuropneumonectomy and chemotherapy [23], any therapy with doxorubicin and radiotherapy as a major component [24], and chemotherapy and more extensive surgery [11] were all predictors of a better survival of the MPM patients. Nevertheless, the retrospective nature of the studies made it impossible to relate the difference in prognosis solely to therapy [41].

As described earlier, performance status is a valuable prognostic factor that can be used to select patients for a particular therapy. Therefore analysis of the factor 'treatment' on survival may be biased by the performance of the patients [24]. For instance, a better outcome for patients receiving chemotherapy might well be due to selection of patients with a better performance status [12]. Patients with better performance status might show better responses to chemotherapy [11]. In some studies the significance of radiotherapy or chemotherapy [10], or radiotherapy and surgery [21], in univariate analysis is lost when performance status is taken into account in the analysis.

Table 5.2 Treatment as a prognostic factor in malignant pleural mesothelioma: summary of papers comparing survival data for different treatment modalities.

Reference	n	Patient selection criteria	Therapies compared	Statistical significance[a]	Prognostic significance of the performance score
Tammilehto [10]	98	Prospective analysis	Debulking surgery vs. none Hemithorax RT vs. none Chemotherapy vs. none	Univariate[b] Univariate Univariate	+
Rusch and Venkatraman [9]	231	Prospective data	EPP vs. pleurectomy/decortication Adjuvant therapy vs. none	– +	Not given
Boutin et al. [12]	125	Prospective series: thoracoscopic diagnosis	Surgery vs. chemotherapy vs. talc pleurodesis vs. none	Univariate	Not given
Antman et al. [23]	180	Pathological database	Pleuropneumonectomy vs. chemotherapy	+	+
Chahinian et al. [11]	69	All patients from department	Partial or complete resection vs. none Radical resection and chemotherapy with response vs. no response	+ +	+
Thylen et al. [30]	100	Clinical data	Any (mainly chemotherapy) vs. none	+	Not given
Spirtas et al. [16]	1475	SEER database, positive histology by life	Any surgery, RT, or chemotherapy	+	Not given
Alberts et al. [24]	262	Histologically confirmed diagnosis	Therapy vs. none Individual treatments	+ –	+
Tammilehto et al. [21]	88	Pleural MM with adequate CT scan	Surgery vs. no surgery Hemithorax RT vs. none chemotherapy vs. not	Univariate Univariate –	+
Chailleux et al. [41]	167	From pathology files	Surgery, chemotherapy or talc pleurodesis vs. none	Univariate	Not given
Edwards et al. [13]	138	Consecutive patients	Surgical resection vs. surgical biopsy	–	+
De Pangher Manzini et al. [25]	80	Consecutive patients	Any surgery or intrapleural or intravenous chemotherapy vs. none	–	Univariate

Table 5.2 *Continued*

Reference	n	Patient selection criteria	Therapies compared	Statistical significance[a]	Prognostic significance of the performance score
Martin-Ucar et al. [26]	51	Patients who had palliative surgery	Pleurectomy vs. decortication	–	Only PS WHO 0 and 1 included
Fusco et al. [27]	113	All patients	Chemotherapy or palliative surgery vs. chemical pleurodesis	–	Not given
Merritt et al. [43]	101	'From a centre'	Pleurodesis, palliative radiotherapy, or chemotherapy vs. none	–	Not given
Ruffie et al. [32]	332	Pathological diagnosis, pleural MM	Chemotherapy vs. none Radical RT vs. palliative or no RT No surgery vs. palliative surgery vs. EPP	+ – –	Not given
Emri et al. [55]	40	Surgically obtained diagnosis	VATS vs. thoracotomy Chemotherapy vs. none	– –	Not tested
Pass et al. [17]	47	From PDT study	EPP vs. pleurectomy/decortication	–	Not given

[a] + Treatment effect proved statistically by multivariate analysis; –treatment effect not statistically significant.

[b] Univariate means that the significance could only be demonstrated by this statistical test. Similarly, a + in the column performance indicates that the performance score was a significant prognostic factor in multivariate analysis.

EPP, extrapleural pneumonectomy; MM, malignant mesothelioma; PDT, photodynamic therapy; PS WHO, performance score according to the WHO classification; RT, radiotherapy; VATS, video-assisted thoracoscopic surgery.

Interpretation of data on the prognostic impact of therapy for MPM is further hampered by different definitions of the 'treatment' between the different studies. This is also illustrated in Table 5.2. Depending on the patient population and the treatment offered in a particular centre, treatment might be defined as any tumour-directed therapy, which sometimes even includes talc pleurodesis [41], whereas in other centres this would be categorized as palliative therapy and not as tumour-directed therapy. Others evaluate different chemotherapy schedules, palliative radiotherapy or high-dose hemithorax irradiation, and surgery either separately or in different therapeutic combinations.

Despite these restrictions, it is likely that a therapy effect is present in malignant mesothelioma. Therefore a description of any tumour-directed therapy that has been given is an indispensable issue for a correct interpretation of survival data of these patients.

Time to diagnosis

Some papers suggest that patients who have a longer interval between the presenting symptoms and the definite diagnosis have a better survival [23, 24, 41]. Although this phenomenon was not apparent in other studies [11, 12, 25, 32], some authors suggest that patients with a longer diagnostic delay may have a more slowly growing tumour [27]. Even if this statement holds, however, the value of diagnostic delay as a prognostic factor seems limited since it relies on the subjectivity of patients and physicians and seems only poorly reproducible.

Prognostic groupings

The CALGB [14] and the EORTC [15] have suggested prognostic scoring systems that discriminate between patients with a good and a poor outlook. The prognostic tree designed by the CALGB uses the performance score, age, haemoglobin, white blood cell count, presence of chest pain, and weight loss to define six patient groups with significantly different survival experiences [14]. They reveal a difference in median survival time from 1.4 to 13.9 months. The EORTC data divided the patients in two groups using the prognostic factors white blood cell count, performance status, histological subtype, probability of histological diagnosis, and gender [15]. The low-risk group comprised patients with no, one, or two poor prognostic factors; the high-risk group had three, four, or five poor prognostic factors. The median survival duration was 5.5 months and 10.8 months for the high-risk and low-risk groups, respectively.

These groupings probably reflect prognosis more precisely than the conventional anatomic staging systems that are available for MPM. The different parameters have the advantage over anatomic staging that they are simple laboratory and clinical indices, and therefore are easy to reproduce and available for all patients. Whether the prognostic factors that form the prognostic groupings mentioned above are optimal remains to be determined. The prognostic value of chest pain and weight loss has not been confirmed irrefutably, and the probability of the histological diagnosis is not documented systematically.

Scoring systems that include parameters other than tumour stage have been proposed for other tumour types, such as small-cell lung cancer [111]. Schemes including performance status and biochemical assessment reflected prognosis more precisely than the classical division between limited and extensive disease [112]. Analogous to this situation, the prognostic grouping proposals of the CALGB and the EORTC seem to reflect the prognosis of mesothelioma patients rather accurately [13, 113]. Figure 5.3 shows an updated analysis of the survival of the patient population from Leicester according to their prognostic grouping. The survival differences are strongly statistically significant.

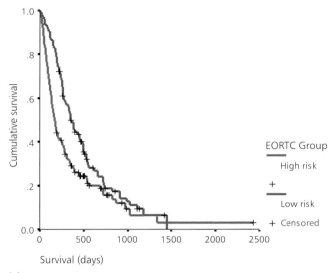

(a)

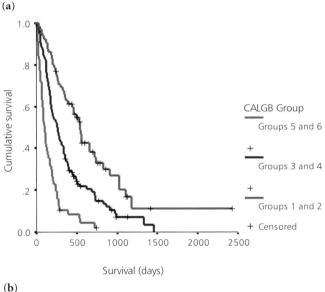

(b)

Figure 5.3 Expanded and updated survival data from the series originally published by Edwards *et al.* [13]. The data are from 240 consecutive patients presenting in Leicester between 1988 and 2002 (a) Survival curves when the patients are stratified according to the EORTC prognostic groups (low risk, *n* = 103; high risk, *n* = 137; *P* = 0.0018). (b) Survival curves when the patients are stratified according to the CALGB prognostic groups (groups 1 and 2, *n* = 65; groups 3 and 4, *n* = 118; groups 5 and 6, *n* = 57; *P* < 0.0001). In the expanded patient population both scoring systems remain useful tools for the prognostic stratification of mesothelioma patients.

There is an obvious need for a simple reproducible prognostic grouping system. If internationally recognized, it will be valuable as an inclusion criterion in clinical trials and as a stratification factor in phase III clinical trials, will make comparison between trials easier, and will provide a better demarcation of the patient group to which the study results are applicable. Examination of the prognostic factors of patient groups may be sufficient to understand the survival differences across phase II trials [113]. Prognostic factors can also be of help in choosing the appropriate therapy for patients who are not eligible for any study protocol and are treated off-study.

Conclusion

Many prognostic factors have been described in MPM. Although only a limited number have been validated by prospective confirmatory studies, clinicians should be aware of their potential importance in deciding on patient management.

The most significant prognostic factors in MPM are histological subtyping, performance status, and tumour stage. Although the majority of studies confirm its prognostic value, tumour stage in general seems less useful clinically as an indicator of prognosis. Proper staging requires surgery and currently there is no consensus on the best staging system. Furthermore, surgical staging is only performed in a minority of patients suitable for radical surgery.

Other factors that are related to a poor prognosis, although the significance was not apparent in all papers, are old age, male gender, the probability of histological diagnosis, weight loss, and high platelet and leucocyte counts. Factors which can be measured simply, cheaply, and routinely in any laboratory, such as C-reactive protein, and which have been proven to be of prognostic significance in many other malignancies, might also be of value in malignant mesothelioma and are worth evaluating [114].

Special attention should be paid to the factor 'treatment'. A treatment effect has been demonstrated repeatedly by numerous, predominantly retrospective, studies. The retrospective studies are obviously biased by patient selection. The loss of statistical significance of the treatment effect when subjected to multivariate analyses illustrates this bias. Nevertheless, evidence of the beneficial effects of therapy on prognosis is growing. The perception that therapeutic interventions have little to offer should be dispelled and early diagnosis and treatment encouraged [9].

The biological prognostic factors need confirmation in larger prospective trials and should be analysed with respect to the existing prognostic factors. In future, they might guide the development of new therapeutic interventions.

The search for better treatments may profit from an accurate and simple prognostic scoring system that is universally accepted. This system will help to identify the individual patient who will benefit from a particular treatment, but will also improve the quality of reporting on clinical trials and facilitate the comparison of therapeutic interventions in mesothelioma [5, 115].

Acknowledgements

The authors would like to thank Dr R. A. M. Damhuis, Comprehensive Cancer Centre, Rotterdam, for helpful and stimulating discussions during the preparation of this chapter, and Ms R. de Wijk-van der Zalm and Ms C. Koopman for their skilful technical assistance.

References

1. Gospodarowicz M, O'Sullivan B. Prognostic factors: principles and application. In: Gospodarowicz M, Henson D, O'Sullivan B, Sobin L, Wittekind C, eds. *Prognostic Factors in Cancer*, 2nd edn. New York: Wiley–Liss, 2001; 17–35.

2. Wong CF, Fung SL, Yew WW, Fu KH. A case of malignant pleural mesothelioma with unexpectedly long survival without active treatment. *Respiration* 2002; **69**: 166–8.

3. Drew PJ, Ilstrup DM, Kerin MJ, Monson JR. Prognostic factors: guidelines for investigation design and state of the art analytical methods. *Surg Oncol* 1998; **7**: 71–6.

4. Simon R. Evaluating prognostic factor studies. In: Gospodarowicz M, Henson D, O'Sullivan B, Sobin L, Wittekind C, eds. *Prognostic Factors in Cancer*, 2nd edn. New York: Wiley–Liss, 2001; 49–56.

5. Shapiro SH, Weijer C, Freedman B. Reporting the study populations of clinical trials. Clear transmission or static on the line? *J Clin Epidemiol* 2000; **53**: 973–9.

6. Huwiler-Muntener K, Juni P, Junker C, Egger M. Quality of reporting of randomized trials as a measure of methodologic quality. *JAMA* 2002; **287**: 2801–4.

7. Steele JP. Prognostic factors in mesothelioma. *Semin Oncol* 2002; **29**: 36–40.

8. Bard M, Ruffie P. Malignant pleural mesothelioma. From diagnosis to prognosis. *Presse Med* 2002; **31**: 406–11.

9. Rusch VW, Venkatraman ES. Important prognostic factors in patients with malignant pleural mesothelioma, managed surgically. *Ann Thorac Surg* 1999; **68**: 1799–804.

10. Tammilehto L. Malignant mesothelioma: prognostic factors in a prospective study of 98 patients. *Lung Cancer* 1992; **8**: 175–84.

11. Chahinian AP, Pajak TF, Holland JF, Norton L, Ambinder RM, Mandel EM. Diffuse malignant mesothelioma. Prospective evaluation of 69 patients. *Ann Intern Med* 1982; **96**: 746–55.

12. Boutin C, Rey F, Gouvernet J. Le mésothéliome malin: facteurs pronostiques dans une série de125 patients étudiés de 1973 à 1987. *Bull Acad Natl Med* 1992; **176**: 105–14.

13. Edwards JG, Abrams KR, Leverment JN, Spyt TJ, Waller DA, O'Byrne KJ. Prognostic factors for malignant mesothelioma in 142 patients: validation of CALGB and EORTC prognostic scoring systems. *Thorax* 2000; **55**: 731–5.

14. Herndon JE, Green MR, Chahinian AP, Corson JM, Suzuki Y, Vogelzang NJ. Factors predictive of survival among 337 patients with mesothelioma treated between 1984 and 1994 by the Cancer and Leukemia Group B. *Chest* 1998; **113**: 723–31.

15. Curran D, Sahmoud T, Therasse P, van Meerbeeck J, Postmus PE, Giaccone G. Prognostic factors in patients with pleural mesothelioma: the European Organization for Research and Treatment of Cancer experience. *J Clin Oncol* 1998; **16**: 145–52.

16. Spirtas R, Connelly RR, Tucker MA. Survival patterns for malignant mesothelioma: the SEER experience. *Int J Cancer* 1988; **41**: 525–30.

17. Pass HI, Temeck BK, Kranda K, Steinberg SM, Feuerstein IR. Preoperative tumor volume is associated with outcome in malignant pleural mesothelioma. *J Thorac Cardiovasc Surg* 1998; **115**: 310–18.

18. O'Sullivan B, Gospodarowicz M, Bristow R. Tumor, host, and environment-related prognostic factors. In: Gospodarowicz M, Henson D, O'Sullivan B, Sobin L, Wittekind C, eds. *Prognostic Factors in Cancer*, 2nd edn. New York: Wiley–Liss, 2001; 71–94.

19. Metintas M, Metintas S, Ucgun I, *et al.* Prognostic factors in diffuse malignant pleural mesothelioma: effects of pretreatment clinical and laboratory characteristics. *Respir Med* 2001; **95**: 829–35.

20. Van Meerbeeck JP. Prognostic factors in malignant mesothelioma: where do we go from here? *Eur Respir J* 1994; **7**: 1029–31.

21. Tammilehto L, Kivisaari L, Salminen US, Maasilta P, Mattson K. Evaluation of the clinical TNM staging system for malignant pleural mesothelioma: an assessment in 88 patients. *Lung Cancer* 1995; **12**: 25–34.

22. Edwards JG, Cox G, Andi A, *et al.* Angiogenesis is an independent prognostic factor in malignant mesothelioma. *Br J Cancer* 2001; **85**: 863–8.

23. Antman K, Shemin R, Ryan L, *et al.* Malignant mesothelioma: prognostic variables in a registry of 180 patients, the Dana–Farber Cancer Institute and Brigham and Women's Hospital experience over two decades, 1965–1985. *J Clin Oncol* 1988; **6**: 147–53.

24. Alberts AS, Falkson G, Goedhals L, Vorobiof DA, Van der Merwe CA. Malignant pleural mesothelioma: a disease unaffected by current therapeutic maneuvers. *J Clin Oncol* 1988; **6**: 527–35.

25. De Pangher Manzini V, Brollo A, Franceschi S, De Matthaeis M, Talamini R, Bianchi C. Prognostic factors of malignant mesothelioma of the pleura. *Cancer* 1993; **72**: 410–17.

26. Martin-Ucar AE, Edwards JG, Rengajaran A, Muller S, Waller DA. Palliative surgical debulking in malignant mesothelioma. Predictors of survival and symptom control. *Eur J Cardiothorac Surg* 2001; **20**: 1117–21.

27. Fusco V, Ardizzoni A, Merlo F, *et al*. Malignant pleural mesothelioma. Multivariate analysis of prognostic factors on 113 patients. *Anticancer Res* 1993; **13**: 683–9.

28. Karnofsky D, Adelmann W, Craver L. The use of nitrogen mustards in the palliative treatment of carcinoma. *Cancer* 1948; **1**: 634–656.

29. World health Organization. *WHO Handbook for Reporting Results of Cancer Treatment.* Geneva: WHO, 1979.

30. Thylen A, Hjerpe A, Martensson G. Hyaluronan content in pleural fluid as a prognostic factor in patients with malignant pleural mesothelioma. *Cancer* 2001; **92**: 1224–30.

31. Ando M, Ando Y, Hasegawa Y, *et al*. Prognostic value of performance status assessed by patients themselves, nurses, and oncologists in advanced non-small cell lung cancer. *Br J Cancer* 2001; **85**: 1634–9.

32. Ruffie P, Feld R, Minkin S, *et al*. Diffuse malignant mesothelioma of the pleura in Ontario and Quebec: a retrospective study of 332 patients. *J Clin Oncol* 1989; **7**: 1157–68.

33. Ross PJ, Ashley S, Norton A, *et al*. Do patients with weight loss have a worse outcome when undergoing chemotherapy for lung cancers? *Br J Cancer* 2004; **90**: 1905–11.

34. van Haarst JM, Baas P, Manegold C, *et al*. Multicentre phase II study of gemcitabine and cisplatin in malignant pleural mesothelioma. *Br J Cancer* 2002; **86**: 342–5.

35. Nash GF, Turner LF, Scully MF, Kakkar AK. Platelets and cancer. *Lancet Oncol* 2002; **3**: 425–30.

36. Pinedo HM, Verheul HM, D'Amato RJ, Folkman J. Involvement of platelets in tumour angiogenesis? *Lancet* 1998; **352**: 1775–7.

37. Higashihara M, Sunaga S, Tange T, Oohashi H, Kurokawa K. Increased secretion of interleukin-6 in malignant mesothelioma cells from a patient with marked thrombocytosis. *Cancer* 1992; **70**: 2105–8.

38. Lip GY, Chin BS, Blann AD. Cancer and the prothrombotic state. *Lancet Oncol* 2002; **3**: 27–34.

39. Ohta Y, Shridhar V, Bright RK, *et al*. VEGF and VEGF type C play an important role in angiogenesis and lymphangiogenesis in human malignant mesothelioma tumours. *Br J Cancer* 1999; **81**: 54–61.

40. Sugarbaker DJ, Flores RM, Jaklitsch MT, *et al*. Resection margins, extrapleural nodal status, and cell type determine postoperative long-term survival in trimodality therapy of malignant pleural mesothelioma: results in 183 patients. *J Thorac Cardiovasc Surg* 1999; **117**: 54–65.

41. Chailleux E, Dabouis G, Pioche D, *et al*. Prognostic factors in diffuse malignant pleural mesothelioma. A study of 167 patients. *Chest* 1988; **93**: 159–62.

42. Van Gelder T, Damhuis RA, Hoogsteden HC. Prognostic factors and survival in malignant pleural mesothelioma. *Eur Respir J* 1994; **7**: 1035–8.

43. Merritt N, Blewett CJ, Miller JD, Bennett WF, Young JE, Urschel JD. Survival after conservative (palliative) management of pleural malignant mesothelioma. *J Surg Oncol* 2001; **78**: 171–4.

44. Swanson GM, Bailar JC, 3rd. Selection and description of cancer clinical trials participants–science or happenstance? *Cancer* 2002; **95**: 950–9.

45. Butchart EG, Ashcroft T, Barnsley WC, Holden MP. Pleuropneumonectomy in the management of diffuse malignant mesothelioma of the pleura. Experience with 29 patients. *Thorax* 1976; **31**: 15–24.

46. Rusch VW. A proposed new international TNM staging system for malignant pleural mesothelioma. From the International Mesothelioma Interest Group. *Chest* 1995; **108**: 1122–8.

47. Sugarbaker DJ, Strauss GM, Lynch TJ, *et al*. Node status has prognostic significance in the multimodality therapy of diffuse, malignant mesothelioma. *J Clin Oncol* 1993; **11**: 1172–8.

48. Benard F, Sterman D, Smith RJ, Kaiser LR, Albelda SM, Alavi A. Prognostic value of FDG PET imaging in malignant pleural mesothelioma. *J Nucl Med* 1999; **40**: 1241–5.

49. Ceresoli GL, Locati LD, Ferreri AJ, *et al*. Therapeutic outcome according to histologic subtype in 121 patients with malignant pleural mesothelioma. *Lung Cancer* 2001; **34**: 279–87.

50. Johansson L, Linden CJ. Aspects of histopathologic subtype as a prognostic factor in 85 pleural mesotheliomas. *Chest* 1996; **109**: 109–14.

51. Nash G, Otis CN. Protocol for the examination of specimens from patients with malignant pleural mesothelioma: a basis for checklists. Cancer Committee, College of American Pathologists. *Arch Pathol Lab Med* 1999; **123**: 39–44.

52. van Gelder T, Hoogsteden HC, Vandenbroucke JP, van der Kwast TH, Planteydt HT. The influence of the diagnostic technique on the histopathological diagnosis in malignant mesothelioma. *Virchows Arch A Pathol Anat Histopathol* 1991; **418**: 315–7.

53. Sturgeon C. Practice guidelines for tumor marker use in the clinic. *Clin Chem* 2002; 48: 1151–9.

54. Bast RC, Jr, Ravdin P, Hayes DF, *et al*. 2000 update of recommendations for the use of tumor markers in breast and colorectal cancer: clinical practice guidelines of the American Society of Clinical Oncology. *J Clin Oncol* 2001; **19**: 1865–78.

55. Emri S, Akbulut H, Zorlu F, *et al*. Prognostic significance of flow cytometric DNA analysis in patients with malignant pleural mesothelioma. *Lung Cancer* 2001; **33**: 109–14.

56. Dazzi H, Hasleton PS, Thatcher N, Wilkes S, Swindell R, Chatterjee AK. Malignant pleural mesothelioma and epidermal growth factor receptor (EGF-R). Relationship of EGF-R with histology and survival using fixed paraffin embedded tissue and the F4, monoclonal antibody. *Br J Cancer* 1990; **61**: 924–6.

57. Isobe H, Sridhar KS, Doria R, *et al*. Prognostic significance of DNA aneuploidy in diffuse malignant mesothelioma. *Cytometry* 1995; **19**: 86–91.

58. Pyrhönen S, Laasonen A, Tammilehto L, *et al*. Diploid predominance and prognostic significance of S-phase cells in malignant mesothelioma. *Eur J Cancer* 1991; **27**: 197–200.

59. Tiainen M, Tammilehto L, Rautonen J, Tuomi T, Mattson K, Knuutila S. Chromosomal abnormalities and their correlations with asbestos exposure and survival in patients with mesothelioma. *Br J Cancer* 1989; **60**: 618–26.

60. Comin CE, Anichini C, Boddi V, Novelli L, Dini S. MIB-1 proliferation index correlates with survival in pleural malignant mesothelioma. Histopathology 2000; **36**: 26–31.

61. Beer TW, Buchanan R, Matthews AW, Stradling R, Pullinger N, Pethybridge RJ. Prognosis in malignant mesothelioma related to MIB 1 proliferation index and histological subtype. *Hum Pathol* 1998; **29**: 246–51.

62. Bongiovanni M, Cassoni P, De Giuli P, *et al*. p27(kip1) immunoreactivity correlates with long-term survival in pleural malignant mesothelioma. *Cancer* 2001; **92**: 1245–50.

63. Esposito V, Baldi A, De Luca A, *et al*. Role of PCNA in differentiating between malignant mesothelioma and mesothelial hyperplasia: prognostic considerations. *Anticancer Res* 1997; **17**: 601–4.

64. Beer TW, Carr NJ, Whittaker MA, Pullinger N. Mitotic and in situ end-labeling apoptotic indices as prognostic markers in malignant mesothelioma. *Ann Diagn Pathol* 2000; **4**: 143–8.

65. Beer TW, Shepherd P, Pullinger NC. p27 immunostaining is related to prognosis in malignant mesothelioma. *Histopathology* 2001; **38**: 535–41.

66. Jongsma J, van Montfort E, Zevenhoven J, *et al*. Development of a conditional malignant mesothelioma model. In: *Abstracts of VII Meeting of the International Mesothelioma Interest Group (IMIG), 24–26 June 2004, Brescia*, 92.

67. Gordon GJ, Jensen RV, Hsiao LL, *et al*. Using gene expression ratios to predict outcome among patients with mesothelioma. *J Natl Cancer Inst* 2003; **95**: 598–605.

68. Prins JB, Williamson KA, Kamp MM, *et al*. The gene for the cyclin-dependent-kinase-4 inhibitor, CDKN2A, is preferentially deleted in malignant mesothelioma. *Int J Cancer* 1998; **75**: 649–53.

69. Bianchi AB, Mitsunaga SI, Cheng JQ, *et al*. High frequency of inactivating mutations in the neurofibromatosis type 2 gene (NF2) in primary malignant mesotheliomas. *Proc Natl Acad Sci USA* 1995; **92**: 10854–8.

70. Cheng JQ, Jhanwar SC, Lu YY, Testa JR. Homozygous deletions within 9p21-p22 identify a small critical region of chromosomal loss in human malignant mesotheliomas. *Cancer Res* 1993; **53**: 4761–3.

71. Isik R, Metintas M, Gibbs AR, *et al.* p53, p21 and metallothionein immunoreactivities in patients with malignant pleural mesothelioma: correlations with the epidemiological features and prognosis of mesotheliomas with environmental asbestos exposure. *Respir Med* 2001; **95**: 588–93.

72. Nakamoto M, Teramoto H, Matsumoto S, Igishi T, Shimizu E. K-*ras* and *rhoA* mutations in malignant pleural effusion. *Int J Oncol* 2001; **19**: 971–6.

73. Burbee DG, Forgacs E, Zochbauer-Muller S, *et al.* Epigenetic inactivation of RASSF1A in lung and breast cancers and malignant phenotype suppression. *J Natl Cancer Inst* 2001; **93**: 691–9.

74. Toyooka S, Pass HI, Shivapurkar N, *et al.* Aberrant methylation and simian virus 40 tag sequences in malignant mesothelioma. *Cancer Res* 2001; **61**: 5727–30.

75. Baldi A, Groeger AM, Esposito V, *et al.* Expression of p21 in SV40 large T antigen positive human pleural mesothelioma: relationship with survival. *Thorax* 2002; **57**: 353–6.

76. Procopio A, Strizzi L, Vianale G, *et al.* Simian virus-40 sequences are a negative prognostic cofactor in patients with malignant pleural mesothelioma. *Genes Chromosomes Cancer* 2000; **29**: 173–9.

77. Carbone M, Kratzke RA, Testa JR. The pathogenesis of mesothelioma. *Semin Oncol* 2002; **29**: 2–17.

78. Folkman J, Shing Y. Angiogenesis. *J Biol Chem* 1992; **267**: 10931–4.

79. Kumar-Singh S, Vermeulen PB, Weyler J, *et al.* Evaluation of tumour angiogenesis as a prognostic marker in malignant mesothelioma. *J Pathol* 1997; **182**: 211–16.

80. Weyn B, Tjalma WA, Vermeylen P, van Daele A, Van Marck E, Jacob W. Determination of tumour prognosis based on angiogenesis-related vascular patterns measured by fractal and syntactic structure analysis. *Clin Oncol (R Coll Radiol)* 2004; **16**: 307–16.

81. Kumar-Singh S, Jacobs W, Dhaene K, *et al.* Syndecan-1 expression in malignant mesothelioma: correlation with cell differentiation, WT1 expression, and clinical outcome. *J Pathol* 1998; **186**: 300–5.

82. Kumar-Singh S, Weyler J, Martin MJ, Vermeulen PB, Van Marck E. Angiogenic cytokines in mesothelioma: a study of VEGF, FGF-1 and -2, and TGF beta expression. *J Pathol* 1999; **189**: 72–8.

83. Kieser A, Weich HA, Brandner G, Marme D, Kolch W. Mutant p53 potentiates protein kinase C induction of vascular endothelial growth factor expression. *Oncogene* 1994; **9**: 963–9.

84. Nicosia RF, Tuszynski GP. Matrix-bound thrombospondin promotes angiogenesis *in vitro*. *J Cell Biol* 1994; **124**: 183–93.

85. Ohta Y, Shridhar V, Kalemkerian GP, Bright RK, Watanabe Y, Pass HI. Thrombospondin-1 expression and clinical implications in malignant pleural mesothelioma. *Cancer* 1999; **85**: 2570–6.

86. Marrogi A, Pass HI, Khan M, Metheny-Barlow LJ, Harris CC, Gerwin BI. Human mesothelioma samples overexpress both cyclooxygenase-2 (COX-2) and inducible nitric oxide synthase (NOS2): *in vitro* antiproliferative effects of a COX-2 inhibitor. *Cancer Res* 2000; **60**: 3696–700.

87. Edwards JG, Faux SP, Plummer SM, *et al.* Cyclooxygenase-2 expression is a novel prognostic factor in malignant mesothelioma. *Clin Cancer Res* 2002; **8**: 1857–62.

88. Baldi A, Santini D, Vasaturo F, *et al.* Prognostic significance of cyclooxygenase-2 (COX-2) and expression of cell cycle inhibitors p21 and p27 in human pleural malignant mesothelioma. *Thorax* 2004; **59**: 428–33.

89. Robinson BW, Creaney J, Lake R, *et al.* Mesothelin-family proteins and diagnosis of mesothelioma. *Lancet* 2003; **362**: 1612–6.

90. Pass HI, Lott D, Lonardo F, Harbut M, Liu Z, Tang N, *et al.* Asbestos exposure, pleural mesothelioma, and serum osteopontin levels. *N Engl J Med* 2005; **353**: 1564–73.

91. Hirano H, Tsuji M, Kizaki T, *et al.* Expression of matrix metalloproteinases, tissue inhibitors of metalloproteinase, collagens, and Ki67 antigen in pleural malignant mesothelioma: an immunohistochemical and electron microscopic study. *Med Electron Microsc* 2002; **35**: 16–23.

92. Edwards JG, McLaren J, Jones JL, Waller DA, O'Byrne KJ. Matrix metalloproteinases 2 and 9 (gelatinases A and B) expression in malignant mesothelioma and benign pleura. *Br J Cancer* 2003; **88**: 1553–9.

93. Schouwink H, Korse CM, Bonfrer JM, Hart AA, Baas P. Prognostic value of the serum tumour markers Cyfra 21–1 and tissue polypeptide antigen in malignant mesothelioma. *Lung Cancer* 1999; **25**: 25–32.

94. Kahlos K, Paakko P, Kurttila E, Soini Y, Kinnula VL. Manganese superoxide dismutase as a diagnostic marker for malignant pleural mesothelioma. *Br J Cancer* 2000; **82**: 1022–9.

95. Kahlos K, Anttila S, Asikainen T, *et al*. Manganese superoxide dismutase in healthy human pleural mesothelium and in malignant pleural mesothelioma. *Am J Respir Cell Mol Biol* 1998; **18**: 570–80.

96. Kinnula K, Linnainmaa K, Raivio KO, Kinnula VL. Endogenous antioxidant enzymes and glutathione S-transferase in protection of mesothelioma cells against hydrogen peroxide and epirubicin toxicity. *Br J Cancer* 1998; **77**: 1097–1102.

97. Kahlos K, Soini Y, Sormunen R, *et al*. Expression and prognostic significance of catalase in malignant mesothelioma. *Cancer* 2001; **91**: 1349–57.

98. Dejmek A, Brockstedt U, Hjerpe A. Optimization of a battery using nine immunocytochemical variables for distinguishing between epithelioid mesothelioma and adenocarcinoma. *APMIS* 1997; **105**: 889–94.

99. Segers K, Kumar-Singh S, Weyler J, *et al*. Glutathione S-transferase expression in malignant mesothelioma and non-neoplastic mesothelium: an immunohistochemical study. *J Cancer Res Clin Oncol* 1996; **122**: 619–24.

100. Beer TW. Immunohistochemical MIB-1 and p27 as prognostic factors in pleural mesothelioma. *Pathol Res Pract* 2001; **197**: 859.

101. Hegmans JP, Radosevic K, Voerman JS, Burgers JA, Hoogsteden HC, Prins JB. A model system for optimising the selection of membrane antigen-specific human antibodies on intact cells using phage antibody display technology. *J Immunol Methods* 2002; **262**: 191–204.

102. Gordon GJ, Jensen RV, Hsiao LL, *et al*. Translation of microarray data into clinically relevant cancer diagnostic tests using gene expression ratios in lung cancer and mesothelioma. *Cancer Res* 2002; **62**: 4963–7.

103. Gordon GJ, Jensen RV, Hsiao LL, *et al*. Using gene expression ratios to predict outcome among patients with mesothelioma. *J Natl Cancer Inst* 2003; **95**: 598–605.

104. Pass HI, Liu Z, Wali A, *et al*. Gene expression profiles predict survival and progression of pleural mesothelioma. *Clin Cancer Res* 2004; **10**: 849–59.

105. Nowak AK, Lake RA, Kindler HL, Robinson BW. New approaches for mesothelioma: biologics, vaccines, gene therapy, and other novel agents. *Semin Oncol* 2002; **29**: 82–96.

106. Schrijvers CT, Coebergh JW, van der Heijden LH, Mackenbach JP. Socioeconomic variation in cancer survival in the southeastern Netherlands, 1980–1989. *Cancer* 1995; **75**: 2946–53.

107. Collette L, Sylvester RJ, Stenning SP, *et al*. Impact of the treating institution on survival of patients with "poor-prognosis" metastatic nonseminoma. European Organization for Research and Treatment of Cancer Genito-Urinary Tract Cancer Collaborative Group and the Medical Research Council Testicular Cancer Working Party. *J Natl Cancer Inst* 1999; **91**: 839–46.

108. Cella DF, Orav EJ, Kornblith AB, *et al*. Socioeconomic status and cancer survival. *J Clin Oncol* 1991; **9**: 1500–9.

109. Campbell NC, Elliott AM, Sharp L, Ritchie LD, Cassidy J, Little J. Impact of deprivation and rural residence on treatment of colorectal and lung cancer. *Br J Cancer* 2002; **87**: 585–90.

110. Vogelzang N, Rusthoven J, Symanowski J, *et al*. Phase III study of pemetrexed in combination with cisplatin versus cisplatin alone in patients with malignant pleural mesothelioma. *J Clin Oncol* 2003; **21**: 2636–44.

111. Cerny T, Blair V, Anderson H, Bramwell V, Thatcher N. Pretreatment prognostic factors and scoring system in 407 small-cell lung cancer patients. *Int J Cancer* 1987; **39**: 146–9.

112. Thatcher N, Anderson H, Burt P, Stout R. The value of anatomic staging and other prognostic factors in small cell lung cancer management: a view of European studies. *Semin Radiat Oncol* 1995; **5**: 19–26.

113. Fennell DA, Parmar A, Shamash J, *et al*. Statistical validation of the EORTC prognostic model for malignant pleural mesothelioma based on three consecutive phase II trials. *J Clin Oncol*. 2005; **23**: 184–9.
114. Mahmoud FA, Rivera NI. The role of C-reactive protein as a prognostic indicator in advanced cancer. *Curr Oncol Rep* 2002; **4**: 250–5.
115. Begg C, Cho M, Eastwood S, *et al*. Improving the quality of reporting of randomized controlled trials. The CONSORT statement. *JAMA* 1996; **276**: 637–9.

Chapter 6

Carcinogenic mechanisms in mesothelioma: effects of asbestos on cell signalling events, transcription factors, and inflammatory cytokines

W. A. Swain and B. T. Mossman

Introduction

Occupational exposure to asbestos fibres, particularly crocidolite asbestos, is associated causally with the vast majority of malignant mesothelioma (MM) [1–3]. The mechanisms of asbestos-induced carcinogenesis have been intensively studied in an effort to establish preventive and therapeutic approaches to MM and other asbestos-related diseases. Studies have largely focused on the properties of asbestos fibres that are important in the development of MM and the mechanisms of action of asbestos in the multistage carcinogenic process. Although asbestos fibres at cytotoxic concentrations cause chromosomal changes, DNA damage, and oxidative DNA lesions in mesothelial cells *in vitro* [4, 5], a more relevant phenomenon leading to alterations in gene expression, proliferation, and transformation may be the stimulation of cell-signalling pathways, including the mitogen-activated protein kinases (MAPKs) and nuclear factor-κB (NF-κB). These pathways may be stimulated through receptor-like mechanisms following fibre–cell interactions [6–8] or via production of reactive oxygen or nitrogen species (ROS or RNS) [9]. Other pathways, such as those mediated by protein kinase C (PKC), may be important in terms of cross-talk or upstream events [9–11].

This chapter focuses on studies suggesting that asbestos-induced cell signalling plays a critical role in MM. The role of MAPK and regulation of the transcription factor activator protein 1 (AP-1) in cell injury, proliferation, and transformation of mesothelial cells by asbestos fibres is reviewed. We then describe pathways leading to the activation of NF-κB, and its role in the resistance of tumour cells to apoptosis and the production of pro-inflammatory cytokines are described. The role of pro-inflammatory cytokines and growth factors, including platelet-derived growth factor (PDGF) and transforming growth factors (TGFs), in growth control of MM are also discussed. Finally, we discuss the potential importance of calcium-signalling pathways and cyclo-oxygenase-2 (COX-2), which is regulated by inflammatory cytokines, in the pathobiology of MM, and the relevance of the overall observations to the treatment of MM.

Role of mitogen-activated protein kinases (MAPKs) and activator protein-1 (AP-1) in mesothelial cell injury, proliferation, and cell transformation

Principles of MAPK activation

MAPK signalling cascades are generally initiated at the cell surface through receptor-dependent or receptor-independent interactions, but their targets are nuclear transcription factors. Different subgroups of MAPK exist. The extracellular signal-regulated protein kinase (ERK) group of MAPKs includes the more widely studied mammalian enzymes ERK1 and ERK2, and other recently characterized family members such as ERK5 or BMK which is induced in epithelial and mesothelial cells by asbestos [12]. The mammalian ERK1 and ERK2 MAPKs are activated by signalling pathways that have a common point of integration, the activation of the small G protein, Ras. Phosphorylated ERKs translocate to the nucleus to phosphorylate the transcription factor, Elk-1, which is essential to the transcriptional activation of c-*fos* [13, 14].

The c-Jun NH$_2$-terminal kinase (JNK) group of MAPKs are cytokine- or stress-activated MAPKs (SAPKs) that are characterized by the dual phosphorylation motif Thr–Pro–Tyr. Three genes that encode mammalian JNK protein kinases are recognized, including the JNK1 and JNK2 genes expressed ubiquitously and the JNK3 gene expressed in brain and testis. Phosphorylation of c-Jun on the NH$_2$-terminal activation domain by JNK leads to increased transcriptional activity [15]. The transcription factors Elk-1 and ATF2 also are regulated by the JNK signalling pathway [16].

The p38 MAPK group with the dual phosphorylation motif Thr–Gly–Try includes four mammalian members (p38α, p38β, p38γ, and p38δ). p38 can be activated by environmental stresses, cytokines, and/or endotoxins, including bacterial lipopolysaccharide [15, 17]. Several studies have established a role of p38 MAPK in gene expression in mammalian cells through activation of the transcription factors activating transcription factor 2 (ATF2) and Elk-1 as well as involvement of other transcription factors (MEF-2C, CHOP, SAP-1) [18].

MAPKs and early-response proto-oncogenes

Regulation of early-response proto-oncogenes, i.e. AP-1 family members, is an important function of MAPK signalling pathways [18]. MAPKs exert regulation at multiple pre-transcriptional, transcriptional, and post-transcriptional steps. Another general mechanism whereby MAPKs regulate gene expression is via regulation of protein degradation. For example, phosphorylation of c-Jun by JNK inhibits its ubiquitination and rapid degradation. Consequently, JNK activation prolongs the half-life of c-Jun [19, 20].

The early-response or AP-1 family proto-oncogenes consist of the *fos* (c-*fos*, *fra*-1, *fra*-2, *fosB*) and *jun* (c-*jun*, *junB*, *junD*) families which encode protein subunits of the AP-1 family of transcription factors [21]. AP-1 complexes consist of Jun–Jun homodimers, Fos–Jun heterodimers, and heterodimers with other basic region leucine zipper (bZIP) proteins such as ATF2 [22]. These complexes control gene expression by recognizing and binding a common DNA sequence element known as the 12-*O*-tetradecanoylphorbol-13-acetate (TPA) response element (TRE) contained in the promoter/enhancer regions of a number of different genes involved in cell proliferation and survival. The specificity of AP-1 function may be dependent on subunit composition of the complexes, as different dimer combinations determine DNA binding affinity and transcriptional activation at different TREs. MAPKs regulate AP-1 transcription factor activity by several mechanisms, including transcriptional regulation of AP-1 genes and phosphorylation of specific Fos and Jun subunit proteins which modulate protein stability and/or transcriptional activity [22].

Activation of extracellular signal-regulated kinases (ERKs), injury, and proliferation of mesothelial cells

In rat pleural mesothelial cells (RPMs), ERK1/2 phosphorylation and ERK2 activity are increased over a protracted time period in response to exposure to chrysotile [$Mg_6Si_4O_{10}(OH)_8$] or crocidolite [$(Na_2(Fe^{3+})_2(Fe^{2+})_3Si_8O_{22}(OH)_2)$] asbestos fibres. In contrast, a number of non-pathogenic particles and glass fibres were found not to transactivate ERK [6]. Activation of ERKs in RPM cells was also seen after addition of epidermal growth factor (EGF) and transforming growth factor α (TGF-α), but not after exposure to PDGF or insulin-like growth factor 1 (IGF-1), suggesting a critical involvement of the EGF receptor (EGFR). Crocidolite asbestos caused autophosphorylation of the EGFR, an event critical to ERK activation in RPM cells, and increased its biosynthesis [7]. To determine the role of oxidant stress in MAPK activation and apoptosis by crocidolite asbestos, patterns of ERK1/2 and JNK1/2 activation by asbestos and H_2O_2 (100–300 µM) were examined in RPM cells [23]. These experiments revealed that transient increases in JNK and ERK activity occurred in a dose-related fashion after exposure to H_2O_2, whereas more protracted activation of ERKs, accompanied by modest increases in JNK1/2, were seen after exposure to asbestos. Both H_2O_2- and asbestos-induced activation of ERKs were inhibited by catalase and chelation of iron from asbestos fibres. Addition of N-acetyl-L-cysteine (NAC) also prevented ERK activation and apoptosis by asbestos. These studies revealed that the MEK1 inhibitor PD98059 abrogated ERK activation and apoptosis by asbestos, confirming a causal relationship between oxidant-induced ERK activation and apoptosis. Immunocytochemistry on the distribution of the extracellular domain of the EGFR in asbestos-exposed human mesothelial cells showed that asbestos fibres also affected EGF binding to the EGFR [8]. Moreover, increased immunoreactivity of EGFR occurred at sites of cell contact with long ($\geq$20 µm) asbestos fibres. A tyrphostin (AG1478) selectively inhibiting the tyrosine kinase activity of the EGFR blocked ERK activation and significantly decreased c-*fos*, but not c-*jun*, mRNA levels in RPM cells as well as apoptosis. These results suggest that ERK1/2 activity is related causally to increased expression of c-*fos* and the development of cell injury and/or cell survival. These results are novel in that they establish a link between ERKs, increased expression/transactivation of c-*fos*, and cell injury, events leading to compensatory cell proliferation in these cell types [24].

ERK1/2-dependent activation of the AP-1 family member *fos*-related antigen 1 (*fra*-1) and links to mesothelioma

Asbestos-induced mesothelial cell transformation is directly linked to increases in AP-1 binding to DNA and the AP-1 component Fra-1 [25]. AP-1 binding to DNA was increased dramatically in rat mesothelioma cell lines in comparison with normal RPM cells. Although elevated levels of AP-1 complexes, including significant increases in c-Jun, JunB and Fra-1, were found in asbestos-exposed RPM cells, only Fra-1 expression was significantly increased and protracted in both asbestos-exposed RPM cells and mesothelioma cell lines. Asbestos-induced Fra-1 expression in RPM cells depended on stimulation of the extracellular signal-regulated kinases (ERKs 1/2). Moreover, inhibition of ERK phosphorylation or transfection with dominant-negative *fra*-1 constructs reversed the transformed phenotype of mesothelioma cells and anchorage-independent growth in soft agar. These studies demonstrate that ERK-dependent Fra-1 is elevated in AP-1 complexes in response to asbestos fibres and is critical to the transformation of mesothelial cells (Figure 6.1).

After oligonucleotide microarray analysis (Affymetrix) of normal RPM cells, RPM cells exposed to crocidolite asbestos, and three rat mesotheliomas, subsets of genes that changed in expression were categorized, including highly upregulated *fra*-1 [26]. Increases in *fra*-1 in both rat and human mesotheliomas and a subset of genes common to both asbestos-exposed RPM cells and mesotheliomas that mimicked *fra*-1 patterns of expression were subsequently confirmed using real-time quantitative polymerase chain reaction (PCR). Using RNA interference technology, we silenced the *fra*-1 gene to determine possible *fra*-1-regulated genes. Results showed that induction of *cd44* and c-*met* were causally linked to *fra*-1 expression, connecting *fra*-1 with genes

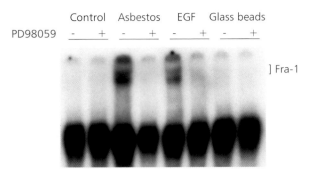

Figure 6.1 Examples of an electrophoretic mobility assay (EMSA) showing DNA binding of the AP-1 transcription factor in rat pleural mesothelial cells. Note that the DNA binding complex is the lower dense band, and the upper complex is Fra-1 as detected with an antibody and supershift analysis. Results show that AP-1 and Fra-1 are increased in the presence of asbestos or EGF and inhibited in the presence of the MEK1/2 inhibitor PD98059 (30 μM). (Reproduced from M. Ramos-Ninos *et al. Cancer Res* 2002; 6 2: 6065–9.)

governing cell motility and invasion in mesothelioma. These studies suggest that inhibition of *fra*-1 signalling pathways may be a strategy for therapy of MM.

Activation of Akt and survival of human mesothelial cells

The phosphotidylinositol 3-kinase (PI3K)/Akt (protein kinase B) pathway plays a central role in the regulation of cell survival. Activation of the pathway and phosphorylation of Akt results in the activation of anti-apoptotic factors such as MDM2 that inhibits p53, and inhibition of a range of pro-apoptotic factors including the forkhead receptor (FKHR) trancription factor, caspase-9 and Bad (see Chapter 8; Figure 8.10). In recent work the capacity of crocidolite asbestos to activate Akt has been studied. Western blot analyses demonstrated that exposure of the SV-40 transformed MET 5A cell line to asbestos resulted in phosphorylation of Akt. This was associated with upregulated tyrosine phosphorylation of EGFR. *In vitro* kinase assays showed criocidolite activated Akt in a time and dose dependent manner. Non-toxic control particulates (polystyrene beads and iron (III) oxide) did not have any effect upon the phosphorylation of Akt [27]. Likewise *in vitro* kinase activity assays demonstrated elevated Akt in human L9/TERT-immortalized human mesothelial cells treated with asbestos (unpublished data).

The activation of Akt in MET 5A cells could be prevented by selective inhibition of PI3K by LY294002 or EGFR/erbB2 tyrosine kinase activity by PKI166. Crocidolite in combination with PKI166 or LY294002 increased the cellular toxicity of crocidolite. The results suggest that the induction of Akt by crocidolite asbestos in MET 5A cells is *via* a signalling pathway linked to EGFR/PI3K activation and this survival signal protects a subpopulation of MET 5A cells from the cellular toxicity of crocidolite [27].

These results were supported by a recently published study in which SV40 was demonstrated to induce cell survival via Akt activation in human mesothelial cells exposed to asbestos. Consequently, prolonged exposure to asbestos fibers progressively induces transformation of SV40-positive mesothelial cells. This has led to a proposed model of SV40/asbestos cocarcinogenesis, in which malignant mesothelioma originates from a subpopulation of transformed stem cells and that Akt signaling plays a key role in this process [28].

Nuclear factor-κB (NF-κB)

Principles of NF-κB activation in inflammation and cancer

NF-κB was first described in 1986 as a transcription factor activated by lipopolysaccharide (LPS) [29]. Since then, the role of NF-κB in both healthy and disease states has become the focus of intense research. NF-κB is a dimeric transcription factor which may be composed of homo- or heterodimers of the Rel family members p65 (RelA), p50 (NF-κB1), p52 (NF-κB2), c-Rel, and RelB [30]. All of these proteins contain a 300 amino acid aminoterminal Rel homology domain (RHD) that is responsible for DNA binding, nuclear localization, and dimerization [31]. p50 and p52 are synthesized as precursors p105 and p100, respectively, from which active transcription factors are released by proteolytic cleavage, whereas p65, RelB and c-Rel contain a transactivation domain [32]. In unstimulated cells, NF-κB is retained in the cytoplasm through its interaction with members of the inhibitors of the NF-κB (IκB) family. Upstream of IκBs are the IκB kinases (IKKs). These proteins are responsible for IκB phosphorylation which leads to its dissociation from NF-κB and subsequent ubiquitin-dependent degradation, allowing NF-κB to enter the nucleus [33].

The complexity of signals upstream of NF-κB allow this transcription factor to be involved in a large number of cellular events including immune and stress responses, inflammation, cell survival, and apoptosis [34]. This is possible through the sheer number of genes containing NF-κB binding sites in their regulatory elements. More than 150 of these genes have been identified to date [35]. These genes fall into a number of categories, but are largely viewed as being important during tissue injury and repair. As a result, NF-κB activation is consistently reported in many models of disease, especially cancers and those involving chronic immune activation.

Many researchers have alluded to the importance of NF-κB in chronic inflammation and cancer. For example, many inflammatory mediators are regulated by NF-κB, and these may be necessary for the development of many cancers. High levels of nuclear NF-κB have also been shown in breast cancer [36], Hodgkin's lymphoma [37], and many other cell lines derived from solid tumours [38]. In these circumstances, it is believed that constitutive activation of NF-κB confers resistance to apoptosis, which may be especially important in allowing tumour cells to resist chemotherapy and radiotherapy [39, 40]. Therefore inhibition of NF-κB in combination with traditional cytotoxic drug regimens may prove to be extremely useful in cancer therapy.

Asbestos-induced activation of NF-κB

Previous studies have shown that crocidolite asbestos induces nuclear accumulation of NF-κB, a phenomenon first noted in hamster tracheal epithelial (HTE) cells, progenitor cells of bronchogenic carcinoma [41]. The presence of both the p65 and p50 subunits within protein–DNA complexes was observed by supershift assays, with the complex containing p65 increasing significantly over time [42]. Moreover, this event was dependent upon production of ROS as incubation with N-acetyl cysteine (NAC) prior to asbestos exposure attenuated the formation of complexes bound to an NF-κB consensus oligonucleotide [44]. This observation was confirmed in a further study, which showed that H_2O_2, a potent source of ROS, could cause increased expression from an NF-κB-dependent luciferase reporter construct in rat lung epithelial (RLE) cells [43]. Moreover, an RNS-generating compound, 3-morpholinosydnonimine (SIN-1), exhibited similar effects in this cell line.

Pulmonary or pleural inflammation often involves the concomitant production of ROS, RNS, and inflammatory cytokines; therefore RLE cells were exposed to H_2O_2/SIN-1 and tumour necrosis factor α (TNF-α) [45]. These combined exposures led to a synergistic increase in the level of NF-κB-dependent transcription, suggesting that a complex set of signals are elicited following exposure to these stimuli, but that they are linked by their convergence on NF-κB. Upon examination of IκB degradation, it was shown that, whilst TNF-α caused rapid degradation of IκB followed by its resynthesis, the ROS/RNS-producing compounds had no such effect. Additionally, a proteosome inhibitor was able to block NF-κB activation induced by TNF-α, but not that induced by SIN-1. However, SIN-1-induced NF-κB activation was blocked by herbimycin, a tyrosine kinase inhibitor. Taken together, these results suggest that the dissociation of IκB from NF-κB may be regulated by two distinct mechanisms: The first is the classically described degradation of the IκB step following exposure to TNF-α and the second involves tyrosine phosphorylation of IκB following exposure to oxidants, a mechanism which has been described by other groups [44].

Later work investigated a role for products of lipid peroxidation in the induction of NF-κB by crocidolite asbestos using a rat lung fibroblast cell line [45]. Preincubation of cells with the membrane-localized antioxidant vitamin E ameliorated the effects of asbestos, a response also noted with an inhibitor of the lipoxygenase pathway, nordihydroguararetic acid (NDGA). These experiments implicate peroxidation of cellular membranes and arachidonic acid metabolism as important steps in asbestos-induced NF-κB activation [45].

Functional consequences of NF-κB DNA binding and activation following asbestos exposure have been demonstrated by a number of groups. For example, crocidolite asbestos upregulates expression of c-*myc* mRNA in HTE cells, as shown by northern blot analysis [42]. In keeping with its role as a pro-inflammatory transcription factor, NF-κB also mediates asbestos-induced TNF-α expression in alveolar macrophages [46]. Subsequent work has shown that RPM and RLE cells exhibit similar responses in NF-κB activation in response to asbestos [47]. Moreover, non-fibrous analogues of crocidolite (riebeckite) and glass beads, which are both non-pathogenic, were unable to mimic the effects of asbestos [47]. Later, Gilmour *et al.* [48] showed that two non-asbestiform fibres, refractory ceramic fibre (RCF)-1 and man-made vitreous fibre (MMVF)-10, were also unable to induce an NF-κB response in macrophages. Additional work from this group tested the ability of a panel of mineral fibres to cause nuclear translocation of NF-κB, which was restricted to cells exposed to carcinogenic fibres, in a lung epithelial tumour cell line [49]. Taken together, these findings strongly suggest that NF-κB DNA binding and activation are common themes in the initial physiological response to carcinogenic fibres. *In vivo* immunoreactivity of p65 also was demonstrated in rat lung bronchiolar epithelial cells following inhalation of either chrysotile or crocidolite as early as 5 days after exposure, an effect that was not seen after 20 days [47]. These findings are crucial as they provide evidence linking observations *in vitro* to those *in vivo*.

NF-κB and mesotheliomas

These observations implicate NF-κB and its associated factors as being crucial in the pathogenesis of malignant mesothelioma, and current studies are underway to investigate a possible role for this factor in resistance of mesothelioma cells to radio- and chemotherapy. The current emergence of targeted biological therapies means that upstream regulators of NF-κB can be targeted specifically. If used either for chemoprevention of this disease or in combination with traditional cytotoxic therapies, targeting of NF-κB in mesotheliomas could represent a means of reducing tumour incidence or minimizing tumour cell resistance to therapy, thus providing new hope for mesothelioma patients.

Pro-inflammatory cytokines induced by asbestos

Recruitment of inflammatory cells following asbestos inhalation is a well-documented phenomenon. A series of rat inhalation experiments have demonstrated the presence of numerous pulmonary immune cells and inflammatory cytokines in bronchial lavage fluid (BALF) from asbestos-exposed animals and from patients with asbestos-associated diseases [50]. However, the significance of these findings is yet to be fully elucidated. Recent years have shown a significant increase in our understanding of these processes, some of which are outlined below.

As its name suggests, TNF-α was initially identified as a factor that had the ability to kill tumour cells [51]. Since then, our knowledge of the role of TNF-α in human carcinogenesis has evolved considerably. A number of studies have now shown that whilst acute high doses of TNF-α are indeed fatal for tumour cells, chronic and lower doses may stimulate growth [52]. This is also true for mesothelial cells. For example, Goldberg et al. [24] demonstrated time-dependent increases in proliferating primary RPM cells following an initial increase in apoptosis after stimulation with 10 ng/ml TNF-α. Moreover, recent studies suggest that the same is true in a simian virus 40 (SV40) transformed human mesothelial cell line (MET5A). Interestingly, a dose–response experiment in this cell line demonstrates that TNF-α has variable effects on cell growth. After 72 h of exposure, doses of 10 and 20 ng/ml induce increases of about 10–15 per cent in cell viability, whereas doses of 50 and 100 ng/ml have no effect [53] (Figure 6.2). Whether the effect of higher doses is cytostatic or a reflection of apoptotic and proliferative processes occurring at equal rates remains to be determined.

Numerous studies have identified the ability of asbestos fibres to upregulate release of TNF-α and/or interleukin 1β (IL-1β) from alveolar macrophages (AMs) [54–58]. This process is believed to arise as a result of 'frustrated phagocytosis', a mechanism employed by AMs when they encounter foreign particles too large to envelope, and is characterized by the release of ROS and pro-inflammatory cytokines such as TNF-α and IL-1β. It may be that frustrated phagocytosis, which one would expect to become more intense with increasing fibre length, may explain the increased pathogenicity of longer fibre preparations *in vivo* [4]. *In vitro* findings by Donaldson *et al.* [54] suggest that this could be the case, as longer amosite fibres induce stronger TNF-α release from AMs than shorter fibres of the same type. A role for fibre opsonization by AMs in this process is demonstrated by elevated TNF-α release following fibre coating with rat immunoglobulin G [54]. Furthermore, the importance of iron-catalysed free radicals in triggering TNF-α release from AMs was demonstrated in a series of experiments by Simeonova and Luster [46]. Incubation with either hydroxyl radical scavengers or deferoxamine, an iron chelator, ameliorated the release of TNF-α, whereas ferrous sulphate and a catalase inhibitor both augmented AM production of TNF-α.

Whilst the relationship between TNF-α and mesothelioma is yet to be fully determined, strong causal evidence exists that provides a link between this cytokine and asbestosis, a form of pulmonary fibrosis. This evidence comes from transgenic experiments in which mice overexpressing TNF-α in alveolar type II epithelial cells spontaneously develop progressive

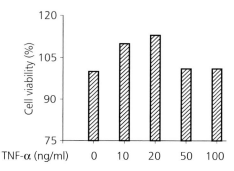

Figure 6.2 Effect of TNF-α on MET5A cell viability.

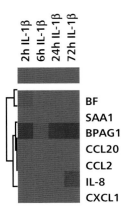

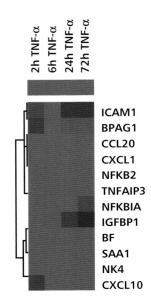

Figure 6.3 Genes expressed more than twofold at all time points.

pulmonary fibrosis [59]. Moreover, in a TNF-α receptor knockout mouse model, no fibroproliferative lesions were noted following exposure to chrysotile asbestos, in contrast with wild-type animals [60].

As with other inflammatory processes, the role of TNF-α and IL-1β release following asbestos exposure is to trigger the production of other cytokines, which in turn recruit further cells of the immune system and maintain the inflammatory response. A recent study investigated the effect of TNF-α and IL-1β when added to mesothelial cells for 72 h using cDNA microarray. Analysis of the data suggests that exposure to these cytokines has a plethora of effects on mesothelial cells [53] (Fig. 6.3). Of particular interest is the sustained increase in expression of genes of the chemokine superfamily. These include CXCL1 (GRO1), which is involved in tumour growth, metastasis, leucocyte infiltration, and angiogenesis [61], CXCL10, which has antiangiogenic properties *in vitro* and is overexpressed in colorectal cancer [62, 63], and CCL20, which may be important in liver tumour cell metastasis [64]. Furthermore, significant elevations in the expression of IL-6 and IL-8 were noted under these conditions. These cytokines have many effects during inflammatory processes; of particular interest to the study of mesothelioma is the ability of IL-8 to induce angiogenesis [65] and proliferation [66]. IL-6 has been shown to be spontaneously produced by mesothelial cells from patients with non-malignant pleural effusions, and addition of a neutralizing monoclonal antibody for IL-6 inhibited growth of these cells *in vitro*, suggesting a role for IL-6 as an autocrine growth factor [67].

A comprehensive study by Simeonova *et al.* [68] examined asbestos-induced IL-6 production in epithelial cells. Asbestos fibres stimulated IL-6 secretion in both A549 malignant and normal human bronchial epithelial cells (NHBE). The induction of IL-6 was dependent on oxidative stress, since intracellular hydroxyl scavengers and NAC abrogated IL-6 secretion by asbestos or H_2O_2 which was mediated through activation of NF-κB. Furthermore, increased IL-6 levels were found in bronchial lavage fluid from patients with occupational exposure to asbestos.

Studies by Driscoll *et al.* [69,70] sought to evaluate the interrelationship between asbestos inhalation and subsequent inflammatory events due to the production of chemotactic cytokines. These studies showed increased release of TNF-α, IL-1β and the chemotactic cytokines macrophage inflammatory protein 2 (MIP-2) and cytokine-induced neutrophil chemoattractant

(CINC) in the bronchoalveolar fluid of asbestos-exposed animals compared with sham treated controls. A study by Tanaka *et al.* [71] demonstrated the direct release of another chemokine, monocyte chemoattractant protein 1 (MCP-1), by rat pleural mesothelial cells both *in vitro* and *in vivo*, an effect that was potentiated by co-stimulation with either TNF-α or IL-1β. Ishihara *et al.* [72] investigated the effect of three types of asbestos dusts on human pulmonary macrophages *ex vivo*. This study focused on the synthesis and release of a number of cytokines, including TNF-α, IL-1β, MIP-1, IL-8, and GROα/CXCL1. All were released in increased quantities in asbestos-exposed cells. However, the production of basic fibroblast growth factor (bFGF), transforming growth factors β_1 and β_2 (TGF-β_1 and TGF-β_2), and platelet-derived growth factors A and B (PDGF-A and PDGF-B) appeared to be unaltered under these conditions in this study, although others have observed increases in these growth factors in other models [50].

PDGF and mesothelioma

PDGF may exist as either a homodimer or heterodimers of A and B chains, which in turn are recognized by either PDGF receptor α (PDGFR-α) or PDGF receptor β (PDGFR-β). A number of studies have alluded to the importance of PDGF and its cognate receptors in the pathogenesis of mesothelioma. PDGF can activate an array of diverse cellular responses which control rates of apoptosis, proliferation, chemotaxis, and survival [73]. Thus PDGF signalling is an attractive target in the study of human carcinogenesis. Gerwin *et al.* [74] performed much of the early research in this area which showed that mesothelioma cell lines expressed higher levels of PDGF-A and PDGF-B chain mRNA than their non-transformed counterparts. These findings were strengthened by further studies showing that the PDGF-B chain was strongly expressed in mesothelioma cell lines, whilst being virtually undetectable in normal cell lines. Furthermore, PDGF-A chain expression was slightly elevated in cancer-derived cells [75, 76]. These observations were mirrored in a study examining the expression of these receptors in serous effusions from patients with either benign disease or MM [77]. Finally, Langerak *et al.* [78] confirmed these trends in examination of normal and malignant mesothelial cells from both cell lines and frozen tissue sections. In another study, examination of PDGFR subtypes showed that human mesothelioma cell lines expressed β receptors almost exclusively, whereas the opposite is true in mesothelial cell lines. These results led to the hypothesis that autocrine stimulation is via PDGF-AA/PDGFR-α in mesothelial cells and PDGF-BB/PDGF-β in mesothelioma cells [76].

Direct evidence linking overexpression of PDGF-A to tumorigenicity has been demonstrated in MET5A cells. Researchers showed that cells overexpressing PDGF-A were able to induce tumours in athymic mice; moreover, PDGF-A overexpression was present in excised tumour specimens [79]. PDGF-A overexpression has recently been shown to have paradoxical effects *in vitro* and *in vivo*. Abrogation of PDGF-A expression in mesothelioma cell lines *in vitro* stimulates growth, whereas overexpression is antiproliferative. However, the opposite is true *in vivo*, where overexpression increases tumour incidence and growth rate while increasing the latency period, and abrogation decreases tumour incidence while increasing latency [80].

Another body of work focused on early events in the disease process by measuring the level of PDGF-A and PDGF-B mRNA and protein in rat lungs following a single 5 h exposure to chrysotile asbestos. The authors reported elevated levels of both PDGF-A and PDGF-B mRNA by *in situ* hybridization and protein by immunohistochemistry at 24 h post-exposure which remained detectable for 2 weeks [81]. Another study using RPM cells showed that transformed cells from this species do not express detectable levels of either PDGF chain, suggesting that PDGF-mediated autocrine signalling is not an important factor in models of rodent mesothelioma [82]. This research is now being extrapolated from the laboratory to the clinic by a phase II trial currently underway to test the efficacy of STI-571 (Gleevec), a PDGF receptor inhibitor, in malignant mesothelioma. This drug is also a highly selective inhibitor of the tyrosine kinases associated with activation of c-Kit and Bcr-Abl.

Transforming growth factors and mesothelioma

Another family of growth factors that are hypothesized to play a role in the mesothelioma disease process are the transforming growth factors (TGFs), of which there are two superfamilies, TGF-α and TGF-β. TGF-α is able to modulate many cellular responses through its ability to bind and activate the epidermal growth factor receptor (EGFR), which in turn activates downstream signalling pathways such as the extracellular signal regulated kinase (ERK) pathway. TGF-β also plays a role in inducing extracellular matrix production, modulating growth and immune responses, and is also known to inhibit the growth of many solid tumours [83].

TGF-α is expressed and secreted by asbestos-transformed rat mesothelial cells and stimulates their growth, Moreover, a neutralizing antibody for TGF-α inhibits growth of these cells [84]. In keeping with these observations, at least one human mesothelioma cell line (ZL34) also has an autocrine growth loop involving TGF-α [85]. TGF-β_1 is growth inhibitory in many epithelial cell types; however, mesothelial cells demonstrate increases in DNA synthesis following stimulation with this cytokine, suggesting that mesothelial cells do not share common epithelial cell-growth regulatory mechanisms [86]. Furthermore, transfection of mesothelioma cells with antisense TGF-β oligonucleotides leads to inhibition of DNA synthesis and proliferation both *in vitro* and *in vivo* [87]. Additionally, downregulation of TGF-β reduces anchorage-independent growth *in vitro* and tumorigenicity *in vivo* of human and murine MM cells [88]. The early involvement of TGF-β following exposure to asbestos has been demonstrated in studies showing its expression in cells at sites of deposition following exposure to asbestos [89]. In this setting, it is believed that TGF-β switches on genes involved in formation of the extracellular matrix and ensuing formation of fibrotic lesions [90].

Ca^{2+}-dependent signalling pathways induced by asbestos

Modulation of intracellular calcium ($[Ca^{2+}]_i$) levels through a variety of mechanisms can regulate a number of cellular processes. The source of calcium may be either from the extracellular compartment or from intracellular stores such as those found in the endoplasmic reticulum. The effects of fluctuating calcium levels are mediated through calcium-binding proteins, such as calmodulin (CaM), which undergo a conformational change when the concentration of intracellular calcium changes. Under these conditions, the affinity of CaM for a discrete subset of proteins [e.g. CaM-dependent kinases (CaMKs) I, II, III, IV, and V, and calcineurin (a protein phosphatase)] increases. In turn, these proteins will act upon their associated effectors and downstream effects will ensue.

The earliest studies of the effect of asbestos exposure on intracellular calcium showed that exposure of polymorphonuclear leucocytes (PMNs) to chrysotile asbestos increased cell membrane permeability. This was demonstrated by the release of lactate dehydrogenase, an effect not observed in the absence of extracellular calcium [91]. Tuomala *et al.* [92] showed that chrysotile, quartz, and formyl-methionyl-leucyl-phenylalanine (fMLP) were all able to induce increases in $[Ca^{2+}]_i$ that were rapid and transient with fMLP, but slow and sustained with the two minerals. Moreover, the authors showed concomitant release of ROS, and suggested that these phenomena may be linked functionally. These data are in keeping with a previous study [93] showing similar effects in alveolar macrophages. However, this study demonstrated a possible link between calcium entry and ROS, as calcium-channel antagonists, such as verapamil, were able to block calcium entry and superoxide anion production at least partially. A link between these events and DNA strand breaks was shown in white blood cells treated with crocidolite asbestos, an effect that was abrogated by the intracellular calcium chelator Quin-2 [94].

Recently, we tested the hypothesis that asbestos-induced calcium influx into cells was functionally related to phosphorylation of ERK1 and ERK2 and the calcium-regulated transcription factor CREB (calcium–cAMP-response element binding protein) in murine epithelial (C10) cells [95]. Ca^{2+} was imaged in single cells using a CaM–FRET construct, and phospho-ERK1/2 and phosphor-CREB were detected by immunocytochemistry. Following exposures to crocidolite asbestos, increases in phospho-CREB were detected as early as 30 minutes, whereas phospho-ERK1 and phospho-ERK2 increased at 4 h. Reducing extracellular Ca^{2+} prevented phosphorylation of CREB but not of ERK1 or ERK2. These results suggest that calcium signalling is important in regulation of some transcription factors.

Given the involvement of calcium in many key cellular processes, it seems likely that it will play a role in functional responses to asbestos, including the carcinogenic process. To date, however, these interactions have not been fully explored and represent an area worthy of future study.

Cyclo-oxygenase-2 in mesothelioma

Cyclo-oxygenase 1 and 2 (COX-1 and COX-2) are isoforms of an enzyme that is involved in prostaglandin synthesis. COX-1 is constitutively expressed in all tissues, whereas COX-2 is inducible, only being expressed following activation of upstream inflammatory elements. Thus these enzymes represent a key point of regulation in the inflammatory process. Moreover, a large body of evidence has shown that abnormal regulation of COX-2 expression is important in solid tumour growth, angiogenesis, and invasiveness. The largest body of research is focused on the role of COX-2 in colorectal carcinogenesis. Transgenic mice which lack the adenomatous polyposis coli (APC) tumour gene are unusually prone to colonic tumours. A series of recent studies have shown that genetic knockout or pharmacological inhibition of COX-2 reduces the numbers of tumours in these animals [96, 97]. As previously mentioned, mesothelioma develops in an environment of chronic inflammatory activation. This knowledge led researchers to investigate a possible role for COX-2 in the pathobiology of this disease.

Initially, COX-2 expression was described in cultured primary mesothelial cells sloughed from the pleural surface. Incubation of these cells with polyunsaturated fatty acids followed by high-performance liquid chromatography (HPLC) demonstrated the presence of reaction products that were indicative of cyclo-oxygenase activity [98]. A later study investigated the regulation of prostaglandin synthesis and the levels of COX-1 and COX-2 mRNA expression in mesothelial cells following exposure to IL-1β or TNF-α. These inflammatory cytokines increased prostaglandin synthesis in a time- and dose-dependent manner, an effect that was inhibited by preincubation with either dexamethasone or neutralizing antibodies. Moreover, COX-1 and COX-2 mRNA expression was increased in a time-dependent manner following stimulation with these cytokines, with the greatest increase seen for COX-2 [99]. COX-2 expression has been observed in human mesothelioma tumour samples, but not in benign tissue. Moreover, mesothelioma cell lines are acutely sensitive to growth arrest by selective COX-2 inhibitors [100]. More recently, elevated COX-2 expression has been associated with poor prognosis in mesothelioma patients [101].

The roles of COX-2 in the progression of mesothelioma and its potential as a therapeutic target are currently subject to further investigation. The findings discussed above and in other experimental systems suggest that future studies to fully elucidate the role of COX-2 in the carcinogenesis of malignant mesothelioma are merited. Moreover, COX-2 inhibition might be advantageous in preventive or therapeutic approaches to mesothelioma.

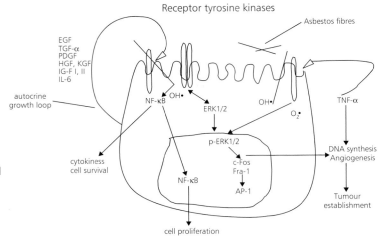

Figure 6.4 The induction of the AP-1 and NF-κB signalling pathways by asbestos in mesothelial cells and their implications in cytokine production, cell survival, and cell proliferation.

Summary and conclusions

The studies summarized in this chapter show that asbestos elicits a number of signalling pathways in mesothelial cells and lung epithelial cells that may be related to the initiation and development of mesotheliomas and/or lung cancers (Fig 6.4). Most notable is the involvement of receptor-dependent signalling pathways (EGFR, PDGF receptors) that may contribute to the growth and survival of these cell types as well as stromal or angiogenic factors contributing to cell invasion or angiogenesis. In addition, the NF-κB pathway may contribute to cell survival as well as resistance to chemotherapy. For these reasons, and because malignant mesotheliomas are known to produce multiple growth factors through autocrine mechanisms, use of cell-signalling-targeted approaches combined with chemotherapy or radiotherapy may be essential in the therapy of mesotheliomas. A number of novel agents are presently being used or advocated for use in clinical trials in the USA and other countries. These include EGFR inhibitors (Iressa, Tarceva), PDGF inhibitors (Gleevec), VEGF inhibitors (SU5416, bevacizumab, thalidomide, PTK 787) and proteosome inhibitors (bortezomib). These are primarily specific for the aforementioned receptor tyrosine kinases but are also known to inhibit other receptor kinases, a potentially attractive aspect. Historically, chemotherapy and ablative surgery have had little impact on survival of patients with MM, but promising new drugs, including novel agents that target signalling cascades, are being developed. Use of these in combination with conventional therapies may provide strategies that will aid in treatment of MM.

Acknowledgements

We acknowledge the assistance of Laurie Sabens, Beth Langford-Corrigan, and Masha Stern in the preparation of this chapter. The research in BM's laboratory is presently supported by grants from NIEHS, NCI, and NHLBI.

References

1. Mossman B, Gee J. Asbestos related disease. *N Engl J Med* 1989; **320**: 1721–30.
2. Mossman B, Bignon J, Corn M, Seaton A, Gee J. Asbestos: scientific developments and implications for public policy. *Science* 1990; **247**: 294–301.

3. Mossman BT, Kamp DW, Weitzman SA. Mechanisms of carcinogenesis and clinical features of asbestos-associated cancers. *Cancer Invest* 1996; **14**: 466–80.

4. *Asbestos in Public and Commercial Buildings: A Literature Reviewed Synthesis of Current Knowledge.* Cambridge, MA: Health Effects Institute, 1991.

5. Fung H, Kow Y, Van Houten B, Mossman B. Patterns of 8-hydroxydeoxyguanosine (8OHdG) formation in DNA and indications of oxidative stress in rat and human pleural mesothelial cells after exposure to crocidolite asbestos. *Carcinogenesis* 1997; **18**: 101–8.

6. Zanella C, Posada J, Tritton T, Mossman B. Asbestos causes stimulation of the ERK-1 mitogen-activated protein kinase cascade after phosphorylation of the epidermal growth factor receptor. *Cancer Res.* 1996; **56**: 5334–8.

7. Zanella C, Timblin C, Cummins A, *et al.* Asbestos-induced phosphorylation of epidermal growth factor receptor is linked to c-*fos* expression and apoptosis. *Am J Physiol* 1999; **277**: L684–93.

8. Pache J, Janssen Y, Walsh E, *et al.* Increased epidermal growth factor-receptor (EGF-R) protein in a human mesothelial cell line in response to long asbestos fibers. *Am J Pathol* 1998; **152**: 333–340

9. Shukla A, Stern M, Lounsbury K, Flanders T, Mossman B. Asbestos-induced apoptosis is protein kinase C delta-dependent. *Am J Respir Cell Mol Biol* 2003; **198**: 205–8.

10. Fung H, Kow Y, Van Houten B, *et al.* Asbestos increases mammalian major AP-endonuclease (APE) gene expression, protein levels and enzyme activity in rat pleural mesothelial cells. *Cancer Res* 1998; **58**: 189–94.

11. Lounsbury KM, Stern M, Taatjes D, Jaken S, Mossman BT. Increased localization and substrate activation of protein kinase C delta in lung epithelial cells following exposure to asbestos. *Am J Pathol* 2002; **160**: 1991–2000.

12. Scapoli L, Ramos-Nino M, Martinelli M, Mossman B. Src-dependent ERK5 and Src/EGFR-dependent ERK1/2 activation is required for cell proliferation by asbestos. *Oncogene* 2004; **23**: 805–13.

13. Gille H, Sharrocks A, Shaw P. Phosphorylation of transcription factor p62TCF by MAP kinase stimulates ternary complex formation at c-*fos* promoter. *Nature* 1992; **358**: 414–17.

14. Marais R, Wynne J, Treisman R. The SRF accessory protein Elk-1 contains a growth factor-regulated transcriptional activation domain. *Cell* 1993; **73**: 381–93.

15. Whitmarsh A, Yang S, Su M, Sharrocks A, Davis R. Role of p38 and JNK mitogen-activated protein kinases in the activation of ternary complex factors. *Mol Cell Biol* 1997; **17**: 2360–71

16. Ip YT, Davis RJ. Signal transduction by the c-Jun N-terminal kinase (JNK)–from inflammation to development. *Curr Opin Cell Biol* 1998; **10**: 205–19.

17. Han J, Lee J, Bibbs L, Ulevitch R. A MAP kinase targeted by endotoxin and hyperosmolarity in mammalian cells. *Science* 1994; **265**: 808–11.

18. Rincón M, Flavell R, Davis R. The JNK and p38 MAP kinase signaling pathways in T-cell mediated immune responses. *Free Radic Biol Med* 2000; **28**: 1328–37.

19. Fuchs S, Dolan L, Davis R, Ronai Z. Phosphorylation-dependent targeting of c-Jun ubiquitination by Jun N-kinase. *Oncogene* 1996; **13**: 1531–5.

20. Musti A, Treier M, Bohmann D. Reduced ubiquitin-dependent degradation of c-Jun after phosphorylation by MAP kinases. *Science* 1997; **275**: 400–2.

21. Reddy S, Mossman B. Role and regulaton of activator protein-1 in toxicant-induced responses of the lung. *Am J Physiol* 2002; **283**: L1161–78.

22. Karin M, Liu A, Zandi E. AP-1 function and regulation. *Curr Opin Cell Biol* 1997; **9**: 240–6.

23. Jimenez L, Zanella C, Fung H, *et al.* Role of extracellular signal-regulated protein kinases in apoptosis by asbestos and H_2O_2. *Am J Physiol* 1997; **273**: L1029–35.

24. Goldberg JL, Zanella CL, Janssen YM, *et al.* Novel cell imaging techniques show induction of apoptosis and proliferation in mesothelial cells by asbestos. *Am J Respir Cell Mol Biol* 1997; **17**: 265–71.

25. Ramos-Ninos M, Timblin C, Mossman B. Mesothelial cell transformation requires increased AP-1 binding activity and ERK-dependent Fra-1 expression. *Cancer Res* 2002; **62**: 6065–9.

26. Ramos-Ninos M, Scapoli L, Martinelli M, Land S, Mossman B. Microarray analysis and RNA silencing link *fra-1* to *cd44* and *c-met* expression in mesothelioma. *Cancer Res* 2003; **63**: 3539–45.

27. Swain W, O'Byrne KJ, Houghton C, Edwards JE, Faux S. EGFR activation of the PI3K/Akt pathway plays a role in human mesothelial cell survival following asbestos exposure. *Proc Am Assoc Cancer Res* 2002; **43**: abstract 1747.

28. Cacciotti P, Barbone D, Porta C, *et al.* SV40-dependent AKT activity drives mesothelial cell transformation after asbestos exposure. *Cancer Res* 2005 Jun 15; **65**(12): 5256–62.

29. Sen R, Baltimore D. Multiple nuclear factors interact with the immunoglobulin enhancer sequences. *Cell* 1986; **46**: 705–16.

30. Mercurio F, Manning AM. NF-kappaB as a primary regulator of the stress response. *Oncogene* 1999; **18**: 6163–71.

31. Kunsch C, Ruben SM, Rosen CA. Selection of optimal kappa B/Rel DNA-binding motifs: interaction of both subunits of NF-kappa B with DNA is required for transcriptional activation. *Mol Cell Biol* 1992; **12**: 4412–21.

32. Zhong H, SuYang H, Erdjument-Bromage H, Tempst P, Ghosh S. The transcriptional activity of NF-kappaB is regulated by the IkappaB-associated PKAc subunit through a cyclic AMP-independent mechanism. *Cell* 1997; **89**: 413–24.

33. Lee FS, Peters RT, Dang LC, Maniatis T. MEKK1 activates both IkappaB kinase alpha and IkappaB kinase beta. *Proc Natl Acad Sci USA* 1998; **95**: 9319–24.

34. Li N, Karin M. Is NF-kappaB the sensor of oxidative stress? *FASEB J* 1999; **13**: 1137–43.

35. Pahl HL. Activators and target genes of Rel/NF-kappaB transcription factors. *Oncogene* 1999; **18**: 6853–66.

36. Nakshatri H, Bhat-Nakshatri P, Martin DA, Goulet RJ Jr, Sledge GW Jr. Constitutive activation of NF-kappaB during progression of breast cancer to hormone-independent growth. *Mol Cell Biol* 1997; **17**: 3629–39.

37. Sovak MA, Bellas RE, Kim DW, *et al.* Aberrant nuclear factor-kappaB/Rel expression and the pathogenesis of breast cancer. *J Clin Invest* 1997; **100**: 2952–60.

38. Visconti R, Cerutti J, Battista S, *et al.* Expression of the neoplastic phenotype by human thyroid carcinoma cell lines requires NFkappaB p65 protein expression. *Oncogene* 1997; **15**: 1987–94.

39. Van Antwerp DJ, Martin SJ, Kafri T, Green DR, Verma IM. Suppression of TNF-alpha-induced apoptosis by NF-kappaB. *Science* 1996; **274**: 787–9.

40. Beg AA, Baltimore D. An essential role for NF-kappaB in preventing TNF-alpha-induced cell death. *Science* 1996; **274**: 782–4.

41. Janssen YM, Heintz NH, Mossman BT. Induction of *c-fos* and *c-jun* proto-oncogene expression by asbestos is ameliorated by *N*-acetyl-L-cysteine in mesothelial cells. *Cancer Res* 1995; **55**: 2085–9.

42. Janssen YM, Barchowsky A, Treadwell M, Driscoll KE, Mossman BT. Asbestos induces nuclear factor kappa B (NF-kappa B) DNA-binding activity and NF-kappa B-dependent gene expression in tracheal epithelial cells. *Proc Natl Acad Sci USA* 1995; **92**: 8458–62.

43. Janssen-Heininger YM, Macara I, Mossman BT. Cooperativity between oxidants and tumor necrosis factor in the activation of nuclear factor (NF)-kappaB: requirement of Ras/mitogen-activated protein kinases in the activation of NF-kappaB by oxidants. *Am J Respir Cell Mol Biol* 1999; **20**: 942–52.

44. Imbert V, Rupec RA, Livolsi A, *et al.* Tyrosine phosphorylation of I kappa B-alpha activates NF-kappa B without proteolytic degradation of I kappa B-alpha. *Cell* 1996; **86**: 787–98.

45. Faux SP, Howden PJ. Possible role of lipid peroxidation in the induction of NF-kappa B and AP-1 in RFL-6 cells by crocidolite asbestos: evidence following protection by vitamin E. *Environ Health Perspect* 1997; **105** (Suppl 5): 1127–30.

46. Simeonova AP, Luster MI. Iron and reactive oxygen species in the asbestos-induced tumor necrosis factor-alpha response from alveolar macrophages. *Am J Respir Cell Mol Biol* 1995; **12**: 676–83.

47. Janssen YM, Driscoll KE, Howard B, *et al*. Asbestos causes translocation of p65 protein and increases NF-kappa B DNA binding activity in rat lung epithelial and pleural mesothelial cells. *Am J Pathol* 1997; **151**: 389–401.

48. Gilmour PS, Brown DM, Beswick PH, MacNee W, Rahman I, Donaldson K. Free radical activity of industrial fibers: role of iron in oxidative stress and activation of transcription factors. *Environ Health Perspect* 1997; **105** (Suppl 5): 1313–17.

49. Brown DM, Beswick PH, Donaldson K. Induction of nuclear translocation of NF-kappaB in epithelial cells by respirable mineral fibres. *J Pathol* 1999; **189**: 258–64.

50. Mossman BT, Churg A. Mechanisms in the pathogenesis of asbestosis and silicosis. *Am J Respir Crit Care Med* 1998; **157**: 1666–80.

51. Carswell EA, Old LJ, Kassel RL, Green S, Fiore N, Williamson B. An endotoxin-induced serum factor that causes necrosis of tumors. *Proc Natl Acad Sci USA* 1975; **72**: 3666–70.

52. Balkwill F. Tumor necrosis factor or tumor promoting factor? *Cytokine Growth Factor Rev* 2002; **13**: 135–41.

53. Swain WA, Sander LS, Gant TW, Faux SP, O'Byrne KJ. Microarray analysis of mesothelial cells treated with crocidolite, erionite, IL-1beta and TNF-alpha. *Lung Cancer* 2003;**41**: S25.

54. Donaldson K, Li XY, Dogra S, Miller BG, Brown GM. Asbestos-stimulated tumour necrosis factor release from alveolar macrophages depends on fibre length and opsonization. *J Pathol* 1992; **168**: 243–8.

55. Dubois CM, Bissonnette E, Rola-Pleszczynski M. Asbestos fibers and silica particles stimulate rat alveolar macrophages to release tumor necrosis factor. Autoregulatory role of leukotriene B4. *Am Rev Respir Dis* 1989; **139**: 1257–64.

56. Geist LJ, Powers LS, Monick MM, Hunninghake GW. Asbestos stimulation triggers differential cytokine release from human monocytes and alveolar macrophages. *Exp Lung Res* 2000; **26**: 41–56.

57. Ljungman AG, Lindahl M, Tagesson C. Asbestos fibres and man made mineral fibres: induction and release of tumour necrosis factor-alpha from rat alveolar macrophages. *Occup Environ Med* 1994; **51**: 777–83.

58. Mongan LC, Jones T, Patrick G. Cytokine and free radical responses of alveolar macrophages *in vitro* to asbestos fibres. *Cytokine* 2000; **12**: 1243–7.

59. Miyazaki Y, Araki K, Vesin C, *et al*. Expression of a tumor necrosis factor-alpha transgene in murine lung causes lymphocytic and fibrosing alveolitis. A mouse model of progressive pulmonary fibrosis. *J Clin Invest* 1995; **96**: 250–9.

60. Liu JY, Brass DM, Hoyle GW, Brody AR. TNF-alpha receptor knockout mice are protected from the fibroproliferative effects of inhaled asbestos fibers. *Am J Pathol* 1998; **153**: 1839–47.

61. Loukinova E, Dong G, Enamorado-Ayalya I, *et al*. Growth regulated oncogene-alpha expression by murine squamous cell carcinoma promotes tumor growth, metastasis, leukocyte infiltration and angiogenesis by a host CXC receptor-2 dependent mechanism. *Oncogene* 2000; **19**: 3477–86.

62. Angiolillo AL, Sgadari C, Taub DD, *et al*. Human interferon-inducible protein 10 is a potent inhibitor of angiogenesis *in vivo*. *J Exp Med* 1995; **182**: 155–62.

63. Zhang R, Zhang H, Zhu W, Pardee AB, Coffey RJ Jr, Liang P. Mob-1, a Ras target gene, is overexpressed in colorectal cancer. *Oncogene* 1997; **14**: 1607–10.

64. Dellacasagrande J, Schreurs OJ, Hofgaard PO, *et al*. Liver metastasis of cancer facilitated by chemokine receptor CCR6. *Scand J Immunol* 2003; **57**: 534–44.

65. Antony VB, Hott JW, Godbey SW, Holm K. Angiogenesis in mesotheliomas. Role of mesothelial cell derived IL-8. *Chest* **109** (Suppl): 21S–2S.

66. Galffy G, Mohammed KA, Dowling PA, Nasreen N, Ward MJ, Antony VB. Interleukin 8: an autocrine growth factor for malignant mesothelioma. *Cancer Res* **59**: 367–71.

67. Fujino S, Yokoyama A, Kohno N, Hiwada K. Interleukin 6 is an autocrine growth factor for normal human pleural mesothelial cells. *Am J Respir Cell Mol Biol* 1996; **14**: 508–15.

68. Simeonova PP, Toriumi W, Kommineni C, *et al.* Molecular regulation of IL-6 activation by asbestos in lung epithelial cells: role of reactive oxygen species. *J Immunol* 1997; **159**: 3921–8.

69. Driscoll KE, Maurer JK, Higgins J, Poynter J. Alveolar macrophage cytokine and growth factor production in a rat model of crocidolite-induced pulmonary inflammation and fibrosis. *J Toxicol Environ Health* 1995; **46**: 155–69.

70. Driscoll KE, Hassenbein DG, Carter JM, Kunkel SL, Quinlan TR, Mossman BT. TNF alpha and increased chemokine expression in rat lung after particle exposure. *Toxicol Lett* 1995; **82–83**: 483–9.

71. Tanaka S, Choe N, Iwagaki A, Hemenway DR, Kagan E. Asbestos exposure induces MCP-1 secretion by pleural mesothelial cells. *Exp Lung Res* 2000; **26**: 241–55.

72. Ishihara Y, Kohyama N, Kagawa J. Contribution of human pulmonary macrohage-derived cytokines to asbestos-induced lung inflammation and fibrosis. *Inhal Toxicol* 1998; **10**: 205–25.

73. Rosenkranz S, Kazlauskas A. Evidence for distinct signaling properties and biological responses induced by the PDGF receptor alpha and beta subtypes. *Growth Factors* 1999; **16**: 201–16.

74. Gerwin BI, Lechner JF, Reddel RR, *et al.* Comparison of production of transforming growth factor-beta and platelet-derived growth factor by normal human mesothelial cells and mesothelioma cell lines. *Cancer Res* 1987; **47**: 6180–4.

75. Versnel MA, Hagemeijer A, Bouts MJ, van der Kwast TH, Hoogsteden HC. Expression of c-*sis* (PDGF B-chain) and PDGF A-chain genes in ten human malignant mesothelioma cell lines derived from primary and metastatic tumors. *Oncogene* 1988; **2**: 601–5.

76. Versnel MA, Claesson-Welsh L, Hammacher A, *et al.* Human malignant mesothelioma cell lines express PDGF beta-receptors whereas cultured normal mesothelial cells express predominantly PDGF alpha-receptors. *Oncogene* 1991; **6**: 2005–11.

77. Ascoli V, Scalzo CC, Facciolo F, Nardi F. Platelet-derived growth factor receptor immunoreactivity in mesothelioma and nonneoplastic mesothelial cells in serous effusions. *Acta Cytol* 1995; **39**: 613–22.

78. Langerak AW, De Laat PA, Van Der Linden-Van Beurden CA, *et al.* Expression of platelet-derived growth factor (PDGF) and PDGF receptors in human malignant mesothelioma *in vitro* and *in vivo*. *J Pathol* 1996; **178**: 151–60.

79. Van der Meeren A, Seddon MB, Betsholtz CA, Lechner JF, Gerwin BI. Tumorigenic conversion of human mesothelial cells as a consequence of platelet-derived growth factor-A chain overexpression. *Am J Respir Cell Mol Biol* 1993; **8**: 214–21.

80. Metheny-Barlow LJ, Flynn B, van Gijssel HE, Marrogi A, Gerwin BI. Paradoxical effects of platelet-derived growth factor-A overexpression in malignant mesothelioma. Antiproliferative effects *in vitro* and tumorigenic stimulation *in vivo*. *Am J Respir Cell Mol Biol* 2001; **24**: 694–702.

81. Liu JY, Morris GF, Lei WH, Hart CE, Lasky JA, Brody AR. Rapid activation of PDGF-A and -B expression at sites of lung injury in asbestos-exposed rats. *Am J Respir Cell Mol Biol* 1997; **17**: 129–40.

82. Walker C, Bermudez E, Stewart W, Bonner J, Molloy CJ, Everitt J. Characterization of platelet-derived growth factor and platelet-derived growth factor receptor expression in asbestos-induced rat mesothelioma. *Cancer Res* 1992; **52**: 301–6.

83. Yue J, Mulder KM. Transforming growth factor-beta signal transduction in epithelial cells. *Pharmacol Ther* 2001; **91**: 1–34.

84. Walker C, Everitt J, Ferriola PC, Stewart W, Mangum J, Bermudez E. Autocrine growth stimulation by transforming growth factor alpha in asbestos-transformed rat mesothelial cells. *Cancer Res* 1995; **55**: 530–6.

85. Morocz IA, Schmitter D, Lauber B, Stahel RA. Autocrine stimulation of a human lung mesothelioma cell line is mediated through the transforming growth factor alpha/epidermal growth factor receptor mitogenic pathway. *Br J Cancer* 1994; **70**: 850–6.

86. Gabrielson EW, Gerwin BI, Harris CC, Roberts AB, Sporn MB, Lechner JF. Stimulation of DNA synthesis in cultured primary human mesothelial cells by specific growth factors. *FASEB J* 1988; **2**: 2717–21.

87. Marzo AL, Fitzpatrick DR, Robinson BW, Scott B. Antisense oligonucleotides specific for transforming growth factor beta2 inhibit the growth of malignant mesothelioma both *in vitro* and *in vivo*. *Cancer Res* 1997; **57**: 3200–7.

88. Fitzpatrick DR, Bielefeldt-Ohmann H, Himbeck RP, Jarnicki AG, Marzo AL, Robinson BW. Transforming growth factor-beta: antisense RNA-mediated inhibition affects anchorage-independent growth, tumorigenicity and tumor-infiltrating T-cells in malignant mesothelioma. *Growth Factors* 1994; **11**: 29–44.

89. Brody AR, Liu JY, Brass D, Corti M. Analyzing the genes and peptide growth factors expressed in lung cells *in vivo* consequent to asbestos exposure and *in vitro*. *Environ Health Perspect* 1997; **105** (Suppl 5): 1165–71.

90. Dai J, Churg A. Relationship of fiber surface iron and active oxygen species to expression of procollagen, PDGF-A, and TGF-beta(1) in tracheal explants exposed to amosite asbestos. *Am J Respir Cell Mol Biol* 2001; **24**: 427–35.

91. Elferink JG, Deierkauf M, Kramps JA, Koerten HK. The involvement of ionic interactions during asbestos-induced enzyme release from polymorphonuclear leukocytes. *Chem Biol Interact* 1989; **72**: 215–27.

92. Tuomala M, Hirvonen MR, Savolainen KM. Changes in free intracellular calcium and production of reactive oxygen metabolites in human leukocytes by soluble and particulate stimuli. *Toxicology* 1993; **80**: 71–82.

93. Kalla B, Hamilton RF, Scheule RK, Holian A. Role of extracellular calcium in chrysotile asbestos stimulation of alveolar macrophages. *Toxicol Appl Pharmacol* 1990; **104**: 130–8.

94. Faux SP, Michelangeli F, Levy LS. Calcium chelator Quin-2 prevents crocidolite-induced DNA strand breakage in human white blood cells. *Mutat Res* 1994; **311**: 209–15.

95. Barlow C, Shukla A, Mossman B, Lounsbury K. Oxidant signals leading to phosphorylation of ERK and CREB in lung epithelial cells: different requirements for Ca^{2+} influx. *Free Radic Biol Med* 2003; **35**: S61.

96. Oshima M, Dinchuk JE, Kargman SL, *et al*. Suppression of intestinal polyposis in Apc delta716 knockout mice by inhibition of cyclooxygenase 2 (COX-2). *Cell* 1996; **87**: 803–9.

97. Oshima M, Murai N, Kargman S, *et al*. Chemoprevention of intestinal polyposis in the Apcdelta716 mouse by rofecoxib, a specific cyclooxygenase-2 inhibitor. *Cancer Res* 2001; **61**: 1733–40.

98. Baer AN, Green FA. Cyclooxygenase activity of cultured human mesothelial cells. *Prostaglandins* 1993; **46**: 37–49.

99. Topley N, Petersen MM, Mackenzie R, *et al*. Human peritoneal mesothelial cell prostaglandin synthesis: induction of cyclooxygenase mRNA by peritoneal macrophage-derived cytokines. *Kidney Int* 1994; **46**: 900–9.

100. Marrogi A, Pass HI, Khan M, Metheny-Barlow LJ, Harris CC, Gerwin BI. Human mesothelioma samples overexpress both cyclooxygenase-2 (COX-2) and inducible nitric oxide synthase (NOS2): *in vitro* antiproliferative effects of a COX-2 inhibitor. *Cancer Res* 2000; **60**: 3696–700.

101. Edwards JG, Faux SP, Plummer SM, *et al*. Cyclooxygenase-2 expression is a novel prognostic factor in malignant mesothelioma. *Clin Cancer Res* 2002; **8**: 1857–62.

Chapter 7

Viral factors in the pathogenesis of malignant mesothelioma

A. Powers, M. Bocchetta, and M. Carbone

Introduction

Simian virus 40 (SV40) is a DNA tumour virus endogenous to Asian macaques that was first isolated in1960. Early studies demonstrated that the virus was highly oncogenic when injected into rodents and was capable of transforming cells from many species in tissue culture. Since then it has been used extensively in medical research because of its potent transforming ability.

SV40 has been reproducibly detected in human mesothelioma samples, and injection of the virus produces mesotheliomas in hamster models. Detailed cellular and molecular mechanisms have also been elucidated which implicate SV40 in mesothelioma oncogenesis. The presence and role that SV40 may play in tumour development presents a unique opportunity for the development of targeted therapies.

General characteristics of SV40

The SV40 genome is a closed circular double-stranded DNA molecule that codes for several proteins, including the large tumour antigen (Tag), the small tumour antigen (tag), 17kT, and the viral capsid proteins (Fig. 7.1) [1,2]. The potent transforming capability of the virus lies in the early region of the genome, which encodes the large and small tumour antigens. Tag, a 90 kDa protein found predominantly in the nucleus of infected cells, but also in the cytoplasm, promotes transformation and oncogenesis through a variety of activities. Tag is directly mutagenic, as it alters the stability and karyotype of the host genome by inducing numerical and structural chromosomal alterations. Tag also binds and inactivates p53 and the pRb family, and through promoter methylation inactivates the tumour suppressor RASSF1A [1]. This, in conjunction with its ability to induce expression of insulin-like growth factor 1 (IGF-1) and its receptor Notch-1, and

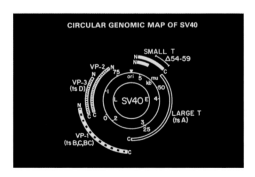

Figure 7.1 Genomic map of SV40 showing large tumour antigen (Tag), small tumour antigen (tag), capsid proteins (VP1–3), and the origin of DNA replication (ori). N, amino terminal; C, carboxy terminal.

Met oncogene activation, allows for unregulated cell growth. The small tumour antigen (tag) is a 17 kDa protein found in the cytoplasm of the host cell. It has been shown to inhibit cellular phosphatase 2A (PP2A), and to increase the production of Tag. Through PP2A inhibition, tag aids Tag in binding and inhibiting tumour suppressor products [1,2].

Although it appears that there is only a single SV40 serotype, different viral strains exist and are distinguishable based on variations in the structure of the viral regulatory region and nucleotide sequence of the C terminus of the Tag gene [1,3]. Non-archetypal, or wild-type, strains have a duplicated 72 bp element in their regulatory region. Non-archetypal strains typically are used in the laboratory, and they were the original strains isolated from the contaminated poliovaccines. In contrast, viruses freshly isolated from monkey tissues or found in human tumours are often archetypal, i.e. they contain no duplications in their regulatory regions. A recent study by Rizzo *et al.* [3] revealed that this strain was also a contaminant of early poliovaccines. The 72 bp duplication is significant because it increases the growth rate of the virus in culture, but the effect of this increased rate of replication in a live host is unclear. It is possible that the slower growth exhibited by the archetypal strains may allow the virus to establish and maintain an infection in a live host more easily by failing to cause cell lysis and elicit a strong immune response [1,3].

Prevalence and origins of SV40 infection in humans

The extent of SV40 infection among the human population is unclear. It is likely that contaminated poliovaccines account for the largest transfer of SV40 from monkeys to humans. Both inactivated and live attenuated poliovaccines distributed between 1955 and 1963 were grown in rhesus monkey kidney cell cultures [1,2]. Many of these cultures were unknowingly produced from SV40-infected monkeys, which resulted in SV40 contamination of many lots of the vaccine. The presence of SV40 in the vaccines escaped detection until African green monkey kidney cells began to be used in culture, since the virus produces cytoplasmic vacuolization in these cells. It was later discovered that the inactivation process used in the vaccine preparation procedure was not sufficient for SV40 inactivation, resulting in the worldwide distribution of vaccines containing live SV40. A recent study by Rizzo *et al.* [3] confirmed that inactivated poliovaccines distributed during this time period contained both archetypal and non-archetypal SV40. In the USA alone, this contamination may have resulted in the inadvertent infection of millions of people with SV40. In fact, it is estimated that 10–30 million of the 98 million people who had received the vaccine by 1961 in the USA had been administered a contaminated lot [1,2]. In the USA, vaccines containing infectious SV40 were distributed until 1963 [1,2].

Infection through contaminated poliovaccines is unlikely to be the only source of the virus in the human population. Serum samples collected prior to 1955, when contaminated vaccines were first distributed, contained varying amounts of SV40 antibodies [1]. For instance, six (11.8 per cent) of 51 serum samples collected from Wisconsin medical students in 1952 contained SV40 antibodies [4]. Furthermore, studies have also shown that people too young to have received the contaminated vaccines are infected with SV40. A recent study performed by Butel and colleagues found that 20 (5.9 per cent) of 377 children born between 1980 and 1995 had SV40-neutralizing antibodies [1]. Molecular studies confirmed that SV40 sequences were present in their peripheral blood cells. These children could not have received contaminated vaccines, indicating that other modes of transfer of the virus, either from monkey to human or from human to human, have occurred. The latter possibility has been supported by data showing that SV40 can be excreted via human faeces, breast milk, semen, and urine [5,6].

Regardless of the mode of transfer, SV40 infection may be widespread among the human population. Serological tests performed on individuals since the 1970s have found SV40-neutralizing antibodies in about 5 per cent of those tested [2]. Laboratory workers who handle live monkeys, primary monkey cell cultures, or SV40 are at high risk, and have been found to have SV40-neutralizing antibodies at rates of 41–55 per cent [1].

Animal models of SV40 oncogenesis

SV40 is highly oncogenic in animals. Experiments by Eddy *et al.* [7] in the early 1960s showed that subcutaneous inoculation of SV40-infected rhesus monkey kidney cells led to fibrosarcomas at the site of injection in newborn hamsters. Weanling and adult animals developed fibrosarcomas when injected subcutaneously with higher doses of the the virus ($>10^9$ pfu), but the tumour incidence was low and development only occurred after a long incubation period [7]. Later studies showed that intracerebral injection of the virus led to ependymomas and choroid plexus tumours in hamsters [8], while intravenous injection led to the development of lymphomas and osteosarcomas [9].

SV40 was first linked to the development of mesotheliomas in 1982, when Lipotich *et al.* [10] reported the development of an SV40-induced hamster mesothelioma cell line (800TU) produced from a newborn hamster following subcutaneous interscapular injection of the virus. The development of mesothelioma in this animal was probably due to accidental intrapleural injection since this was the only mesothelioma observed among hundreds of hamsters who otherwise developed subcutaneous fibrosarcomas (R. Mayer, personal communication). Subsequently, in 1991, Carbone *et al.* [11] observed that 60 per cent of 21-day-old hamsters injected intracardially with wild-type SV40 developed malignant mesotheliomas within 6 months. All of those injected intrapleurally developed the tumour in 3–6 months [12,13], and 67 per cent of 21-day-old hamsters injected in the peritoneum with SV40 developed mesothelioma in 3–6 months. In contrast, in parallel experiments, intracardial injection of SV40 small t mutants led to the development of mesothelioma in only a single animal, suggesting that tag is important in mesothelioma tumorigenesis [12]. Interestingly, mesotheliomas do not occur in hamsters following intracerebral or subcutaneous injection, indicating that that the route of inoculation determines the type of tumour which develops, and that only certain cells are susceptible to transformation by SV40.

The SV40-induced hamster mesotheliomas produced in these experiments spread along the serosal surfaces and infiltrated the diaphragm and chest wall. Distant metastases were not observed. Histologically, epithelioid, biphasic, and sarcomatous variants were observed, and immunohistochemical studies revealed results similar to those seen in human mesotheliomas [1,2]. Southern blot hybridization of DNA extracted from the tumours showed SV40 sequences, and cell lines derived from these tumours contained and expressed SV40 early region DNA. Intranuclear Tag was observed in both the tumours and cell lines following immunohistochemical staining [11,12].

SV40 and human mesotheliomas

The preferential induction of specific tumour types in animals following SV40 infection led to the analysis of these same tumour types in humans for the presence of the virus. In an initial study, polymerase chain reaction (PCR) analysis of 48 human mesotheliomas showed that SV40 sequences were present in 29 (60 per cent) of the samples [14]. Sequence analysis confirmed that the sequences were homologous to SV40. The presence of SV40 in human mesotheliomas was later confirmed by numerous other laboratories and by a multilaboratory study sponsored by the International Mesothelioma Interest Group [15]. Overall, more than 40 laboratories have detect-

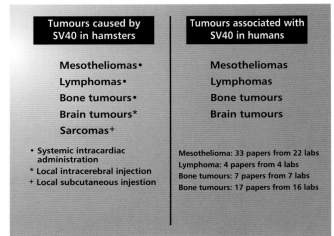

Tumours caused by SV40 in hamsters	Tumours associated with SV40 in humans
Mesotheliomas•	Mesotheliomas
Lymphomas•	Lymphomas
Bone tumours•	Bone tumours
Brain tumours*	Brain tumours
Sarcomas+	
• Systemic intracardiac administration * Local intracerebral injection + Local subcutaneous injestion	Mesothelioma: 33 papers from 22 labs Lymphoma: 4 papers from 4 labs Bone tumours: 7 papers from 7 labs Bone tumours: 17 papers from 16 labs

Figure 7.2 Tumour types caused by SV40 in hamsters compared with tumor types in which SV40 has been reproducibly detected in humans.

ed SV40 in mesotheliomas or other human tumours, including lymphomas, brain tumours, and bone tumours (Fig. 7.2) [13,16,17].

A variety of techniques, including PCR, Southern blot hybridization, viral rescue, Tag immunofluorescence, Tag immunohistochemistry, DNA sequencing, mRNA *in situ* hybridization, Tag immunoprecipitation and Western blot analysis, antisense Tag, co-precipitation of cellular p53 and Rb with Tag, and electron microscopy, have been used to confirm that SV40 is present in these tumours [17]. Furthermore, Shivapurkar *et al.* [18] microdissected malignant mesothelioma cells and nearby stromal cells from paraffin sections, and found SV40 sequences in 57 per cent of samples of epithelial mesothelioma tumour cells using PCR and DNA sequencing. These sequences were not present in matched adjacent lung tissue samples microdissected in parallel. SV40 was also found in both the pre-invasive and invasive components of these tumours, indicating that it is present in the early stages of tumour development [18].

The overwhelming number of positive reports from different laboratories using different techniques proves that SV40 is present in some human tumours. At an international consensus meeting on SV40 and human tumours held at the University of Chicago in 2001, experts in the field of SV40 and mesothelioma reviewed all the published data linking SV40 to human tumours. George Klein and Carlo Croce, who chaired the final panel discussion stated that 'the presence of SV40 in human tumours has been convincingly demonstrated' [19]. Similar conclusions were subsequently reached at a workshop organized by the Biological Carcinogenesis Branch of the National Cancer Institute, Bethesda, MD [20].

While it is certain that SV40 is present in some human mesotheliomas and brain tumours, data on lymphomas and bone tumours are still preliminary [1]. It remains to be demonstrated that SV40 is present in the tumour cells, rather than in nearby non-malignant cells such as macrophages and osteoclasts that are always present in lymphoma or bone tumour biopsies, respectively. Functional studies are currently in progress to determine whether SV40 acts as a pathogen or a passenger in lymphomas and bone tumours.

While most laboratories have been able to detect SV40 in some human tumours, a number of negative studies have also been reported which have caused considerable controversy. It appears that geographical differences account for the majority of these discrepant studies. For example, Hirvonen *et al.* [21] failed to detect SV40 in 49 Finnish mesotheliomas, but detected the virus in three out of five mesothelioma specimens from the USA. Emri *et al.* [22] failed to detect SV40 in

29 Turkish mesotheliomas, but found SV40 in an Italian osteosarcoma and mesothelioma specimen [22]. De Rienzo et al. [23] did not detect SV40 in 9 Turkish mesotheliomas, but found it in four out of 11 specimens from the USA [23]. Leithner et al. [24] found SV40 in three out of three American and Italian mesotheliomas, but did not detect the virus in eight Austrian mesotheliomas and 24 Austrian bone tumours. The negative results obtained from the Finnish, Austrian, and Turkish samples have been attributed to the fact that SV40-contaminated vaccines were not used in Finland, Austria, or Turkey [22–24]. In a study in the former Federal Republic of Germany, Weggen et al. [25] detected SV40 in two out of 27 ependymomas. The two positive cases were from American patients treated in Germany, while all negative samples were obtained from German patients. The overall exposure of Germans to SV40-contaminated poliovaccines is unclear, because the German Democratic Republic and the Federal Republic of Germany received different batches and types of vaccines. Taken together, these studies argue for true geographical differences in the occurrence of SV40-positive tumours, which appear to be closely linked to distribution of contaminated vaccine.

Apart from geographical differences, other unknown factors probably play a role in some negative reports. For example, although Mayall et al. [27] reported the presence of SV40 in human mesotheliomas using PCR in 1999 [26], they were unable to detect SV40 in English and New Zealand mesotheliomas using real-time PCR in a later study in 2003 [27]. The reasons for these different results were not stated. Technical differences probably account for some discrepancies in the literature. For instance, Gordon et al. [28] reported the presence of SV40 in two out of 35 mesothelioma biopsies and three out of seven mesothelioma cell lines. However, the authors stated that they originally failed to detect the virus in all specimens and obtained positive results only after modification of their original technique. The true number of false-negative studies in the literature is difficult to estimate, but it is likely that they may account for a small number of the reported negative studies.

Finally, the presence of SV40 in human tumours has been repeatedly challenged by the Viral Epidemiology Branch at the National Cancer Institute (USA) and their contracting testing laboratory headed by K. Shah. Together, this team has consistently reported negative findings in human mesotheliomas [29,30]. However, the group have acknowledged that the sensitivity of Shah's original assay for SV40 detection, published in 1996 [reported in 29], was too low at times, as he failed to detect SV40 in positive controls using the same technique in later assays. The group subsequently reported possible irregularities in the purported blinded 2001 multi-laboratory study [30,31]. This raised serious concerns among several of Shah's co-authors, and a number of them expressed their desire to retract their association with the manuscript in a series of letters to Anticancer Research [32]. Furthermore, the 2001 study was flawed because half the negative water controls were reported as positive, raising further questions about the validity of its conclusions. Moreover, in a 2002 paper by Engels et al. [33], some members of this same team reported that SV40 was not present in brain tumours from India. This study was flawed by technical errors that invalidate its negative conclusions. Further discussion of these errors is described by Carbone et al. [17]. Overall, technical errors and recent information regarding the sensitivity of the assays used by this group raise concerns about the validity of these negative reports.

Mechanisms of SV40 pathogenesis in human mesotheliomas

Although SV40 is found in human tumours, its presence alone does not prove causality. A variety of mechanisms by which SV40 could play a pathogenic role in human mesothelial cell transformation have been demonstrated. (Fig. 7.3).

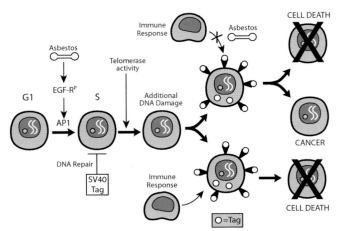

Figure 7.3 Working model of the pathogenic mechanisms of SV40 and asbestos. Arrowheads indicate a stimulatory effect and crossed bars indicate an inhibitory effect. Tag, SV40 large T antigen; tag, SV40 small t antigen; ROS, reactive oxygen species; TSG, tumour suppressor gene; PP2A, phosphatase 2A. Asbestos causes autophosphorylation of the epidermal growth factor receptor (EGF-R) which activates the mitogen-activated protein (MAP) kinases, leading to AP1 induction, cell mitosis, and apoptosis. In mesothelial cells containing alterations of the cyclin-dependent kinase inhibitor p16, or of the related p14 ARF, which inactivates MDM2 and interferes with p53 and pRb activity, cell division may ensue. Mesotheliomas often contain alterations of p16 and p14 ARF. If the mesothelial cell is infected with SV40, Tag-mediated inhibition of apoptotic pathways may also lead to cell division. In addition, tag inhibits PP2A, which normally dephosphorylates and inactivates the MAP kinases. This may increase the effects of asbestos on AP1. Phagocytosis of asbestos fibres produces mutagenic ROS, which may also contribute to genetic damage. Damaged cells should undergo apoptosis, but occasionally may divide and continue to develop additional mutations in essential genes, including tumour suppressors, to become malignant.

Experiments have shown that SV40 Tag inhibits tumour suppressor products in human mesothelioma cells. Immunostaining and *in situ* mRNA hybridization experiments by Carbone *et al.* [34] in 1997 revealed that Tag and p53 were often coexpressed in human mesotheliomas (Fig. 7.4). Normally, wild-type p53 should not be detectable in human mesotheliomas, as its levels are too small to be shown through staining. However, single-strand conformational polymorphism analysis of the exons encoding p53 demonstrated that p53 was wild type in 23 of 25 samples. This finding suggested that its detection was not due to mutation. Instead, immunoprecipitation reactions indicated that Tag binds and stabilizes p53 in mesotheliomas, allowing its detection. Furthermore, tumours expressing Tag failed to induce p21, indicating that p53 was also inactivated by its interactions with Tag. Treatment of SV40+ mesothelioma cell lines with Tag antisense restored the p53 pathway, and induced p21 expression and growth arrest [35]. Apart from p53, Tag was also shown to bind, stabilize, and inactivate members of the retinoblastoma tumour suppressor family (pRb, p107, and pRb2/p130) in both mesotheliomas and brain tumours [36].

The ability of SV40 to induce mesotheliomas preferentially in hamsters, its presence in human mesotheliomas, and the capacity of Tag to bind and inhibit tumour suppressors in these malignancies strongly suggested a link between SV40 and the development of malignant mesothelioma. Nevertheless, a number of observations remained unexplained [2]. Among them, SV40

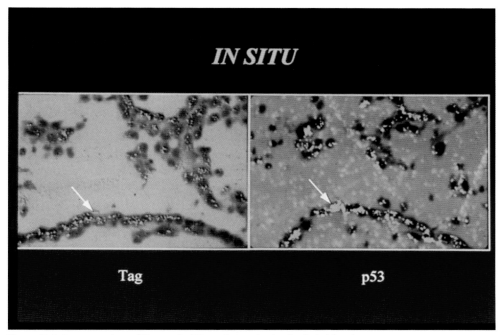

Figure 7.4 Co-expression of Tag and p53 as shown by *in situ* hybridization.

transformation of human cells was thought to be a very rare event which occurred only when the virus became integrated into the host cell genome [37]. However, viral integration had not been demonstrated in human mesotheliomas. Furthermore, SV40-transformed mesothelial cells should have expressed viral antigens, and therefore should have been targeted and eliminated by the host immune system [2].

The long-held belief that SV40 transformation of human mesothelial cells was a rare event was based on the assumption that all human cells were semi-permissive to SV40 infection, i.e. only a fraction of all exposed human cells were infected by SV40. Normally, these infected cells expressed Tag, allowed the production of numerous SV40 particles, and were lysed [37]. Transformation could occur only if the SV40 genome became integrated in the host cell DNA. However, integration was a very rare event, as indicated by the rare foci that developed following SV40 infection of human cells in culture [37]. The majority of cells from these foci were not fully transformed. In about 95 per cent of cases, these rare 'transformed' cells demonstrated a period of extended lifespan followed by a crisis stage of decreased growth and cell death [37]. Only about 5 per cent of these foci contained a small subpopulation of cells which occasionally escaped death and became immortal [37]. SV40 infection of hamster cells, in contrast, was described as non-permissive [37]. Blockade of the lytic cycle in non-permissive cells leads to prolonged exposure to the mutagenic effects of SV40 Tag, integration on the host cell genome, and malignant transformation. Thus SV40 is highly oncogenic in hamsters. SV40 infection of primate cells was described as permissive, since the virus caused a lytic infection and was not thought to induce tumour development because cells were lysed before they could be transformed [37].

Similar to what has been observed in hamster cells, transformation of human cells by SV40 was thought to be due to the integration of SV40 DNA into the host cell genome and prolonged expression of the viral oncogenes in the absence of viral replication and cell lysis. However, SV40

DNA was thought to remain episomal in most human cells where it was free to replicate actively and cause cell lysis before transformation could occur. The notion that all human cells are equally semi-permissive to SV40 was challenged by O'Neill and Carroll [38] who found differences in the type of SV40 infection among different cell types. While most of the cell types they tested were semi-permissive, some human kidney carcinoma, glioblastoma, and rhabdomyosarcoma cell lines were permissive to SV40 infection. One human glioblastoma cell line was non-permissive [38]. However, despite this study, the notion that all human cells were semi-permissive to SV40 continued to be accepted.

The specific effects of SV40 infection in human mesothelial cells were unknown until recently, when Bocchetta et al. [39] observed that human mesothelial cells were uniquely susceptible to SV40 infection and transformation. These authors found that human mesothelial cells normally contained high levels of wild-type p53. These levels were four to five times higher than those observed in human fibroblasts, and therefore p53 was easily detectable by immunostaining. Bocchetta and colleagues revealed that, in human mesothelial cells, SV40 Tag binds and inactivates cellular p53, favouring malignant transformation. At the same time, the interaction between p53 and Tag inhibits the ability of Tag to sustain SV40 replication. Thus, when mesothelial cells are infected with SV40, viral replication occurs, but at a slow rate. This slow rate of replication is compatible with cell survival in the presence of episomal SV40 [1]. When mesothelial cells were treated with antisense p53 (which reduced p53 levels by about a factor of 4) and infected with SV40 48 h later, viral replication occurred at a rate similar to that in fibroblasts and the cells were lysed [39].

In addition to this finding, Bocchetta et al. [39] demonstrated that mesothelial cells exhibited a second unique characteristic. Specifically, almost all the mesothelial cells exposed to SV40 were infected and expressed Tag. In contrast, when human fibroblasts were infected, only a minority of the cells (5–20 per cent) expressed Tag. Thus, when SV40 infects mesothelial cells, viral particles are produced and released from infected cells (permissive infection), but this occurs in the absence of marked cell lysis. In other words, mesothelial cells and SV40 have a type of parasitic relationship, and it seems possible that even if a small amount of virus reaches mesothelial cells through the bloodstream, this may lead to virus production in the infected cells, release of viral particles, and infection of nearby mesothelial cells [1]. In mesothelial cells, prolonged expression of SV40 Tag and tag was observed in the absence of cell lysis in most cells. In fibroblasts, in contrast, only a small portion of the cells were infected and were soon lysed before transformation could occur [1]. Accordingly, Bocchetta et al. [39] found that the rate of transformation was extremely high (>1000 higher) in human mesothelial cells infected with SV40 than in human fibroblasts. Of interest, all the SV40-transformed mesothelial clones (16/16) could be established in tissue culture compared with ≤5 per cent for fibroblasts in parallel infections. Furthermore, 14/16 of these clones appeared to be immortal from the start. They never entered a crisis and were passed in tissue culture more than 80 times. The other two clones entered a crisis around passage 30–35 and died. Human mesothelial cell clones contained episomal SV40 and supported low levels of viral replication, releasing small amounts of infectious SV40 even after 55 passages. Rapid replication and lysis in these cells was probably prevented by the high levels of p53. Thus this study demonstrated that integrated SV40 DNA is not required for transformation in human mesothelial cells [39]. In summary, the data of Bocchetta and colleagues prove that SV40 can preferentially transform mesothelial cells, which may lead to the development of mesotheliomas. Human mesothelial cells are more susceptible to SV40 infection, and the high levels of p53 expressed inhibit cell lysis leading to prolonged exposure of the cells to the mutagenic effects of Tag [39].

Data which further elucidate a role for SV40 in tumour development were reported by Foddis et al. [40], who demonstrated that SV40 induction of telomerase activity may also lead to the development of mesothelioma. They revealed that SV40 induces telomerase in mesothelial cells following infection. The telomerase activity observed is directly proportional to the level of SV40 Tag expressed in the cell. In contrast, SV40 does not induce detectable telomerase activity in fibroblasts. Mesothelial cells infected with SV40 tag mutants did not express telomerase activity, indicating that SV40 tag is necessary for the induction of telomerase. Induction of telomerase following SV40 infection may partly account for the increased susceptibility and high rate of mesothelial cell transformation by SV40 [40].

Apart from telomerase, SV40 has also been shown to induce hepatocyte growth factor receptor and Met oncogene activation in mesotheliomas [41]. Interestingly, Met activation was found only in SV40-positive mesotheliomas, and it was not activated in SV40-negative human mesotheliomas, which suggests that Met activation may contribute to the development of SV40-positive mesotheliomas but is not essential for the induction of all mesotheliomas [41].

Toyooka *et al.* [42] found that the frequency of aberrant methylation of RASSF1A, a tumour suppressor gene, is significantly higher in SV40-positive mesotheliomas than in SV40-negative mesotheliomas. This suggests that SV40 oncogenesis may involve methylation and silencing of RASSF1A and other tumour suppressor genes.

Finally, Bocchetta *et al.* [43] found that SV40 induces Notch-1 oncogene activation upon infection of human mesothelial cells. Notch-1 activity was required for the growth of SV40-transformed human mesothelial cells, and SV40-positive mesotheliomas were found to express high levels of active Notch-1. These findings link Notch-1 activation by SV40 to the growth of mesotheliomas [43] (Fig. 7.3).

SV40 epidemiology

In vivo, cellular, and molecular studies have provided convincing evidence supporting a link between SV40 and tumour development (Fig. 7.3). Several epidemiological studies have been conducted to determine whether SV40 infection could be linked to the development of mesotheliomas or other human cancers. Most studies have focused on whether SV40-contaminated vaccines have been linked to higher rates of tumour development in populations who probably received contaminated lots. It is known that poliovaccines and adenovaccines distributed between 1955 and 1963 were prepared in cell cultures grown on monolayers of infected rhesus monkey kidney cells. Because the virus produces no cytopathic effects in these cells, SV40 contamination went unrecognized until 1960 when high titres of the virus were found in some lots of the vaccine [2]. Despite this finding, contaminated lots were distributed until 1963. It is now estimated that a significant proportion of the millions of people who received the vaccine during this period were exposed to infectious SV40 [2].

Following the finding in the early 1960s that SV40 induced tumours when injected into hamsters, initial epidemiological studies were undertaken to determine whether the administration of SV40-contaminated poliovaccines was associated with increased cancer incidence. No increase in cancer incidence in children was detected in the years immediately following vaccine distribution. However, only one long-term follow-up of vaccinated children in the USA was conducted [5]. Mortimer and colleagues analysed 1073 children born between 1960 and 1962 who received either oral or inactivated poliovaccine shortly after birth and followed them for 17–19 years. Overall, the group showed no increased cancer incidence. In fact, only one child developed a malignancy [5]. Thus it was suggested that SV40 posed no increased cancer risk. However, the authors and critics have cautioned that the 17–19 year follow-up period may have been inadequate, since other carcinogens can take 20–40 years to cause cancer [5,19]. In addition, the small number of children studied would not have been sufficient to detect increases in the rare

SV40-associated tumours [5,19]. Studies conducted by the Viral Epidemiology Branch, National Cancer Institute, comparing cohorts born prior to 1963 (and thus likely to have been infected by contaminated vaccines) with cohorts born after 1963 (presumably not exposed to contaminated vaccines) have also failed to detect an increase in SV40-associated cancer [44–46].

However, a number of studies have shown a possible association between SV40 exposure and cancer development. A study by Geissler [47] in 1990 detected an increase in the incidence of certain types of brain tumours in SV40-exposed cohorts compared with non-exposed cohorts. SV40 was detected by Southern blot hybridization in some of the brain tumours in the exposed cohorts, and not in the brain tumours of the unexposed cohorts. A prospective study of 50 000 pregnant women who did or did not receive poliovaccines between 1959–1965 showed a twofold greater rate of malignancies, particularly neural tumours, in the children of mothers who received SV40-contaminated vaccines during pregnancy [48]. A case–control study of Australian children hospitalized with malignancies had a higher rate of previous polio vaccination than matched controls [49].

Overall, the available data from these epidemiological studies are conflicting and inconclusive. They are limited by a lack of data drawn from large samples of confirmed SV40-exposed and unexposed cohorts. The length of follow-up has also been inadequate for most of these SV40-associated tumours, which typically have long latency periods. In an attempt to address these shortcomings, Fisher *et al.* [50] used data from the Surveillance, Epidemiology, and End Results (SEER) database to analyse the incidence of mesotheliomas, bone tumours, and brain tumours between 1973 and 1993 and the association of these tumours with the administration of contaminated poliovaccines. The SEER Program represents approximately 12 per cent of the US population. It provides population-based tumour-specific data on all tumours occurring in specific geographical areas in the USA. Fisher *et al.* [50] demonstrated that since 1973–1974 the age-adjusted incidence of ependymomas has increased by 25 per cent, the rate of osteogenic sarcomas has increased by 2.4 per cent, and the incidence of other bone and joint tumours has increased by 22.9 per cent. The incidence of mesothelioma has increased by 90 per cent. Fisher and colleagues also performed a more specific analysis to make a direct comparison of cancer incidence in a birth cohort highly likely to have been exposed to SV40-contaminated vaccines (1955–1959) with that in a cohort unlikely to have been exposed to the contaminated vaccines (1963–1967). The overall cancer incidence rate was 11 per cent lower in the exposed cohort than in the unexposed cohort. However, the incidence of ependymoma and choroid plexus tumours was approximately 20 per cent greater in the exposed than in the unexposed cohort, and the incidence of bone malignancies was also higher in the exposed cohort. Interestingly, the incidence of mesothelioma, an unusual finding given the young age of the participants at the time of the analysis, was higher in the exposed cohort (six cases) than in the unexposed cohort (two cases) [50].

While the study by Fisher and colleagues examines a longer follow-up period, it compares 'assumed' SV40-exposed with 'assumed' unexposed cohorts. Many studies have shown that people too young to have received contaminated vaccines (members of the 'assumed' unexposed cohort) have been infected with SV40. This indicates that other routes of exposure are present, and that the presumed unexposed cohort probably contained exposed individuals. For this reason, it is currently not possible to establish SV40-positive and SV40-negative cohorts that are large enough for a statistically significant study. In 2002, the Vaccine Safety Review Committee of the Institute of Medicine (IOM), National Academy of Sciences, USA, reviewed all the epidemiological studies concerning SV40 and human tumours. The IOM concluded that 'the evidence was inadequate to conclude whether or not the contaminated polio vaccine caused cancer because the epidemiological studies are sufficiently flawed' [51].

SV40 as a co-carcinogen

Because the development of most cancers is multifactorial, it is likely that SV40 acts with other agents or factors to cause mesothelioma. SV40 is highly immunogenic and induces both an antibody and a cytotoxic T-cell response [1]. Thus it is likely that SV40 tumours develop under circumstances in which early transformed cells are able to escape immune detection and continue to proliferate. *In vivo* models show that mesotheliomas and other tumours are most successfully induced by SV40 in newborn animals. For instance, newborn animals will develop fibrosarcomas following subcutaneous innoculation of low-dose SV40 [7]. In contrast, weanling and adult animals will develop fibrosarcomas only when injected with higher loads of SV40 [7]. Tumour incidence in these mature animals is typically lower, and latency periods are generally longer [7]. The increased sensitivity of newborn animals to SV40-induced tumorigenesis may be a result of their more immature immune systems. Immunosuppression may also make humans more susceptible to the carcinogenic effects of SV40.

Experiments have suggested that asbestos and SV40 may act as co-carcinogens in the induction of some mesotheliomas. Asbestos may act as an immunosuppressant, increasing the likelihood of mesothelial cell transformation by SV40 in SV40-infected individuals [2] (Fig. 7.3). Furthermore, asbestos and SV40 have been shown to act as co-carcinogens *in vitro* as human fibroblasts transfected with ori–SV40 constructs in the presence of crocidolite produced a greater number of foci than either factor alone [39]. In addition, foci developed in human fibroblasts and mesothelial cells transfected with SV40 tag mutants in the presence of crocidolite, while the same cells did not produce foci when transfected with SV40 tag mutants alone [39].

The possibility that SV40 and asbestos may also act as co-carcinogens *in vivo* is important, since SV40 is frequently found in mesothelioma patients with a history of asbestos exposure. Figure 7.3 provides a working model of the possible interactions between SV40 and asbestos in mesothelioma production. A study by Mayall *et al.* [26] reported that SV40 was present in New Zealand mesotheliomas, and suggested that there is a relationship between the presence of SV40 and asbestos exposure in human mesotheliomas. Eleven mesotheliomas were analysed for the presence of SV40 and history of asbestos exposure. Seven of the tumours were associated with a high level of asbestos exposure and five were SV40 positive. Four of the tumours were not associated with high levels of asbestos exposure, and none of these four contained SV40 sequences. Thus Mayall *et al.* [26] suggested that a synergistic relationship between asbestos and SV40 may exist in mesothelioma development.

SV40- and asbestos-induced mesotheliomas: a comparison

Asbestos, especially crocidolite asbestos, is a widely accepted cause of human mesothelioma. Interestingly, SV40 is a more potent carcinogen than asbestos both *in vitro* and *in vivo*. Mesotheliomas have been induced following inhalation or injection of various forms of asbestos in only ≤65 per cent of animals after a mean latency period of 1 year or more [2]. In contrast, the intrapleural injection of SV40 in hamsters has led to mesothelioma development in 100 per cent of the animals in 3–6 months [12]. Furthermore, experiments performed by Bocchetta *et al.* [39] demonstrated that crocidolite asbestos, the most carcinogenic form of asbestos in humans, failed to induce foci formation in human mesothelial cells and fibroblasts at all concentrations tested, confirming similar observations carried out in other laboratories. As previously discussed, Bocchetta *et al.* [39] demonstrated that SV40 is capable of transforming and immortalizing human mesothelial cells in culture at a very high frequency.

McConnell and Carbone [52] directly compared the development and histological characteristics of pleural mesotheliomas induced by intrapleural injection of SV40 and inhalation of amosite asbestos in hamsters. Asbestos-induced tumours typically had a longer latency period (>12 months) than SV40-induced mesotheliomas (3–6 months). The asbestos-induced mesotheliomas were rarely a cause of death even after 18 months. In contrast, SV40-induced mesotheliomas were invariably a cause of death in 100 per cent of the hamsters within 3–6 months of SV40 injection. Asbestos-induced tumours were smaller (a third were discovered after necropsy on histological examination only) and were rarely accompanied by effusions. SV40-induced tumours were typically multicentric, covered large areas of the pleura, and were accompanied by large pleural effusions. Microscopically, SV40-induced mesotheliomas were uniformly biphasic with areas containing tubulopapillary formations next to areas of sarcomatous change. Invasion of surrounding structures was common, and occasional metastases outside the thorax were observed. Fibrosis did not occur. The cells were small and basophilic, had little cytoplasm, rare pseudovacuoles, and numerous mitotic figures. The asbestos-induced mesotheliomas were also tubulopapillary, but sarcomatous change was less frequent. Invasion of surrounding tissue and metastasis was rare, but lung fibrosis was common. The tumour cells were large, less basophilic, and contained more cytoplasm. Pseudovacuoles were common, but mitotic figures were rare [52].

The more rapid growth and aggressive nature of the SV40-induced tumours observed by McConnell and Carbone [52] may be due to differences in the mechanisms by which SV40 and asbestos induce mesotheliomas. It has been proposed that, as in hamsters, SV40-associated human mesotheliomas may be more aggressive than SV40-negative tumours. A study by Procopio et al. [53] proposed that the presence of SV40 is a negative prognostic factor in human mesotheliomas, regardless of histotype.

Conclusion

A considerable amount of new data on SV40 and mesothelioma has accumulated in the literature in the past 10 years. SV40 is present in some human mesotheliomas [19], and its presence in the tumour cells but not in the surrounding stroma indicates that the virus is a pathogen rather than a passenger in these tumours [18]. The prevalence of SV40-positive mesotheliomas varies in different countries. SV40 is present in about 50 per cent of US mesotheliomas [19], but is not present, or is rarely present, in mesotheliomas from Finland [21], Turkey [22,23], Austria [24], and Sweden [54]. The different prevalence of SV40-positive mesotheliomas has been linked to the distribution of SV40-contaminated vaccines; Finland, Turkey, Austria, and Sweden did not receive SV40-contaminated vaccines [21–24,54]. It is likely that SV40 alone, or more frequently together with asbestos, contributes to the development of human mesothelioma [13]. The presence of SV40 in mesothelioma cells but not in the nearby stroma [18] offers a potential target for immunotherapeutic and molecular approaches aimed at eliminating SV40-positive tumour cells [55,56].

Acknowledgements

This work was supported by grant RO-1 CA92657 to M.C.

References:

1. Gazdar A, Butel J, Carbone M. SV40 and human tumours: myth, association or causality? *Nat Rev Cancer* 2002; **2**: 957–64.
2. Rizzo P, Bocchetta M, Powers A, *et al*. SV40 and the pathogenesis of malignant mesothelioma. *Semin Cancer Biol* 2001; **11**: 63–71.

3. Rizzo P, Di Resta I, Powers A, *et al.* Unique strains of SV40 in commercial poliovaccines from 1955 not readily identifiable with current testing for SV40 infection. *Cancer Res* 1999; **59**: 6103–8.

4. Geissler E, Konzer P, Scherneck S, Zimmermann W. Sera collected before introduction of contaminated poliovaccine contain antibodies against SV40. *Acta Virol* 1985; **29**: 420–3.

5. Carbone M, Rizzo P, Pass HI. Simian virus 40, poliovaccines, and human tumors: a review of recent developments. *Oncogene* 1997; **15**: 1877–88.

6. Li R, Branton M, Tanawattanacharoen S, *et al.* Molecular identification of SV40 infection in human subjects and possible association with kidney disease. *J Am Soc Nephrol* 2002; **13**: 2320–30.

7. Eddy BE, Borman GS, Grubbs GE, Young RD. Identification of the oncogenic substance in rhesus monkey cell cultures as simian virus 40. *Virology* 1962; **17**: 65–75.

8. Kirschstein RL, Gerber P. SV40 induced ependymomas in newborn hamsters. *Virology* 1962; **18**; 582–8.

9. Diamandopoulous GT). Leukemia, lymphoma, and osteosarcoma induced in syrian golden hamsters by simian virus 40. *Science* 1972; **40**: 73–5.

10. Lipotich G, Moyer M, Moyer R (1982). Rescue of SV40 following transfection of TC 7 cells with cellular DNAs containing complete and partial SV40 genomes. *Mol Gen Genet* 1982; **186**: 78–81.

11. Carbone M, Pompetti F, Cicala C. The role of small t antigen in SV40 oncogenesis. In: Nicolini C, ed. *Molecular Basis of Human Cancer.* New York: Plenum, 1991; 191–206.

12. Cicala C, Pompetti F, Carbone M. SV40 induces mesotheliomas in hamsters. *Am J Pathol* 1993; **142**: 1524–33.

13. Carbone M, Kratzke R, Testa J. The pathogenesis of mesothelioma. *Semin Oncol* 2002; **29**: 2–17.

14. Carbone M, Pass HI, Rizzo P, *et al.* Simian virus 40 like DNA sequences in human pleural mesothelioma. *Oncogene* 1994; **9**: 1781–90.

15. Testa JR, Carbone M, Hirvonen A, *et al.* A multi-institutional study confirms the presence and expression of simian virus 40 in human malignant mesotheliomas. *Cancer Res* 1998; **58**: 4505–9.

16. Jasani B, Cristaudo A, Emri SA, *et al.* Association of SV40 with human tumours. *Semin Cancer Biol* 2001; **11**: 49–61.

17. Carbone M, Pass HI, Miele L, Bocchetta M. New developments about the association of SV40 with human mesothelioma. *Oncogene* 2003; **22**: 5173–80.

18. Shivapurkar N, Wiethege T, Wishuba II, *et al.* Presence of SV40 in malignant mesothelioma and mesothelial cell proliferations. *J Cell Biochem* 1999; **76**: 181–8.

19. Klein G, Powers A, Croce C. Meeting review. Malignant mesothelioma: therapeutic options and the role of SV40. *Oncogene* 2002; **21**: 1141–9.

20. Wong JM, Kusdra L, Collins K. Subnuclear shuttling of human telomerase induced by transformation and DNA damage. *Nat Cell Biol* 2002; **4**: 731–6.

21. Hirvonen A, Mattson K, Karjalainen A, *et al.* Simian Virus 40 (SV40)-like DNA sequences not detectable in Finnish mesothelioma patients not exposed to SV40-contaminated polio vaccines. *Mol Carcinog* 1999; **26**: 93–9.

22. Emri S, Kocagoz T, Olut A, *et al.* Simian virus 40 is not a cofactor in the pathogenesis of environmentally induced malignant pleural mesothelioma in Turkey. *Anticancer Res.* 2000; **20**: 891–4.

23. De Rienzo A, Tor M, Sterman D, *et al.* Detection of SV40 DNA sequences in malignant mesothelioma specimens from the United States, but not from Turkey. *J Cell Biochem* 2002; **84**: 455–9.

24. Leithner A, Weinhaeusel A, Windhager R, *et al.* Absence of SV40 in Austrian tumors correlates with low incidence of mesotheliomas. *Cancer Biol Ther* 2002; **1**: 375–9.

25. Weggen S, Bayer TA, von Deimling A, *et al.* Low frequency of SV40, JC, and BK polyomavirus sequences in human medulloblastomas, meningiomas and ependymomas. *Brain Pathol* 2000; **10**: 85–92.

26. Mayall FG, Jacobson G, Wilkins R. Mutations of p53 gene and SV40 sequences in asbestos associated and non-asbestos associated mesotheliomas. *J Clin Pathol* 1999; **52**: 291–3.

27. Mayall F, Barratt K, Shanks J. The detection of simian virus 40 in mesotheliomas from New Zealand and England using the real time FRET probe PCR protocols. *J Clin Pathol* 2003; **56**: 728–30.

28. Gordon GJ, Chen CJ, Jaklitsch MT, *et al.* Detection and quantification of SV40 large T antigen DNA in mesothelioma tissues and cell lines. *Oncol Rep* 2002; **9**: 631–4.

29. Strickler HD, Goedert JJ, Fleming M, *et al.* Simian virus 40 and pleural mesothelioma in humans. *Cancer Epidemiol Biomarkers Prev* 1996; **5**: 473–5.

30. Strickler HD and The International SV40 Working Group. A multicenter evaluation of assays for detection of SV40 DNA and results in masked mesothelioma specimens. *Cancer Epidemiol Biomarkers Prev* 2001; **10**: 523–32.

31. MacLachlan DS (2002). SV40 in human tumors: new documents shed light on the apparent controversy. *Anticancer Res* 22, 3495–3500.

32. Delinassios JG. Responses to the article: MacLachlan DS: SV40 in human tumors: new documents shed light on the apparent controversy. *AntiCancer Res* 2003; **23**: 3109–18.

33. Engles AE, Sarkar C, Daniel RW, *et al.* Absence of simian virus 40 in human brain tumors from Northern India. *Int J Cancer* 2002; **101**: 348–52.

34. Carbone M, Rizzo P, Grimely PM, *et al.* Simian virus 40 large T antigen binds p53 in human mesotheliomas. *Nat Med* 1997; **8**: 908–12.

35. Waheed I, Guo S, Chen GA, *et al.* Antisense to SV40 early gene region induces growth arrest and apoptosis in T-antigen-positive human pleural mesothelioma cells. *Cancer Res* 1999; **59**: 6068–73.

36. De Luca A, Baldi A, Esposito V, *et al.* The retinoblastoma gene family pRb/p105, p107, pRb2/p130, and simian virus 40 large T antigen in human mesotheliomas. *Nat Med* 1997; **8**: 913–16.

37. Bryan TM, Reddel RR. SV40-induced immortilization of human cells. *Crit Rev Oncog* 1994; **5**: 331–57.

38. O'Neil F, Carroll D. Amplification of papovavirus defectives during serial low multiplicity infections. *Virology* 1981; **112**; 800–3.

39. Bocchetta M, Di Resta I, Powers A, *et al.* Human mesothelial cells are unusually susceptible to SV40 mediated transformation and asbestos co-carcinogenicity. *Proc Natl Acad Sci USA* 2000; **97**: 10214–19.

40. Foddis R, De Rienzo A, Broccoli D, *et al.* SV40 infection induces telomerase activity in human mesothelial cells. *Oncogene* 2002; **21**: 1434–42.

41. Cacciotti P, Libener R, Betta P, *et al.* SV40 replication in human mesothelial cells induces HGF/Met receptor activation: a model for viral-related carcinogenesis in human malignant mesothelioma. *Proc Natl Acad Sci USA* 2001; **98**: 12032–7.

42. Toyooka S, Pass H, Shivapurkar N, *et al.* Aberrant methylation and simian virus 40 tag sequences in malignant mesothelioma. *Cancer Res* 2001; **10**: 5727–30.

43. Bocchetta M, Miele L, Pass H, Carbone M. Notch-1 induction, a novel activity of SV40 required for growth of SV40-transformed human mesothelial cells. *Oncogene* 2003; **22**: 81–9.

44. Fraumeni JF, Ederer F, Miller RW. An evaluation of the carcinogenicity of simian virus 40 in man. *JAMA* 1963; **185**: 713–18.

45. Strickler HD, Goedert JJ. Exposure to SV40 contaminated poliovirus vaccine and the risk of cancer—a review of the epidemiological evidence. *Dev Biol Stand* 1998; **94**: 235–44.

46. Carrol-Pankhurst C, Engels EA, Strickler HD, *et al.* Thirty-five year mortality following receipt of SV40 contaminated polio vaccine during the neonatal period. *Br J Cancer* 2001; **85**: 1295–7.

47. Geiseler E. SV40 and human brain tumors. *Prog Med Virol* 1990; **37**: 211–22.

48. Heinonen OP, Shapiro S, Monson RR, *et al.* Immunization during pregnancy against poliomyelitis and influenza in relation to childhood malignancy. *Int J Epidemiol* 1973; **2**: 229–34.

49. Innis MD. Oncogenesis and poliomyelitis vaccine. *Nature* 1968; **219**: 972–3.

50. Fisher S, Weber L, Carbone M. Cancer risk associated with simian virus 40 contaminated poliovaccine. *Anticancer Res* 1999; **19**: 2173–80.

51. Starton K, Almario DA, McCormick M, eds. *Immunization Safety Review: SV40 Contamination of Poliovaccine and Cancer.* Washington, DC: National Academy of Sciences, 2002. Available online at http://www.nap.edu/catalog/10534.html

52. McConnell EE, Carbone M. A comparison of pleural mesotheliomas induced by asbestos or SV40 virus in Syrian golden hamsters. *Inhal Toxicol* 2000; **12**: 173–81.

53. Procopio A, Strizzi L, Vianale G, *et al.* Simian virus 40 sequences are a negative prognostic cofactor in patients with malignant pleural mesothelioma. *Genes Chromosomes Cancer* 2000; **29**: 173–9.

54. Priftakis P, Bodganovic G, Hjerpe A, Dalianis T. Presence of simian virus 40 (SV40) is not frequent in Swedish malignant mesotheliomas. *Anticancer Res* 2002; **22**: 1357–60.

55. Schrump D, Waheed I. Strategies to circumvent SV40 oncoprotein expression in malignant pleural mesotheliomas. *Cancer Biol* 2001; **11**: 73–80.

56. Imperiale M, Pass H, Sanda M. Prospects for an SV40 vaccine. *Cancer Biol* 2001; **11**: 81–5.

Chapter 8

Growth and survival factors in malignant pleural mesothelioma

J. G. Edwards, U. Zangemeister-Wittke, and K. J. O'Byrne

Introduction

Growth factors play a key role in the evolution and progression of malignant pleural mesothelioma (MPM) through the induction of increasingly well understood cell-signalling cascades (Fig. 8.1). Inhalation of asbestos or exposure to viral agents associated with transformation of

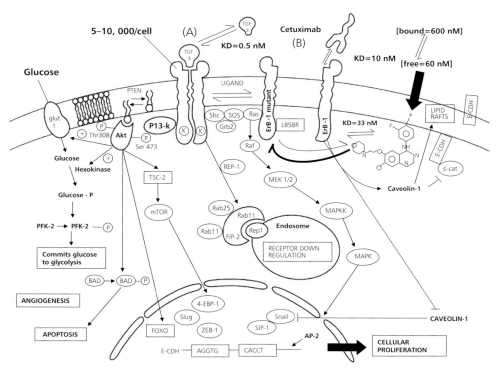

Figure 8.1 Cell signalling events that may occur on activation of a tyrosine kinase growth factor receptor in mesothelioma cells. This example demonstrates homodimerisation of the epidermal growth factor receptor (EGFR) (A) following TGF-α binding which induces a cascade of intracellular signalling events resulting in cell survival and proliferation. The ligand-receptor interaction may be blocked by selective anti-EGFR monoclonal antibodies such as cetuximab (B). Courtesy of Prof David Ferry, Wolverhampton, UK.

mesothelial cells results in the induction of a number of growth factors and cytokines, which induce angiogenesis and a relative downregulation of cell-mediated immunity that may precede the development of malignancy [1,2]. In this regard, the resultant chronic exposure of mesothelial cells to growth factors may give rise to an environment favourable for the development of MPM. The surrounding stromal cells, particularly macrophages, play a crucial role in the secretion of and responses to growth factors and cytokines, acting in concert with the exposed mesothelial cells themselves. With the development of frank malignancy, paracrine and autocrine growth factors (Table 8.1) play a crucial role in the maintenance, local progression, and dissemi-

Table 8.1 Autocrine and paracrine growth factors and cytokines with a role in the pathogenesis of malignant pleural mesothelioma

Growth factor/cytokine	Pathophysiological functions
PDGF-A, PDGF-B, and receptors	Autocrine tumour growth loop Angiogenesis Tumour invasion
IGF-I, IGF-II, and receptors	Autocrine tumour growth loop Suppression of cell-mediated immunity Angiogenesis
bFGF and receptor	Autocrine tumour growth loop Angiogenesis Tissue repair and remodelling
VEGF and receptors	Autocrine growth factor loop Angiogenesis
HGF/SF and *met*	Autocrine growth factor loop Angiogenesis Chemotaxis
TGF-α and EGFR	Autocrine tumour growth loop Angiogenesis
IL-1	Pro-inflammatory cytokine
IL-2	Induction of cell-mediated immune response
IL-6	Angiogenesis Humoral immunity
IL-8	Angiogenesis Humoral immunity
IL-10	Humoral immunity
IL-12	Cell-mediated immunity Inhibition of angiogenesis
TNF-α	Pro-inflammatory cytokine
M-CSF and GM–CSF	Macrophage differentiation and activation
TGF-β1, TGF-β2, TGF-β3, and receptors	Autocrine tumour growth loop Anchorage-dependent growth of mesothelioma cells Angiogenesis Humoral immunity.

PDGF, platelet-derived growth factor; IGF, insulin-like growth factor; bFGF, basic fibroblast growth factor; VEGF, vascular endothelial growth factor; HGF/SF, hepatocyte growth factor/scatter factor; TGF, transforming growth factor; EGFR, epidermal growth factor receptor; IL, interleukin; TNF, tumour necrosis factor; M-CSF, macrophage colony-stimulating factor; GM-CSF, granulocyte–macrophage colony-stimulating factor.

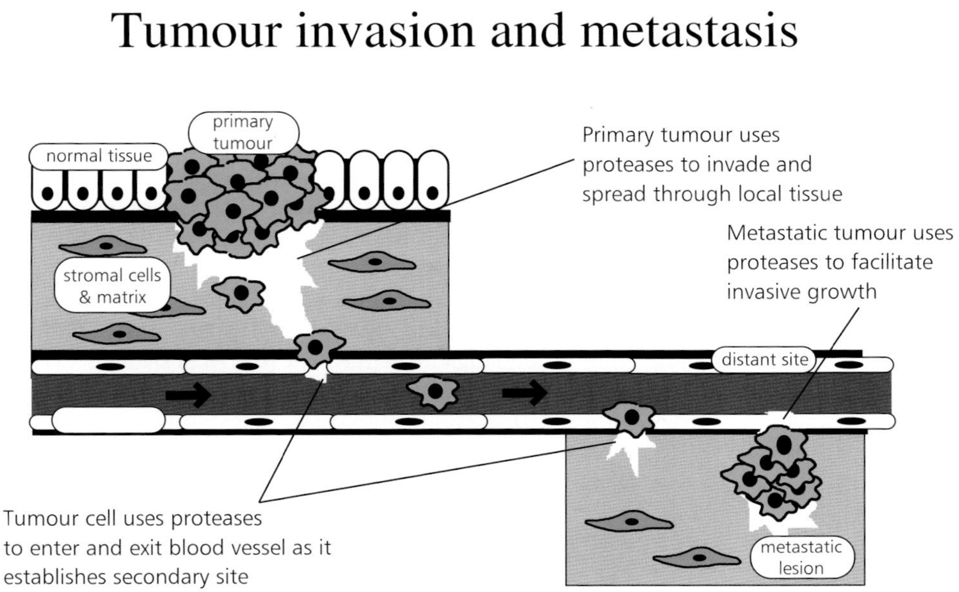

Tumour invasion and metastasis

Figure 8.2 Growth factors and protease enzymes play a central role in the pathogenesis of solid tumours including MPM.

nation of MPM (Fig. 8.2). This chapter discusses the role that growth factors, cytokines, proteases and their inhibitors, apoptosis regulators, and cell survival signalling play in MPM.

Type 1 growth factor receptor family

The type 1 growth factor receptor (GFR) family includes epidermal growth factor receptor (EGFR, HER1, ErbB-1), ErbB-2 (HER2, neu), ErbB-3 (HER3), and ErbB-4 (HER4) [3]. These are cell-membrane-situated receptors, which have an extracellular ligand binding domain, a transmembrane domain, and an internal domain with tyrosine kinase enzyme activity. They are central to cell proliferation, differentiation, migration, adhesion, and survival [4]. Inappropriate over-expression may contribute to tumour growth and invasion [3]. Immunoreactivity may reflect gene amplification, upregulated transcription, increased translation, and/or reduced degradation of the protein, all of which may be present in tumours [4–7]. Aberrant activation of the EGFR family as a result of these processes is well recognized as a predictor of poor prognosis in solid tumours [8].

In comparison to other solid tumours, there are relatively few reports investigating expression of type 1 GFRs in MPM. Amplification of the EGFR gene has been examined by the differential polymerase chain reaction (PCR) technique in three cases of malignant mesothelioma (MM), with one case representing each of the main histological cell types [9]. Amplification of the EGFR gene was found in the biphasic and sarcomatoid samples, with an additional band suggesting gene rearrangement in the sarcomatoid case.

There have been a number of studies investigating EGFR expression in mesothelioma tumour samples by immunohistochemistry. Dazzi *et al.* [10] found EGFR expression in 23 of 34 (68 per cent) cases examined, with positivity more common in the epithelioid cell type. In contrast with studies in many other tumours, Dazzi and colleagues found that the loss of EGFR staining was associated with a worse outcome, but that this was not independent of the effect of cell type. Ramael *et al.* [11] described both cytoplasmic and nuclear immunoreactivity in mesothelial cells of all 32 mesothelioma specimens. Govindan *et al.* [12] examined paraffin-embedded sections of 24 cases of mesothelioma (21 MPMs) by immunohistochemistry and detected EGFR in 14 (58 per cent). Cai *et al.* [13] compared the expression of EGFR in 30 reactive mesothelial proliferations and 39 epithelioid MMs. They found that only 3 per cent of the former, but 45 per cent of the latter, were positive. In a larger series, the expression of EGFR in 171 cases was examined by immunohistochemistry (Fig. 8.3) [14]. EGFR correlated strongly with cell type: 58 of 98 epithelioid cases, compared with three of 27 sarcomatoid cases (11 per cent), were positive. EGFR positivity correlated with absence of chest pain, good performance status and prognostic groups, and early IMIG Tumour–Nodes–Metastasis (TNM) stage. Interestingly, expression of EGFR was more common in tumours displaying TN, although no perinecrotic pattern of staining was seen. Although EGFR positivity was associated with good prognosis in univariate analysis, it was not found to be an independent prognostic factor. Two further studies have confirmed that EGFR

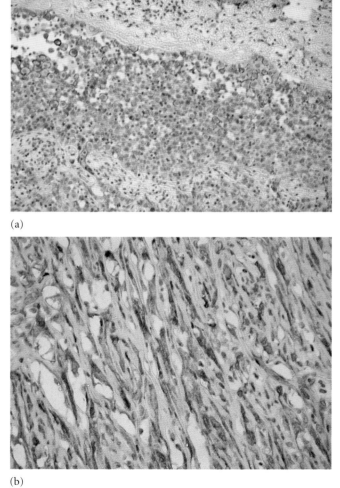

(a)

(b)

Figure 8.3 Epidermal growth factor receptor expression in (a) epithelioid and (b) sarcomatoid pleural mesothelioma.

expression is associated with a favourable outcome [15,16]. Furthermore Destro *et al.* demonstrated a significant correlation between EGFR protein and mRNA levels indicating that the quantification method of EGFR membrane expression used in their study was reliable [16].

With regard to other type 1 GFRs in MPM, Govindan *et al.* [12] did not detect HER-2 in their immunohistochemical study of 24 cases. Similarly, Ascoli *et al.* [17] did not find HER-2 positivity in MM cells obtained from pleural fluid aspirates. However, Thirkettle *et al.* [18] found HER-2 expression in 28 of 29 cases. Horvai *et al.* [19] reported a study correlating HER-2 immunoreactivity in 37 tumour samples with gene amplification by fluorescence *in situ* hybridization and RT-PCR [19]. Cytoplasmic staining was seen in 26 cases (70 per cent) but no membranous staining was evident. However, examination of the three most positive cases revealed no significant evidence of gene amplification or increase in mRNA.

Membranous EGFR expression has also been noted in four mesothelioma cell lines [20]. In this study, the four mesothelioma cell lines were examined for their responses to EGF and TGF-α. The investigators found evidence for an autocrine growth loop via TGF-α, a known ligand of EGFR, in one of the four cell lines.

There is emerging evidence of a second putative autocrine growth loop involving EGFR, which may act via cyclo-oxygenase 2 (COX-2). EGFR has been shown to stimulate COX-2 transcription in squamous carcinoma cells [21] and cholangiocarcinoma cells [22]. COX-2 activation can induce EGFR transcription, an effect abolished by addition of the non-selective COX inhibitor indomethacin [23]. Furthermore, prostaglandin E_2 (PGE_2) is capable of transactivation of EGFR [24]. This loop has not been investigated directly in MPM, although it is clear that EGFR and COX-2 (see below) are both important in the pathogenesis of MPM.

Insulin-like growth factors I and II

Insulin-like growth factor I (IGF-I) has well-established roles in cell transformation and tumour growth [25]. Crocidolite fibres induce the expression of both IGF-I [26] and the IGF-I receptor (IGF-IR) by alveolar macrophages [27]. There is compelling evidence that IGF-I may act as an autocrine growth factor in normal proliferating mesothelial cells. One study demonstrated that five human mesothelial cell samples and 11 human mesothelioma cell lines expressed IGF-I, IGF binding protein 3 (IGFBP-3) and IGF-IR mRNA. Furthermore, administration of exogenous IGF-I stimulated growth of the mesothelial cells, suggesting a possible role for IGF-I in malignant transformation [28].

In addition to its proliferative effects in mesothelial cells, IGF-I may contribute to the epithelial to mesenchymal transformation of mesothelioma cells. Exposure to IGF-I, in common with EGF, stimulated conversion of epithelioid MPM cells into a sarcomatoid phenotype [29]. This was associated with the synthesis of chondroitin sulphate containing proteoglycans. Expression of hyaluronan and other proteoglycans, such as those containing heparan sulphate, may also be induced by IGF-I [30].

As with EGFR, IGF-I is also involved in the regulation of COX-2, enhancing induction of the immunomodulatory enzyme by the pro-inflammatory cytokine IL-1β [31]. As discussed previously, high IGF-I expression may downregulate Th1 cell-mediated immune responses with inhibition of T-cell activation and reduce cytotoxic T-cell activity. These effects may be in part related to the upregulation of COX-2 [32]. IGF-I is a pro-angiogenic growth factor which stimulates the migration and tube-forming activity of endothelial cells [33] and promotes the expression of MMP-2 [34]. IGF-IR has attracted interest as a possible therapeutic target in MPM. Pass *et al.* [35] found that an antisense IGF receptor transcript reduced the proliferation and tumorigenicity of the hamster mesothelioma cell line H9A.

High levels of IGF-II mRNA have been noted in MPM [36,37]. Rutten *et al.* [38] found that cell lines derived from normal rat mesothelium and spontaneous mesotheliomas. In contrast, IGF-II was not expressed in asbestos-induced rat mesotheliomata in this study. All cell lines co-expressed IGF-II receptors. The biological activity of secreted IGF-II was abrogated by the action of an IGF-II-specific antibody in a dose-dependent fashion that could be partially reversed by the addition of IGF-II to the cell cultures [37]. IGF-II expression is also seen in human MPM cell lines [38]. These observations suggest that IGF-II is an autocrine growth factor in MPM and a further potential target for therapy [37].

Hepatocyte growth factor/scatter factor

Hepatocyte growth factor/scatter factor (HGF/SF) is a cytokine which stimulates the proliferation and motility of epithelial cells and tumour cells [39]. Its secretion is upregulated by basic fibroblast growth factor (bFGF) [40], and cleavage by urokinase plasminogen activator (uPA) is required for its activation [41]. HGF/SF may stimulate all three aspects of metastasis: growth, invasion, and angiogenesis. These effects are mediated via a tyrosine kinase receptor, *met*, resulting in endothelial cell proliferation, secretion of proteases, and invasion. HGF/SF stimulates production of matrix metalloproteinases (MMPs) in colorectal cancer cell lines [42] and induces synthesis of MMP-1 and MMP-3, but not MMP-9, in keratinocytes [43]. It may also be implicated in the activation of the angiogenic integrin $\alpha_v\beta_3$ [44]. HGF/SF is over-secreted in a range of tumours [39].

Mesothelioma samples stain strongly for HGF/SF and *met* with immunohistochemical techniques [18,45,46]. HGF/SF has been found in the pleural effusions of patients with MPM [47]. It stimulates chemotactic and chemokinetic mobility in mesothelioma cell lines [45] and has been associated with increased microvessel density in MPM tumours [48]. Of further interest is that Adamson *et al.* [49] found that HGF levels increased in bronchoalveolar and pleural lavage fluid following asbestos exposure in crocidolite-exposed rats. Exposure of mesothelial cells in culture to pleural lavage fluid induced mitogenic activity significantly inhibited by antibodies to HGF [49].

Keratinocyte growth factor

As with HGF/SF there is emerging evidence that keratinocyte growth factor (KGF) is released from mesothelial cells in response to crocidolite exposure in rats [49]. Adamson *et al.* [50] administered crocidolite fibres into the trachea of rats, and cultured mesothelial cells and fibroblasts in the presence of pleural lavage fluid from the animals. Mesothelial cell proliferation was blocked by an antibody to KGF. KGF expression has not been investigated in established MPM, either in cell lines or in tumour samples.

Transforming growth factors α and β

Members of the transforming growth factor (TGF) family play important roles in the pathogenesis of MPM. TGF-α, a ligand of EGFR, appears to be an autocrine growth factor in transformed rat mesothelial cells [51]. Although EGFR expression was noted in both asbestos-transformed and spontaneously transformed cells in this study, the asbestos-transformed cells also expressed TGF-α. TGF-α was shown to stimulate their growth, the effect of which was abolished by a neutralizing antibody. A similar effect was noted in a study of mesothelioma cell lines [20]. All four mesothelioma cell lines investigated expressed EGFR, whereas two secreted TGF-α and expressed its membrane-bound precursor pro-TGF-α. In ZL-34 cells, administration of neutralizing antibodies to TGF-α reduced TGF-α synthesis, suggesting its potential role as an autocrine growth factor. Cai *et al.* [13] demonstrated TGF-α expression by immunohistochemistry in 26 of 38 (76 per cent) cases of mesothelioma. TGF-α, in common with the other EGFR ligands, EGF, and heparin-binding epidermal growth factor, may also act as a chemotactic agent for normal human mesothelial cells [52].

TGF-β elicits different responses from different cell types. It usually inhibits growth of haematopoietic cells and enhances mesenchymal growth. In the progression from transformed to malignant cells, TGF-β may switch from mediating inhibition of cell proliferation to being a mitogenic factor [53]. It is one of several factors secreted by normal mesothelial cells or macrophages *in vitro* after exposure to asbestos fibres and by mesothelioma cells *in vivo* [54]. Kumar-Singh *et al.* [55] examined the expression of TGF-β in 52 cases of MPM. Tumour cell immunoreactivity for TGF-β was noted in 96 per cent of cases, with strong stromal positivity also being seen, whereas TGF-β was present in only 10 per cent of samples of non-neoplastic pleura. TGF-β expression was not associated with prognosis. However, co-expression of TGF-β with vascular endothelial growth factor (VEGF), aFGF, and bFGF (see below and Chapter 9) correlated with poor survival. A second immunohistochemical study by Jagirdar *et al.* [56] investigated the expression of the TGF-β_1 and TGF-β_2 isoforms, finding expression of the former predominantly in the stromal and the latter in tumour cells. Constitutive expression of TGF-β_2 was found by Orengo *et al.* [57] in the four mesothelioma cell lines that they examined, whilst Fitzpatrick *et al.* [58] found that both TGF-β_1 and TGF-β_2 were produced by human mesothelioma cells. Administration to the cells of blocking antisense oligonucleotides against mRNA of either TGF isoform reduced expression of both TGF-β_1 and TGF-β_2 proteins. TGF-β_2 inhibition reduced anchorage-independent growth *in vitro* and tumorigenicity *in vivo*. Furthermore, blocking the effects of TGF-β_2 by intratumoral administration of the antisense oligonucleotides increased infiltration into the tumours by T lymphocytes [58,59]. Thus TGF-β, as well as TGF-α, appears to act as an autocrine growth factor in MM.

TGF-β modulates angiogenic factors; administration of TGF-β_2 stimulated VEGF production by mesothelial cells both *in vitro* and *in vivo* [59]. TGF-β was also found to be partially responsible for the induction of uPA receptor (uPAR) by asbestos. Human and rabbit mesothelial cell uPAR expression was upregulated by the media from monocytes cultured with chrysotile and crocidolite asbestos. The use of blocking antibodies to TGF-β demonstrated that this effect was mediated in part by TGF-β [61]. In addition, in mesothelioma TGF-β upregulates the expression of a number of matrix proteins, including tenascin and fibronectin [61], proteoglycans and hyaluronan [63], syndecan-1 [29], and MMPs [64], all of which play important roles in the pathogenesis of the disease.

Vascular endothelial growth factor

Vascular endothelial growth factor (VEGF) represents a family of proteins implicated in both angiogenesis and lymphangiogenesis and includes VEGF-A, -B, -C ,and -D. The most important pro-angiogenic growth factor of the family is VEGF-A which itself has at least four isoforms (see Chapter 9). However, recent evidence suggests that VEGF-A and its receptors VEGFR-1 (flt-1), VEGFR-2 (KDR, flk-1), and the neuropilin receptors 1 and 2 (NP-1, NP-2) may also act as growth and survival factors for many solid tumours.

Human mesothelioma cell lines have recently been found to produce VEGF, VEGFR-1 and VEGFR-2. VEGF has been demonstrated to induce a dose-dependent increase in cellular proliferation and phosphorylation of both VEGFR-1 and VEGFR-2 tyrosine kinase receptors. This effect is blocked by both anti-VEGF and anti-VEGFR antibodies, suggesting a potential autocrine growth factor function for VEGF in MM. Furthermore MPM biopsies were found to express VEGF and both receptors [65]. These data collectively indicate that VEGF and its receptors are potential targets for therapy in MM.

Unlike VEGF-A, the closely related molecule VEGF-C is a lymphangiogenic growth factor. However, evidence that VEGF-C may also have an autocrine growth factor role in MPM has recently emerged. VEGF-C and its receptor VEGFR-3 are co-expressed in MPM, and the expression of VEGF-C correlates with the degree of lymphangiogenesis seen in tumour specimens [66]. A VEGF antisense oligonucleotide that inhibited both VEGF and VEGF-C expression has recently been found to inhibit MPM cell growth [67]. Selective antibodies to both flk-1 and VEGFR-3 had synergistic antitumour activity. These findings suggest that targeting VEGF and VEGF-C simultaneously may be an effective therapeutic approach for the management of this disease.

Platelet-derived growth factor

It has long been recognized that high platelet counts are associated with a poor prognosis in solid tumours, including MPM. Whilst there are a number of reasons for this, there is clear evidence that platelets are carriers of a number of potent growth factors that may be released at the site of a tumour. One such factor originally isolated from platelets is platelet-derived growth factor (PDGF) [68,69]. PDGF is a potent mitogen of cells of mesenchymal origin, including normal mesothelial cells *in vitro* and *in vivo* [70,71]. It consists of A and B chain subunits, which form homo- or heterodimers activating the PDGF receptors (PDGFR) α and β [72]. PDGFR-α and PDGFR-β activate a wide range of both common and separate pathways affecting cell proliferation, chemotaxis, survival, and apoptosis [73].

In *in vivo* experiments increased expression of PDGF and its receptors has been implicated in the stimulation of fibroblasts and development of pulmonary fibrosis following asbestos administration, a condition associated with the development of MPM in humans [74]. This pathology may be related to the upregulation of the expression of PDGF subunits and PDGFR by alveolar macrophages and bronchoalveolar epithelial cells seen in response to asbestos fibre exposure [75]. Simian virus 40 (SV40) has also been implicated in the pathogenesis of MPM. SV 40 Tag immortalized mesothelial cells are not tumorigenic but become so after transfection with the PDGF-A chain gene [76]. In this study, the resultant tumours in athymic mice themselves overexpressed PDGF-A. This suggests that constitutive expression of PDGF-A is an essential step in the malignant transformation of mesothelial cells.

Tumour cells from asbestos-induced mesotheliomata in rats expressed increased levels of PDGFR-β, but the PDGF isoforms could not be detected [77]. In comparison with normal human mesothelial cells, mesothelioma cell lines over-express PDGF A and B subunits [78–80]. Most mesothelioma cell lines and tumour tissue samples express PDGFR-β but not PDGFR-α mRNA; the latter is the transcript expressed predominantly by normal mesothelial cells. The data suggest that autocrine stimulation of growth may occur with a positive loop for normal mesothelial cells being established between PDGF-A and PDGFR-α, whilst in malignant cells the feedback loop is between PDGF-B and PDGFR-β [80–81]. The downregulation of PDGFR-α in mesothelioma may be due in part to the action of TGF-β_1 [83]. There is some evidence to suggest that activation of PDGFR-α modulates an antiproliferative effect *in vitro* in conjunction with the PDGF-A subunit. However, PDGF-A expression *in vivo* is associated with tumour formation and growth [84].

Further evidence that the PDGF-B may function as an autocrine growth factor in mesothelioma comes from growth-inhibition studies. Interruption of the PDGFR-β-mediated autocrine growth loop has been demonstrated in human mesothelial cells *in vitro* with a hammerhead c-*sis* ribozyme [85]. Furthermore, the PDGF-BB homodimer has been shown to act as a chemoattractant for mesothelioma cells in a Boyden chamber model, an action mediated via PDGFR-β in conjunction with integrin $\alpha_3\beta_1$ [86].

Interleukins and colony-stimulating factors

As has been discussed in Chapter 6, both IL-6 and IL-8 are upregulated in SV40-transformed human mesothelial cells exposed to the pro-inflammatory cytokines TNF-α and IL-1β. IL-6 is also produced by MM cell lines [87], whilst IL-8 has been demonstrated in the supernatant of mesothelioma cell lines and localized to MPM cells of pleural biopsies [88]. Both IL-6 and IL-8 levels are raised significantly in pleural effusions due to MPM compared with other malignant pleural effusions [88,89]. Serum IL-6 levels in MPM patients correlate with elevated platelet counts, a poor prognostic feature in this disease [66,67]. The direct effects of IL-6 and IL-8 on mesothelioma cells remain to be characterized. Nonetheless there is clear evidence that both are pro-angiogenic and induce a relative suppression of the cell-mediated immune response [1,32]. Therefore both factors may play a role in carcinogenesis and tumour growth and metastasis.

Granulocyte–macrophage colony-stimulating factor (GM-CSF) and granulocyte colony-stimulating factor (G-CSF) may be expressed by normal human mesothelial cells exposed to EGF and TNF-α *in vitro* and by mesothelioma cells *in vivo* [90,91]. Although the prognostic and clinical relevance of GM-CSF and G-CSF expression in MPM remain to be established, there is clear evidence that both factors play a role in angiogenesis and the progression of solid tumours [92]. Interestingly, gene therapy with GM-CSF is being evaluated in MPM for its potential antitumour immunomodulatory effects [93,94].

Growth factors and extracellular matrix proteolysis

Proteolysis of the extracellular matrix (ECM) and basement membrane by proteinases such as matrix metalloproteinases, cathepsins, and enzymes of the fibrinolytic system is a central part of metastasis. These enzymes facilitate not only tumour cell mobility and extravasation but also the stromal remodelling around endothelial cells as a central part of angiogenesis. Expression and activity of the ECM proteolytic enzymes are induced by a number of different growth factors.

Matrix metalloproteinases

Matrix metalloproteinases (MMPs) are a family of zinc-dependent enzymes which are implicated in the growth of primary and secondary tumours [95]. Between them, they are capable of digesting all the components of the ECM and basement membrane. They have a distinctive PRCGVPD sequence in the pro-enzyme domain with an unpaired cysteine residue which co-binds the zinc atom. Disruption of this sulphur–zinc bond activates the enzyme. MMP family members differ in their structure and substrate specificity and interactions with their inhibitors. Most MMPs are secreted as latent pro-enzymes which undergo extracellular proteolytic activation by cleavage of their N-terminal sequence. For example, MMP-2 activation occurs at the cell surface, with pro-MMP-2 interacting with TIMP-2 bound to membrane type 1 MMP (MT1-MMP), forming a ternary complex. Free MT1-MMP, located close to the ternary complex, then activates pro-MMP-2 on the cell surface [96,97]. MMPs may be secreted by stromal cells near to tumour cells, rather than by tumour cells themselves, with diffusion through the tissue to the site of action [98,99].

MMPs are regulated in a number of different ways [100,101]. They are inhibited directly by the tissue inhibitors of metalloproteinase (TIMPs) [95,102], with the balance between activated MMPs and TIMPs determining the net MMP activity. At low levels, TIMP-2 promotes complex formation with MT1-MMP and pro-MMP-2 as described above. However, at high concentrations, TIMP-2 inhibits MMP-2 activation [103]. TIMPs inhibit the extravasation of metastatic tumour cells, reduce the growth of both the primary and secondary tumours, and also reduce angiogenesis [102,104]. With regard to upregulation of MMPs, growth and angiogenic factors, such as TGF-α and TGF-β, aFGF and bFGF, EGF, VEGF, and TNF-α have been shown to increase expression of MMPs [96,100,101,105–109]. Specific growth factors increase the expression of some, but not all, MMPs. For example, bFGF upregulates the expression of the gelatinases MMP-2 and MMP-9 and interstitial collagenase (MMP-1) but not MMP-3 [106], whereas TNFα increases expression of MMP-1, MMP-3, and MMP-9, but not MMP-2 [107–109]. COX-2 is implicated in the activation of MMP-2. In colorectal cancer, COX-2-expressing cells were associated with activation of MMP-2 whereas sulindac sulphide, a COX-2 inhibitor, blocked the increase in RNA levels of the MMP-2 activator MT-MMP-1 [110]. PGE_2 may also regulate expression of MMP-9 [111]. Over-expression of MMPs and their relation to disease progression has been described in many solid tumours, including non-small-cell lung cancer [112], breast cancer [113], and colorectal cancer [114]. However, the pattern of over-expression varies greatly between tumour types.

MMPs in mesothelioma

Hirano *et al.* [115] described the expression of MMP-1, MMP-2, MMP-3, MMP-7, MMP-9, TIMP-1, and TIMP-2 in 16 cases of MPM by immunohistochemistry. MMP-1 was expressed by most tumour cells in all cases and MMP-2 was detected in two cases (13 per cent), but the other MMPs were not expressed. This contrasts with another study, where homogenized tumour supernatants were analysed by semiquantitative gelatin zymography in 35 cases of MPM and 26 benign controls [116]. MMP-2 was found to be the predominant gelatinase expressed in MPM, with both latent and active forms detectable in all tumours (Fig. 8.4). Although latent MMP-9 was noted in all tumours, the active isoform was not detected by the assay in nine cases (26 per cent). MMP-2

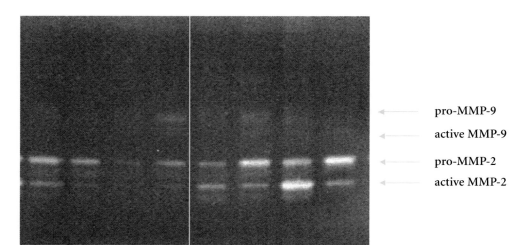

Figure 8.4 (a) Zymography and (b, c) immunohistochemistry detection of MMP-2 and MMP-9 in malignant pleural mesothelioma.

correlated with extrapleural nodal metastasis; however, the number undergoing pathological nodal staging was small (13 cases). No correlations between MMP activity and COX-2 protein levels (as assessed by western blotting) were found. Although just missing statistical significance in univariate analysis, the gelatinolytic activity of pro-MMP-2 and total MMP-2 were significant independent prognostic factors, together with weight loss, in respective multivariate analyses.

MMPs in mesothelioma cell lines: patterns of expression and upregulation by growth factors

Rubins *et al.* [117] examined the activity of the gelatinases in mesothelioma cell lines by semi-quantitative gelatin zymography and found that all nine lines expressed MMP-2 and MMP-9 constitutively, with increased activity of the former in the sarcomatoid line and the latter in the epithelioid line. TGF-β increased the activity of MMP-2 in all lines. TNF-α increased MMP-9 activity in five cell lines. Harvey *et al.* [118] investigated the expression of MMP-1, MMP-2, MMP-3, MMP-9 , MT1-MMP, TIMP-1, and TIMP-2 in three cell lines in response to the administration of HGF/SF. HGF/SF was found to increase the expression of MMP-1, MMP-9, and MT1-MMP, and also enhanced motility and invasion of the mesothelioma cells. Liu *et al.* [119] assessed the expression (by RT-PCR and western blotting) and activity (by substrate zymography) of MMPs and TIMPS in eight mesothelioma cell lines. It was found that all lines expressed MMP-1, MMP-2, MMP-3, MMP-9, and TIMP-1, TIMP-2, and TIMP-3, and six cell lines expressed MMP-10, but MMP-11 was detected in none. The same investigators have examined the regulation of MMPs in mesothelioma cell lines [120]. Using substrate zymography, they found that a number of different factors, including EGF, TGF-α, amphiregulin, heparin binding EGF, β-cellulin (BTC), stem cell factor, IGF-I and IGF-II, aFGF, bFGF, and HGF increased the secretion of MMP-3 and/or MMP-9 into the culture medium. This increase was blocked by the tyrosine kinase inhibitor genistein. However, the expression of MMP-2 was not affected by these growth factors. These findings suggest that MMPs play a role in MPM, although their interactions, control by growth factors, and prognostic significance require further investigation.

Fibrinolytic enzymes

The balance of the fibrinolytic enzymes uPA and tissue plasminogen activator (tPA), and their regulator plasminogen activator inhibitor 1 (PAI-1), is important in tumour invasion and angiogenesis. Plasmin is an enzyme implicated in the proteolysis of the major protein components of the ECM [53], enabling invasion of tumour cells and angiogenesis. tPA binds strongly to fibrin and is involved primarily in fibrinolysis; however, uPA is associated more with tissue remodelling and cellular invasion. Migrating endothelial cells express elevated levels of uPA *in vitro*. Anti-uPA antibodies and blockade of uPAR have been observed to reduce tumour growth and metastasis *in vivo* [121,122]. uPA is secreted as a pro-enzyme and activated by plasmin and cathepsins, among other enzymes. Induction of uPA activity may be mediated by TNF-α and TGF-β, which also activate the uPA receptor *in vitro* [123]. uPA is also implicated in the activation of metalloproteinases such as MMP-2 and MMP-9 [124,125]. uPA is produced by a number of tumours and its expression can be linked to tumour size, lymph node metastasis, and angiogenesis [122,126,127]. Lung cancers which do not express PAI activity are associated with a poor prognosis [128].

MPM often produces a fibrinous pleural effusion. However, although the levels of uPA, tPA, and PAI-1 are increased in the plasma of MPM patients, the activity of the enzymes is not significantly greater than normal [129]. Activity of uPA appears to be higher in the pleural fluid of these patients, but the importance of this is unclear. This 'balance' of the fibrinolytic system seen with MPM is absent in lung carcinoma [128], which may explain the relatively increased metastatic potential of the latter.

Hyaluronic acid

Hyaluronic acid (HA) is a glycosaminoglycan of the ECM [53] which plays a role in angiogenesis and may be involved in the pathogenesis of MM. HA degrades to form oligosaccharide fragments which are angiogenic; this process is inhibited by native HA [130]. HA oligosaccharides have synergistic angiogenic effects with VEGF *in vitro* [131]. PDGF, TGF-β, and bFGF, produced by mesothelial cells, stimulate HA synthesis [132,133]. CD44 is a widely expressed cell surface glycoprotein which acts as an adhesion molecule in cell–ECM and cell–cell interactions and is a receptor for HA. It is produced by reactive mesothelium and mesothelioma cells [134], but HA receptors are not a feature of normal mesothelial cells [135]. The interaction between HA and CD44 may be involved in the mobility of mesothelioma cells through the ECM. The expression of CD44 is a poor prognostic factor in a number of tumours, including gastric, colorectal, and breast cancers [136–138], although this has not yet been established in MPM. CD44 expression is also upregulated in tumour endothelial cells compared with those of surrounding vessels, and these cells are a target for anti-CD44 cytotoxic therapy with immunotoxins [139].

Cyclo-oxygenase-2

Epidemiological evidence links a reduction in the risk of colorectal cancer to the use of aspirin. This has led to investigation of the role of the cyclo-oxygenase (COX) enzymes in carcinogenesis. COX-1 and COX-2 both catalyse the first two steps of prostanoid synthesis. COX-1 is constitutively expressed in nearly all cell types and plays a central role in homeostatic processes through the synthesis of prostaglandins and prostacyclin. COX-2 is expressed in response to inflammatory stimuli, being upregulated by cytokines including IL-1β, IL-2, interferon α (IFN-α), IFN-β, IFN-γ, and TNF-α. The particular prostaglandin synthesized following COX-2 activity is cell specific. PGE_2, which is synthesized by PGE_2 synthase, may stimulate cell growth, alter cell adhesion, and inhibit apoptosis [1,32].

Recent evidence suggests that the over-expression of COX-2 plays an important role in the pathogenesis of a wide range of solid tumours. COX-2 is associated with the altered balance of the immune response seen in solid tumours through the induction of cyclic adenosine monophosphate (cAMP) [140]. PGE_2 downregulates the cell-mediated immune response by inhibiting the production by T lymphocytes of the T-helper lymphocyte (Th_1) cytokines IL-2, IFN-γ, and TNF-α, whereas it upregulates cytokines associated with the humoral immune (Th_2) response such as IL-6 [1,32].

Although there has been little investigation of the immunological roles of COX-2 in MPM, there is evidence suggestiing COX-2 activity in this regard. The transcription factor, nuclear factor κB (NF-κB), has two binding sites on the promoter region of the COX-2 gene. Exposure of rat mesothelial cells to asbestos causes translocation of the p65 protein and increases NF-κB DNA-binding activity in rat lung epithelial and pleural mesothelial cells [141]. Asbestos causes release of PGE_2 from alveolar macrophages and inhibition of mediated cytotoxicity [142,143]. Indomethacin, a COX-2 inhibitor, restored cell-mediated immune responses in an *ex vivo* mesothelioma model [144] and those mediated by alveolar macrophages [142]. A recent report has suggested that COX-2 inhibition with the specific COX-2 inhibitor rofecoxib enhances the efficacy of IFN-β immunotherapy in a murine model of MPM [145]. Administration of rofecoxib alone slowed the growth of small tumours, with no effect on large tumours. Rofecoxib in combination with IFN-β gene therapy led to cures in small tumours, reduced growth in large tumours, and inhibited the growth of metastatic tumour foci after surgical debulking had been performed.

COX-2 has also been shown to play a central role in angiogenesis [146]. Expression of a number of angiogenic growth factors, including VEGF, bFGF, TGF-β, and PDGF, is upregulated by COX-2-expressing colorectal cancer cells. Synthesis and release of these angiogenic factors is inhibited by aspirin and selective COX-2 inhibitors [147]. COX-2 expression has been correlated with angiogenesis, as assessed by microvessel density, in non-small cell lung cancer [148], breast cancer [149], gastric cancer [150], and colorectal cancer [151], but the evidence for this association is mixed. Furthermore, hypoxia induces COX-2 transcription in human umbilical vein endothelial cells [152]. COX-2 inhibition may reduce angiogenesis, stimulate apoptosis [153,154], and reduce tumour invasion [110,155].

There have been two reports of COX-2 expression in MPM. Marrogi *et al.* [156] demonstrated that COX-2 was expressed in all 30 cases of mesothelioma examined by immunohistochemistry. Similarly, we have demonstrated COX-2 expression by immunofluorescence (Fig. 8.5(a)) and western blotting (Fig. 8.5(b)) in 48 tumour samples [157]. Using a semiquantitive assay, we found that increasing levels of COX-2 protein correlated with weight loss and the presence of tumour necrosis [158]. A high COX-2 level was associated with poorer survival and was an independent prognostic factor in multivariate analysis.

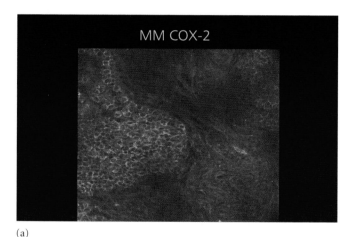

(a)

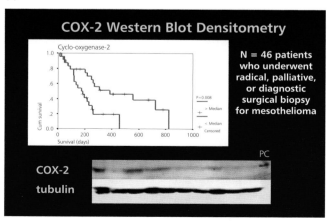

(b)

Figure 8.5 (a) Fluorescent immunohistochemistry and (b) western blot detection of COX-2 expression in MPM.

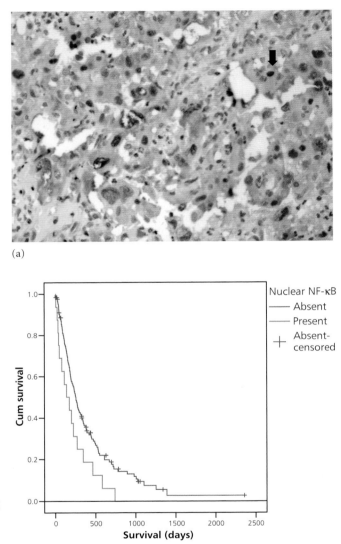

Figure 8.6 (a) Nuclear (arrow) and cytoplasmic expression of transcription factor NF-κB in MPM. (b) The presence of nuclear NF-κB staining in MPM is associated with a poor outcome.

In keeping with this observation, a recent immunohistochemistry study evaluated the expression of NF-κB in MPM [159]. Preliminary results indicate that any expression of NF-κB is associated with a poor outcome (Fig. 8.6).

Hypoxia and necrosis

Tumour cell hypoxia has been associated with resistance to radiotherapy and a poor outcome for many years. In 1958, Gray *et al.* [160] demonstrated that the absence of oxygen at the time of irradiation reduced tumour cell sensitivity to radiotherapy. Hypoxia occurs frequently in tumours because of the imbalance between the increased oxygen demand of the rapidly proliferating cells and a relatively poor oxygen supply by the neovasculature. Hypoxia induces a number

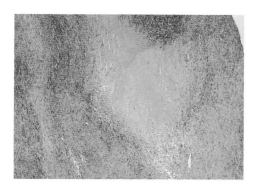

Figure 8.7 Tumour necrosis in MPM.

of angiogenic growth factors, such as VEGF, bFGF, PDGF, platelet-derived endothelial cell growth factor (PD-ECGF) and COX-2 [161–165]. Surrogate markers of hypoxia, such as carbonic anhydrase IX (CA-IX) and hypoxia inducible factor 1α (HIF-1α), have been correlated with microvessel density in solid tumours [166–168].

Coagulative necrosis, which is caused by chronic ischaemic injury, is a common feature of solid tumours and reflects the level of intratumoral hypoxia. Tumour necrosis (TN) has been correlated with poor prognosis in a number of solid tumours [169–170]. TN has been studied extensively in breast cancer and correlates with stage, grade, and both angiogenesis and macrophages which secrete angiogenic growth factors [171–172].

Although MPM is recognized clinically to be a fast growing tumour which responds poorly to radiotherapy, tumour hypoxia and its associated growth factors and cytokines have not been fully characterized. Until relatively recently there was little mention of TN in MPM in the literature beyond that it may be used in the differentiation of malignant from benign pleural proliferations [173]. In a recent study investigating the clinical and pathological correlations of TN in 171 cases of MPM, we found that the presence of intratumoral TN (Fig. 8.7) was a poor prognostic factor in univariate analysis [174]. TN correlated with thrombocytosis, lower haemoglobin, and a high microvessel density. Furthermore, TN was more likely to be present in EGFR-positive tumours [14] and was associated with higher levels of COX-2 protein in homogenized tumour tissue supernatants [174].

A recent study has identified the expression of CA-IX in 200 MPM tumour samples (Fig. 8.8). Standard immunohistochemical techniques were used and expression was scored according to the percentage of tumour cell staining seen. There is variable expression of CA-IX in MPM tissue, with membranous staining being most distinct. Membranous or cytoplasmic CA-IX tumour immunostaining was detected in 97.5 per cent of cases, with the majority (95 per cent) of tumour samples displaying both patterns of staining. Patients with MPM showing increased expression of CA-IX on biopsy tissue tend to fall into favourable prognostic groups. CA-IX expression above median value correlated with the absence of chest pain ($P < 0.0001$), no significant weight loss ($P = 0.01$), epithelial cell type ($P < 0.0001$), ECOG performance status 0–1 ($P < 0.0007$), and low-risk EORTC prognostic group ($P < 0.0001$). CA-IX expression above the median value was a good prognostic factor in univariate analysis ($P = 0.0065$), but not in multivariate analyses or if epithelial histology alone was considered [175]. CA-IX is regulated by HIF-1α [176]. HIF-1α induces the transcription of a number of target genes involved in angiogenesis, glycolysis, and erythropoiesis. It has been correlated with the expression of the angiogenic growth factors VEGF, bFGF and PD-ECGF in non-small cell lung cancer [177]. HIF- is commonly overexpressed in MPM but not in normal mesothelium, consistent with the prtesence of hypoxia [178].

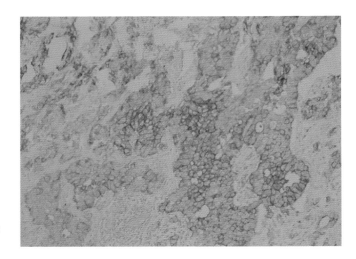

Figure 8.8 CA-IX expression in MPM.

Thus it is possible to hypothesize that, because of the high proliferative rate of MPM, the tumour growth outstrips its metabolic demand on the neovasculature, with the induction of angiogenic growth factors by hypoxia through factors such as CA-IX. However, the growth factors induced by MPM tumour cell hypoxia, their clinicopathological correlations, and the pathways involved remain to be elucidated.

Apoptosis and survival signalling in malignant pleural mesothelioma

Apoptosis signalling in MPM

Apoptosis proceeds via two converging cascades: the extrinsic pathway which is induced by members of the TNF family of ligands, and the intrinsic pathway which includes the mitochondria and is induced by DNA damage and other cellular stress stimuli. Both pathways trigger a cascade of proteolytic events culminating in the activation of the effector caspases 3, 6, and 7, which themselves cleave a variety of death substrates to initiate nuclear fragmentation and cellular disassembly [179]. Binding of TNF-α, tumour necrosis factor-related apoptosis-induced ligand (TRAIL), or Fas ligand (FasL) to their cognate receptors on the cell surface triggers extrinsic apoptosis. This initiates a cascade of events by activation of caspase-8 that either activates caspase-3 directly or, as demonstrated in the majority of cells, links to the intrinsic death pathway by cleavage of the pro-apoptotic BH3-only protein Bid [180]. The process can be blocked by c-FLIP, which inhibits caspase-8 activation, and by inhibitor of apoptosis proteins (IAPs), which inhibit processing and activation of initiator and effector caspases downstream of the mitochondria [181].

DNA damage and cellular stress are sensed by proteins such as ataxia-telangiectasia mutated (ATM) and Chk2 which stabilize p53. Once activated, p53 induces the expression of the pro-apoptotic Bcl-2 family members Bax and Bak as well as the regulatory BH3-only proteins Puma and Noxa. These factors contribute to changes in mitochondrial physiology, resulting in the release of cytochrome-c and Smac/DIABLO. Cytochrome-c binds apoptosis protease activating factor (Apaf)-1 in the presence of ATP to form the apoptosome, which recruits and activates initiator caspase-9. Caspase-9 then recruits and activates effector caspases that execute cell death. Anti-apoptotic members of the Bcl-2 family, such as Bcl-2, Bcl-xL, and Mcl-1, negatively control apoptosis on the level of mitochondrial integrity, whereas activation of caspase-9 and downstream effector caspases is controlled by IAPs that include XIAP, cIAP-1, cIAP-2, and survivin [181].

Altered expression of apoptosis regulators in mesothelioma

Cancer cells may loose their capacity to undergo apoptosis by reduced expression of p53 and pro-apoptotic members of the cell death machinery (Apaf-1, caspase-8, Bax, death receptors) because of genetic or epigenetic alterations, or by increased expression of Bcl-2, Bcl-xL, and IAPs. Expression of Bcl-xL and/or Bcl-2 has been detected in the majority of solid tumours including MPM, and several reports have shown a correlation between Bcl-2 and Bcl-xL expression and drug resistance, indicating resistance to apoptosis [182]. Recent work has shown that downregulation of Bcl-2 and Bcl-xL by antisense oligonucleotides sensitizes MPM cells to cisplatin and gemcitabine [183].

Similarly, IAPs are frequently upregulated in cancer cells [184]. Survivin is a 17 kDa protein that contains only a single baculovirus IAP repeat domain (BIR) and no really interesting new gene (RING) domain. In the nucleus, survivin binds to microtubules and assists in chromosomal segregation and cytokinesis during mitosis. In the cytoplasm, survivin inhibits apoptosis by interacting with caspase-9 in the presence of the HBXIP cofactor [185], binding to Smac [186], or associating with XIAP [187]. Survivin is expressed in normal proliferating haematopoietic cells as well as in terminally differentiated neutrophils, where it inhibits apoptosis independent of the cell cycle. Survivin expression has been demonstrated in a range of solid tumours, and in MPM correlates with a poor prognosis. Of particular importance, survivin expression has been demonstrated to correlate with resistance to conventional cytotoxic chemotherapeutic agents routinely used in the management of MPM [188]. In this regard the observation that targeted suppression of survivin can increase the sensitivity of cancer cells to chemotherapy may have clinical relevance for the future management of the disease [189].

Survival pathways that attenuate apoptosis signalling

In normal cells survival signals provided by activation of mitogen-activated protein (MAP) kinases and phosphatidyl-inositol 3 kinase (PI3K)/Akt (protein kinase B) pathways are responsible for reducing cell death and promoting proliferation, thereby controlling cellular homeostasis. Inappropriate activation of these pathways favours tumorigenesis by upregulation of anti-apoptotic proteins and downregulation of pro-apoptotic proteins. Growth factors that bind to receptor tyrosine kinases on the cell surface can trigger a variety of growth and survival responses. In MPM these receptors include EGFR, HGF, and VEGFR which have all been reported to initiate mitogenic and cytoprotective responses by activating MAP kinases and PI3K/Akt [190–192] (Fig. 8.9).

Binding of growth factors to receptor tyrosine kinases leads to activation of PI3K which produces PI-3,4,5-P3, leading to membrane attachment and subsequent phosphorylation and activation of Akt, a second-messenger-regulated subfamily of protein kinases [193] (Fig. 8.9). This latter step can be inhibited by the phosphatase and tensin homolog deleted on chromosome ten (PTEN) tumour suppressor, which is frequently deleted in human tumours. Transfection of MPM cells with PTEN engenders apoptosis, suggesting that activation of the PI3K/Akt pathway is indeed an active survival strategy of these tumours [194]. Akt can also be activated by nicotinic cholinergic receptors expressed in a variety of non-neuronal tissues including MPM [195].

Activated Akt is implicated in glucose metabolism, transcriptional control, and the regulation of apoptosis in many different cell types. Akt acts on the genomic level by regulating transcription factors and on the proteomic level by regulating post-translational modification of proteins involved in apoptosis control. Specifically, it promotes transcription of Bcl-xL and XIAP, and at

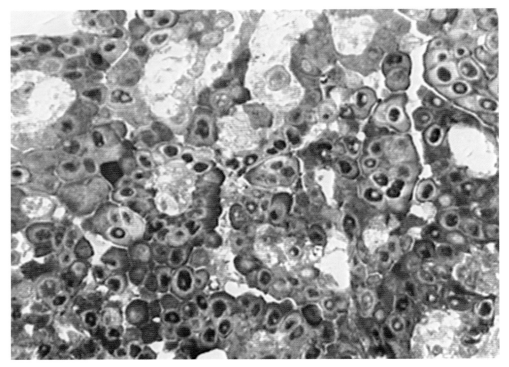

Figure 8.9 Cytoplasmic and nuclear phospo-Akt expression in malignant pleural mesothelioma.

the same time inactivates the proapoptotic proteins BAD and caspase-9. Recent work has also identified murine double minute-2 (MDM2) and the IAP survivin as targets positively regulated by Akt. Akt also phosporylates and thus inactivates glycogen synthase kinase-3 (GSK-3), a component of the canonical Wnt signalling pathway which promotes β-catenin degradation [196] (Fig. 8.10). This results in increased translocation of β-catenin to the nucleus and transcriptional activation of oncogenes engaged in cell survival, proliferation, and angiogenesis. To what extent activated Akt triggers Wnt signalling in MPM remains to be determined. A hypothetical model suggesting how the link between the PI3K/Akt and the Wnt signalling pathway may be established is illustrated in Figure 8.11. The importance of Wnt signalling in MPM cell survival was described by You *et al.* [197] who demonstrated that inhibition of this survival pathway also induces apoptosis in MPM cells by involving the non-canonical Wnt/JNK pathway. Thus, by providing cells with cytoprotective function, Akt is a central player in a survival signalling network which involves many components that have been linked to tumorigenesis [198,199].

Collectively, these observations demonstrate that MPM is a highly malignant disease in which defects in apoptosis regulation and execution underpin the development of the disease. Understanding the molecular events and identifying the molecular targets and signalling pathways that contribute to intrinsic apoptosis provides new avenues for improved cancer diagnostics and therapy. To develop more effective therapies for drug-resistant tumours including MPM, in forthcoming studies rational strategies must be devised to specifically manipulate cell death and survival programmes by targeted molecular intervention.

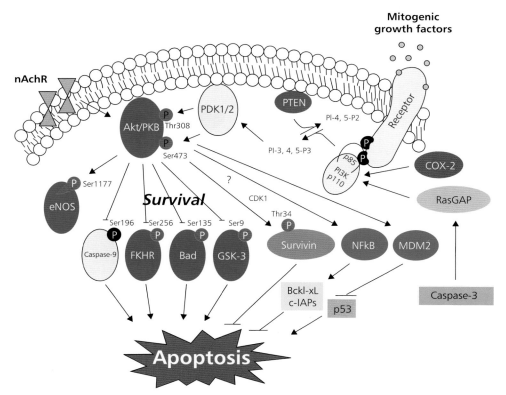

Figure 8.10 Regulation of cell survival by activation of the PI3K/Akt pathway. Upon binding to their cognate receptors on the cell surface, growth factors activate PI3K which further activates the second-messenger-regulated kinase Akt. This step can be inhibited by the PTEN tumour suppressor gene which is frequently deleted in human tumours. The stress kinase Akt is the central player in this pro-survival signalling network, which can also be activated by various other stimuli. Akt has several downstream targets and exerts its cytoprotective function by inhibiting pro-apoptotic pathways whilst at the same time activating anti-apoptotic pathways.

Microarray technology

Microarray is a powerful new technique which is able to identify increased expression in several thousand genes, which may include many growth factors (see Chapters 3 and 5). Expression profiles in mesothelial cells exposed to asbestos, MPM cell lines, and tumour samples have been reported by a number of different research groups. Sandhu *et al.* [200] investigated microarray expression profiles in mesothelial cells, which had been exposed to asbestos, at various stages of carcinogenesis. Upregulation of c-*myc*, *fra*-1, and EGFR was demonstrated following asbestos exposure. Rihn *et al.* [201] investigated gene expression ratios between human mesothelioma and mesothelial cells and identified, out of 6500 genes assessed, less than 300 which were upregulated. The function of some of these concerned cell division, migration, and invasiveness. Singhal *et al.* [202] examined 16 MM cases, validating results with quantitative RT-PCR. Amongst the genes over-expressed were several involved with pathways of energy, protein translation, and cytoskeleton remodelling. Interestingly, HIF-1 was also upregulated. Mohr *et al.* [203] attempted to avoid bias from the inherent tissue heterogeneity in MPM by using laser capture microdissection to

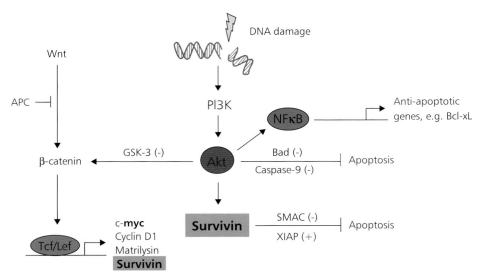

Figure 8.11 Proposed model of inducible cancer drug resistance. Apart from the signalling events illustrated in Figure 8.10, activated Akt also favours anti-apoptotic decisions by inactivation of GSK-3, which links to the canonical Wnt signalling pathway. Cytoplasmic and finally nuclear accumulation of β-catenin results in increased expression of oncogenes engaged in cell survival, proliferation, and angiogenesis.

select the cancer cells alone from tumour samples. Comparing the expression of 10 000 genes between MPM and *ex vivo* mesothelial cells, they found upregulation of 302. IGF-BP7 was one of eight genes particularly over-expressed. Gordon *et al.* [204] developed a model predicting survival using gene expression ratio data from 17 patients. They validated their technique in a separate dataset of 29 cases. It is anticipated that further studies using this technology will produce data pertaining to growth factor function in MPM.

Conclusions

There are a number of well-characterized growth factors in MPM, but many more which have yet be investigated to the same degree as they have in other solid tumours. Data regarding growth factor function and activity provide important insights into the carcinogenesis in response to asbestos fibres and SV40, the pathology of the histological MM subtypes, the prognosis of the disease, and the efficacy of novel therapies.

References

1. O'Byrne KJ, Dalgleish AG, Browning MJ, Steward WP, Harris AL. The relationship between angiogenesis and the immune response in carcinogenesis and the progression of malignant disease. *Eur J Cancer* 2000; **36**: 151–69.
2. O'Byrne KJ, Dalgleish AG. Chronic immune activation and inflammation as the cause of malignancy. *Br J Cancer* 2001; **85**: 473–83.
3. Walker R. The erbB/HER type 1 tyrosine kinase receptor family. *J Pathol* 1998; **185**: 234–5.
4. Yarden Y. The EGFR family and its ligands in human cancer. signalling mechanisms and therapeutic opportunities. *Eur J Cancer* 2001; **37** (Suppl 4): S3–8.

5. Arteaga CL. The epidermal growth factor receptor: from mutant oncogene in nonhuman cancers to therapeutic target in human neoplasia. *J Clin Oncol* 2001; **19**(Suppl): 32S–40S.

6. Slichenmyer WJ, Fry DW. Anticancer therapy targeting the erbB family of receptor tyrosine kinases. *Semin Oncol* 2001; **28** (Suppl 16): 67–79.

7. Gill GN, Bertics PJ, Santon JB. Epidermal growth factor and its receptor. *Mol Cell Endocrinol* 1987; **51**: 169–86.

8. Nicholson RI, Gee JM, Harper ME. EGFR and cancer prognosis. *Eur J Cancer* 2001; **37** (Suppl 4): S9–15.

9. Ramael M, Stinissen P, Segers K, Van Broeckhoven C, Van Marck E. Structural and quantitative aberrations in the epidermal growth factor receptor (EGF-R) gene in human malignant mesothelioma of the pleura. *Eur Respir Rev* 1993; **3**: 161–2.

10. Dazzi H, Hasleton PS, Thatcher N, Wilkes S, Swindell R, Chatterjee AK. Malignant pleural mesothelioma and epidermal growth factor receptor (EGF-R). Relationship of EGF-R with histology and survival using fixed paraffin embedded tissue and the F4, monoclonal antibody. *Br J Cancer* 1990; **61**: 924–6.

11. Ramael M, Segers K, Buysse C, Van den Bossche J, Van Marck E. Immunohistochemical distribution patterns of epidermal growth factor receptor in malignant mesothelioma and non-neoplastic mesothelium. *Virchows Arch A Pathol Anat Histopathol* 1991; **419**: 171–5.

12. Govindan R, Ritter J, Suppiah R. EGFR and HER-2 overexpression in malignant mesothelioma. *Proc Am Soc Clin Oncol* 2001; **20**: 3106 (abstract).

13. Cai YC, Roggli V, Mark E, Cagle PT, Fraire AE. Transforming growth factor alpha and epidermal growth factor receptor in reactive and malignant mesothelial proliferations. *Arch Pathol Lab Med* 2004; **128**: 68–70.

14. Edwards JG, Swinson DEB, Jones JL, Waller DA, O'Byrne KJ. EGFR expression in malignant mesothelioma—correlation with clinical, pathological and biological variables. *Lung Cancer* (in press).

15. Govindon R, Kratze RA, Herndon JE 2nd, *et al.* (CALGB 30101). Gefitinib in patients with malignant mesothelioma: a phase II study by the Cancer and Leukaemia Group B. *Clin Cancer Res* 2005; **11**: 2300–4.

16. Destro A, Ceresoli GL, Falleni M, *et al.* EGFR overexpression in malignant pleural mesothelioma. An immunohistochemical and molecular study with clinico-pathological correlations. *Lung Cancer* 2006: **51**: 207–15.

17. Ascoli V, Scalzo CC, Nardi F. C-erbB-2 oncoprotein immunostaining in serous effusions. *Cytopathology* 1993; **4**: 207–18.

18. Thirkettle I, Harvey P, Hasleton PS, Ball RY, Warn RM. Immunoreactivity for cadherins, HGF/SF, *met*, and erbB-2 in pleural malignant mesotheliomas. *Histopathology* 2000; **36**: 522–8.

19. Horvai AE, Xu Z, Kramer MJ, Jablons DM, Treseler PA. Malignant mesothelioma does not demonstrate overexpression or gene amplification despite cytoplasmic imunohistochemical staining for c-Erb-B2. *Arch Pathol Lab Med* 2003; **127**: 465–9.

20. Morocz IA, Schmitter D, Lauber B, Stahel RA. Autocrine stimulation of a human lung mesothelioma cell line is mediated through the transforming growth factor alpha/epidermal growth factor receptor mitogenic pathway. *Br J Cancer* 1994; **70**: 850–6.

21. Mestre JR, Subbaramaiah K, Sacks PG, *et al.* Retinoids suppress epidermal growth factor-induced transcription of cyclooxygenase-2 in human oral squamous carcinoma cells. *Cancer Res* 1997; **57**: 2890–5.

22. Yoon JH, Higuchi H, Werneburg NW, Kaufmann SH, Gores GJ. Bile acids induce cyclooxygenase-2 expression via the epidermal growth factor receptor in a human cholangiocarcinoma cell line. *Gastroenterology* 2002; **122**: 985–93.

23. Kinoshita T, Takahashi Y, Sakashita T, Inoue H, Tanabe T, Yoshimoto T. Growth stimulation and induction of epidermal growth factor receptor by overexpression of cyclooxygenases 1 and 2 in human colon carcinoma cells. *Biochim Biophys Acta* 1999; **1438**: 120–30.

24. Pai R, Soreghan B, Szabo IL, Pavelka M, Baatar D, Tarnawski AS. Prostaglandin E2 transactivates EGF receptor: a novel mechanism for promoting colon cancer growth and gastrointestinal hypertrophy. *Nat Med* 2002; **8**: 289–93.

25. Baserga R, Hongo A, Rubini M, Prisco M, Valentinis B. The IGF-I receptor in cell growth, transformation and apoptosis. *Biochim Biophys Acta* 1997; **1332**: F105–26.

26. Noble P, Henson P, Riches D. Insulin-like growth factor-1 (IGF-1) mRNA expression in bone marrow derived macrophages is stimulated by chrysotile asbestos and bleomycin. *Chest* 1991; **99** (Suppl): 79S–80S.

27. Rom WN, Paakko P. Activated alveolar macrophages express the insulin-like growth factor-I receptor. *Am J Resp Cell Mol Biol* 1991; **4**: 432–9.

28. Lee TC, Zhang Y, Aston C, *et al.* Normal human mesothelial cells and mesothelioma cell lines express insulin-like growth factor I and associated molecules. *Cancer Res* 1993; **53**: 2858–64.

29. Dobra K, Nurminen M, Hjerpe A. Growth factors regulate the expression profile of their syndecan co-receptors and the differentiation of mesothelioma cells. *Anticancer Res* 2003; **23**: 2435–44.

30. Syrokou A, Tzanakakis GN, Hjerpe A, Karamanos NK. Proteoglycans in human malignant mesothelioma. Stimulation of their synthesis induced by epidermal, insulin and platelet-derived growth factors involves receptors with tyrosine kinase activity. *Biochimie* 1999; **81**: 733–44.

31. Guan Z, Buckman S, Baier L, Morrison A. IGF-I and insulin amplify IL-1 beta-induced nitric oxide and prostaglandin biosynthesis. *Am J Physiol* 1998; **274**: F673–9.

32. O'Byrne KJ, Dalgleish AG. Chronic immune activation and inflammation as the cause of malignancy. *Br J Cancer* 2001; **85**: 473–83.

33. Nakao-Hayashi J, Ito H, Kanayasu T, Morita I, Murota S. Stimulatory effects of insulin and insulin-like growth factor I on migration and tube formation by vascular endothelial cells. *Atherosclerosis* 1992; **92**: 141–9.

34. Long L, Navab R, Brodt P. Regulation of the Mr 72,000 type IV collagenase by the type I insulin-like growth factor receptor. *Cancer Res* 1998; **58**: 3243–7.

35. Pass HI, Mew DJ, Carbone M, *et al.* Inhibition of hamster mesothelioma tumorigenesis by an antisense expression plasmid to the insulin-like growth factor-1 receptor. *Cancer Res* 1996; **56**: 4044–8.

36. Hodzic D, Delacroix L, Willemsen P, *et al.* Characterization of the IGF system and analysis of the possible molecular mechanisms leading to IGF-II overexpression in a mesothelioma. *Horm Metab Res* 1997; **29**: 549–55.

37. Rutten AA, Bermudez E, Stewart W, Everitt JI, Walker CL. Expression of insulin-like growth factor II in spontaneously immortalized rat mesothelial and spontaneous mesothelioma cells: a potential autocrine role of insulin-like growth factor II. *Cancer Res* 1995; **55**: 3634–9.

38. Langerak AW, Williamson KA, Miyagawa K, Hagemeijer A, Versnel MA, Hastie ND. Expression of the Wilms' tumor gene WT1 in human malignant mesothelioma cell lines and relationship to platelet-derived growth factor A and insulin-like growth factor 2 expression. *Genes Chromosomes Cancer* 1995; **12**: 87–96.

39. Rosen E, Goldberg I. Regulation of angiogenesis by scatter factor. *EXS* 1997; **79**: 193–208.

40. Roletto F, Galvani AP, Cristiani C, Valsasina B, Landonio A, Bertolero F. Basic fibroblast growth factor stimulates hepatocyte growth factor/scatter factor secretion by human mesenchymal cells. *J Cell Physiol* 1996; **166**: 105–11.

41. Naldini L, Tamagnone L, Vigna E, *et al.* Extracellular proteolytic cleavage by urokinase is required for activation of hepatocyte growth factor/scatter factor. *EMBO J* 1992; **11**: 4825–33.

42. Aparicio T, Kermorgant S, Lewin M, Lehy T. [Effects of HGF on the production of matrix metalloproteinases by colonic cancer cells DHD/K12]. *C R Seances Soc Biol Fil* 1998; **192**: 311–15.

43. Dunsmore S, Rubin J, Kovacs S, Chedid M, Parks W, Welgus H. Mechanisms of hepatocyte growth factor stimulation of keratinocyte metalloproteinase production. *J Biol Chem* 1996; **271**: 24576–82.

44. Trusolino L, Serini G, Cecchini G, *et al.* Growth factor-dependent activation of alphavbeta3 integrin in normal epithelial cells: implications for tumour invasion. *J Cell Biol* 1998; **142**: 1145–56.

45. Klominek J, Baskin B, Liu Z, Hauzenberger D. Hepatocyte growth factor/scatter factor stimulates chemotaxis and growth of malignant mesothelioma cells through c-*met* receptor. *Int J Cancer* 1998; **76**: 240–9.

46. Harvey P, Warn A, Newman P, Perry L, Ball R, Warn R. Immunoreactivity for hepatocyte growth factor/scatter factor and its receptor, *met*, in human lung carcinomas and malignant mesotheliomas. *J Pathol* 1996; **180**: 389–94.

47. Eagles G, Warn A, Ball R, *et al.* Hepatocyte growth factor/scatter factor is present in most pleural effusion fluids from cancer patients. *Br J Cancer* 1996; **73**: 377–81.

48. Tolnay E, Kuhnen C, Wiethege T, Konig JE, Voss B, Muller KM. Hepatocyte growth factor/scatter factor and its receptor c-*met* are overexpressed and associated with an increased microvessel density in malignant pleural mesothelioma. *J Cancer Res Clin Oncol* 1998; **124**: 291–6.

49. Adamson IY, Bakowska J. KGF and HGF are growth factors for mesothelial cells in pleural lavage fluid after intratracheal asbestos. *Exp Lung Res* 2001; **27**: 605–16.

50. Adamson IY, Prieditis H, Young L. Lung mesothelial cell and fibroblast responses to pleural and alveolar macrophage supernatants and to lavage fluids from crocidolite-exposed rats. *Am J Respir Cell Mol Biol* 1997; **16**: 650–6.

51. Walker C, Everitt J, Ferriola PC, Stewart W, Mangum J, Bermudez E. Autocrine growth stimulation by transforming growth factor alpha in asbestos-transformed rat mesothelial cells. *Cancer Res* 1995; **55**: 530–6.

52. Palmer U, Liu Z, Broome U, Klominek J. Epidermal growth factor receptor ligands are chemoattractants for normal human mesothelial cells. *Eur Respir J* 1999; **14**: 405–11.

53. Price JT, Bonovich MT, Kohn EC. The biochemistry of cancer dissemination. *Crit Rev Biochem Mol Biol* 1997; **32**: 175–253.

54. Bielefeldt-Ohmann H, Jarnick A, Fitzpatrick D. Molecular pathobiology and immunology of malignant mesothelioma. *J Pathol* 1996; **178**: 369–78.

55. Kumar-Singh S, Weyler J, Martin MJ, Vermeulen PB, Van Marck E. Angiogenic cytokines in mesothelioma: a study of VEGF, FGF-1 and -2, and TGF beta expression. *J Pathol* 1999; **189**: 72–8.

56. Jagirdar J, Lee TC, Reibman J, *et al.* (1997) Immunohistochemical localization of transforming growth factor beta isoforms in asbestos-related diseases. *Environ Health Perspect* 1997; **105** (Suppl 5): 1197–1203.

57. Orengo AM, Spoletini L, Procopio A, *et al.* Establishment of four new mesothelioma cell lines: characterization by ultrastructural and immunophenotypic analysis. *Eur Respir J* 1999; **13**: 527–34.

58. Fitzpatrick DR, Bielefeldt-Ohmann H, Himbeck RP, Jarnicki AG, Marzo AL, Robinson BW. Transforming growth factor-beta: antisense RNA-mediated inhibition affects anchorage-independent growth, tumorigenicity and tumor-infiltrating T-cells in malignant mesothelioma. *Growth Factors* 1994; **11**: 29–44.

59. Marzo AL, Fitzpatrick DR, Robinson BW, Scott B. Antisense oligonucleotides specific for transforming growth factor beta2 inhibit the growth of malignant mesothelioma both *in vitro* and *in vivo*. *Cancer Res* 1997; **57**: 3200–7.

60. Lee YC, Melkerneker D, Thompson PJ, Light RW, Lane KB. Transforming growth factor beta induces vascular endothelial growth factor elaboration from pleural mesothelial cells *in vivo* and *in vitro*. *Am J Respir Crit Care Med* 2002; **165**: 88–94.

61. Perkins RC, Broaddus VC, Shetty S, Hamilton S, Idell S. Asbestos upregulates expression of the urokinase-type plasminogen activator receptor on mesothelial cells. *Am J Resp Cell Mol Biol* 1999; **21**: 637–46.

62. Kinnula VL, Linnala A, Viitala E, Linnainmaa K, Virtanen I. Tenascin and fibronectin expression in human mesothelial cells and pleural mesothelioma cell-line cells. *Am J Respir Cell Mol Biol* 1998; **19**: 445–52.

63. Tzanakakis GN, Hjerpe A, Karamanos NK. Proteoglycan synthesis induced by transforming and basic fibroblast growth factors in human malignant mesothelioma is mediated through specific receptors and the tyrosine kinase intracellular pathway. *Biochimie* 1997; **79**: 323–32.

64. Ma C, Tarnuzzer RW, Chegini N. Expression of matrix metalloproteinases and tissue inhibitor of matrix metalloproteinases in mesothelial cells and their regulation by transforming growth factor-beta1. *Wound Repair Regen* 1999; **7**: 477–85.

65. Strizzi L, Catalano A, Vianale G, *et al*. Vascular endothelial growth factor is an autocrine growth factor in human malignant mesothelioma. *J Pathol* 2001; **193**: 468–75.

66. Ohta Y, Shridhar V, Bright RK, *et al*. VEGF and VEGF type C play an important role in angiogenesis and lymphangiogenesis in human malignant mesothelioma tumours. *Br J Cancer* 1999; **81**: 54–61.

67. Masood R, Kundra A, Zhu S, *et al*. Malignant mesothelioma growth inhibition by agents that target the VEGF and VEGF-C autocrine loops. *Int J Cancer* 2003; **104**: 603–10.

68. Ruffie P, Feld R, Minkin S, *et al*. Diffuse malignant mesothelioma of the pleura in Ontario and Quebec: a retrospective study of 332 patients. *J Clin Oncol* 1989; **7**: 1157–68.

69. Edwards JG., Abrams KR, Leverment JN, Spyt TJ, Waller DA, O'Byrne KJ. Prognostic factors for malignant mesothelioma in 142 patients: validation of CALGB and EORTC prognostic scoring systems. *Thorax* 2000; **55**: 731–5.

70. Gabrielson EW, Gerwin BI, Harris CC, Roberts AB, Sporn MB, Lechner JF. Stimulation of DNA synthesis in cultured primary human mesothelial cells by specific growth factors. *FASEB J* 1988; **2**: 2717–21.

71. Mutsaers S, McNulty R, Laurent G, Versnel M, Whitaker D, Papadimitriou J. Cytokine regulation of mesothelial cell proliferation *in vitro* and *in vivo*. *Eur J Cell Biol* 1997; **72**: 24–9.

72. Heldin CH, Ostman A, Eriksson A, Siegbahn A, Claesson-Welsh L, Westermark B. Platelet-derived growth factor: isoform-specific signalling via heterodimeric or homodimeric receptor complexes. *Kidney Int* 1992; **41**: 571–4.

73. Heldin CH, Ostman A, Ronnstrand L. Signal transduction via platelet-derived growth factor receptors. *Biochim Biophys Acta* 1998; **1378**: F79–113.

74. Lasky J, Friedman M, Zhou Y, Liu J.-Y, Poovey H, Brody A. Platelet-derived growth factor receptors are essential in the development of asbestos-induced fibrosis. *Chest* 2001; **120** (Suppl): 61S.

75. Liu JY, Morris GF, Lei WH, Hart CE, Lasky JA, Brody AR. Rapid activation of PDGF-A and -B expression at sites of lung injury in asbestos-exposed rats. *Am J Respir Cell Mol Biol* 1997; **17**: 129–40.

76. Van der Meeren A, Seddon MB, Betsholtz CA, Lechner JF, Gerwin BI. Tumorigenic conversion of human mesothelial cells as a consequence of platelet-derived growth factor-A chain overexpression. *Am J Resp Cell Mol Biol* 1993; **8**: 214–21.

77. Walker C, Bermudez E, Stewart W, Bonner J, Molloy CJ, Everitt J. Characterization of platelet-derived growth factor and platelet-derived growth factor receptor expression in asbestos-induced rat mesothelioma. *Cancer Res* 1992; **52**: 301–6.

78. Gerwin BI, Lechner JF, Reddel RR, *et al*. Comparison of production of transforming growth factor-beta and platelet-derived growth factor by normal human mesothelial cells and mesothelioma cell lines. *Cancer Res* 1987; **47**: 6180–4.

79. Pogrebniak HW, Lubensky IA, Pass HI. Differential expression of platelet derived growth factor-beta in malignant mesothelioma: a clue to future therapies? *Surg Oncol* 1993; **2**: 235–40.

80. Versnel MA, Claesson-Welsh L, Hammacher A, *et al*. Human malignant mesothelioma cell lines express PDGF beta-receptors whereas cultured normal mesothelial cells express predominantly PDGF alpha-receptors. *Oncogene* 1991; **6**: 2005–11.

81. Ramael M, Buysse C, van den Bossche J, Segers K, van Marck E. Immunoreactivity for the beta chain of the platelet-derived growth factor receptor in malignant mesothelioma and non-neoplastic mesothelium. *J Pathol* 1992; **167**: 1–4.

82. Langerak AW, De Laat PA, Van Der Linden-Van Beurden CA, *et al*. Expression of platelet-derived growth factor (PDGF) and PDGF receptors in human malignant mesothelioma *in vitro* and *in vivo*. *J Pathol* 1996; **178**: 151–60.

83. Langerak AW, van der Linden-van Beurden CA, Versnel MA. Regulation of differential expression of platelet-derived growth factor alpha- and beta-receptor mRNA in normal and malignant human mesothelial cell lines. *Biochim Biophys Acta* 1996; **1305**: 63–70.

84. Metheny-Barlow LJ, Flynn B, van Gijssel HE, Marogi A, Gerwin BI. Paradoxical effects of platelet-derived growth factor-A overexpression in malignant mesothelioma. Antiproliferative effects *in vitro* and tumorigenic stimulation *in vivo. Am J Respir Cell Mol Biol* 2001; **24**: 694–702.

85. Dorai T, Kobayashi H, Holland JF, Ohnuma T. Modulation of platelet-derived growth factor-beta mRNA expression and cell growth in a human mesothelioma cell line by a hammerhead ribozyme. *Mol Pharmacol* 1994; **46**: 437–44.

86. Klominek J, Baskin B, Hauzenberger D. Platelet-derived growth factor (PDGF) BB acts as a chemoattractant for human malignant mesothelioma cells via PDGF receptor beta-integrin alpha3beta1 interaction. *Clin Exp Metastasis* 1998; **16**: 529–39.

87. Schmitter D, Lauber B, Fagg B, Stahel RA. Hematopoietic growth factors secreted by seven human pleural mesothelioma cell lines: interleukin-6 production as a common feature. *Int J Cancer* 1992; **51**: 296–301.

88. Antony VB, Hott JW, Godbey SW, Holm K. Angiogenesis in mesotheliomas. Role of mesothelial cell derived IL-8. *Chest* 1996; **109** (Suppl): 21S–2S.

89. Nakano T, Chahinian AP, Shinjo M, *et al.* Interleukin 6 and its relationship to clinical parameters in patients with malignant pleural mesothelioma. *Br J Cancer* 1998; **77**: 907–12.

90. Demetri GD, Zenzie BW, Rheinwald JG, Griffin JD. Expression of colony-stimulating factor genes by normal human mesothelial cells and human malignant mesothelioma cells lines *in vitro. Blood* 1989; **74**: 940–6.

91. Kasuga I, Ishizuka S, Minemura K, Utsumi K, Serizawa H, Ohyashiki K. Malignant pleural mesothelioma produces functional granulocyte-colony stimulating factor. *Chest* 2001; **119**: 981–3.

92. Bussolino F, Colotta F, Bocchieto E, Guglielmetti A, Mantovani A. Recent developments in the cell biology of granulocyte–macrophage colony-stimulating factor and granulocyte colony-stimulating factor: activities on endothelial cells. *Int J Clin Lab Res* 1993; **23**: 8–12.

93. Mukherjee S, Nelson D, Loh S, *et al.* The immune anti-tumor effects of GM-CSF and B7-1 gene transfection are enhanced by surgical debulking of tumor. *Cancer Gene Ther* 2001; **8**: 580–8.

94. Nowak AK, Lake RA, Kindler HL, Robinson BW. New approaches for mesothelioma: biologics, vaccines, gene therapy, and other novel agents. *Semin Oncol* 2002; **29**: 82–96.

95. Chambers AF, Matrisian LM. Changing views of the role of matrix metalloproteinases in metastasis. *J Natl Cancer Inst* 1997; **89**: 1260–70.

96. Corcoran ML, Hewitt RE, Kleiner DE Jr, Stetler-Stevenson WG. MMP-2: expression, activation and inhibition. *Enzyme Protein* 1996; **49**: 7–19.

97. Nagase H. Cell surface activation of progelatinase A (proMMP-2) and cell migration. *Cell Res* 1998; **8**: 179–86.

98. Heppner KJ, Matrisian LM, Jensen RA, Rodgers WH. Expression of most matrix metalloproteinase family members in breast cancer represents a tumor-induced host response. *Am J Pathol* 1996; **149**: 273–82.

99. Pyke C, Ralfkiaer E, Tryggvason K, Dano K. Messenger RNA for two type IV collagenases is located in stromal cells in human colon cancer. *Am J Pathol* 1993; **142**: 359–65.

100. Cox G, Steward W, O'Byrne K. The plasmin cascade and matrix metalloproteinases in non-small cell lung cancer. *Thorax* 1999; **54**: 169–79.

101. Jones, J.L., Walker, R.A., Control of matrix metalloproteinase activity in cancer. *J Pathol* 1997. **183**(4): 377–379.

102. Johnson MD, Choi Kim H-R, Chesler L, Tsao-Wu G, Bouck N, Polverini PJ. Inhibition of angiogenesis by tissue inhibitor of metalloproteinase. *J Cell Physiol* 1994; **160**: 194–202.

103. Strongin AY, Collier I, Bannikov G, Marmer BL, Grant GA, Goldberg GI. Mechanism of cell surface activation of 72-kDa type IV collagenase. Isolation of the activated form of the membrane metalloprotease. *J Biol Chem* 1995; **270**: 5331–8.

104. Gomez D, Alonso D, Yoshiji H, Thorgeirsson U. Tissue inhibitors of metalloproteinases: structure, regulation and biological functions. *Eur J Cell Biol* 1997; **74**: 111–22.

105. Lamoreaux WJ, Fitzgerald ME, Reiner A, Hasty KA, Charles ST. Vascular endothelial growth factor increases release of gelatinase A and decreases release of tissue inhibitor of metalloproteinases by microvascular endothelial cells *in vitro*. *Microvasc Res* 1998; **55**: 29–42.

106. Mignatti P, Tsuboi R, Robbins E, Rifkin DB. *In vitro* angiogenesis on the human amniotic membrane: requirement for basic fibroblast growth factor-induced proteinases. *J Cell Biol* 1989; **108**: 671–82.

107. Hanemaaijer R, Koolwijk P, le Clercq L, de Vree WJ, van Hinsbergh VW. Regulation of matrix metalloproteinase expression in human vein and microvascular endothelial cells. Effects of tumour necrosis factor alpha, interleukin 1 and phorbol ester. *Biochem J* 1993; **296**: 803–9.

108. Esteve PO, Tremblay P, Houde M, St-Pierre Y, Mandeville R. *In vitro* expression of MMP-2 and MMP-9 in glioma cells following exposure to inflammatory mediators. *Biochim Biophys Acta* 1998; **1403**: 85–96.

109. Qin H, Moellinger JD, Wells A, Windsor LJ, Sun Y, Benveniste EN. Transcriptional suppression of matrix metalloproteinase-2 gene expression in human astroglioma cells by TNF-alpha and IFN-gamma. *J Immunol* 1998; **161**: 6664–73.

110. Tsujii M, Kawano S, DuBois R. Cyclooxygenase-2 expression in human colon cancer cells increases metastatic potential. *Proc Natl Acad Sci USA* 1997; **94**: 3336–40.

111. Zeng L, An S, Goetzl E. Regulation of matrix metalloproteinase-9 in early human T cells of the HSB.2 cultured line by the EP_3 subtype of prostaglandin E_2 receptor. *J Biol Chem* 1996; **271**: 27744–50.

112. Cox G, Jones JL, O'Byrne KJ. Matrix metalloproteinase 9 and the epidermal growth factor signal pathway in operable non-small cell lung cancer. *Clin Cancer Res* 2000; **6**: 2349–55.

113. Jones JL, Glynn P, Walker RA. Expression of MMP-2 and MMP-9, their inhibitors, and the activator MT1-MMP in primary breast carcinomas. *J Pathol* 1999; **189**: 161–8.

114. Baker EA, Bergin FG, Leaper DJ. Matrix metalloproteinases, their tissue inhibitors and colorectal cancer staging. *Br J Surg* 2000; **87**: 1215–21.

115. Hirano H, Tsuji M, Kizaki T, *et al.* Expression of matrix metalloproteinases, tissue inhibitors of metalloproteinase, collagens, and Ki67 antigen in pleural malignant mesothelioma: an immunohistochemical and electron microscopic study. *Med Electron Microsc* 2002; **35**: 16–23.

116. Edwards JG, McLaren J, Jones JL, Waller DA, O'Byrne KJ. Matrix metalloproteinases 2 and 9 (gelatinases A and B) expression in malignant mesothelioma and benign pleura. *Br J Cancer* 2003; **88**: 1553–9.

117. Rubins J, Charboneau D, Wilson M, Kratzke R. Matrix metalloproteinase expression by human malignant mesothelioma cell lines *in vitro*. *Chest* 2000; **118** (Suppl): 231S–2S.

118. Harvey P, Clark IM, Jaurand MC, Warn RM, Edwards DR. Hepatocyte growth factor/scatter factor enhances the invasion of mesothelioma cell lines and the expression of matrix metalloproteinases. *Br J Cancer* 2000; **83**: 1147–53.

119. Liu Z, Ivanoff A, Klominek J. Expression and activity of matrix metalloproteases in human malignant mesothelioma cell lines. *Int J Cancer* 2001; **91**: 638–43.

120. Liu Z, Klominek J. Regulation of matrix metalloprotease activity in malignant mesothelioma cell lines by growth factors. *Thorax* 2003; **58**: 198–203.

121. Ossowski L, Russo-Payne H, Wilson E. Inhibition of urokinase-type plasminogen activator by antibodies: the effect on dissemination of a human tumor in the nude mouse. *Cancer Res* 1991; **51**: 274–81.

122. Rabbani S. Metalloproteinases and urokinase in angiogenesis and tumour progression *in vivo*. 1998; **12**: 135–42.

123. Shetty S, Kumar A, Johnson A, Pueblitz S, Idell S. Urokinase receptor in human malignant mesothelioma cells: role in tumor cell mitogenesis and proteolysis. *Am J Physiol* 1995; **268**: L972–982.

124. Mignatti P, Rifkin D. Plasminogen activators and matrix metalloproteinases in angiogenesis. *Enzyme Protein* 1996; **49**: 117–37.

125. Mazzieri R, Masiero L, Zanetta L, *et al.* Control of type IV collagenase activity by components of the urokinase–plasmin system: a regulatory mechanism with cell-bound reactants. *EMBO J* 1997; **16**: 2319–32.

126. Bolon I, Devouassoux M, Robert C, Moro D, Brambilla C, Brambilla E. Expression of urokinase-type plasminogen activator, stromelysin 1, stromelysin 3, and matrilysin genes in lung carcinomas. *Am J Pathol* 1997; **150**: 1619–29.

127. Rifkin D, Gleizes P, Harpel J, *et al.* Plasminogen/plasminogen activator and growth factor activation. *Ciba Found Symp* 1997; **212**: 105–18.

128. Gris J, Schved J, Marty Double C, Mauboussin J, Balmes P. Immunohistochemical study of tumour cell-associated plasminogen activators and plasminogen activator inhibitors in lung carcinomas. *Chest* 1993; **104**: 8–13.

129. Ozdemir O, Emri S, Karakoca Y, *et al.* Fibrinolytic system in plasma and pleural fluid in malignant mesothelioma. *Thromb Res* 1996; **84**: 121–8.

130. Deed R, Rooney P, Kumar P, *et al.* Early-response gene signalling is induced by angiogenic oligosaccharides of hyaluronan in endothelial cells. Inhibition by non-angiogenic, high-molecular-weight hyaluronan. *Int J Cancer* 1997; **71**: 251–6.

131. Montesano R, Kumar S, Orci L, Pepper M. Synergistic effect of hyaluronan oligosaccharides and vascular endothelial growth factor on angiogenesis *in vitro*. *Lab Invest* 1996; **75**: 249–62.

132. Asplund T, Versnel MA, Laurent TC, Heldin P. Human mesothelioma cells produce factors that stimulate the production of hyaluronan by mesothelial cells and fibroblasts. *Cancer Res* 1993; **53**: 388–92.

133. Jacobson A, Brinck J, Briskin MJ, Spicer AP, Heldin P. Expression of human hyaluronan synthases in response to external stimuli. *Biochem J* 2000; **348** Pt 1: 29–35.

134. Attanoos R, Webb R, Gibbs A. CD44H expression in reactive mesothelium, pleural mesothelioma and pulmonary adenocarcinoma. *Histopathology* 1997; **30**: 260–3.

135. Asplund T, Heldin P. Hyaluronan receptors are expressed on human malignant mesothelioma cells but not on normal mesothelial cells. *Cancer Res* 1994; **54**: 4516–23.

136. Mulder J, Wielenga V, Pals S, Offerhaus G. p53 and CD44 as clinical markers of tumour progression in colorectal carcinogenesis. *Histochem J* 1997; **29**: 439–52.

137. Streit M, Schmidt R, Hilgenfeld R, Thiel E, Kreuser E. Adhesion receptors in malignant transformation and dissemination of gastrointestinal tumours. *Recent Results Cancer Res* 1996; **142**: 19–50.

138. Sleeman J, Moll J, Sherman L, *et al.* The role of CD44 splice variants in human metastatic cancer. *Ciba Found Symp* 1995; **189**: 142–56, 174–6.

139. Griffoen A, Coenen M, Damen C, *et al.* CD44 is involved in tumor angiogenesis; an activation antigen on human endothelial cells. *Blood* 1997; **90**: 1150–9.

140. Uotila P. The role of cyclic AMP and oxygen intermediates in the inhibition of cellular immunity in cancer. *Cancer Immunol Immunother* 1996; **43**: 1–9.

141. Janssen Y, Driscoll K, Howard B, *et al.* Asbestos causes translocation of p65 protein and increases NF-κB DNA binding activity in rat lung epithelial and pleural mesothelial cells. *Am J Pathol* 1997; **151**: 389–401.

142. Bissonnette E, Carre B, Dubois C, Rola-Pleszczynski M. Inhibition of alveolar macrophage cytotoxicity by asbestos: possible role of prostaglandins. *J Leukoc Biol* 1990; **47**: 129–34.

143. Leikauf GD, Fink SP, Miller ML, Lockey JE, Driscoll KE. Refractory ceramic fibers activate alveolar macrophage eicosanoid and cytokine release. *J Appl Physiol* 1995; **78**: 164–71.

144. Manning LS, Bowman RV, Davis MR, Musk AW, Robinson BW. Indomethacin augments lymphokine-activated killer cell generation by patients with malignant mesothelioma. *Clin Immunol Immunopathol* 1989; **53**: 68–77.

145. DeLong P, Tanaka T, Kruklitis R, *et al.* Use of cyclooxygenase-2 inhibition to enhance the efficacy of immunotherapy. *Cancer Res* 2003; **63**: 7845–52.

146. Fosslien E. Review: molecular pathology of cyclooxygenase-2 in cancer-induced angiogenesis. *Ann Clin Lab Sci* 2001; **31**: 325–48.

147. Tsujii M, Kawano S, Tsuji S, Sawaoka H, Hori M, DuBois RN. Cyclooxygenase regulates angiogenesis induced by colon cancer cells. *Cell* 1998; **93**: 705–16.

148. Marrogi AJ, Travis WD, Welsh JA, *et al.* Nitric oxide synthase, cyclooxygenase 2, and vascular endothelial growth factor in the angiogenesis of non-small cell lung carcinoma. *Clin Cancer Res* 2000; **6**: 4739–44.

149. Costa C, Soares R, Reis-Filho JS, Leitao D, Amendoeira I, Schmitt FC. Cyclo-oxygenase 2 expression is associated with angiogenesis and lymph node metastasis in human breast cancer. *J Clin Pathol* 2002; **55**: 429–34.

150. Uefuji K, Ichikura T, Mochizuki H. Cyclooxygenase-2 expression is related to prostaglandin biosynthesis and angiogenesis in human gastric cancer. *Clin Cancer Res* 2000; **6**: 135–8.

151. Masunaga R, Kohno H, Dhar DK, *et al.* Cyclooxygenase-2 expression correlates with tumor neovascularization and prognosis in human colorectal carcinoma patients. *Clin Cancer Res* 2000; **6**: 4064–8.

152. Ji YS, Xu Q, Schmedtje JF Jr. Hypoxia induces high-mobility-group protein I(Y) and transcription of the cyclooxygenase-2 gene in human vascular endothelium. *Circ Res* 1998; **83**: 295–304.

153. Seed M, Brown J, Freemantle C, *et al.* The inhibition of colon-26 adenocarcinoma development and angiogenesis by topical diclofenac in 2.5% hyaluronan. *Cancer Res* 1997; **57**: 1625–9.

154. Tsujii M, DuBois RN. Alterations in cellular adhesion and apoptosis in epithelial cells overexpressing prostaglandin endoperoxide synthase 2. *Cell* 1995; **83**: 493–501.

155. Reich R, Martin GR. Identification of arachidonic acid pathways required for the invasive and metastatic activity of malignant tumor cells. *Prostaglandins* 1996; **51**: 1–17.

156. Marrogi A, Pass HI, Khan M, Metheny-Barlow LJ, Harris CC, Gerwin BI. Human mesothelioma samples overexpress both cyclooxygenase-2 (COX-2) and inducible nitric oxide synthase (NOS2): *in vitro* antiproliferative effects of a COX-2 inhibitor. *Cancer Res* 2000; **60**: 3696–700.

157. Edwards JG, Faux SP, Plummer SM, *et al.* Cyclooxygenase-2 expression is a novel prognostic factor in malignant mesothelioma. *Clin Cancer Res* 2002; **8**: 1857–62.

158. Edwards JG. *Angiogenesis, cyclooxygenase-2 and matrix metalloproteinases in malignant mesothelioma in Department of Oncology.* Leicester: University of Leicester 2003; 193.

159. Jennions E, Stewart DJ, Edwards JG, Waller DA, O'Byrne KJ, Walker R. NFêB: the impact of active nuclear factor-kappa B in malignant mesothelioma. Presented at 3rd Annual Meeting of the British Thoracic Oncology Group, 2005.

160. Gray LH, Conger AD, Ebert M, Hornsey S, Scott OC. Concentration of oxygen dissolved in the tissues at the time of irradiation as a factor in radiotherapy. *Br J Radiol* 1953; **26**: 638–48.

161. Griffiths L, Dachs GU, Bicknell R, Harris AL, Stratford IJ. The influence of oxygen tension and pH on the expression of platelet-derived endothelial cell growth factor/thymidine phosphorylase in human breast tumor cells grown *in vitro* and *in vivo*. *Cancer Res* 1997; **57**: 570–2.

162. Kuwabara K, Ogawa S, Matsumoto M, *et al.* Hypoxia-mediated induction of acidic/basic fibroblast growth factor and platelet-derived growth factor in mononuclear phagocytes stimulates growth of hypoxic endothelial cells. *Proc Natl Acad Sci USA* 1995; **92**: 4606–10.

163. Shweiki D, Itin A, Soffer D, Keshet E. Vascular endothelial growth factor induced by hypoxia may mediate hypoxia-initiated angiogenesis. *Nature* 1992; **359**: 843–5.

164. Harris AL. Hypoxia—a key regulatory factor in tumour growth. *Nat Rev Cancer* 2002; **2**: 38–47.

165. Chiarugi V, Magnelli L, Chiarugi A, Gallo O. Hypoxia induces pivotal tumor angiogenesis control factors including p53, vascular endothelial growth factor and the NFkappaB-dependent inducible nitric oxide synthase and cyclooxygenase-2. *J Cancer Res Clin Oncol* 1999; **125**: 525–8.

166. Beasley NJ, Wykoff CC, Watson PH, *et al.* Carbonic anhydrase IX, an endogenous hypoxia marker, expression in head and neck squamous cell carcinoma and its relationship to hypoxia, necrosis, and microvessel density. *Cancer Res* 2001; **61**: 5262–7.

167. Giatromanolaki A, Koukourakis MI, Sivridis E, *et al.* Expression of hypoxia-inducible carbonic anhydrase-9 relates to angiogenic pathways and independently to poor outcome in non-small cell lung cancer. *Cancer Res* 2001; **61**: 7992–8.

168. Birner P, Gatterbauer B, Oberhuber G, *et al.* Expression of hypoxia-inducible factor-1 alpha in oligodendrogliomas: its impact on prognosis and on neoangiogenesis. *Cancer* 2001; **92**: 165–71.

169. Swinson D, Jones J, Richardson D, Cox G, Edwards J, O'Byrne K. Tumour necrosis is an independent prognostic marker in non-small cell lung cancer: correlation with biological variables. *Lung Cancer* 2002; **37**: 235–40.

170. Llombart-Bosch A, Contesso G, Henry-Amar M, *et al.* Histopathological predictive factors in Ewing's sarcoma of bone and clinicopathological correlations. A retrospective study of 261 cases. *Virchows Arch A Pathol Anat Histopathol* 1986; **409**: 627–40.

171. Leek RD, Landers RJ, Harris AL, Lewis CE. Necrosis correlates with high vascular density and focal macrophage infiltration in invasive carcinoma of the breast. *Br J Cancer* 1999; **79**: 991–5.

172. Lewis JS, Landers RJ, Underwood JC, Harris AL, Lewis CE. Expression of vascular endothelial growth factor by macrophages is up-regulated in poorly vascularized areas of breast carcinomas. *J Pathol* 2000; **192**: 150–8.

173. Churg A, Colby TV, Cagle P, *et al.* The separation of benign and malignant mesothelial proliferations. *Am J Surg Pathol* 2000. **24**: 1183–1200.

174. Edwards JG, Swinson DE, Jones JL, Muller S, Waller DA, O'Byrne KJ. Tumor necrosis correlates with angiogenesis and is a predictor of poor prognosis in malignant mesothelioma. *Chest* 2003; **124**: 1916–23.

175. Stewart D, Edwards JG, Richardson D, Swinson DEB, O'Byrne KJ. Expression of carbonic anhydrase-IX in malignant mesothelioma—clinicopathological correlations. *Proc 7th Meeting Int Mesothelioma Interest Group*, 2004; 104.

176. Wykoff CC, Beasley NJ, Watson PH, *et al.* Hypoxia-inducible expression of tumor-associated carbonic anhydrases. *Cancer Res* 2000; **60**: 7075–7083.

177. Giatromanolaki A, Koukourakis MI, Sivridis E, *et al.* Relation of hypoxia inducible factor 1 alpha and 2 alpha in operable non-small cell lung cancer to angiogenic/molecular profile of tumours and survival. *Br J Cancer* 2001; **85**: 881–90.

178. Klabatsa A, Sheaff MT, Steele JP, Evans MT, Rudd RM, Fennell DA. Expression and prognostic significance of hypoxia-inducible factor 1alpha (HIF-1alpha) in malignant pleural mesothelioma (MPM). *Lung Cancer* 2006; **51**: 53–9.

179. Okada H, Mak TW. Pathways of apoptotic and non-apoptotic death in tumour cells. *Nat Rev Cancer* 2004; **4**: 592–603.

180. Friesen C, Fulda S, Debatin KM. Deficient activation of the CD95 (APO-1/Fas) system in drug-resistant cells. *Leukemia* 1997; **11**: 1833–41.

181. Vaux DL, Silke J. IAPs, RINGs and ubiquitylation. *Nat Rev Mol Cell Biol* 2005; **6**: 287–97.

182. Fennell DA, Corbo MV, Dean NM, Monia BP, Cotter FE. *In vivo* suppression of Bcl-XL expression facilitates chemotherapy-induced leukaemia cell death in a SCID/NOD-Hu model. *Br J Haematol* 2001; **112**: 706–13.

183. Hopkins-Donaldson S, Cathomas R, Simoes-Wust AP, *et al.* Induction of apoptosis and chemosensitization of mesothelioma cells by Bcl-2 and Bcl-xL antisense treatment. *Int J Cancer* 2003; **106**: 160–6.

184. LaCasse EC, Baird S, Korneluk RG, MacKenzie AE. The inhibitors of apoptosis (IAPs) and their emerging role in cancer. *Oncogene* 1998; **17**: 3247–59.

185. Marusawa H, Matsuzawa S, Welsh K, *et al.* HBXIP functions as a cofactor of survivin in apoptosis suppression. *EMBO J* 2003; **22**: 2729–40.

186. Song Z, Yao X, Wu M. Direct interaction between survivin and Smac/DIABLO is essential for the anti-apoptotic activity of survivin during taxol-induced apoptosis. *J Biol Chem* 2003; **278**: 23130–40.

187. Dohi T, Okada K, Xia F, *et al.* An IAP–IAP complex inhibits apoptosis. *J Biol Chem* 2004; **279**: 34087–90.

188. Zangemeister-Wittke U, Simon HU. An IAP in action: the multiple roles of survivin in differentiation, immunity and malignancy. *Cell Cycle* 2004; **3**: 1121–3.

189. Olie RA, Simoes-Wust AP, Baumann B, *et al.* A novel antisense oligonucleotide targeting survivin expression induces apoptosis and sensitizes lung cancer cells to chemotherapy. *Cancer Res* 2000; **60**: 2805–9.

190. Janne PA, Taffaro ML, Salgia R, Johnson BE. Inhibition of epidermal growth factor receptor signaling in malignant pleural mesothelioma. *Cancer Res* 2002; **62**: 5242–7.

191. Catalano A, Romano M, Martinotti S, Procopio A. Enhanced expression of vascular endothelial growth factor (VEGF) plays a critical role in the tumor progression potential induced by simian virus 40 large T antigen. *Oncogene* 2002; **21**: 2896–900.

192. Masood R, Kundra A, Zhu S, *et al.* Malignant mesothelioma growth inhibition by agents that target the VEGF and VEGF-C autocrine loops. *Int J Cancer* 2003; **104**: 603–10.

193. Jimenez C, Jones DR, Rodriguez-Viciana P, *et al.* Identification and characterization of a new oncogene derived from the regulatory subunit of phosphoinositide 3-kinase. *EMBO J* 1998; **17**: 743–53.

194. Mohiuddin I, Cao X, Ozvaran MK, Zumstein L, Chada S, Smythe WR. Phosphatase and tensin analog gene overexpression engenders cellular death in human malignant mesothelioma cells via inhibition of AKT phosphorylation. *Ann Surg Oncol* 2002; **9**: 310–16.

195. Trombino S, Cesario A, Margaritora S, *et al.* Alpha7-nicotinic acetylcholine receptors affect growth regulation of human mesothelioma cells: role of mitogen-activated protein kinase pathway. *Cancer Res* 2004; **64**: 135–45.

196. Huelsken J, Behrens J. The Wnt signalling pathway. *J Cell Sci* 2002; **115**: 3977–8.

197. You L, He B, Xu Z, *et al.* An anti-Wnt-2 monoclonal antibody induces apoptosis in malignant melanoma cells and inhibits tumor growth. *Cancer Res* 2004; **64**: 5385–9.

198. Chan TO, Rittenhouse SE, Tsichlis PN. AKT/PKB and other D3 phosphoinositide-regulated kinases: kinase activation by phosphoinositide-dependent phosphorylation. *Annu Rev Biochem* 1999; **68**: 965–1014.

199. Brognard J, Clark AS, Ni Y, Dennis PA. Akt/protein kinase B is constitutively active in non-small cell lung cancer cells and promotes cellular survival and resistance to chemotherapy and radiation. *Cancer Res* 2001; **61**: 3986–97.

200. Sandhu H, Dehnen W, Roller M, Abel J, Unfried K. mRNA expression patterns in different stages of asbestos-induced carcinogenesis in rats. *Carcinogenesis* 2000; **21**: 1023–9.

201. Rihn BH, Mohr S, McDowell SA, *et al.* Differential gene expression in mesothelioma. *FEBS Lett* 2000; **480**: 95–100.

202. Singhal S, Wiewrodt R, Malden LD, *et al.* Gene expression profiling of malignant mesothelioma. *Clin Cancer Res* 2003; **9**: 3080–97.

203. Mohr S, Bottin MC, Lannes B, *et al.* Microdissection, mRNA amplification and microarray: a study of pleural mesothelial and malignant mesothelioma cells. *Biochimie* 2004; **86**: 13–19.

204. Gordon GJ, Jensen RV, Hsiao LL, *et al.* Using gene expression ratios to predict outcome among patients with mesothelioma. *J Natl Cancer Inst* 2003; **95**: 598–605.

Chapter 9

Vascularization in malignant mesothelioma

P. B. Vermeulen, R. Salgado, and E. A. Van Marck

Introduction

Angiogenesis is, by definition, the development of new blood vessels from the wall of an existing blood vessel. Angiogenesis implies proliferation of endothelial cells and, in certain conditions, maturation of the new blood vessel walls by recruitment of mural cells or pericytes. Malignant and physiological growth processes need a system of patent channels that transports blood and is connected with the circulation of the patient/host [1,2]. Although angiogenesis is one of the mechanisms that fulfil this need, several other mechanisms have been described [3–7]. Their existence has an important impact on the quantification of 'vascularization' in tumour tissue sections and has urged researchers to develop tools to detect the prevailing mechanism of vascularization in the tumours of individual patients [8].

Angiogenesis-independent tumour growth, in its most simple form, is based upon the co-option of the vasculature of the host tissue. Obviously, this pathway is expected to be used by tumour cells residing in densely vascularized tissue, such as the liver and the lungs. In some primary non-small-cell lung carcinomas and metastases of tumours to the lung as well as the liver, angiogenesis-independent growth patterns have been described in studies based on patient material. These growth patterns, the 'alveolar' growth pattern in the lung and the 'replacement' growth pattern in the liver, are characterized by low or absent endothelial cell proliferation, by conservation of the host tissue architecture within the tumours and by a stable non-activated endothelial cell phenotype within the co-opted blood vessels [9,10]. Hypoxia is not as prevalent in liver metastases with the non-angiogenic growth pattern as in those with angiogenic growth patterns (unpublished data).

Other mechanisms of angiogenesis-independent growth are based upon recruitment of angioblasts or endothelial precursor cells from the bone marrow (vasculogenesis) or are based on an epithelial-to-mesenchymal phenotypical switch of tumour cells (vasculogenic mimicry) [4,6]. Both types of tumour vascularization appear to occur more frequently in human cancer than previously thought and are not based upon the proliferation of endothelial cells from a 'mother' vessel. Although the tumour cells involved in vasculogenic mimicry start expressing some endothelial cell markers, they cannot be regarded as true endothelial cells [11].

Intussusceptive vascular growth is a another, albeit more difficult to study, angiogenesis-independent mechanism of vascularization which is based upon the partitioning of existing blood vessels by interstitial tissue columns. It does not involve endothelial cell proliferation [12,13]. The importance or prevalence of intussusceptive vascular growth in human cancer is not clear.

Finally, animal experiment data suggest that, owing to mutations of oncogenes and tumour suppressor genes, tumour cells in angiogenic or non-angiogenic tumours may become independent of the vascular tree and may survive and even proliferate in hypoxic areas because of a defective hypoxia-driven apoptosis pathway [14].

Although angiogenesis quantification has been performed in tissue sections of patients with malignant mesothelioma, there have been no investigations of the possibility of vascularization in these tumours being established by the alternative non-angiogenic mechanisms.

In this chapter we aim to review the studies reporting on the measurement of vascular parameters in tissue from malignant mesothelioma patients and on the growth factors involved in the vascularization of this tumour. We shall also try to provide a framework for future translational research projects concerning angiogenesis or other mechanisms of vascularization in malignant mesothelioma.

Quantification of vascularization in malignant mesothelioma

In all published studies, angiogenesis, a process based on endothelial cell proliferation, has been studied and quantified suboptimally in malignant mesothelioma tissue sections. As was stated in the report by Vermeulen *et al.* [8], microvessel density (MVD) assessed by counting CD34-immunostained blood vessels in vascular 'hot spots', i.e. areas with elevated numbers of blood vessels recognized at low magnification, is not necessarily a measure of ongoing angiogenesis. Tumours that co-opt pre-existing vessels may have a high MVD, but not as a result of angiogenesis. The fraction of proliferating endothelial cells, measured after double immunostaining of tumour tissue sections with antibodies directed at an endothelial cell marker (CD34 or CD31) and at a marker of proliferating cells, reflects ongoing angiogenesis more accurately. This technique also allows the simultaneous assessment of tumour cell proliferation. The ratio of tumour to endothelial cell proliferation is increased in tumours growing independently of angiogenesis [7]. A parameter reflecting the functional status of the microvascular bed is the degree of pericyte recruitment [15]. In prostate cancer, this pericyte coverage index has been shown to predict the response to anticancer treatment by an anti-VEGF strategy. Immature blood vessels without surrounding pericytes regressed, while mature blood vessels remained intact [16].

The results of the histological studies of vascularization in malignant mesothelioma are summarized in Table 9.1. Estimation of the relative vascular area by Chalkley morphometry, the proposed standard methodology, yields high counts in malignant mesothelioma (range 13–29; median 23) [17]. This is much higher than the Chalkley counts of inflammatory breast cancer. Inflammatory breast cancer has a significantly higher endothelial cell proliferation fraction (19 per cent) than non-inflammatory breast cancer (11 per cent), indicative of more intense ongoing angiogenesis in the former tumour type ($P = 0.014$) [18]. The fraction of proliferating endothelial cells has not been determined in malignant mesothelioma samples. Therefore no conclusions can be drawn concerning the degree of angiogenesis-dependent growth of these tumours. The high Chalkley count may be, at least in part, the consequence of co-option of blood vessels, vasculogenic mimicry or true vasculogenesis.

An interesting paradox arises when comparing malignant mesothelioma, which has a high Chalkley count, with inflammatory breast cancer, which has a lower Chalkley count, given the opposite ways of progression of both tumours. Inflammatory breast cancer is characterized by extensive lymphovascular permeation by tumour cell nests [19]. Despite its high Chalkley count, malignant mesothelioma is characterized by local spread and not by its metastatic propensity. Comparing gene expression profiles of both tumours might yield interesting information about genes involved in the first steps of the metastatic cascade.

In five studies mentioned in Table 9.1, the prognostic value of MVD or Chalkley count was assessed [17,20–26]. In all five studies, a high MVD or Chalkley count was associated with a

Table 9.1 Summary of studies of the quantification of the vascularization of malignant mesothelioma by immunohistochemistry with endothelial-specific antibodies and morphometry

Reference	No. of patients	Method[a]/antigen	Consensus[b]	Result	Δepi/sarc	Univariate	Multivariate	Correlation[c]
Edwards et al. [17]	104	Chalkey/CD34	Yes (2nd)	23 (med); 13–29(range)	epi = sarc	Prognostic	Prognostic	ND
König et al. [20]	103	MVD/FVIII	No	10 (epi); 8 (biph); 6 (sarc) (vessels/mm2)	epi > sarc	ND	ND	+VEGF IHC
Ohta et al. [21]	54	MVD/FVIII	No	11 (mean) (vessels/field (400×))	Not mentioned	Prognostic	Prognostic	+VEGF mRNA (extracted)
Kumar-Singh et al. [23]	52	MVD/CD34	Yes (lst)	Not mentioned	Not mentioned	Prognostic	Prognostic	+cumulative IHC, aFGF, bFGF, VEGF, TGF-β
Tolnay et al [24]	39	MVD/FVIII	No	20 (med) (vessels/mm2)	epi > sarc	ND	ND	+HGF/SF IHC
Soini et al. [24]	36	MVD/FVIII	No	9 (epi); 9 (biph); 11 (sarc) (vessels/HPF)	epi = sarc	ND	ND	No (eNOS, VEGF, FLK1,FLT1;IHC)
Edwards et al. [70]	29	Chalkey/CD34	Yes (2nd)	Not mentioned	Not mentioned	Prognostic	Not prognostic	No (COX-2 IHC, PGE2 EIA)
Kumar-Singh [22]	25	MVD/CD34	Yes (lst)	127 (mean) (vessels/field (0.7 mm2))	ND	Prognostic	Prognostic	ND
Strizzi et al. [26]	12	MVD/FVIII	No	25 (mean) (vessels/field (400×))	ND	ND	ND	No (serum and pleural exudate EGF(ELISA))

[a] MVD, microvessel density assessed according to the method of Weidner in vascular hot spots; Chalkley, the Chalkley point overlap morphometric technique for quantifying the relative area of blood vessels in the tumour tissue. Both techniques are discussed in the text.

[b] This column indicates whether a consensus methodology to quantify vascularization was adopted (1st, First International Consensus Report [133]; 2nd, Second International Consensus Report [8]).

[c] The + sign indicates a significant positive correlation with the factors following the sign.

HPF, high-power field; epi, epithelial; biph, biphasic; sarc, sarcomatoid malignant mesothelioma; IHC, immunohistochemical detection technique for expression of the factor mentioned; EIA, enzyme immunoassay.

worse outcome in univariate analysis. In four of the studies this was still true after multivariate analyses [17,21–23]. This confirms the general trend observed in other tumours that high 'vascularity' predicts shorter survival. In the largest study, in which the Chalkley morphometry methodology was adopted as suggested in the Second Internal Consensus Report [8], the prognostic value was independent of the histological type (epithelial or non-epithelial) and of the currently used prognostic scoring systems (EORTC and CALGB) [17]. Furthermore, tumour vascularization was assessed by the microvessel count (MVC) of CD34-immunostained sections in relation to tumour necrosis in a series of 171 patients. Tumour necrosis was identified in 22.8 per cent of cases and correlated with thrombocytosis ($P = 0.04$) and high MVC ($P = 0.02$) [27].

In two studies summarized in Table 9.1, the parameter reflecting vascular density was higher in the epithelial type of malignant mesothelioma than in the non-epithelial type. Given the poorer prognosis associated with the sarcomatoid cell type [17] and the general association of high vascular density with short survival, the results of these two studies are surprising [20,24].

An explanation can be found in the concept of 'vascular independence' described by Yu et al. [14] in a genetically engineered animal model of tumour growth. Briefly, p53$^{-/-}$ or HIF$^{-/-}$ tumour cells were found to be able to survive and proliferate in hypoxic regions of the tumour at a distance from blood vessels. This state of vascular independence was the result of a defective apoptotic response to hypoxia. Both HIF and p53 are necessary for hypoxia-induced apoptosis [28–30]. In sarcomatoid malignant mesothelioma, which is a less differentiated tumour because of a more developed mutator phenotype, more oncogenes might be activated and more tumour suppressor genes mutated, resulting in the failure of hypoxia response, leading to less angiogenesis and less apoptosis. The findings of Stewart and colleagues (personal communication) that the tumour cell expression of the hypoxia marker CAIX is more pronounced in epitheloid than in non-epitheloid tumours supports the aforementioned hypoxia-independent growth of sarcomatoid tumours. Moreover, this hypothesis ties in with the study by König et al. [20]. Vascular endothelial growth factor (VEGF) immunostaining was negative in 54 per cent of the sarcomatoid tumours compared with 21 per cent and 16 per cent of the biphasic and epithelioid tumours, respectively. VEGF is the prototype of a hypoxia-driven angiogenic factor and the most important factor in tumour angiogenesis since it combines vascular leakage and the formation of a fibrin matrix with endothelial cell migration and proliferation. In the study by Soini et al. [25], the degree of VEGF immunoreactivity was the same in epithelioid and sarcomatoid malignant mesotheliomas, but expression of two VEGF-receptors, flk-1 and flt-1, was more pronounced in the epithelioid tumours. Fibrin, detected by phosphotungstic acid haematoxylin (PTAH) histochemical staining, was demonstrated at the invasive margins of all epithelial and all but one of the mixed epithelioid–sarcomatoid tumours in a study comprising 12 malignant mesotheliomas [31]. Almost none of the purely sarcomatoid malignant mesotheliomas contained fibrin. Immunohistochemically, coagulation and fibrinolytic reactants were detected in all epitheloid and epitheloid–sarcomatoid tumours, being equally expressed in both epithelioid and sarcomatoid regions. In the one mixed tumour with predominantly sarcomatoid areas, the expression of these antigens was weak, in contrast with all other tumours which were purely epithelioid or mixed with a predominantly epithelial component. The purely sarcomatoid malignant mesotheliomas did not express coagulation and fibrinolytic reactants. This study strongly supports the hypothesis of a state of 'vascular independence' of sarcomatoid malignant mesotheliomas and the aforementioned results of lower vascularity and lower VEGF expression frequently encountered in these tumours (Fig. 9.1). In uterine sarcomatoid carcinomas, uncommon neoplasms consisting of a carcinoma component and a sarcomatoid, transdifferentiated component, a comparable difference in vascularity, expressed as MVD, has been found between both components

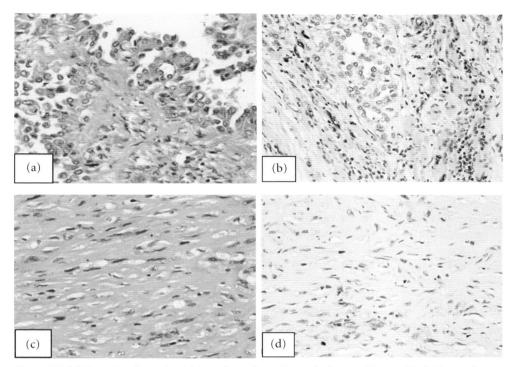

Figure 9.1 (a) Haematoxylin–eosin staining of a malignant mesothelioma with an epithelioid growth pattern. (b) CD34 staining of a vascular hot spot demonstrating intense vascularization of the tumour stroma. (c) Haematoxylin–eosin staining of a malignant mesothelioma with a biphasic growth pattern. (d) CD34 staining demonstrating minimal vascularization in these tumours.

[32]. MVD assessed in vascular hot spots after immunostaining for CD34 was 121 vessels/mm^2 in the carcinoma component of the 10 tumours, and 67 vessels/mm^2 in the sarcomatoid component ($P = 0.003$).

Growth factors involved in vascularization in malignant mesothelioma

Vascular endothelial growth factor A (VEGF)

Several studies discussed in Table 9.1 describe a positive correlation between VEGF expression measured at the protein level by immunohistochemistry or at the RNA level by *in situ* hybridization and parameters of vascularity. A topographical correlation of areas of highest vascular density (vascular 'hot spots') with areas of increased anti-VEGF antibody immunoreactivity has been reported by König *et al.* [20]. In different studies, VEGF expression was localized in tumour cells, in endothelial cells and in activated alveolar macrophages. Several studies have investigated the expression and localization of the VEGF receptors flt-1 and flk-1. Co-expression of VEGF and its receptors on malignant mesothelial cells was demonstrated by Soini *et al.* [25], Strizzi *et al.* [26] and König *et al.* [20]. Malignant mesothelioma cell lines have been reported to produce 5- to 10-fold higher VEGF levels than normal mesothelial cells [26]. Incubating these cell lines with increasing concentrations of rhVEGF induced a dose-dependent stimulation of cellular proliferation and of the phosphorylation of both tyrosine kinase receptors. Anti-VEGF neutralizing antibodies as well as VEGF-receptor blocking antibodies reduced these effects. Elevated serum levels and pleural fluid levels of VEGF in patients with malignant mesothelioma are common [26,33,34]. In a study of 132 patients with metastatic solid tumours of various histology which were untreated at the time of serum sampling, including breast cancer, ovarian cancer, cervical carcinoma, sarcoma, renal cell carcinoma, colon cancer and malignant mesothelioma, serum VEGF levels were strikingly higher in malignant mesothelioma patients compared with all other patients, with the median serum level for malignant mesothelioma being 1260 pg/ml compared with 664, 720, 324, 498, 540 and 570 pg/ml for the other tumours [34].

The results of the aforementioned studies are compatible with potential autocrine growth factor function for VEGF in malignant mesothelioma. Although VEGF is known as a potent endothelial cell growth factor, the common mesenchymal embryological origin of endothelium and mesothelium supports a regulatory role for VEGF in malignant mesothelioma. The practical implications of this dual effect of VEGF in malignant mesothelioma, stimulating angiogenesis and directly affecting tumour cell proliferation, is that malignant mesotheliomas are good candidates for anti-angiogenic trials. Several angiogenesis inhibitors are being assessed in clinical studies [35]. Masood and colleagues (http://www.mesorfa.org/study.htm) have tested both a VEGF antisense oligonucleotide and a diphteria toxin–VEGF fusion protein in a malignant mesothelioma xenograft model in athymic mice. Both therapeutic strategies very effectively inhibited mesothelioma cell growth *in vitro* and in tumour xenografts.

Production of other angiogenic growth factors together with expression of their respective receptors in malignant mesothelioma cells has also been reported for PDGF [36] and HGF/SF [24]. Selective inhibitors of the PDGF receptor tyrosine kinase are being tested for their antitumour activity in clinical trials including patients with malignant mesothelioma [35].

Interleukin 6

Interleukin-6 (IL-6) has a pleothrophic function during tumour growth. The stimulatory effects of IL-6 on tumour-related angiogenesis have been studied extensively and mainly occur through the upregulation of VEGF. Treatment of various cell lines (e.g. derived from human carcinomas and gliomas) with IL-6 results in the induction of VEGF mRNA [37]. The effect of IL-6 on VEGF expression is mediated by specific DNA motifs located on the putative promotor region of VEGF as well as by specific elements in the 5′-untranslated region. Transient expression of IL-6 mRNA was shown in endothelial cells during physiological angiogenic processes associated with the development of ovarian follicles and with the embryonic implantation in maternal decidua [38]. IL-6 expression is elevated in healing wounds [39]. It is also produced by melanoma and other malignant tumour cells [40,41]. IL-6 is upregulated by hypoxia [42]. IL-6 can thus be regarded as an indirect angiogenic factor produced by stromal cells and tumour cells. Transient tumour-stimulating effects have been observed during IL-6 treatment of cancer patients [43], and high IL-6 serum levels have been associated with an adverse prognosis in metastatic renal cell carcinoma [44,45] and in benign angiogenic diseases such as Crohn's disease [46].

IL-6 has potent thrombopoietic effects [47]. In advanced cancer patients (80 blood samples from 50 patients), serum IL-6 levels correlated with platelet count, with serum VEGF levels and with the calculated load of VEGF per platelet [48]. Patients with thrombocytosis had a median

VEGF serum concentration which was 3.2 times higher ($P < 0.0001$) and a median IL-6 serum level which was 5.8 times higher ($P = 0.03$) than those of other patients. Other studies have shown that, after induction of platelet aggregation, VEGF concentration increases in the supernatant of a platelet suspension of cancer patients [49–51]. Salgado et al. [52] have subsequently demonstrated the storage of VEGF in platelets of cancer patients by immunoelectron microscopy.

Given the observation that thrombocytosis is the most frequent paraneoplastic syndrome associated with malignant mesothelioma [53], Nakano et al. [54] have investigated the relationship between serum IL-6 levels and clinical parameters in 25 patients with malignant mesothelioma. Median serum IL-6 levels of mesothelioma patients (29 pg/ml; range 4–322 pg/ml) were significantly higher than the serum levels of patients with lung adenocarcinoma and cytology-positive pleural effusion ($n = 17$; 6.3 pg/ml) ($P < 0.05$). The levels in malignant mesothelioma patients are much higher than the IL-6 serum levels of advanced non-mesothelioma cancer patients ($n = 80$; median IL-6 serum level 3 pg/ml; range 2–170 pg/ml) [48]. The pleural fluid levels of the malignant mesothelioma patients were 60–1400 times higher than the serum levels and tended to correlate with the serum IL-6 levels. A comparable difference between serum and pleural fluid levels of IL-6 was reported by Monti et al. [55] in 17 patients. Numerous cells in the pleural fluid with a malignant morphology had immunoreactivity with antibodies directed at IL-6. Thrombocytosis was observed in 12 of the 25 malignant mesothelioma patients (48 per cent) in the study by Nakano et al. [54] compared with 28 per cent of the patients with advanced cancer [48]. Serum IL-6 levels of the malignant mesothelioma patients correlated significantly with platelet counts ($r = 0.8$; $P < 0.01$). However, there was no significant survival difference between patients with serum IL-6 levels above and below 100 pg/ml. Several human and murine mesothelioma cell lines have been found to produce bioactive IL-6 in vitro and to express IL-6 mRNA [56]. In a murine model using one of the IL-6-producing cell lines, treatment with anti-IL-6 antibodies or rhIFN-α curtailed the clinical symptoms associated with tumour growth.

In the context of the role of IL-6 in the biology of malignant mesothelioma, an interesting comparison can be made with the biphasic function of IL-6 in malignant melanoma. Mesothelial hyperplasia is characterized by the lack of invasion through the elastic layer of the pleura into the underlying chest wall or lung tissue. The invasive state shows similarities with the vertical growth phase of advanced malignant melanoma as opposed to the horizontal growth phase of early lesions [40,57]. Although the early malignant mesothelioma lesion is difficult to define, it is conceivable that some kind of horizontal growth phase might exist prior to overt invasion. In malignant melanoma, the progression from horizontal growth to vertical growth is accompanied by dramatic changes in the effect of IL-6 on the tumour cells. In early melanoma lesions, tumour cell proliferation is inhibited by IL-6 secreted by stromal cells [40,41,58,59]. Upon progression, this paracrine inhibitory effect is lost and converted into a paracrine stimulatory effect. In advanced melanoma lesions, the tumour cells start producing IL-6, resulting in an autocrine growth-stimulating pathway. Given the extensive production of IL-6 by tumour cells in clinically detectable malignant mesothelioma, the same autocrine mitogenic switch might occur in malignant mesothelioma.

Interleukin 8

Interleukin 8 (IL-8) induces migration and proliferation of endothelial cells [60,61] and is also involved in adhesion, diapedesis and activation of leucocytes during inflammation [62]. VEGF is able to upregulate the expression of IL-8 [63]. IL-8 is also positively associated with vascularity in colon cancer [64].

Elevated levels of IL-8 are detectable in the pleural fluid of malignant mesothelioma patients. Mesothelioma cell lines also produce detectable levels of IL-8 without stimulation [65,66]. In contrast, normal mesothelial cells do not produce IL-8. By immunohistochemistry, cellular anti-genic IL-8 is expressed by mesothelioma cell lines and not by mesothelial cell lines. IL-8 has been shown to have a mitogenic effect on some mesothelioma cell lines. This stimulation by IL-8 in an autocrine fashion is again comparable to the effect of IL-8 on melanoma cells [67,68]. In a human xenograft mesothelioma model in athymic mice, intrapleural injection of IL-8 antibodies resulted in lower IL-8 levels in serum and pleural fluid of the mice and in a decreased rate of tumour growth [66]. Effects of anti-IL-8 antibodies on ongoing angiogenesis (e.g. by assessing the fraction of proliferating endothelial cells in pre- and post-treatment biopsies) was not investigated. When IL-8 levels in pleural effusions were determined in six patients with malignant mesothelioma and 12 patients with pleural metastases of other tumours, the pleural fluid of mesothelioma patients contained significantly more IL-8 than the pleural fluids of the other patients (9 ng/ml compared with 1 ng/ml).

Cyclo-oxygenase 2

The cyclo-oxygenases are the catalysts of the first rate-limiting steps of prostaglandin synthesis from arachidonic acid [69]. The isoform cyclo-oxygenase 2 (COX-2) also promotes angiogenesis and overexpression of COX-2 has been observed in many solid tumour types. COX-2 expression was quantified by western blot analysis and densitometry of the gels in 30 epithelioid, 10 biphasic and eight sarcomatoid malignant mesotheliomas (see Chapter 8) [70]. Strong cytoplasmic staining was observed in all cases after immunohistochemistry with anti-COX-2 antibodies, mainly in the tumour cells and variably in the stroma. High COX-2 band densitometry values correlated with poor survival in both univariate and multivariate analysis. COX-2 expression levels did not correlate with Chalkley counts [71]. Areas of mesotheliomas containing normal mesothelial cells did not express COX-2, detected by immunohistochemistry, in another study encompassing 30 tumours [72]. Neither the studies of Edwards et al. [70,71], nor the study of Marrogi et al. [72] showed a difference in the level of COX-2 expression between epithelioid and sarcomatoid malignant mesotheliomas.

Fibroblast growth factor 2

Three studies have analysed the expression of basic-fibroblast growth factor (FGF-2) in malignant mesothelioma. FGF-2 is a mitogen for endothelial and mesothelial cells [73,74]. Immunoreactivity for antibodies directed at FGF-2 was present in 92 per cent of 52 mesothelioma specimens and in only 40 per cent of 20 cases of non-neoplastic mesothelium, 16 of which contained hyperplastic mesothelium [23]. High FGF-2 expression correlated with worse prognosis. Serum FGF-2 levels in 15 malignant mesothelioma patients had a mean value of 36 pg/ml [75]. Tumour vascularity measured in vascular hot spots after immunostaining for factor VIII/von Willebrand factor antigen did not correlate with the FGF-2 serum levels. Above average serum FGF-2 levels or pleural exudate FGF-2 levels were associated with reduced survival. The serum FGF-2 levels of five malignant mesothelioma patients (median 21 pg/ml; range 3–108) were higher than the levels measured in 127 patients with metastatic solid tumours of various histology [34].

Methionine aminopeptidase (MetAPs)

Methionine aminopeptidases (MetAPs) are enzymes responsible for the cleavage of the N-terminal methionine from peptides and proteins. Concerning angiogenesis, it was shown that MetAP-2 is the prime target of the angiogenesis inhibitors fumagillin and ovalacin in endothelial cells [76–78]. MetAP-2 is also highly expressed in malignant mesothelioma cells and modulates the anti-apoptotic protein bcl-2 [79]. Normal mesothelial cells show very low levels of MetAP-2 mRNA. MetAP-2 inhibition resulted in reduced bcl-2 protein levels and reduced telomerase activity, suggesting that MetAPs might be suitable targets for the treatment of malignant mesothelioma since this strategy combines an anti-angiogenic action with a direct antitumour action.

Angiogenesis, asbestos and simian virus 40

Asbestos and angiogenesis

It is well established that about 80 per cent of malignant mesotheliomas develop in individuals with higher than background exposure to asbestos [80,81]. When asbestos fibres reach the alveolus, the initial response of the body is a macrophage-mediated attempt to remove them. Eventually, if the fibres are too long or the asbestos exposure is too overwhelming, removal becomes inadequate. The fibres may then reach the pleural space via the lymphatics or by direct spread, and fibrosis, pleural plaques and eventually mesothelioma can develop [82].

One of the main initial responses to asbestos fibre inhalation is a wound-healing response. It has been demonstrated in *in vivo* models that intraperitoneal injection of crocidolite asbestos fibres produced mesotheliomas in 20–30 per cent of animals after 30–50 weeks [83]. Initially, nodular lesions developed composed of activated macrophages and proliferating mesenchymal cells. Endothelial cells surrounded 7 per cent of these lesions 14 days after a single intraperitoneal injection of 200 mg of crocidolite asbestos fibres. After six weekly injections neo-angiogenesis occurred in about 30 per cent of these lesions. It has also been demonstrated that the length of the asbestos fibres is important when inducing angiogenesis. Shorter fragments induced less angiogenesis than longer fragments. Activated macrophages and platelets associated with the wound-healing response persist around fibres until tumours develop. Macrophages and platelets are a rich source of angiogenic factors (e.g. VEGF) and therefore may promote neo-angiogenesis in pleural sites [49,52,81–84].

Considering these results it can be suggested that angiogenesis associated with the wound-healing response could facilitate the emergence of malignant mesothelioma lesions later. There is indeed evidence that the angiogenic process associated with wound healing precedes and contributes significantly to the tumorigenic process itself in other tumours (e.g. chronic hepatitis and cirrhosis of the liver following hepatitis B and C infection leading to the development of hepatocellular carcinoma) [85–87]. Similarly, chronic asbestos exposure triggers a chronic inflammatory response, inducing a highly angiogenic environment in pleural plaques and facilitating mesothelioma formation [82].

As well as inducing a wound-healing response associated with local release of angiogenic factors, asbestos is also able to stimulate the autophosphorylation of the epidermal growth factor receptor (EGFR) in mesothelial cells [88–92]. This in turn triggers the extracellular-regulated kinase (ERK) pathway, leading to an increased activity of the transcription factor AP-1 which in turn leads to either mitosis or apoptosis depending on the ability of the cell to repair the DNA damage caused by the asbestos fibres. Moreover, autophosphorylation of the EGFR stimulates a number of signal transduction pathways including not only the ERK pathway but also the RAS–RAF–MAP kinase pathway, the PI3-kinase pathway, the Janus kinase and the JNK and p38 pathways, which may all be involved in the transcriptional regulation of angiogenesis factors [93–97]. It is not clear to what extent these pathways contribute to the angiogenic phenotype of the mesothelial cells.

An additional pathway by which asbestos may promote angiogenesis-dependent tumorigenesis is by both local and systemic immunosuppression. Macrophages that phagocytize asbestos fibres produce lymphokines that depress the function of immune cells [98]. Specifically, asbestos decreases the cell-mediated immune response (Th_1) and increases the humoural immune response (Th_2). A decreased Th_1-response is associated with decreased IL-2, IFN-γ, IL-12 and IL-18 secretion. Since these cytokines have all been associated with anti-angiogenic properties, a decreasing Th_1 response would then be associated with an environmental pro-angiogenic change [82,99–102]. This coincides with the above-mentioned local Th_2-induced macrophage infiltration early in asbestos-induced lesions promoting angiogenesis. Indeed, several lines of study suggest that in most human tumours a shift occurs from a Th_1-dominant immune response associated with anti-angiogenic and tumoricidal properties to a Th_2-dominant phenotype that promotes angiogenesis and tumour growth [85].

In addition, tumour growth induces hypoxia [103] which in turn depresses the immune system and induces angiogenesis by modulating the HIF-1 pathway in tumour cells [85,103–106]. Hypoxia-inducible factor 1 (HIF-1) promotes production of angiogenic growth factors (e.g. VEGF) by binding to hypoxia-response elements located upstream of the promotor site of the angiogenic growth factor gene in several tumour cells. To what extent hypoxia develops in malignant mesothelioma cells is unknown. Moreover, it has been shown that growth factors may induce HIF-1 expression in areas without hypoxia, inducing a hypoxia-related gene expression profile [107]. Whether this HIF–hypoxia mismatch occurs in malignant mesothelioma needs to be investigated.

Macrophages have other pathways, in addition to angiogenic growth factor release and modulating the immune response by releasing lymphokines, that may contribute to angiogenesis. Upon ingestion of asbestos fibres macrophages release nitric oxide (NO) which is synthesized by inducible, endothelial and neuronal NO synthases (iNOS, eNOS and nNOS, respectively). eNOS and nNOS are constitutively expressed while iNOS can be induced by growth factors [108]. Several studies have investigated the expression of iNOS in malignant mesothelioma and whether it is associated with the expression of angiogenic growth factors and their receptors. iNOS expression is found in mesothelial cells both *in vitro* and *in vivo* [109]. With respect to angiogenesis, NO is able to induce the expression of VEGF in endothelial cells. In addition, VEGFR-2 activation induces both eNOS and iNOS expression, resulting in local release of NO by VEGFR-2-carrying cells [110–112]. The expression of eNOS, VEGF, VEGFR-1 and VEGFR-2 and their association with vascular density has been investigated in a series of 36 mesothelioma samples [25]. Reverse transcriptase–polymerase chain reaction (RT–PCR) analysis showed that mesothelioma cells express eNOS *in vitro*. Immunoreactivity of eNOS was found in 89 per cent of tumours, whereas VEGF expression was found in 45 per cent. VEGFR and VEGFR-2 expression was found in 69 per cent and 71 per cent of cases, respectively. No significant associations were found between eNOS expression and VEGFR-1, VEGFR-2 and VEGF expression. Therefore the importance of this pathway in the pathogenesis of malignant mesothelioma is not clear.

Furthermore, crocidolite asbestos induces the oncogenes *c-fos* and *c-jun* [113,114]. Transfection of these genes in tumour cells enhances angiogenic growth factor production by these cells (e.g. VEGF) [115]. Not only are oncogenes induced in malignant mesothelioma cells, but tumour suppressor genes are deleted in malignant mesothelioma cells. The CDKN2A locus encoding the tumour suppressor genes p16^{INK4a} and p14^{ARF} is found in the 9p21 region. Most malignant mesothelioma cells exhibit homozygous deletion of this region [116]. This has functional cell-cycle consequences since both are involved in the regulation of the cyclin-dependent kinase CDK4. With respect to angiogenesis in malignant mesothelioma, no arguments are known that might involve upregulation of angiogenic growth factor production upon loss of these tumour suppressor genes. However, such associations have been described in other tumours. For example, the expression of VEGF was significantly reduced in p16-negative glioma cells transfected with a recombinant replication-defective adenovirus vector containing the cDNA of wild-type p16 [117]. This finding suggests that p16 is implicated in the modulation of angiogenesis in gliomas. It may be assumed, considering the high frequency of p16 deletions in malignant mesothelioma cells, that similar mechanisms also occur. However, this has not been investigated thoroughly yet.

In summary, asbestos fibres may initially induce a wound-healing response involving mainly platelets and macrophages. This is associated with the local release of angiogenic molecules and angiogenesis. Furthermore, in addition to the induction of a wound-healing response in the pleura, asbestos fibres induce molecular alterations involving the activation of oncogenes and the inactivation of tumour suppressor genes that results in the activation of signalling pathways, which in turn may enhance the expression levels of angiogenic growth factors.

Simian virus 40 and angiogenesis

Simian virus 40 (SV40) is a double-stranded circular DNA virus capable of inducing malignant mesothelioma in hamsters. The SV40 DNA molecule encodes three transforming proteins: the large T-antigen (Tag), the small t-antigen (tag) and 17kT. These proteins are responsible for the transformation-inducing capability of the virus. SV40 nucleic acids and proteins have been observed in malignant mesothelioma cells (see Chapter 7). One of the major characteristics of Tag is that it can bind and inhibit several tumour suppressor genes such as p53 and pRb, and induce chromosomal alterations in the genome of affected cells [118,119].

Catalano *et al.* [120] have recently studied relationships between SV40-related proteins and VEGF expression in human malignant mesothelioma cells (HMMCs). An SV40-Tag expression vector (pw2dl) was transfected into an SV40-negative HMMC (MPP89). A time-dependent relationship was observed between SV40-Tag transfection and VEGF expression. Interestingly, the expression of several other angiogenesis factors (e.g. FGF-2 and PDGF) was not increased. This temporal relationship between SV40-Tag and VEGF could be blocked by cycloheximide. Moreover, both small and large T-antigen oncoproteins act synergistically in activating the VEGF promotor. Whole small t-antigen alone did not activate the VEGF promotor. Carbone *et al.* [121] have demonstrated that SV40 can bind and inactivate p53 in human malignant mesothelioma cells. Using meniodine, a drug which explicitly disrupts the Tag–p53 complex, they showed that the activation of the VEGF promotor was drastically reduced, suggesting intricate links between SV40, p53 and VEGF expression.

p53 is one of the main modulators of VEGF expression in tumour cells [122]. Volpert *et al.* [123] have reported that loss of wild-type p53 resulted in the reduced expression of the presumed anti-angiogenic factor thrombospondin, and in the upregulation of VEGF expression in fibroblasts. The reduced VEGF expression by mutant p53 is attributed to a reduced binding of Sp-1 to the VEGF promotor region. In malignant mesothelioma this is somewhat different. A characteristic of mesothelioma cells is that wild-type p53 levels are about five times higher than in fibroblasts. Moreover, p53 is rarely mutated in mesothelioma [124]. Therefore additional mechanisms of p53 regulation must occur in mesothelioma cells.

Moreover, not only p16, as already mentioned, but also members of the Rb family, which are also frequently found to be altered in malignant mesothelioma lesions [125–127], are able to reduce the VEGF expression in tumour cells [128].

Lymphangiogenesis and malignant mesothelioma

The concept of lymphangiogenesis, defined as the formation of new lymphatic vessels from the wall of pre-existing ones, is currently a controversial topic in cancer research. However, the study of lymphangiogenesis is hampered by a lack of suitable and specific markers for lymphatic endothelial cells.

Nevertheless, there is accumulating evidence that lymphangiogenesis may occur in human tumours [129]. It has been shown in animal models that lymphatic vessels are present at the rim of the tumour and are not functionally active [130]. This raises concerns as to whether these are indeed newly formed vessels or are merely pre-existing ones that are incorporated at the rim of the tumour by the tumour cells.

Malignant mesothelioma is clinically rarely associated with lymphatic spread. However, lymphatic metastases may occur at an advanced disease stage. Moreover, in autopsy series lymphatic metastases have been detected in about 70 per cent of patients with malignant mesothelioma.

In a series of 54 human malignant mesothelioma tissues the expression of VEGF, VEGF-C and the VEGF-receptors flt-1, KDR and flt-4 was analysed and compared with expression levels in normal pleural tissue. VEGF-C and flt-4 are of prime importance for lymphangiogenesis. Compared with normal pleural tissues, the expression levels of VEGF, flt-1 and KDR were higher in 31.5 per cent, 20.4 per cent and 42.6 per cent, respectively, of malignant mesothelioma cases. VEGF-C and flt-4 were elevated in 66.7 per cent and 59.3 per cent of cases, respectively. The lymphatic vessel density (LVD) was analysed using the expression of 5′-nucleotidase on presumably lymphatic endothelial cells. A strong association was found between VEGF-C expression and LVD and between LVD and flt-4. In contrast with what might be expected, no correlation was found between LVD and nodal metastasis [131].

Although there is some controversy as to whether these markers are specific enough to detect lymphangiogenesis, the results reported by Ohta *et al.* [131] indicate that higher concentrations of lymphangiogenic factors (VEGF-C) are found in malignant mesothelioma lesions. VEGF-D expression levels have yet not been investigated in malignant mesothelioma lesions.

Considering the common ontogenic origin of mesothelioma cells and endothelial cells and the expression of both VEGF-C and its receptor flt-4 on mesothelioma cells, an autocrine importance of VEGF-C can be postulated. This was investigated in a more recent study. Targeting of VEGF-C or its receptor flt-4 were shown to inhibit mesothelioma cell growth *in vitro*. A synergistic effect was noted when targeting both VEGF and VEGF-C [132].

In conclusion, the presence of lymphatic metastases does not seem to be of clinical importance in patients with malignant mesothelioma lesions. The presence or absence of lymph node metasastases is not considered to be a prognostic factor. The data so far do not explictly support the occurrence of lymphangiogenesis in malignant mesothelioma lesions. Identifying proliferating lymphatic endothelial cells by double staining of membranous molecules (e.g. LYVE-1) and nuclear markers (e.g. Ki-67) might be useful when evaluating lymphangiogenesis in malignant mesothelioma lesions. The lymphangiogenic factor-mediated autocrine growth-stimulating loops seem to be of importance for mesothelioma cell growth. Therefore both lymphangiogenic factors and angiogenic factors appear to be plausible therapeutic targets for controlling mesothelioma cell growth.

Conclusions

The process of angiogenesis seems to be intricately linked with the propagation of malignant mesothelioma. Nevertheless, angiogenesis has been suboptimally quantified in human mesothelioma tissue sections, and the degree of angiogenesis-independent vascularization of this tumour type is not known. Malignant mesotheliomas of the sarcomatoid type have a less-developed vascular bed and are associated with a worse prognosis, indicating that the tumour cells might be in a state of vascular independence with concomitant resistance to hypoxia-induced apoptosis.

Table 9.2 *Angiogenesis* in malignant mesothelioma: future translational research topics

Determine the degree of angiogenesis-independent growth of malignant mesothelioma

Are areas of sarcomatoid type malignant mesotheliomas vascular independent?

What is the role of hypoxia in angiogenesis of malignant mesothelioma?

Compare gene expression profiles of metastasis-incompetent malignant mesotheliomas with highly metastatic inflammatory breast cancer

Is IL-6 involved in the progression of early (precursor) lesion to overt malignant mesothelioma (inhibition of tumour cells by stromal-component-derived IL-6 in early lesions vs. autocrine stimulation of tumour cells by IL-6 in advanced lesions)?

Efficacy of anti-angiogenic treatment that targets both the endothelial cells and the malignant mesothelium?

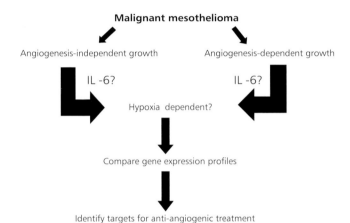

Figure 9.2 Future translational research topics.

Both asbestos fibre inhalation and SV40 infection, with consequent activation of oncogenes and inactivation of tumour suppressor genes, appear to be implicated in the pathogenesis of mesothelioma-associated angiogenesis. Moreover, the autocrine stimulatory loop of several angiogenic factors in mesothelioma cells, the expression of receptors for angiogenic growth factors on mesothelial cells and the common ontogenetic origin of both endothelial cells and mesothelial cells renders malignant mesotheliomas theoretically very suitable for anti-angiogenic agents aimed at targeting endothelial cells as well as mesothelial cells (e.g. anti-VEGF antibodies and fumagillin).

Future translational research on angiogenesis in malignant mesothelioma is necessary. A framework is presented in Table 9.2 and in the flow diagram in Figure 9.2.

References

1. Carmeliet P, Jain RK. Angiogenesis in cancer and other diseases. *Nature* 2000; **407**: 249–57.
2. Carmeliet P. Mechanisms of angiogenesis and arteriogenesis. *Nat Med* 2000; **6**: 389–95.
3. Chang YS, di Tomaso E, McDonald DM, Jones R, Jain RK, Munn LL. Mosaic blood vessels in tumors: frequency of cancer cells in contact with flowing blood. *Proc Natl Acad Sci USA* 2000; **97**: 14608–13.
4. Asahara T, Masuda H, Takahashi T, *et al.* Bone marrow origin of endothelial progenitor cells responsible for postnatal vasculogenesis in physiological and pathological neovascularization. *Circ Res* 1999; **85**: 221–8.

5. Maniotis AJ, Folberg R, Hess A, *et al.* Vascular channel formation by human melanoma cells *in vivo* and *in vitro*: vasculogenic mimicry. *Am J Pathol* 1999; **155**: 739–52.

6. Folberg R, Hendrix MJ, Maniotis AJ. Vasculogenic mimicry and tumor angiogenesis. *Am J Pathol* 2000; **156**: 361–81.

7. Vermeulen PB, Colpaert C, Salgado R, *et al.* Liver metastases from colorectal adenocarcinomas grow in three patterns with different angiogenesis and desmoplasia. *J Pathol* 2001; **195**: 336–42.

8. Vermeulen PB, Gasparini G, Fox SB, *et al.* Second international consensus on the methodology and criteria of evaluation of angiogenesis quantification in solid human tumours. *Eur J Cancer* 2002; **38**: 1564–79.

9. Passalidou E, Trivella M, Singh N, *et al.* Vascular phenotype in angiogenic and non-angiogenic lung non-small cell carcinomas. *Br J Cancer* 2002; **86**: 244–9.

10. Pezzella F, Pastorino U, Tagliabue E, *et al.* Non-small-cell lung carcinoma tumor growth without morphological evidence of neo-angiogenesis. *Am J Pathol* 1997; **151**: 1417–23.

11. McDonald DM, Foss AJ. Endothelial cells of tumor vessels: abnormal but not absent. *Cancer Metastasis Rev* 2000; 19: 109–120.

12. Patan S. Vasculogenesis and angiogenesis as mechanisms of vascular network formation, growth and remodeling. *J Neurooncol* 2000; **50**: 1–15.

13. Patan S, Munn LL, Jain RK. Intussusceptive microvascular growth in a human colon adenocarcinoma xenograft: a novel mechanism of tumor angiogenesis. *Microvasc Res* 1996; **51**: 260–72.

14. Yu JL, Rak JW, Carmeliet P, Nagy A, Kerbel RS, Coomber BL. Heterogeneous vascular dependence of tumor cell populations. *Am J Pathol* 2001; **158**: 1325–34.

15. Eberhard A, Kahlert S, Goede V, Hemmerlein B, Plate KH, Augustin HG. Heterogeneity of angiogenesis and blood vessel maturation in human tumors: implications for antiangiogenic tumor therapies. *Cancer Res* 2000; **60**: 1388–93.

16. Benjamin LE, Golijanin D, Itin A, Pode D, Keshet E. Selective ablation of immature blood vessels in established human tumors follows vascular endothelial growth factor withdrawal. *J Clin Invest* 1999; **103**: 159–65.

17. Edwards JG, Cox G, Andi A, *et al.* Angiogenesis is an independent prognostic factor in malignant mesothelioma. *Br J Cancer* 2001; **85**: 863–8.

18. Colpaert CG, Vermeulen PB, Benoy I, *et al.* Inflammatory breast cancer shows angiogenesis with high endothelial proliferation rate and strong E-cadherin expression. *Br J Cancer* 2003; **88**: 718–25.

19. Kleer CG, van Golen KL, Merajver SD. Molecular biology of breast cancer metastasis. Inflammatory breast cancer: clinical syndrome and molecular determinants. *Breast Cancer Res* 2000; **2**: 423–9.

20. König JE, Tolnay E, Wiethege T, Muller KM. Expression of vascular endothelial growth factor in diffuse malignant pleural mesothelioma. *Virchows Arch* 1999; **435**: 8–12.

21. Ohta Y, Shridhar V, Bright RK, *et al.* VEGF and VEGF type C play an important role in angiogenesis and lymphangiogenesis in human malignant mesothelioma tumours. *Br J Cancer* 1999; **81**: 54–61.

22. Kumar-Singh S, Vermeulen PB, Weyler J, *et al.* Evaluation of tumour angiogenesis as a prognostic marker in malignant mesothelioma. *J Pathol* 1997; **182**: 211–16.

23. Kumar-Singh S, Weyler J, Martin MJ, Vermeulen PB, Van Marck E. Angiogenic cytokines in mesothelioma: a study of VEGF, FGF-1 and -2, and TGF beta expression. *J Pathol* 1999; **189**: 72–8.

24. Tolnay E, Kuhnen C, Wiethege T, König JE, Voss B, Muller KM. Hepatocyte growth factor/scatter factor and its receptor c-Met are overexpressed and associated with an increased microvessel density in malignant pleural mesothelioma. *J Cancer Res Clin Oncol* 1998; **124**: 291–6.

25. Soini Y, Puhakka A, Kahlos K, Saily M, Paakko P, Koistinen P, Kinnula V. Endothelial nitric oxide synthase is strongly expressed in malignant mesothelioma but does not associate with vascular density or the expression of VEGF, FLK1 or FLT1. *Histopathology* 2001; **39**: 179–86.

26. Strizzi L, Catalano A, Vianale G, *et al.* Vascular endothelial growth factor is an autocrine growth factor in human malignant mesothelioma. *J Pathol* 2001; **193**: 468–75.

27. Edwards JG, Swinson DE, Jones JL, Muller S, Waller DA, O'Byrne KJ. Tumor necrosis correlates with angiogenesis and is a predictor of poor prognosis in malignant mesothelioma. *Chest* 2003; **124**: 1916–23.

28. Shimamura A, Fisher DE. p53 in life and death. *Clin Cancer Res* 1996; **2**: 435–40.

29. Wykoff CC, Pugh CW, Harris AL, Maxwell PH, Ratcliffe PJ. The HIF pathway: implications for patterns of gene expression in cancer. *Novartis Found Symp* 2001; **240**: 212–25.

30. Piret J, Mottet D, Raes M, Michiels C. Is HIF-1alpha a pro- or an anti-apoptotic protein? *Biochem Pharmacol* 2002; **64**: 889.

31. Idell S, Pueblitz S, Emri S, *et al*. Regulation of fibrin deposition by malignant mesothelioma. *Am J Pathol* 1995; **147**: 1318–29.

32. Yoshida Y, Kurokawa T, Fukuno N, Nishikawa Y, Kamitani N, Kotsuji F. Markers of apoptosis and angiogenesis indicate that carcinomatous components play an important role in the malignant behavior of uterine carcinosarcoma. *Hum Pathol* 2000; **31**: 1448–54.

33. Zebrowski BK, Yano S, Liu W, *et al*. Vascular endothelial growth factor levels and induction of permeability in malignant pleural effusions. *Clin Cancer Res* 1999; **5**: 3364–8.

34. Vermeulen PB, LD, De Pooter, C, *et al*. Serum levels of bFGF and VEGF in patients with metastatic solid tumors. *Proc Annu Meet Am Assoc Cancer Res* 1996; **15**: 90.

35. Nowak AK, Lake RA, Kindler HL, Robinson BW. New approaches for mesothelioma: biologics, vaccines, gene therapy, and other novel agents. *Semin Oncol* 2002; **29**: 82–96.

36. Versnel MA, Claesson-Welsh L, Hammacher A, , *et al*. Human malignant mesothelioma cell lines express PDGF beta-receptors whereas cultured normal mesothelial cells express predominantly PDGF alpha-receptors. *Oncogene* 1991; **6**: 2005–11.

37. Cohen T, Nahari D, Cerem LW, Neufeld G, Levi BZ. Interleukin 6 induces the expression of vascular endothelial growth factor. *J Biol Chem* 1996; **271**: 736–41.

38. Motro B, Itin A, Sachs L, Keshet E. Pattern of interleukin 6 gene expression *in vivo* suggests a role for this cytokine in angiogenesis. *Proc Natl Acad Sci USA* 1990; **87**: 3092–6.

39. Mateo RB, Reichner JS, Albina JE. Interleukin-6 activity in wounds. *Am J Physiol* 1994; **266**: R1840–4.

40. Rak JW, Hegmann EJ, Lu C, Kerbel RS. Progressive loss of sensitivity to endothelium-derived growth inhibitors expressed by human melanoma cells during disease progression. *J Cell Physiol* 1994; **159**: 245–55.

41. Lu C, Sheehan C, Rak JW, Chambers CA, Hozumi N, Kerbel RS. Endogenous interleukin 6 can function as an *in vivo* growth-stimulatory factor for advanced-stage human melanoma cells. *Clin Cancer Res* 1996; **2**: 1417–25.

42. Yan SF, Tritto I, Pinsky D, *et al*. Induction of interleukin 6 (IL-6) by hypoxia in vascular cells. Central role of the binding site for nuclear factor-IL-6. *J Biol Chem* 1995; **270**: 11463–71.

43. Ravoet C, DeGreve J, Vandewoude K, *et al*. Tumour stimulating effects of recombinant human interleukin-6. *Lancet* 1994; **344**: 1576–7.

44. Blay JY, Negrier S, Combaret V, *et al*. Serum level of interleukin 6 as a prognosis factor in metastatic renal cell carcinoma. *Cancer Res* 1992; **52**: 3317–22.

45. Blay JY, Schemann S, Favrot MC. Local production of interleukin 6 by renal adenocarcinoma *in vivo*. *J Natl Cancer Inst* 1994; **86**: 238.

46. Bross DA, Leichtner AM, Zurakowski D, Law T, Bousvaros A. Elevation of serum interleukin-6 but not serum-soluble interleukin-2 receptor in children with Crohn's disease. *J Pediatr Gastroenterol Nutr* 1996; **23**: 164–71.

47. Clarke D, Johnson PW, Banks RE, *et al*. Effects of interleukin 6 administration on platelets and haemopoietic progenitor cells in peripheral blood. *Cytokine* 1996; **8**: 717–23.

48. Salgado R, Vermeulen PB, Benoy I, *et al*. Platelet number and interleukin-6 correlate with VEGF but not with bFGF serum levels of advanced cancer patients. *Br J Cancer* 1999; **80**: 892–7.

49. Salven P, Orpana A, Joensuu H. Leukocytes and platelets of patients with cancer contain high levels of vascular endothelial growth factor. *Clin Cancer Res* 1999; **5**: 487–91.

50. Verheul HM, Hoekman K, Luykx-de Bakker S, *et al.* Platelet: transporter of vascular endothelial growth factor. *Clin Cancer Res* 1997; **3**: 2187–90.

51. Vermeulen PB, Salven P, Benoy I, Gasparini G, Dirix LY. Blood platelets and serum VEGF in cancer patients. *Br J Cancer* 1999; **79**: 370–3.

52. Salgado R, Benoy I, Bogers J, *et al.* Platelets and vascular endothelial growth factor (VEGF): a morphological and functional study. *Angiogenesis* 2001; **4**: 37–43.

53. Chahinian AP, Pajak TF, Holland JF, Norton L, Ambinder RM, Mandel EM. Diffuse malignant mesothelioma. Prospective evaluation of 69 patients. *Ann Intern Med* 1982; **96**: 746–55.

54. Nakano T, Chahinian AP, Shinjo M, *et al.* Interleukin 6 and its relationship to clinical parameters in patients with malignant pleural mesothelioma. *Br J Cancer* 1998; **77**: 907–12.

55. Monti G, Jaurand MC, Monnet I, *et al.* Intrapleural production of interleukin 6 during mesothelioma and its modulation by gamma-interferon treatment. *Cancer Res* 1994; **54**: 4419–23.

56. Bielefeldt-Ohmann H, Marzo AL, Himbeck RP, Jarnicki AG, Robinson BW, Fitzpatrick DR. Interleukin-6 involvement in mesothelioma pathobiology: inhibition by interferon alpha immunotherapy. *Cancer Immunol Immunother* 1995; **40**: 241–50.

57. Rak JW, St Croix BD, Kerbel RS. Consequences of angiogenesis for tumor progression, metastasis and cancer therapy. *Anticancer Drugs* 1995; **6**: 3–18.

58. Lu C, Vickers MF, Kerbel RS. Interleukin 6: a fibroblast-derived growth inhibitor of human melanoma cells from early but not advanced stages of tumor progression. *Proc Natl Acad Sci USA* 1992; **89**: 9215–19.

59. Lu C, Kerbel RS. Interleukin-6 undergoes transition from paracrine growth inhibitor to autocrine stimulator during human melanoma progression. *J Cell Biol* 1993; **120**: 1281–8.

60. Strieter RM, Kunkel SL, Elner VM, *et al.* Interleukin-8. A corneal factor that induces neovascularization. *Am J Pathol* 1992; **141**: 1279–84.

61. Koch AE, Polverini PJ, Kunkel SL, *et al.* Interleukin-8 as a macrophage-derived mediator of angiogenesis. *Science* 1992; **258**: 1798–1801.

62. Peveri P, Walz A, Dewald B, Baggiolini M. A novel neutrophil-activating factor produced by human mononuclear phagocytes. *J Exp Med* 1988; **167**: 1547–59.

63. Lee TH, Avraham H, Lee SH, Avraham S. Vascular endothelial growth factor modulates neutrophil transendothelial migration via up-regulation of interleukin-8 in human brain microvascular endothelial cells. *J Biol Chem* 2002; **277**: 10445–51.

64. Haraguchi M, Komuta K, Akashi A, Matsuzaki S, Furui J, Kanematsu T. Elevated IL-8 levels in the drainage vein of resectable Dukes' C colorectal cancer indicate high risk for developing hepatic metastasis. *Oncol Rep* 2002; **9**: 159–65.

65. Galffy G, Mohammed KA, Dowling PA, Nasreen N, Ward MJ, Antony VB. Interleukin 8: an autocrine growth factor for malignant mesothelioma. *Cancer Res* 1999; **59**: 367–71.

66. Galffy G, Mohammed KA, Nasreen N, Ward MJ, Antony VB. Inhibition of interleukin-8 reduces human malignant pleural mesothelioma propagation in nude mouse model. *Oncol Res* 1999; **11**: 187–94.

67. Detmers PA, Powell DE, Walz A, Clark-Lewis I, Baggiolini M, Cohn ZA. Differential effects of neutrophil-activating peptide 1/IL-8 and its homologues on leukocyte adhesion and phagocytosis. *J Immunol* 1991; **147**: 4211–17.

68. Moser B, Schumacher C, von Tscharner V, Clark-Lewis I, Baggiolini M. Neutrophil-activating peptide 2 and gro/melanoma growth-stimulatory activity interact with neutrophil-activating peptide 1/interleukin 8 receptors on human neutrophils. *J Biol Chem* 1991; **266**: 10666–71.

69. Taketo *et al.*

70. Edwards JG, Faux SP, Plummer SM, *et al.* Cyclooxygenase-2 expression is a novel prognostic factor in malignant mesothelioma. *Clin Cancer Res* 2002; **8**: 1857–62.

71. Edwards JG, Faux S, Plummer S.M., Walker R, Waller D, O'Byrne K. Cyclooxygenase-2 and angiogenesis in malignant mesothelioma. *Proc Annu Meet Am Assoc Cancer Res* 2001.

72. Marrogi A, Pass HI, Khan M, Metheny-Barlow LJ, Harris CC, Gerwin BI. Human mesothelioma samples overexpress both cyclooxygenase-2 (COX-2) and inducible nitric oxide synthase (NOS2): *in vitro* antiproliferative effects of a COX-2 inhibitor. *Cancer Res* 2000; **60**: 3696–700.

73. Pepper MS, Ferrara N, Orci L, Montesano R. Potent synergism between vascular endothelial growth factor and basic fibroblast growth factor in the induction of angiogenesis *in vitro*. *Biochem Biophys Res Commun* 1992; **189**: 824–31.

74. Mutsaers SE, McAnulty RJ, Laurent GJ, Versnel MA, Whitaker D, Papadimitriou JM. Cytokine regulation of mesothelial cell proliferation *in vitro* and *in vivo*. *Eur J Cell Biol* 1997; **72**: 24–29.

75. Strizzi L, Vianale G, Catalano A, Muraro R, Mutti L, Procopio A. Basic fibroblast growth factor in mesothelioma pleural effusions: correlation with patient survival and angiogenesis. *Int J Oncol* 2001; **18**: 1093–8.

76. Griffith EC, Su Z, Turk BE, *et al.* Methionine aminopeptidase (type 2) is the common target for angiogenesis inhibitors AGM-1470 and ovalicin. *Chem Biol* 1997; **4**: 461–71.

77. Griffith EC, Su Z, Niwayama S, Ramsay CA, Chang YH, Liu JO. Molecular recognition of angiogenesis inhibitors fumagillin and ovalicin by methionine aminopeptidase 2. *Proc Natl Acad Sci USA* 1998; **95**: 15183–8.

78. Sin N, Meng L, Wang MQ, Wen JJ, Bornmann WG, Crews CM. The anti-angiogenic agent fumagillin covalently binds and inhibits the methionine aminopeptidase, MetAP-2. *Proc Natl Acad Sci USA* 1997; **94**: 6099–103.

79. Catalano A, Romano M, Robuffo I, Strizzi L, Procopio A. Methionine aminopeptidase-2 regulates human mesothelioma cell survival: role of Bcl-2 expression and telomerase activity. *Am J Pathol* 2001; **159**: 721–31.

80. Britton M. The epidemiology of mesothelioma. *Semin Oncol* 2002; **29**: 18–25.

81. Carbone M, Kratzke RA, Testa JR. The pathogenesis of mesothelioma. *Semin Oncol* 2002; **29**: 2–17.

82. Bielefeldt-Ohmann H, Jarnicki AG, Fitzpatrick DR. Molecular pathobiology and immunology of malignant mesothelioma. *J Pathol* 1996; **178**: 369–78.

83. Branchaud RM, MacDonald JL, Kane AB. Induction of angiogenesis by intraperitoneal injection of asbestos fibers. *FASEB J* 1989; **3**: 1747–52.

84. Craighead JE. Current pathogenetic concepts of diffuse malignant mesothelioma. *Hum Pathol* 1987; **18**: 544–57.

85. O'Byrne KJ, Dalgleish AG, Browning MJ, Steward WP, Harris AL. The relationship between angiogenesis and the immune response in carcinogenesis and the progression of malignant disease. *Eur J Cancer* 2000; **36**: 151–69.

86. El-Assal ON, Yamanoi A, Soda Y, *et al.* Clinical significance of microvessel density and vascular endothelial growth factor expression in hepatocellular carcinoma and surrounding liver: possible involvement of vascular endothelial growth factor in the angiogenesis of cirrhotic liver. *Hepatology* 1998; **27**: 1554–62.

87. Mazzanti R, Messerini L, Monsacchi L, *et al.* Chronic viral hepatitis induced by hepatitis C but not hepatitis B virus infection correlates with increased liver angiogenesis. *Hepatology* 1997; **25**: 229–34.

88. Zanella CL, Posada J, Tritton TR, Mossman BT. Asbestos causes stimulation of the extracellular signal-regulated kinase 1 mitogen-activated protein kinase cascade after phosphorylation of the epidermal growth factor receptor. *Cancer Res* 1996; **56**: 5334–8.

89. Jimenez LA, Zanella C, Fung H, *et al.* Role of extracellular signal-regulated protein kinases in apoptosis by asbestos and H_2O_2. *Am J Physiol* 1997; **273**: L1029–35.

90. Zanella CL, Timblin CR, Cummins A, *et al.* Asbestos-induced phosphorylation of epidermal growth factor receptor is linked to c-*fos* and apoptosis. *Am J Physiol* 1999; **277**: L684–93.

91. Robledo RF, Buder-Hoffmann SA, Cummins AB, Walsh ES, Taatjes DJ, Mossman BT. Increased phosphorylated extracellular signal-regulated kinase immunoreactivity associated with proliferative and morphologic lung alterations after chrysotile asbestos inhalation in mice. *Am J Pathol* 2000; **156**: 1307–16.

92. Buder-Hoffmann S, Palmer C, Vacek P, Taatjes D, Mossman B. Different accumulation of activated extracellular signal-regulated kinases (ERK 1/2) and role in cell-cycle alterations by epidermal growth factor, hydrogen peroxide, or asbestos in pulmonary epithelial cells. *Am J Respir Cell Mol Biol* 2001; **24**: 405–13.

93. Zachary I, Gliki G. Signaling transduction mechanisms mediating biological actions of the vascular endothelial growth factor family. *Cardiovasc Res* 2001; **49**: 568–81.

94. Lamorte L, Park M. The receptor tyrosine kinases: role in cancer progression. *Surg Oncol Clin N Am* 2001; **10**: 271–88.

95. Jimenez B, Volpert OV. Mechanistic insights on the inhibition of tumor angiogenesis. *J Mol Med* 2001; **78**: 663–72.

96. Baselga J. The EGFR as a target for anticancer therapy—focus on cetuximab. *Eur J Cancer* 2001; **37** (Suppl 4): S16–22.

97. Fleming I. Cytochrome p450 and vascular homeostasis. *Circ Res* 2001; **89**: 753–62.

98. Rosenthal GJ, Simeonova P, Corsini E. Asbestos toxicity: an immunologic perspective. *Rev Environ Health* 1999; **14**: 11–20.

99. Watanabe M, McCormick KL, Volker K, *et al.* Regulation of local host-mediated anti-tumor mechanisms by cytokines: direct and indirect effects on leukocyte recruitment and angiogenesis. *Am J Pathol* 1997; **150**: 1869–80.

100. Dinney CP, Bielenberg DR, Perrotte P, *et al.* Inhibition of basic fibroblast growth factor expression, angiogenesis, and growth of human bladder carcinoma in mice by systemic interferon-alpha administration. *Cancer Res* 1998; **58**: 808–14.

101. Coughlin CM, Salhany KE, Gee MS, *et al.* Tumor cell responses to IFNgamma affect tumorigenicity and response to IL-12 therapy and antiangiogenesis. *Immunity* 1998; **9**: 25–34.

102. Coughlin CM, Salhany KE, Wysocka M, *et al.* Interleukin-12 and interleukin-18 synergistically induce murine tumor regression which involves inhibition of angiogenesis. *J Clin Invest* 1998; **101**: 1441–52.

103. Harris AL. Hypoxia—a key regulatory factor in tumour growth. *Nat Rev Cancer* 2002; **2**: 38–47.

104. Knowles HJ, Harris AL. Hypoxia and oxidative stress in breast cancer. Hypoxia and tumorigenesis. *Breast Cancer Res* 2001; **3**: 318–22.

105. Lewis JS, Lee JA, Underwood JC, Harris AL, Lewis CE. Macrophage responses to hypoxia: relevance to disease mechanisms. *J Leukoc Biol* 1999; **66**: 889–900.

106. Durnova GN, Kaplanskii AS, Portugalov VV. [The effect of hypoxia on the function and metabolism of alveolar macrophages.] *Biull Eksp Biol Med* 1975; **79**: 113–15.

107. Semenza GL, Agani F, Feldser D, *et al.* Hypoxia, HIF-1, and the pathophysiology of common human diseases. *Adv Exp Med Biol* 2000; **475**: 123–30.

108. Nathan C, Xie QW. Regulation of biosynthesis of nitric oxide. *J Biol Chem* 1994; **269**: 13725–8.

109. Soini Y, Kahlos K, Puhakka A, *et al.* Expression of inducible nitric oxide synthase in healthy pleura and in malignant mesothelioma. *Br J Cancer* 2000; **83**: 880–6.

110. Jenkins DC, Charles IG, Thomsen LL, *et al.* Roles of nitric oxide in tumor growth. *Proc Natl Acad Sci USA* 1995; **92**: 4392–6.

111. Kroll J, Waltenberger J. VEGF-A induces expression of eNOS and iNOS in endothelial cells via VEGF receptor-2 (KDR). *Biochem Biophys Res Commun* 1998; **252**: 743–6.

112. Kroll J, Waltenberger J. A novel function of VEGF receptor-2 (KDR): rapid release of nitric oxide in response to VEGF-A stimulation in endothelial cells. *Biochem Biophys Res Commun* 1999; **265**: 636–9.

113. Robledo R, Mossman B. Cellular and molecular mechanisms of asbestos-induced fibrosis. *J Cell Physiol* 1999; **180**: 158–66.

114. Mossman BT, Churg A. Mechanisms in the pathogenesis of asbestosis and silicosis. *Am J Respir Crit Care Med* 1998; **157**: 1666–80.

115. Hu YL, Tee MK, Goetzl EJ, Auersperg N, Mills GB, Ferrara N, Jaffe RB. Lysophosphatidic acid induction of vascular endothelial growth factor expression in human ovarian cancer cells. *J Natl Cancer Inst* 2001; **93**: 762–8.

116. Murthy SS, Testa JR. Asbestos, chromosomal deletions, and tumor suppressor gene alterations in human malignant mesothelioma. *J Cell Physiol* 1999; **180**: 150–7.

117. Harada H, Nakagawa K, Iwata S, *et al*. Restoration of wild-type p16 down-regulates vascular endothelial growth factor expression and inhibits angiogenesis in human gliomas. *Cancer Res* 1999; **59**: 3783–9.

118. Butel JS, Lednicky JA. Cell and molecular biology of simian virus 40: implications for human infections and disease. *J Natl Cancer Inst* 1999; **91**: 119–34.

119. Ali SH, DeCaprio JA. Cellular transformation by SV40 large T antigen: interaction with host proteins. *Semin Cancer Biol* 2001; **11**: 15–23.

120. Catalano A, Romano M, Martinotti S, Procopio A. Enhanced expression of vascular endothelial growth factor (VEGF) plays a critical role in the tumor progression potential induced by simian virus 40 large T antigen. *Oncogene* 2002; **21**: 2896–900.

121. Carbone M, Rizzo P, Grimley PM, *et al*. Simian virus-40 large-T antigen binds p53 in human mesotheliomas. *Nat Med* 1997; **3**: 908–12.

122. Rak J, Yu JL, Klement G, Kerbel RS. Oncogenes and angiogenesis: signaling three-dimensional tumor growth. *J Invest Dermatol Symp Proc* 2000; **5**: 24–33.

123. Volpert OV, Dameron KM, Bouck N. Sequential development of an angiogenic phenotype by human fibroblasts progressing to tumorigenicity. *Oncogene* 1997; **14**: 1495–1502.

124. Metcalf RA, Welsh JA, Bennett WP, *et al*. p53 and Kirsten-*ras* mutations in human mesothelioma cell lines. *Cancer Res* 1992; **52**: 2610–15.

125. Modi S, Kubo A, Oie H, Coxon AB, Rehmatulla A, Kaye FJ. Protein expression of the RB-related gene family and SV40 large T antigen in mesothelioma and lung cancer. *Oncogene* 2000; **19**: 4632–9.

126. Testa JR, Giordano A. SV40 and cell cycle perturbations in malignant mesothelioma. *Semin Cancer Biol* 2001; **11**: 31–8.

127. De Luca A, Baldi A, Esposito V, *et al*. The retinoblastoma gene family pRb/p105, p107, pRb2/p130 and simian virus-40 large T-antigen in human mesotheliomas. *Nat Med* 1997; **3**: 913–16.

128. Claudio PP, Stiegler P, Howard CM, *et al*. RB2/p130 gene-enhanced expression down-regulates vascular endothelial growth factor expression and inhibits angiogenesis *in vivo*. *Cancer Res* 2001; **61**: 462–8.

129. He Y, Karpanen T, Alitalo K. Role of lymphangiogenic factors in tumor metastasis. *Biochim Biophys Acta* 2004; **1654**: 3–12.

130. Padera TP, Kadambi A, di Tomaso E, *et al*. Lymphatic metastasis in the absence of functional intratumor lymphatics. *Science* 2002; **296**: 1883–6.

131. Ohta Y, Shridhar V, Bright RK, *et al*. VEGF and VEGF type C play an important role in angiogenesis and lymphangiogenesis in human malignant mesothelioma tumours. *Br J Cancer*. 1999; **81**: 54–61.

132. Masood R, Kundra A, Zhu S, *et al*. Malignant mesothelioma growth inhibition by agents that target the VEGF and VEGF-C autocrine loops. *Int J Cancer* 2003; **104**: 603–10.

133. Vermeulen PB, Gasparini G, Fox SB, *et al*. Quantification of angiogenesis in solid human tumours: an international consensus on the methodology and criteria of evaluation. *Eur J Cancer* 1996; **32A**: 2474–84.

Chapter 10

Immunobiology of malignant mesothelioma

A. M. Smith, S. Lansley, C. Jackaman, B. Koloska,
S. Broomfield, B. W. S. Robinson, and D. J. Nelson

Introduction

Exactly how malignant mesothelioma (MM) tumours arise, both at the molecular level, as a result of genetic mutation(s), and subsequently at the cellular level, remains poorly defined. The lengthy period between asbestos exposure and the manifestation of obvious disease makes tracking immune responses to developing MM tumours difficult in humans. Furthermore, the lack of obvious early symptoms means that MM remains undetectable until characteristic clinical symptoms manifest; even then, rigorous histopathological and/or cytopathological examination is required for confirmation of disease. As a result, MM is diagnosed late in disease progression and is associated with a rapid decline in health. Despite these limitations, a number of experimental approaches have been utilized to characterize MM-specific and non-specific immune responses to the progressing disease. In this chapter we briefly review the cell types involved in the innate and adaptive immune systems, current thinking regarding the interplay between these cells, and their immunobiological roles during the development of MM.

The goal of tumour immunology is to induce, or enhance, an antitumour immune response such that this response will mediate tumour regression. A number of studies of MM have been undertaken with this in mind but, although there have been some promising data, to date the clinical outcomes have generally been disappointing. The reason for this may be that our knowledge of the immune system is still evolving, and it is significantly more complex than first thought. Even less is known about the role the immune system plays during MM tumour progression. Without this knowledge it seems unlikely that we will be able to determine which components of the immune system to target for therapeutic purposes.

Brief overview of the immune system

The immune system has evolved to protect the body from constant challenge by environmental pathogens. These foreign agents, including viruses, bacteria, and even inert allergens like pollen, constantly enter the body and evoke an immune response. The immune system also protects the body from diseases and removes damaged or dead cells. The host response to invading pathogens has been extensively studied and is classically viewed as a two-tier system comprising innate (inflammatory) and acquired (adaptive) immune mechanisms (Table 10.1). Unlike the innate immune system, the adaptive immune system is able to recognize specific components of the elements it encounters; these are usually small portions of proteins derived from foreign bodies, or from one's own cells, and are referred to as antigens. Antigens can subsequently be identified by the immune system as self (belonging to the body, e.g. dead cells) or non-self (foreign agents).

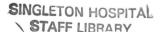

Table 10.1 Cellular components of the innate and adaptive immune responses

Innate response	Adaptive response
Phagocytic cells	Professional antigen-presenting cells:
Monocytes/macrophages, dendritic cells	Macrophages, B cells & dendritic cells
Granulocytes	T cells
Neutrophils, eosinophils, mast cells	$CD4^+$ (helper, regulator, suppressor), $CD8^+$ (cytotoxic)
Cytolytic cells	B cells
NK cells, NK T cells, LAK cells	Antibody producing
ϒ T cells	

NK, natural killer; LAK, lymphokine-activated killer.

Innate immunity

The innate immune system is the primary defence system of humans; it is present at birth and is effective without prior exposure to any form of antigen. Innate immunity consists of a multitude of protective mechanisms including the skin and mucous membranes, interferons, and inflammation. At the cellular level, innate immunity consists primarily of specialized cells such as macrophages, natural killer (NK) cells and polymorphonuclear cells (PMNs), i.e. neutrophils, eosinophils and mast cells, as well as professional antigen presenting cells (APCs), referred to as dendritic cells (DC) [1]; all these cell types can directly kill pathogens.

Innate immune responses are mediated by receptors expressed on the cell surface that are not diversified by genetic recombination events and mutations [2]. Toll receptors are now believed to be an important part of the innate immune response, as they function as cytokine receptors in insects and as pattern-recognition receptors in mammals [3]. Toll receptors in mammalian species are known as toll-like receptors (TLRs) [3]; they play an important role in the detection of microbial infection and activate the inflammatory and antimicrobial arms of the innate immune response [4].

Whilst the magnitude and kinetics of the innate response to pathogens continues to be studied, the role of these cellular components during infection is better characterized than their corresponding role in tumour immunology. A first line of defence to infection is provided by the rapid recruitment of PMNs to sites of tissue injury in response to locally produced chemotactic factors. It is now clear that a transient wave of dendritic cells (DCs) coincides with this PMN response, and that the DCs may function not only as members of both the innate and adaptive immune systems, but also as a link between the two. The PMN–DC response is followed up to 48 h later by a second wave of mononuclear cells containing large numbers of macrophages which are effective in pathogen destruction, removal of infected, damaged, or dead cells, and antigen uptake. It may well be that these events (particularly those involved in chronic inflammation) are also critical in providing the local milieu essential for the evolution and progression of a MM tumour (discussed in more detail below).

Whilst the innate immune system is the first system to be provoked by a pathogen, it may also be the initiator/activator of the adaptive immune system via a range of soluble mediators as well as through cell–cell contact. It is also becoming increasingly clear that the adaptive and innate immune systems cooperate at several levels to ensure an optimal immune response, and any decline in adaptive immunity will impact upon the function of the innate immune system and vice versa (see below). However, the role of these two systems and their interplay is less well defined in MM tumour immunology.

Adaptive immunity

Once the innate immune system is activated, the adaptive (or acquired) immune system may also be initiated via interaction with professional APC. Adaptive immunity is characterized by defined 'memory' responses to previously encountered antigens. The adaptive immune system comprises lymphocytes, either T cells or B cells, which specifically recognize antigens and actively destroy them or, in the case of B cells, generate specific antibodies against them. Lymphocytes recognize antigens in the body via interaction with professional APCs; the most effective APC is the DC, but macrophages and B cells are also capable of presenting antigen to T cells. In fact, naive T cells can only recognize and act upon antigens in this way. Once T cells and B cells have encountered the antigen and received appropriate activation signals, either a T-cell-mediated response or a B-cell dependent antibody (humoral) response is initiated.

Whilst understanding the generation of adaptive immune responses to foreign antigens represents continuing studies, this area is still better defined than the induction and maintenance of anti-tumour immune responses. Nonetheless, there is evidence to suggest that a similar mechanism is operating in anticancer immunity. It is becoming clear that although solid tumours, including MM tumours, are recognized by the immune system, the host antitumour immune response is ineffective at preventing tumour development (discussed in detail below). Figure 10.1 shows how the cellular players of the immune system must operate within a tumour and in tumour-draining lymph nodes such that the adaptive immune system can recognize and react to a solid tumour.

Tumour immunity can be initiated by effectors of innate immunity and further developed by cells of adaptive immunity, with DCs playing a central regulatory role. Several steps are involved, including activation of macrophages, capture of tumour molecules by DC precursors, direct and interferon-γ-mediated killing of transformed cells by NK/NK T cells that have been activated by DCs, cross-presentation (described in more detail below) of tumour-associated antigens by immature DCs, selection and activation of tumour-specific T cells, and homing of these T cells to

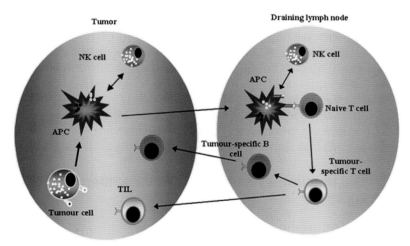

Figure 10.1 Events required to generate an anti-MM tumour immune response. APC must encounter MM tumour antigens in the tumour, process these antigens, traffic them to draining lymph node and present the antigens to naive T cells. MM-specific CD4$^+$ and CD8$^+$ T cells can be generated that have to infiltrate the tumour before they can be effective. CD4$^+$ T cells can provide help to B cells, whilst NK cells may engage in bidirectional cross-talk with APC such that the APC is further activated and the NK cell is conditioned to kill tumour cells. However, these NK cells may also kill the APC in the tumour or the lymph node, thereby attenuating the immune response. B cells may produce antitumour antibodies and/or suppress T cells.

the tumour where they recognize their cognate antigen, leading to lysis of tumour cells. Tumours may escape immune surveillance by avoiding some of these steps. Release of cytokines such as IL-6, IL-10, macrophage colony stimulating factor (M-CSF), and vascular endothelial growth factor (VEGF) can prevent DC differentiation and/or APC function.

Cross-talk between the innate and adaptive immune systems

Studies of immune responses to infectious agents have clearly demonstrated that immune cells cooperate via direct cell–cell interactions, as well as through the release of soluble mediators, and that this is critical for activating an appropriate immune response. For example, helper T (Th) cells bind to macrophages via the T cell's antigen receptor (TCR). This union, aided by DC, makes immune cells cluster and stimulates macrophages and Th cells to exchange chemical messages between themselves and other cells of the immune system. Interestingly, TLRs expressed on DCs recognize microbial products and trigger the functional maturation of DCs, leading to antigen-specific immune responses of adaptive immunity [5]. Activated DC can form immune cell clusters and stimulate Th cells to release several lymphokines, including interleukin-2 (IL-2). IL-2, in turn, causes T cells to secrete interferon-γ (IFN-γ, which activates NK cells and macrophages and instructs other Th cells and cytotoxic T lymphocytes (CTLs) to multiply. Proliferating Th cells release substances that signal B cells to begin multiplying and differentiating into antibody-producing cells. Antibodies can bind to surface antigens, making it easier for macrophages and NK cells to destroy infectious agents or host cells expressing that antigen. The binding of antibodies to foreign antigens also signals complement proteins that can mediate direct killing. Finally, suppressor T cells are activated that can 'switch off' B cells, DCs, Th cells, and cytotoxic T cells.

Recent reports have shown that the generation and maintenance of immune response to infectious agents are more complex than originally thought. It is now clear that NK cells engage in cross talk with DCs [6–9]. NK cells can be activated by immature and mature DCs, and these NK cells may act with more specificity than was previously believed [8]. DC-activated NK cells proliferate, secrete IFN-γ and acquire cytolytic activity [8]. Similar results are seen with IL-2-activated NK cells. Activated NK cells can promote DC maturation via CD40, thereby enhancing the immune response [8,9]. However, DC-activated NK cells can surround DCs, leading to NK cell-mediated DC death which switches off antigen presentation [9], thereby attenuating the immune response. Thus *in vivo* expansion of both NK cells and DCs may be required before a fully effective antitumour response can be induced.

The important 'take home' message is that there is considerable cross-talk occurring between different cellular members of the immune system. Our understanding of this cross-talk, and the cells involved, is limited in the immunobiology of MM.

The role of the immune system in the development of malignant mesothelioma

Inflammation and malignant mesothelioma

MM is a cancer of the serosal cavities, generally originating in the pleural space following inhalation of asbestos fibres. One of the first events that may lead to the development of many solid tumours is local inflammation induced by a virus, a chemical, or, in the case of MM, asbestos fibres lodged in the lungs. Animal models have shown that the initial injury caused by asbestos appears to be dependent upon the chemical and physical properties of asbestos fibres. Short fibres are cleared by the local mucociliary transport system such that asbestos is coughed up. Alternatively, phagocytic macrophages carry short asbestos fibres to the lymph nodes or spleen where they may dissolve or degrade [10,11]. However, longer fibres (>10 μm) lodge in the upper airways and are then mobilized to the terminal bronchioles or the pleura or penetrate through the alveolar wall; this process can happen between 5 h and 21 days after inhalation [12–15]. A rat model showed that the earliest response to intrapleural inoculation of asbestos was haemorrhage followed by pleural inflammation and localized destruction of the elastic membrane under the visceral pleura. As a result, asbestos fibres were able to penetrate into the lung, and chronic stimulation of the pleura eventually led to the development of MM [16].

The role of polymorphonuclear neutrophils in the evolution of malignant mesothelioma

Despite their ability to destroy tumour cells, PMNs may in fact play a role in altering the local tissue milieu such that a tumour can develop, become invasive, and metastasize. A number of studies have shown that the inhalation of asbestos generates an inflammatory response characterized by elevated lung cell proliferation, a PMN infiltrate, and release of lactate dehydrogenase, possibly PMN derived [17], as well as persistent abnormal macrophage–fibre clumps in the lungs [11,18–20]. PMN may be directly recruited by transformed mesothelial cells which constitutively produce IL-8 [21].

Although PMNs can be found in the lung interstitium 2 years after asbestos exposure [22], their role in the development of MM is unclear. Interestingly, in humans there is evidence that patients with chronic inflammation may also develop MM. Non-asbestos-exposed patients with familial Mediterranean fever (a hereditary serositis) have an increased risk of developing MM [25]. PMN may assist in the establishment of solid tumours by releasing serine proteinases, such as elastase, cathepsin G, and protease 3, that activate matrix metalloproteinases (MMPs), including MMP-2, which then degrade a variety of basement membrane components essential for tumour invasion [26,27].

The role of macrophages in the evolution of malignant mesothelioma

Macrophages are postulated to be crucial players in the development of MM. Studies have shown that inflammatory cells, in particular macrophages, surround the wound site within 48 h of injury to serosal surfaces. Depletion of circulating monocytes in a murine model resulted in significantly delayed serosal healing. In contrast, addition of peritoneal macrophages to the wound site 36 h before injury increased the healing rate. These findings suggest that macrophages play a major role in serosal repair by stimulating mesothelial cell proliferation [28]. However, the presence of asbestos fibres may complicate the healing process.

A number of studies have shown that asbestos fibres activate macrophages *in vitro* [29,30] and *in vivo* [11,18,19]. Increased numbers of macrophages are recovered from bronchoalveolar lavages (BALs) of patients and experimental animals for up to 93 weeks after asbestos injury [22]. Multinucleated macrophages with increased phagocytic activity have been recovered from human BAL following asbestos exposure. After inhalation, the majority of asbestos fibres deposited in the lungs are initially phagocytosed by alveolar macrophages [31]. These macrophages serve as scavengers that are attempting to remove asbestos from the airways. It is believed that once in the airspace macrophages cannot re-enter the interstitium and that, after having ingested fibres, they migrate, by amoeboid movement, to the terminal bronchioles where they are mobilized by muco-ciliary clearance towards the mouth and are subsequently swallowed or expectorated [12]. Following exposure to asbestos, alveolar macrophages display increased expression of Fc receptors for IgG, surface ruffles, and filopodia [32].

Only some macrophages succeed in clearing asbestos as, although fibre-laden macrophages accumulate in draining lymph nodes, others remain within alveolar walls and the lung interstitium. Trapped asbestos fibres were seen in mouse diaphragms less than 6 h after intraperitoneal injections of long crocidolite asbestos. The majority of fibres were rapidly cleared (within 3 days) followed by an intense local inflammatory reaction with accumulation of activated macrophages. However, 6 months later clusters of fibres partially covered by mesothelium, but surrounded by macrophages and regenerating mesothelial cells, could be readily visualized [18].

Whilst it is becoming increasingly clear that the processes of inflammation, fibrosis, and carcinogenesis are closely intertwined, the role of macrophages in the development of MM remains unclear. One hypothesis is that asbestos induces apoptosis of alveolar macrophages, resulting in the development of an inflammatory state; this is supported by studies showing that low doses of asbestos fibres cause apoptosis in cultured human alveolar macrophages [33]. Significantly, macrophages have been shown to accelerate the process of mesothelial cell transformation [34]. The development of angiogenesis may be also mediated by activated macrophages, and evidence of angiogenesis was seen in inflammatory lesions 14 days after a single exposure to crocidolite asbestos fibres. After six weekly injections, lesions containing asbestos fibres were surrounded by a capillary network that radiated toward the centre of the lesion. Hence this process may provide transformed cells with the ideal microenvironment that facilitates the later emergence of MM at these sites [19].

Innate immune responses to malignant mesothelioma

PMN and malignant mesothelioma

Several murine models of MM have been developed by inoculating mice with asbestos fibres, excising the consequent tumours, and cloning the tumour cells *in vitro*. Re-inoculation of cloned tumour cells into syngeneic mice results in progressing tumours, confirmed by histopathology to be representative of human MM. In an MM model referred to as AE17 [35], PMNs can be found scattered throughout established tumours in low numbers (2–5 per cent) (unpublished data). These cells are also seen collected around areas of necrosis in larger tumours. The role of these cells, whether it be enhancing or delaying tumour growth, has yet to be determined. PMNs could be involved in the inhibition of tumour growth through their ability to respond to and produce cytokines, or through their involvement in the cross-talk between non-specific and specific immune cells [36]. Alternatively, PMNs could contribute to the tumour environment by the release of soluble factors that mediate angiogenesis and/or inhibit antitumour effector cells. Recently, murine MM tumours have been treated with IL-2 and activating anti-CD40 antibody. This treatment resulted in a marked PMN infiltrate, followed by necrosis and destruction of the tumour. Whether PMN cells are important for IL-2/anti-CD40-induced tumour regression, or whether the PMN infiltrate is seen as a by-product of other effects, is currently being investigated.

Macrophages and malignant mesothelioma

Once MM tumours become established, macrophages continue to play a crucial role in tumorigenesis. Both human and murine MM tumours are heavily infiltrated by macrophages, which can comprise up to 50 per cent of the tumour cellularity (Fig. 10.2). Expression of major histocompatibility complex (MHC) class II (Fig. 10.2), CD11b, and CD18 are restricted to macrophages newly recruited at the tumour site. Whilst some CD11b+ tumour-infiltrating macrophages (TIMs) are found near the edge of the necrotic foci, the majority express few to none of these markers and are distributed throughout the intact tumour tissue [37]. Hence they are no longer activated macrophages and, rather than present MHC-class II-restricted antigens (discussed in more detail below) or exert cytotoxic activity against tumour cells, they may pro-

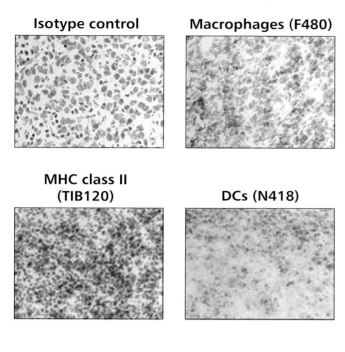

Isotype control

Macrophages (F480)

MHC class II (TIB120)

DCs (N418)

Figure 10.2 APCs in solid MM tumours. Immunohistochemistry using monoclonal antibodies on cryopreserved sections of MM tumours revealed significant numbers of tumour-infiltrating macrophages (TIMs), dendritic cells (DCs), and cells expressing MHC class II molecules, i.e. cells that have the capacity to present antigens to CD4$^+$ T cells; note that the tumour cells do not express MHC class II molecules on their surface.

vide many of the soluble factors required to promote matrix components, tumour cell proliferation, and angiogenesis. Importantly, macrophages may also suppress immune cells, such as professional APCs (DCs in particular), NK cells, and T cells, via the production of transforming growth factor β (TGF-β), nitric oxide (NO), and hydrogen peroxide (H$_2$O$_2$).

Natural killer cells and malignant mesothelioma

NK cells represent a distinct population of large granular lymphocytes that play an important role in innate immunity and form a first line of defence against a variety of host cells that are infected, stressed, and/or cancerous in an MHC unrestricted manner. NK cells can act against tumour initiation, growth, and metastasis in rodents and humans [38]. NK cells are activated by interferon-α (IFN-α) and their cytotoxic function is greatly enhanced by IL-2. NK cells provide IFN-γ to control infections and tumour cells, but also use other effector mechanisms including the perforin/granzyme-containing granule-mediated and death-receptor pathways. The mechanisms of their regulation and delivery of antitumour effects are not completely understood. However, it is clear that NK activity is regulated by signals generated by both inhibitory and stimulatory receptors expressed by target cells. MHC class I molecules expressed on target cells inhibit NK lytic activity by engaging surface inhibitory receptors, whilst co-stimulatory molecules, such as B7–1, B7–2, and CD40, are able to trigger NK activity. The local cytokine microenvironment serves to define the differentiation and proliferation of NK cells. Very little has been reported with regard to the role of NK cells during early events in the development of MM.

There is controversy as to whether NK cells are functionally abnormal in asbestosis, as smoking is a confounding factor in human studies. A recent study of retired healthy asbestos workers showed that asbestos exposure of 10 years or more generated an increased number of circulating NK cells but their effectiveness was diminished relative to non-asbestos-exposed controls [39]. Similarly, asbestos fibres have been shown to decrease NK activity *in vitro* [40]. However, smoking and asbestos exposure appear to interact and decrease NK activity, which may help explain the increased risk of neoplasia in this population [41]. Similarly, in one study 14 of 20 MM patients had significantly depressed NK cell activity [42].

Preliminary experiments have been conducted comparing the numbers and location of NK cells in small and large MM tumours using the AE17 murine model of MM. In these experiments mice were subcutaneously injected with AE17 tumour cells. The MM tumours were removed at different time points and examined using immunohistochemistry or single-cell suspensions were prepared, stained, and analysed via flow cytometry.

Preliminary experiments using antibodies for fluorescence-activated cell sorter (FACS) analysis and/or immunhistochemistry showed that a number of subpopulations of NK cells could infiltrate solid MM tumours [43]. NK1.1 is a widely used NK cell marker for FACS analysis; however, NKT cells also express NK1.1 (see below). Consistent NK1.1$^+$ cell percentages (6.4 ± 0.4 per cent of the total viable cells in the intratumoral lymphocyte population) were detected within solid MM tumours throughout tumour growth. The DX5 antibody detects the recently discovered CD49b antigen on the surface of NK cells [44], whilst the 4D11 antibody reacts with an inhibitory receptor, known as Ly-49G2, on the surface of NK cells and mediates negative regulation of NK cytolytic activity [45]. Low numbers of DX5$^+$ and 4D11$^+$ NK cells could be seen within MM tumours at all time points when examined by FACS.

Immunohistochemistry showed that NK cells could be seen trafficking through MM tumour-associated blood vessels, as well as being located within the tumour itself. Interestingly, some NK cells were juxtaposed against B cells and investigations are ongoing regarding the significance of the potential cross-talk between NK and B cells in MM tumours.

Whilst the antibodies confirmed the presence of NK cells in solid MM tumours, there was a considerable difference in the expression levels of each marker. Dual staining revealed that a number of different NK subsets can be found in MM tumours; however, their function in MM tumour growth has yet to be determined. Importantly, using the same model it was found that MM tumour growth was accelerated in NK-depleted or NK knockout mice [43], implying that NK cells can retard but not prevent MM tumour growth.

MM is an intracavity disease and therefore an intraperitoneal model may resemble disease progression more closely. Odaka *et al.* [46] examined the lymphocyte population of peritoneal exudate cells (PECs) in tumour-bearing mice. They found that NK cells account for 16.9 per cent of the PECs in normal mice; however, after intraperitoneal injection with a murine MM tumour cell line, NK cells comprised 29.6 per cent of PECs 6 days later but then decreased to 5 per cent by day 14 after tumour inoculation. Analysis of the intraperitoneal tumour lesions mirrored the PEC data with an early NK cell infiltration followed by a gradual decline 14 days after tumour cell inoculation.

Therefore NK cells may respond rapidly at the onset of malignant cell formation and may even exert some control of tumour growth. However, they are unable to halt disease progression.

Natural killer T cells and malignant mesothelioma

A second NK cell population from within T cell populations, natural killer T cells (NKT), that coexpress the NK receptors NK1.1 [47] or NKR-P1A (CD161) and a T-cell receptor (TCR or CD3) [48] has recently been identified. NKT cell responses occur at very early times after viral infection and upon stimulation secrete large quantities of immunoregulatory cytokines, including IFN-γ and IL-4; thus NKT cells may be important for the initiation and regulation of immune responses [49]. In preliminary studies, low numbers of NKT cells (~4 per cent of the NK cell population) have been detected by flow cytometry in murine MM tumours [43]; however, the role of these infiltrating NKT cells in MM is unknown.

Lymphokine-activated killer cells and malignant mesothelioma

Lymphokine-activated killer (LAK) cells are IL-2-activated cytolytic lymphocytes which can effectively kill many NK-resistant tumour cells in a non-MHC-restricted manner [50]. Early work showed that this was true for human and murine MM tumour cell lines which are susceptible to non-MHC restricted lysis *in vitro* by LAK cells and δ T lymphocytes, but not by NK cell lysis [50–52]. Like NK cell activity, LAK cell activity is diminished in the presence of asbestos [52], but the role of this cell type *in vivo* remains unclear. Studies have shown that whilst patients with MM maintain normal white cell counts, total serum proteins, and immunoglobulin levels, their LAK cell activity against MM tumour targets is depressed to about 60 per cent of that of healthy controls [53,54].

These data imply that 'rescuing' or generating LAK cells, but not NK cells, may be clinically significant. However, studies that have systemically administered IL-2 to activate NK and LAK cells in patients have generally been disappointing, and intrapleural delivery of LAK cells and IL-2 to MM patients caused severe side effects. Others studies have reported that the prolonged use of low doses of IL-2 given subcutaneously to MM patients can activate discrete T and NK cell subpopulations [55]. Recent work has shown that IL-2 can be successfully used to induce complete tumour regression in murine MM models, but only if the tumours are small when treatment begins and the IL-2 is administered in high doses directly into the tumour; however, neither NK nor LAK cells were solely responsible for this tumour destruction [35; unpublished data].

Adaptive immune responses to malignant mesothelioma

MM is generally considered to be 'non-immunogenic', or at best only partially immunogenic, because vaccination of mice with irradiated tumour cells confers little to no protection from subsequent tumour challenge. However, this definition may now be outdated as it has become increasingly clear that many tumours considered to be non-immunogenic are in fact recognized by the immune system (see below). There is even evidence that this immune response is able to restrain MM tumours until an event occurs that allows the tumour to progress. In one case, a 40-year-old woman was diagnosed with MM after routine radiography; however, the tumour spontaneously regressed only to emerge in a different location 2 months later [56]. This may be true for many cancers, as autopsies of individuals who have died of trauma often reveal microscopic colonies of cancer cells, referred to as *in situ* tumours. Indeed, virtually all autopsied individuals aged 50–70 years have *in situ* carcinomas in the thyroid gland, whereas only 0.1 per cent of individuals in this age group are diagnosed with thyroid cancer [57].

Cell-mediated (T-cell) responses to malignant mesothelioma tumours

T cells are the critical mediators of tumour immunity and consist of two major subtypes based upon their expression of CD markers, i.e. $CD4^+$ and $CD8^+$ T cells. Both these cell types only recognize antigen bound to self-MHC proteins and therefore are referred to as MHC restricted. T cells originate from the bone marrow and initially migrate to the thymus to mature before circulating through the blood, tissues, and lymphatics. Upon completing maturation and activation, T cells differentiate into effector cells which function by becoming cytolytic cells, helper cells which offer 'help' to T and B cells, or suppressor cells which regulate the function of other T and B cells. Importantly, many studies have shown that T-cell-mediated immunity is critical for the rejection of tumours in both animal models and humans.

There is evidence that MM patients mount a tumour-specific immune response as the majority of MM patients have detectable antitumour antibodies (see below). Furthermore, 10–20 per cent of patients treated with immune-enhancing agents such as IL-2, IFN-α or granulocyte–macrophage colony-stimulating factor (GM-CSF) have an improved clinical outcome [58,59]. Similarly, animal models have shown that use of IL-12 and IL-2 can induce regression of established MM tumours [35,60]. However, dissecting out the critical components involved in a specific immune response directed against MM has been hampered because of the current lack of known MM tumour antigens.

Several studies have reported simian virus 40 (SV40) sequences in MM [61–63]. SV40 is a DNA tumour virus encoding two transforming proteins, the large tumour antigen (Tag) and the small tumour antigen (tag), and three capsid proteins (VP1–3). Tag is the replicase of SV40 and its expression can lead to cellular transformation, principally through inhibition of cellular p53 and retinoblastoma (Rb) family proteins [64]. SV40 infects cells from different species. It causes lytic infection in the cells of its natural primate host where it does not induce tumours. In contrast, it is non-lytic and highly oncogenic in rodents [65]. Crucially, infection is semipermissive in human cell lines, and up to 60 per cent of human MMs contain SV40 DNA. Hence SV40 Tag may represent an MM-associated tumour antigen.

Whilst identifying human MM-specific tumour antigens represents work in progress, one experimental approach that has been employed to overcome this obstacle is the construction of defined model systems using mouse MM tumour cell lines transfected with nominal marker antigens such as influenza haemagglutinin (HA) [66,67] and ovalbumin (OVA) [35,68]. Importantly, the expression of either HA or OVA as potentially potent neo-tumour antigens does not induce tumour rejection in the majority of syngeneic immunologically intact animals. In both systems the class I and II peptide reactivities are well defined, and anti-HA as well as anti-OVA T-cell receptor (TCR) transgenic mice are available with MHC class I and II specificities. The advantage of using these TCR transgenic mice is that they provide a monoclonal source of cells with known specificities. Thus it is possible to investigate whether MM-associated tumour antigens are presented *in vivo* during tumour progression, whether or not a tumour-specific T-cell and/or B-cell response is induced, and whether specific CD8$^+$ and CD4$^+$ T cells have a role in modulating the anti-MM immune response.

Antigen-presenting cells and malignant mesothelioma

As described above and shown in Figure 10.1, the first event that is required to induce an anti-MM adaptive immune response is the transport of tumour antigens from the tumour itself to regional draining lymph nodes. Immunohistochemical analysis of solid MM tumours shows that professional APCs can be found residing in human and murine MM tumours. These include macrophages, B cells and DCs [69]. Figures 10.2, 10.3, and 10.4 show the distribution of B cells, macrophages, and DCs in MM tumours. Hence these cells represent potential APCs which can transport tumour antigens to the lymph nodes and present them to T cells.

The transfection/transgenic mouse models of MM described above were used to determine whether or not MM tumour antigens are presented in secondary lymphoid organs. To do this, CD8$^+$ cells from TCR transgenic mice were labelled with CFSE (a fluorescent dye) and adoptively transferred into mice bearing the HA-transfected MM tumour cell lines, the OVA-transfected MM tumour cell lines or the parental cell line (i.e. non-transfected controls). This labelling procedure allows subsequent monitoring and identification of proliferating cells which is a measure of antigen recognition [70–72]. Three days after transfer, cells from secondary lymphoid organs are re-isolated and the relative fluorescent intensity of the labelled cells is analysed by FACS. To examine the kinetics of tumour antigen presentation and the relationship of antigen load, animals were inoculated with either a high or low tumour antigen expressing MM tumour cell line and the mice were killed 7, 14, 21, and 28 days after tumour inoculation. As

Day 7

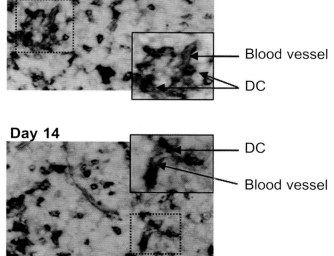

Blood vessel

DC

Day 14

DC

Blood vessel

Figure 10.3 DCs in solid MM tumours. Immunohistochemistry using monoclonal antibodies on cryopreserved sections of MM tumours revealed significant numbers of tumour-associated DCs at days 7 and 14 after tumour cell inoculation. These DCs could be seen trafficking through blood vessels, as well as located within the tumour itself.

Isotype control

B cells (blue) and blood vessels (brown)

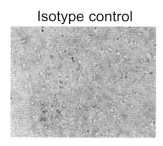

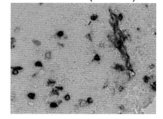

Figure 10.4 B cells in solid MM tumours. Immunohistochemistry using monoclonal antibodies on cryopreserved sections of MM tumours revealed significant numbers of tumour B cells, NK cells and CD4$^+$ cells. These B cells could be seen trafficking through blood vessels, as well as located within the tumour itself. B cells were occasionally found juxtaposed against NK or CD4$^+$ cells, suggesting that intratumoral B cells may engage in cell–cell cross-talk with these cells.

B cells (blue) and NK cells (brown)

B cells (blue) and CD4$^+$ T cells (brown)

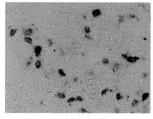

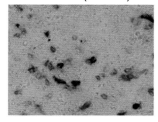

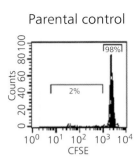
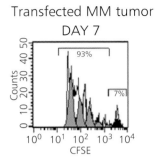
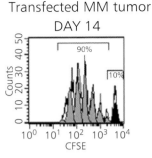

Figure 10.5 MM tumour antigens are presented to T cells in the draining lymph node. Mice were inoculated with a MM tumour cell line expressing a neo-tumour antigen. CFSE (a fluorescent marker) labelled tumour-specific CD8$^+$ T cells were adoptively transferred intravenously into mice at different time points of tumour growth, re-isolated from the draining lymph nodes 3 days after transfer and analysed by FACS. It is clear that the MM neo-tumour antigen is presented to these CD8$^+$ T cells 7 and 14 days after MM tumour cell inoculation at sufficient levels to promote T-cell proliferation.

shown in Figure 10.5, adoptively transferred CFSE-labelled CD8$^+$ TCR cells isolated from the draining lymph node of tumour-bearing animals had proliferated by day 14 after tumour inoculation [66,68].

This work clearly showed that MM tumour antigens are not only transported to draining lymph nodes, and occasionally to the spleen and non-draining lymph nodes, in the apparent absence of metastatic spread of tumour, but are also presented to naive T cells prepared from TCR mice. These APCs induce a strong proliferative response in the adoptively transferred tumour-specific T cells (Fig. 10.5). Interestingly, in the odd instance when a mouse did not develop a solid tumour, *in vivo* tumour antigen presentation was also detectable in the 'tumour-draining' lymph nodes for up to 6 months after tumour cell inoculation (Fig. 10.6), implying that either the immune system kept tumour growth in check or the tumour antigen was somehow trapped and persisted within the draining lymph nodes [66].

Malignant mesothelioma cells as inducers of an immune response

The ability of tumour cells to generate an immune response or to act as targets for antigen-specific immune effector cells is primarily influenced by expression of cell surface antigens. Studies of human and murine MM cell lines showed that 85 per cent of these cells express surface MHC class I at levels comparable to normal cells, and that these levels can be upregulated by treatment with either IFN-γ [73,74] or IFN-α [75,76]. Expression of accessory molecules involved in antigen presentation appears to differ between established MM cell lines and primary cultures. Phenotypic analysis revealed the presence of MHC class I and class II (DR) molecules, as well as ICAM-1 and B7.2 on primary cultures of MM. In contrast, evaluation of established MM cell lines did not show the presence of B7.1, B7.2 or MHC-II(DR). However, following IFN-γ treatment, MHC-II(DR) molecules were detectable whilst MHC class I expression levels increased [77] Despite the presence of molecules involved in adhesion, recognition, and co-stimulation, MM derived from primary cultures are not effective in presenting self-antigens to the immune system and thus escape a local immune response [77]. This is supported by the observation that after transduction of B7.1 into MM tumour cells cytotoxic CD8$^+$ T cells are generated which recognize and destroy both the transfectant and the untransfected parental cell line [78]. Hence MM tumour cells are not able to induce a class I restricted response by directly presenting their own antigens to CD8$^+$ T cells during *in vivo* growth.

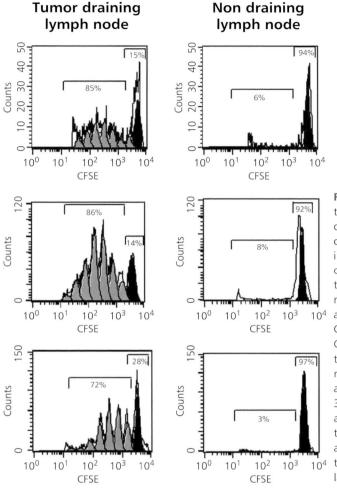

Tumor draining lymph node

Non draining lymph node

Figure 10.6 Proliferation of tumour-specific CD8$^+$ T cells occurs in the absence of obvious tumour. Mice were inoculated with a MM tumour cell line expressing a neo-tumour antigen. Three mice did not develop tumours 32, 72 and 179 days after inoculation. CFSE-labelled tumour-specific CD8$^+$ T cells were adoptively transferred intravenously and re-isolated from the draining and non-draining lymph nodes 3 days after transfer and analysed by FACS. It is clear that the MM neo-tumour antigen is still presented to these CD8$^+$ T cells despite the lack of a palpable tumour.

Malignant mesothelioma tumour antigen presentation pathways

The observations of MM tumour antigen presentation cells in the secondary lymphoid organs highlights an ongoing controversy regarding the mechanisms underlying tumour antigen presentation to CD8$^+$ T cells. T lymphocytes recognize target cells via their antigen-specific T-cell receptor for antigen (TcR). The TcR is a membrane-anchored molecule specific for antigen that is associated with other protein molecules known as the CD3 complex. The TcR–CD3 complex interacts with antigen bound to an MHC-encoded molecule on the APC or target cell. CD8$^+$ T lymphocytes recognize antigen bound to class I MHC molecules, whilst CD4$^+$ T helper lymphocytes (Th cells) recognize antigen bound to class II MHC molecules.

CD8$^+$ CTL can recognize antigens via two pathways: the classical class I pathway and the cross-presentation pathway

The antigen bound by the MHC and TcR is a peptide fragment isolated from the larger intact protein. Class I MHC bound peptides are usually derived from intracellular endogenously synthesized proteins within the APC that are processed within the proteosome complex into 8–11 amino acid peptides and transported into the endoplasmic reticulum (ER) by the transporter molecules TAP-1 and TAP-2. Here they are bound to synthesized MHC class I molecules and this complex is translocated to, and expressed on, the APC surface.

However, another antigen presentation pathway exists whereby CD8[+] T cells can recognize protein antigens from non-haemopoietic cells that are captured and re-presented on bone-marrow-derived APCs, i.e. the cross-presentation pathway [79]. Cross-presentation defines the capacity of APCs to take up exogenous antigen and shunt them into the class I pathway for presentation to CD8[+] T cells. Cross-presentation of exogenous antigens via the MHC class I pathway is believed to be important for its role in self-tolerance, vaccine development, and tumour immunity. Many self-antigens may be cross-presented under healthy conditions, as well as in diseases such as cancer [66,80,81] and autoimmunity [82]. In cross-presentation, APCs collect antigen in peripheral tissues and transfer antigen, by an undefined mechanism, from endocytic vesicles to the cytosol and/or to the endolysosomal ER fusion compartments [83]. The proteosome degrades cytosolic antigen to peptides and the class I pathway as described above is followed. Effective CD8[+] T-cell responses to cross-presented antigens may be facilitated via help from CD4[+] T cells [84].

Cross-presentation is believed to be the major pathway for activation of tumour-specific CD8[+] T cells, and use of the transfection/transgenic models described above has confirmed that MM tumour antigens are indeed cross-presented to CD8[+] T cells [66,68,81] (Fig. 10.6). DCs are the most likely APCs involved in eliciting this response, although this has not yet been confirmed *in vivo*.

As mentioned above, the presence of SV40-like Tag in nearly 60 per cent of human MM represents a potential target for the induction of anti-MM immunity, and CTLs from the peripheral blood of a MM patient were able to recognize and respond to the dominant epitope of SV40 Tag, as well as MM tumour cells that expressed SV40 Tag [85].

CD4[+] T lymphocytes recognize exogenous antigens processed and presented via the class II pathway

CD4[+] T cells also recognize processed peptide fragments of antigen; in this case the antigens are usually of foreign (exogenous), rather than self, origin. The peptides seen by CD4[+] T cells are larger than those seen by CD8[+] T cells, and they associate with MHC class II molecules using a different pathway to peptides presented by MHC class I molecules. MHC class II molecules are expressed on B lymphocytes, DCs, macrophages, and Langerhans cells, and these cells can efficiently present antigen to CD4[+] T lymphocytes. The APCs phagocytose or endocytose soluble antigen and then process the antigen into peptides within endosomes, where peptides bind to class II molecules with the assistance of a chaperone molecule called the invariant (Ii) chain. The resultant peptide–MHC class II complex is transported and inserted into the plasma membrane where it can be recognized by CD4[+] T cells.

CD4[+] T cells and malignant mesothelioma

When evaluating antitumour responses, the main effector cell examined is usually the CD8[+] T cell; however, there is accumulating evidence that CD4[+] T cells play an important role in facilitating the eradication of tumours [86]. CD4[+] T cells have been implicated indirectly in experiments that replace 'help' by introducing IL-2 [87]. It has also been shown that tumours transduced with syngeneic class II molecules can induce protection against parental class II negative tumours [88]. Once again the transfection/transgenic models of MM were used to evaluate the role of CD4[+] T cells in MM. Interestingly, even though MM tumour cell lines are class II negative, when CD4[+] T cells are labelled with CFSE and adoptively transferred into MM-tumour-bearing animals, these CD4[+] T cells proliferated in the draining lymph nodes [67]. This proliferation occurs in the absence of any detectable tumour and is not observed in the non-draining lymph nodes.

More recently, CD4+ T cells have been shown to have an important role in determining the magnitude and persistence of a CTL response in chronic viral infections and models of autoimmunity [89–91]. Therefore the transfection/transgenic models were used to determine the effect that tumour-specific CD4+ T cells have with CD8+ T cells on MM tumour growth. Direct visualization of MM-specific CD8+ CTL was achieved using peptide–MHC tetramers. Co-injection of tumour antigen-specific CD4+ and CD8+ T cells did not cause an obvious change in CD8+ T cell numbers, and MM-specific CD4+ T cells were not required for the generation of CTLs. However, CD4+ T cells were critically required for the maintenance of CD8+ T-cell numbers and for CD8+ T-cell infiltration into MM tumours. Importantly, the co-transfer of class I (CD8+) and class II (CD4+) restricted tumour antigen-specific T cells (from TCR transgenic mice) offered complete protection from tumour growth and induced regression of established MM tumours. It was only in the presence of CD4+ T cells that MM tumours exhibited upregulation of MHC class II and ICAM expression which may be necessary to generate an effective antitumour immune response.

T cells can infiltrate malignant mesothelioma tumours (Figs 10.7 and 10.8)

The extent of lympocytic infiltration in human MM is variable and depends on the individual tumour, but a significant infiltrate is believed to correlate with a better prognosis for survival. In a study conducted by Leigh and Webster [92] the majority of MM patients showed a minimal number of tumour-infiltrating lymphocytes (TILs) with a mean survival of 9 months; in contrast, 10 of the 15 patients with a significant lymphocytic infiltrate survived for more than 18 months. However, lymphohistiocytoid MM, a rare histological subtype of MM, is characterized by an intense lymphoplasmocytic infiltrate of predominantly reactive mature T cells that do not offer an improved clinical outcome [93].

Few studies have analysed the number and cytokine phenotype of TILs throughout MM development. However, preliminary experiments conducted in our laboratory using a murine model of MM reveal CD8+ and CD4+ T cells constitute approximately 2–5 per cent of the total cell population, with the majority of CD8+ T cells staining positive for intracellular IFN-γ (C. Jackaman, unpublished data), indicative of activation. However, like its human counterpart, the CD4-to-CD8 ratio of TILs is found to vary between MM tumour lines [37]. Selective downregulation of CD2 and CD3 expression on lymphocytes infiltrating murine MM tumours and the inability of these cells to respond to most stimuli in vitro suggests a functional deactivation of lymphocytes in the local tumour environment [37]. This will be discussed in more detail below.

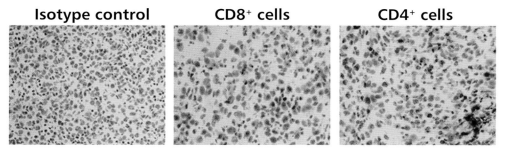

Figure 10.7 T cells in solid MM tumours. Immunohistochemistry using monoclonal antibodies on cryopreserved sections of MM tumours revealed low numbers of tumour-infiltrating T cells. These cells could be seen in MM tumours at all time points examined.

CD8+ T cells (blue) and blood vessels (brown)

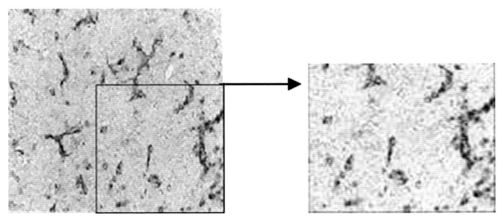

Figure 10.8 CD8$^+$ T cells in solid MM tumours. (a) Immunohistochemistry using monoclonal antibodies on cryopreserved sections of MM tumours revealed significant numbers of tumour-infiltrating CD8+ T cells trafficking through blood vessels. (b) Magnified view of the area outlined in (a).

Malignant mesothelioma and humoral immunity

B lymphocytes are generated in the bone marrow and upon maturation leave and circulate through blood and the lymphatic system. After antigen encounter in the periphery, B lymphocytes differentiate into plasma cells capable of secreting antigen-specific immunoglobulins of a single class. The secreted antibody is the major effector molecule of the humoral immune system.

Tumour-infiltrating B cells

B cells can be seen within many solid tumours, including MM, at different time points and can comprise up to 40 per cent of the TIL population [94,95]. Importantly, B cells have been reported to suppress T-cell-dependent tumour immunity by disabling the CD4$^+$ T-cell help required for CD8$^+$ CTLs [96].

Preliminary data using the B220 antibody (a pan-B-cell marker) shows that several distinct B-cell subpopulations may exist in murine MM tumours [43; S. Lansley, unpublished data]. Interestingly, the percentages of B cells in the tumour-draining lymph nodes increased during tumour progression; these B cells may transport tumour antigens to regional draining lymph nodes for cross-presentation to T cells. A B220$^+$NK1.1$^+$ cell subset was detected in MM tumours which may represent NK cell progenitors [97]. Another two B220$^+$ cell populations were also observed in solid MM tumours; i.e. high and low B220 expression (B220^{+high} and B220^{+low}); these cells could represent mature B or pre-B cells, respectively [98,99]. As the tumours progressed, the proportion of B220^{+low} cells increased. B220 downregulation can also occur when B cells become plasma cells [97]. This suggests that, in tumours, B220^{+low} B cells represent either immature B cells or plasma cells.

Activated B cells express CD40 and their presence in tumours would indicate that interactions may occur between Th cells and B cells, or that the therapeutic use of anti-CD40 (or CD40L) could activate intratumoural (i.t.) B cells. Preliminary data show that B220$^+$CD40$^+$ cells can be detected in MM tumours. No studies to date have systematically examined the expression of CD40 on tumour-infiltrating B cells, or the consequences of activating these B cells *in vivo* via anti-CD40.

Humoral immunity and malignant mesothelioma

As mentioned above, no MM-specific antigens have been identified to date; therefore studies examining sera from MM patients were undertaken in order to understand antibody responses to MM, and to define potential target antigens expressed by MM tumours. These MM antigens may have a diagnostic or immunotherapeutic value.

A significant proportion of MM patients were found to have a humoral immune response against a number of previously established human MM cell lines [100]. In this study, western blot analysis showed that MM patients had serum antibodies of the IgG class in high titre, and each antiserum recognized different protein antigens. Sequential analysis of these sera showed that the antibody titre increased with disease progression. It was found that 28 per cent of patients screened had serum antibodies recognizing only one, or a restricted number of antigenic determinants [100]. Sera from these patients were studied further and six of the antigen complexes were expressed (at least) partially in the nucleus, whilst two showed some specificity for MM tumours, i.e. they discriminated antigens that were highly expressed in all human MM cell lines but were not expressed in a human SV40-transformed mesothelial line. Four of the antisera recognized a homologue in mouse tissue and each of these had a different pattern of expression. Collectively, these antisera define a subset of nuclear autoantigens that are overexpressed in dividing cells. However, the presence of anti-MM antibodies was not a prognostic indicator of survival.

A technique referred to as the serological analysis of recombinant complementary DNA (cDNA) expression libraries (SEREX) has been used to identify antigens in MM. This technique identifies antibody responses generated in patients by using sera from MM patients to probe tumour cDNA libraries to identify specific antigens. The most prevalent MM tumour antigens recognized were self-antigens (i.e. U2AF, Siah binding protein, topoisomerase IIb (TOPIIb), ZFM1, mire1 and pendulin) [101]. Thirteen of 14 MM patients had a strong antibody response to topoisomerase IIb, suggesting that there are shared tumour antigens in this disease. Importantly, only 37 per cent of healthy volunteers were weakly positive to topoisomerase IIb. However, with the exception of TOPIIb and U2AF, each of the autoantibody specificities was associated with a single patient. Interestingly, the mean survival time from diagnosis was the longest in those patients manifesting more than one serum reactivity. None of the antigens detected in this study was uniquely expressed in MM.

Although SV40 antigenic sequences have been detected in MM, the role of this virus in the disease pathogenesis is still controversial. Nonetheless, SV40 Tag-specific humoral immunity was demonstrated by the detection of IgG titres against Tag in serum samples from one out of three patients examined [85]. SV40 Tag has been used in a murine tumour model, with a vaccinia virus vaccine construct encoding only immunogenic domains of this antigen [102]. Immunization of mice with a single dose of this vaccine protected against a murine cancer expressing SV40 Tag.

Other antigens expressed in MM include MAGE-2 and MAGE-6 [103]. Despite some early indications that p53 mutation could be a feature of this disease [104], numerous subsequent studies have failed to confirm this [105–107]. Anti-p53 antibodies are observed only at a low frequency (~10 per cent) in the sera of MM patients as an early event that is probably unrelated to antigen load [108].

Whilst identification of a MM-specific antigens has been met with little success, a reliable serum marker for MM has recently been described [109]. Serum concentrations of soluble mesothelin-related proteins (SMRPs) were determined using ELISA in a blinded study of serum samples from 44 patients with MM. Of the patients screened, 84 per cent had significantly higher concentrations of SMRP at all serum dilutions compared with asbestos-exposed and non-asbestos-exposed individuals [109]. Only 2 per cent of patients with inflammatory, pleural or malignant pulmonary diseases contained a raised serum concentration of SMRP, indicating that the marker is relatively specific to MM. Furthermore, SMRP concentrations were significantly higher in patients with the greatest tumour bulk and tended to increase with disease progression. Seven of the 40 healthy asbestos-exposed controls had increased serum concentrations of SMRP, with three of these seven going on to develop MM within 5 years of measurement [109]. Therefore determination of SMRP levels in serum could be a useful marker for diagnosis of MM and screening at-risk individuals. However, the level of anti-SMRP immune reactivity in MM patients has yet to be worked out.

Overall, the data discussed above show that, despite the presence of tumour-infiltrating B lymphocytes and the ability of patients to develop an antitumour antibody response, MM tumour progression is not prevented.

Mechanisms of immune escape by malignant mesothelioma

An effective immune response to a tumour can only occur by successful transition through a series of checkpoints, each of which consists of a sophisticated sequence of events (discussed above and illustrated in Fig. 10.1). The resulting cellular response must be of an adequate magnitude and must also persist long enough to slow tumour growth. It is helpful if the tumour burden is low and does not outpace the immune response. Numerous hypotheses have been suggested to explain how tumours manage to evade the antitumour immune response, embracing defects at many points in this complex sequence of events. There is considerable evidence that patients with MM have impaired immune responsiveness. Although they maintain normal white cell counts, total serum proteins, and immunoglobulin levels, mitogen responsiveness is reduced and LAK cell activity against MM tumour targets is depressed to about 60 per cent of normal [52–54]. The CD4$^+$ subset of lymphocytes is reduced in number whilst the CD8$^+$ subset remains unchanged; NK cell activity is reduced; and abnormal humoral and cell-mediated antibody-dependent cellular toxicity have also been demonstrated [42]. T cells within murine MM have been shown to have features of downregulation, such as low surface expression of CD3 which is directly involved in T-cell activation, and asbestos itself suppresses the function of NK cells and LAK cells *in vitro* [40,52,110].

Various studies have examined potential mechanisms by which tumours evade the immune response. These include lack of tumour antigen expression, downregulation of surface MHC molecules or loss of peptide processing [111,112], lack of co-stimulatory molecules [113,114], production of suppressor factors [115,116], and physical exclusion of immune cells from the tumour site [117,118]. MM is similar to other tumours in that it can avoid immune-mediated destruction. Human and murine MM tumour cell lines have been intensively studied for their soluble factor secreting profiles. Several cytokines and growth factors are produced by MM cells, including platelet derived growth factors A and B, insulin-like growth factors I and II, TGF-α and TGF-β, GM-CSF, IL-6, IL-10, leukaemia inhibitory factor, VEGF, and other mitogenic factors that have not yet been defined [37,103].

Transforming growth factor β

TGF-β is a particularly powerful immunosuppressant which can inhibit priming of CD8$^+$ T lymphocytes, downregulate MHC class II expression on lymphoid and non-lymphoid cells, and suppress nitric oxide and TNF-α production by macrophages [119]. High levels of TGF-β have been detected in pleural effusions from MM patients [120] and most cultured MM cell lines express and secrete significant amounts of the various TGF-β isoforms [115,121]. In a murine model of MM, low TIL numbers in TGF-β-producing tumours correlated with selective downregulation of the T-cell signal transduction molecule CD3 [122]. Analysis of TILs revealed a decrease in CD3γ, CD3δ, and CD3ζ/η mRNA expression throughout tumour progression, whereas CD3ε subunit expression remained constant. However, this profound downregulation of CD3 could be partially reversed by stably transfecting tumour cells with an inducible TGF-β antisense construct, which leads to increased numbers of TILs [115,122]. Clearly, TGF-β confers a survival advantage on MM cells.

Furthermore, TGF-β can recruit and activate resting monocytes [123], hence the large number of TIMs in MM tumours. However, TGF-β may then modulate the cytokines and chemokines produced by the TIMs. TGF-β has been shown to induce a cytokine cascade, resulting in the release of TGF-β, IL-1β and IL-6 by macrophages. These cytokines then lead to the downregulation of CD2 and CD3 mRNA by TILs, as well as a reduced surface MHC class II molecule and integrin expression by TIMs [124].

Interleukin 6

IL-6 has pro-inflammatory, immunoregulatory, and haemopoietic effects, is produced by the majority of MM cell lines [125–127], and can be isolated in large amounts from MM pleural effusions [128]. Its role in the pathogenesis of human MM is unclear, but it is likely to be involved in the development of MM-associated fever, thrombocytosis, and cachexia. *In vivo* studies in a murine MM model (AB22) reported that detectable serum IL-6 levels preceded macroscopically detectable tumour growth, clinical signs such as cachexia, abdominal distension, diarrhoea, and changes in the peripheral lymphoid organs including cell depletion and functional depression. Treatment with either anti-IL-6 antibody or recombinant IFN-α curtailed the clinical symptoms [129]. The latter treatment attenuated both IL-6 mRNA expression in the tumours and serum IL-6 levels, ameliorated the depression of lymphocyte activities, and enhanced the number of TILs and macrophages implying a palliative role for combination therapy using rIFN-α and anti-IL-6 for MM patients [129,130].

Whilst it is clear that MM tumours secrete a number of soluble mediators that can affect the immune system, their influence on tumour progression and on the development of an anti-MM immune response is yet to be fully elucidated. The role of potent immunomodulatory factors, particularly those that are released systemically, can only be realistically evaluated using *in vivo* models.

Summary

For the induction of an effective anti-MM immune response it is essential that MM-specific antigen(s) are presented appropriately by APCs that activate the effector arm of the antitumour response (i.e. CD8+ and CD4+ T cells), which then traffic into MM tumours, overcome local tolerance mechanisms, and eradicate tumour cells. The data discussed above show that APCs continuously present MM tumour antigens to effector CD8+ T cells in tumour draining lymph nodes. However, in the absence of fully operational CD4 T cells, and perhaps other cell types such as NK and B cells, this CD8+ T-cell response is unable to restrain MM tumours. This failure may be overcome by offering the appropriate immune-activating agents that target cellular members of both the innate and adaptive immune systems. This area is the subject of ongoing studies in laboratories around the world.

References

1. McWilliam A, Nelson D, Thomas J, Holt P. Rapid dendritic cell recruitment is a hallmark of the acute inflammatory response at mucosal surfaces. *J Exp Med* 1994; **179**: 1331–6.

2. Medzhitov R, Janeway Jr. CA. Innate immune recognition and control of adaptive immune responses. *Semin Immunol* 1998; **10**: 351–3.

3. Imler J-L, Hoffmann JA. Toll receptors in innate immunity. *Trends Cell Biol* 2001; **11**: 304–11.

4. Medzhitov R. Toll-like receptors and innate immunity. *Nat Rev Immunol* 2001; **1**: 135–45.

5. Hertz CJ, Kiertscher SM, Godowski PJ, *et al.* (2001). Microbial lipopeptides stimulate dendritic cell maturation via toll-like receptor 2. *J Immunol* 2001; **166**: 2444–50.

6. Andrews D, Scalzo A, Yokoyama W, Smyth M, Degli-Esposti M. Functional interactions between dendritic cells and NK cells during viral infection. *Nat Immunol* 2001; **4**: 175–81.

7. Fernandez N, Lozier A, Flament C, *et al.* Dendritic cells directly trigger NK cell functions: cross-talk relevant in innate anti-tumour immune responses *in vivo*. *Nat Med* 1999; **5**: 405–11.

8. Ferlazzo G, Tsang ML, Moretta L, Melioli G, Steinman RM, Munz C. Human dendritic cells activate resting natural killer (NK) cells and are recognized via the NKp30 receptor by activated NK cells. *J Exp Med* 2002; **195**: 343–51.

9. Zitvogel L. Dendritic and natural killer cells cooperate in the control/switch of innate immunity. *J Exp Med* 2002; **195**: F9–14.

10. Auerbach O, Conston A, Garfinkel L, Parks V, Kaslow H, Hammond E. Presence of asbestos bodies in organs other than the lung. *Chest* 1980; **77**: 133–7.

11. Bernstein D, Drew R, Kuschner M. Experimental approaches for exposure to sized glass fibers. *Environ Health Perspect* 1980; **34**: 47–57.

12. Malhotra A, Kradin R. The pulmonary immune response to asbestos. In: Peters G, Peters B, ed. *Asbestos and Cancer*. Charlottesville, VA: Lexis Law Publishing, 1997; 1–16.

13. Churg A, Wright J, Gilks B, DePaoli L. Rapid short-term clearance of chrysotile compared with amosite asbestos in the guinea pig. *Am Rev Respir Dis* 1989; **139**: 885–90.

14. Costabel U, Bross K, Huck E, Guzman J, Matthys H. Lung and blood lymphocyte subsets in asbestosis and in mixed dust pneumoconiosis. *Chest* 1987; **91**: 110–12.

15. Doll R. Mineral fibres in the non-occupational environment: concluding remarks. *IARC Sci Publ* 1989; **90**: 511–18.

16. Hill R, Edwards R, Carthew P. Early changes in the pleural mesothelium following intrapleural inoculation of the mineral fibre erionite and the subsequent development of mesotheliomas. *J Exp Pathol* 1990; **71**: 105–18.

17. Saint-Remy P, Buret J, Radermecker M. Significance of lactate dehydrogenases in pleural effusions. *Rev Pneumol Clin* 1986; **42**: 74–81.

18. Moalli P, MacDonald J, Goodglick L, Kane A. Acute injury and regeneration of the mesothelium in response to asbestos fibers. *Am J Pathol* 1987; **128**: 426–45.

19. Branchaud R, MacDonald J, Kane A. Induction of angiogenesis by intraperitoneal injection of asbestos fibers. *FASEB J* 1989; **3**: 1747–52.

20. Hesterberg T, Axten C, McConnell E, *et al.* Studies on the inhalation toxicology of two fiberglasses and amosite asbestos in the Syrian golden hamster. Part I. Results of a subchronic study and dose selection for a chronic study. *Inhal Toxicol* 1999; **11**: 747–84.

21. Galffy G, Mohammed KA, Dowling PA, Nasreen N, Ward MJ, Antony VB. Interleukin 8: an autocrine growth factor for malignant mesothelioma. *Cancer Res* 1999; **59**: 367–71.

22. Sjostrand M, Rylander R, Bergstrom R. Lung cell reactions in guinea pigs after inhalation of asbestos (amosite). *Toxicology* 1989; **57**: 1–14.

23. Berger H. Of asbestosis, smoking, and mesothelioma. *Hosp Pract (Off Ed)* 1988; **23**: 17.

24. Berry G, Newhouse ML, Antonis P. Combined effect of asbestos and smoking on mortality from lung cancer and mesothelioma in factory workers. *Br J Ind Med* 1985; **42**: 12–18.

25. Livneh A, Langevitz P, Pras M. Pulmonary associations in familial Mediterranean fever. *Curr Opin Pulm Med* 1999; **5**: 326–31.

26. Shamamian P, Pocock BJZ, Schwartz JD, *et al*. Neutrophil-derived serine proteinases enhance membrane type-1 matrix metalloproteinase-dependent tumour cell invasion. *Surgery* 2000; **127**: 142–7.

27. Shamamian P, Schwartz J, Pocock B, *et al*. Activation of progelatinase A (MMP-2) by neutrophil elastase, cathepsin G, and proteinase-3: a role for inflammatory cells in tumour invasion and angiogenesis. *J Cell Physiol* 2001; **189**: 197–206.

28. Mutsaers SE, Whitaker D, Papadimitriou JM. Stimulation of mesothelial cell proliferation by exudate macrophages enhances serosal wound healing in a murine model. *Am J Pathol* 2002; **160**: 681–92.

29. Lipkin L. Cellular effects of asbestos and other fibers: Correlations with *in vivo* induction of pleural sarcoma. *Environ Health Perspect* 1980; **34**: 91–102.

30. Bignon J, Jaurand M. Biological *in vitro* and *in vivo* responses of chrysotile versus amphiboles. *Environ Health Perspect* 1983; **51**: 73–80.

31. Rom WN, Travis WD, Brody AR. Cellular and molecular basis of the asbestos-related diseases. *Am Rev Respir Dis* 1991; **143**: 408–22.

32. Takemura T, Rom W, Ferrans V, Crystal R. Morphologic characterization of alveolar macrophages from subjects with occupational exposure to inorganic particles. *Am J Respir Cell Mol Biol* 1989; **140**: 1674–85.

33. Hamilton R, Iyer L, Holian A. Asbestos induces apoptosis in human alveolar macrophages. *Am J Physiol* 1996; **271**: L813–9.

34. Kravchenko I, Furalyov V, Vasylieva L, Pylev L. Inhibition of asbestos-induced transformation of rat pleural mesothelial cells in co-culture with rat macrophages. *Teratog Carcinog Mutagen* 2001; **21**: 315–23.

35. Jackaman C, Bundell CS, Kinnear BF, *et al*. IL-2 intratumoral immunotherapy enhances CD8[+] T cells that mediate destruction of tumour cells and tumour-associated vasculature: a novel mechanism for IL-2 *J Immunol* 2003; **171**: 5051–63.

36. Di Carlo E, Forni G, Lollini P, Colombo MP, Modesti A, Musiani P. The intriguing role of polymorphonuclear neutrophils in antitumor reactions. *Blood* 2001; **97**: 339–45.

37. Bielefeldt-Ohmann H, Fitzpatrick DR, Marzo AL, *et al*. Patho- and immunobiology of malignant mesothelioma: Characterisation of tumour infiltrating leucocytes and cytokine production in a murine model. *Cancer Immunol Immunother* 1994; **39**: 347–59.

38. Smyth MJ, Hayakawa Y, Takeda K, Yagita H. New aspects of natural-killer-cell surveillance and therapy of cancer. *Nat Rev Cancer* 2002; **2**: 850–61.

39. Froom P, Lahat N, Kristal-Boneh E, Cohen C, Lerman Y, Ribak J. Circulating natural killer cells in retired asbestos cement workers. *J Occup Environ Med* 2000; **42**: 19–24.

40. Robinson B. Asbestos and cancer: human natural killer cell activity is suppressed by asbestos fibers but can be restored by recombinant interleukin-2. *Am Rev Respir Dis* 1989; **139**: 897–901.

41. deShazo R, Morgan J, Bozelka B, Chapman Y. Natural killer cell activity in asbestos workers. Interactive effects of smoking and asbestos exposure. *Chest* 1988; **94**: 482–5.

42. Lew F, Tsang P, Holland JF, Warner N, Selikoff IJ, Bekesi JG. High frequency of immune dysfunctions in asbestos workers and in patients with malignant mesothelioma. *J Clin Immunol* 1986; **6**: 225–33.

43. Lansley S. The characterisation of tumour infiltrating natural killer cells and tumour infiltrating B cells during cancer progression. Unpublished thesis. Perth, Australia: Curtin University of Technology, 2003.

44. Arase H, Saito T, Phillips JH, Lanier LL. Cutting edge: the mouse NK cell-associated antigen recognized by DX5 moncoclonal antibody is CD49b (α2 integrin, very late antigen-2). *J Immunol* 2001; **167**: 1141–4.

45. Ortaldo J, Mason A, Winkler-Pickett R, Raziuddin A, Murphy W, Mason L. Ly-49 receptor expression and functional analysis in multiple mouse strains. *J Leukoc Biol* 1999; **66**: 512–20.

46. Odaka M, Wiewrodt R, DeLong PA, *et al.* Analysis of the immunologic response generated by Ad.IFN-β during successful intraperitoneal tumour gene therapy. *Mol Ther* 2002; **6**: 210–18.

47. Slifka MK, Pagarigan RR, Whitton JL. NK markers are expressed on a high percentage of virus-specific CD8$^+$ and CD4$^+$ T cells. *J Immunol* 2000; **164**: 2009–15.

48. Wiltrout RH. Regulation and antimetastatic functions of liver-associated natural killer cells. *Immunol Rev* 2000; **174**: 63–76.

49. Kronenberg M, Gapin L. The unconventional lifestyle of NKT cells. *Nat Rev Immunol* 2002; **2**: 557–68.

50. Manning LS, Bowman RV, Darby SB, Robinson BW. Lysis of human malignant mesothelioma cells by natural killer (NK) and lymphokine-activated killer (LAK) cells. *Am Rev Respir Dis* 1989; **139**: 1369–74.

51. Yanagawa H, Sone S, Fukuta K, Nishioka Y, Ogura T. Local adoptive immunotherapy using lymphokine-activated killer cells and interleukin-2 against malignant pleural mesothelioma: report of two cases. *Jpn J Clin Oncol* 1991; **21**: 377–83.

52. Manning LS, Davis MR, Robinson BW. Asbestos fibres inhibit the *in vitro* activity of lymphokine-activated killer (LAK) cells from healthy individuals and patients with malignant mesothelioma. *Clin Exp Immunol* 1991; **83**: 85–91.

53. Garlepp M, Fitzpatrick D, Mutsaers S, Bielefeldt-Ohmann H, David M, Robinson B. Mesothelioma: recent studies of growth regulation. In: Peters G, ed. *Sourcebook on Asbestos Diseases: Asbestos Medical Research*. New York: Garland, 1992.

54. Haslam P, Lukoszek A, Merchant J, M T-W. Lymphocyte responses to phytohaemagglutinin in patients with asbestosis and pleural mesothelioma. *Clin Exp Immunol* 1978; **31**: 178–88.

55. Kaiser LR. New therapies in the treatment of malignant pleural mesothelioma. *Semin Thorac Cardiovasc Surg* 1997; **9**: 383–90.

56. Robinson BWS, Robinson C, Lake RA. Localised spontaneous regression in mesothelioma—possible immunological mechanism. *Lung Cancer* 2001; **32**: 197–201.

57. Folkman J, Kalluri R. Cancer without disease. *Nature* 2004; **427**: 787–8.

58. Upham JW, Musk AW, van Hazel G, Byrne M, Robinson BW. Interferon alpha and doxorubicin in malignant mesothelioma: a phase II study. *Aust NZ J Med* 1993; **23**: 683–7.

59. Davidson JA, Musk AW, Wood BR, *et al.* Intralesional cytokine therapy in cancer: a pilot study of GM-CSF infusion in mesothelioma. *J Immunother* 1998; **21**: 389–98.

60. Caminschi I, Venetsanakos E, Leong CC, Garlepp MJ, Scott B, Robinson BWS. Interleukin-12 induces an effective antitumor response in malignant mesothelioma. *Am J Respir Cell Mol Biol* 1998; **19**: 738–46.

61. Ke Y, Reddel R, Gerwin B, *et al.* Establishment of a human *in vitro* mesothelial cell model system for investigating mechanisms of asbestos-induced mesothelioma. *Am J Pathol* 1989; **134**: 979–91.

62. Procopio A, Strizzi L, Vianale G, *et al.* Simian virus-40 sequences are a negative prognostic cofactor in patients with malignant pleural mesothelioma. *Genes Chromosomes Cancer* 2000; **29**: 173–9.

63. McLaren BR, Haenel T, Stevenson S, Mukherjee S, Robinson BW, Lake RA. Simian virus (SV) 40 like sequences in cell lines and tumour biopsies from Australian malignant mesotheliomas. *Aust NZ J Med* 2000; **30**: 450–6.

64. Bryan T, Reddel R. SV40-induced immortalization of human cells. *Crit Rev Oncol Hematol* 1994; **5**: 331–57.

65. Cicala C, Pompetti F, Carbone M. SV40 induces mesotheliomas in hamsters. *Am J Pathol* 1993; **142**: 1524–33.

66. Marzo AL, Lake RA, Lo D, *et al.* Tumour antigens are constitutively presented in the draining lymph nodes. *J Immunol* 1999; **162**: 5838–45.

67. Marzo AL, Lake RA, Robinson BWS, Scott B. T-cell receptor transgenic analysis of tumour-specific CD8 and CD4 responses in the eradication of solid tumours. *Cancer Res* 1999; **59**: 1071–9.

68. Nelson DJ, Mukherjee S, Bundell C, Fisher S, van Hagen D, Robinson B. Tumour progression despite efficient tumour antigen cross-presentation and effective 'arming' of tumour antigen-specific CTL. *J Immunol* 2001; **166**: 5557–66.

69. Friedlander PL, Delaune CL, Abadie JM, *et al*. Efficacy of CD40 ligand gene therapy in malignant mesothelioma. *Am J Respir Cell Mol Biol* 2003; **29**: 321–30.

70. Lyons A, Parish C. Determination of lymphocyte division by flow cytometry. *J Immunol Methods* 1994; **171**: 131–7.

71. Kurts C, Heath W, Carbone F, Allison J, Miller J, Kosaka H. Constitutive class I-restricted exogenous presentation of self antigens *in vivo*. *J Exp Med* 1996; **184**: 923–30.

72. Hodgkin P, Lee J, Lyons A. B cell differentiation and isotype switching is related to division cycle number. *J Exp Med* 1996; **184**: 277–81.

73. Phan-Bich L, Buard A, Petit J, *et al*. Differential responsiveness of human and rat mesothelioma cell lines to recombinant interferon-gamma. *Am J Respir Cell Mol Biol* 1997; **16**: 178–86.

74. Zeng L, Buard A, Monnet I, *et al*. In vitro effects of recombinant human interferon gamma on human mesothelioma cell lines. *Int J Cancer* 1993; **55**: 515–20.

75. Christmas TI, Manning LS, Garlepp MJ, Musk AW, Robinson BW. Effect of interferon-alpha 2a on malignant mesothelioma. *J Interferon Res* 1993; **13**: 9–12.

76. Wadler S, Wersto R, Weinberg V, Thompson D, Schwartz E. Interaction of fluorouracil and interferon in human colon cancer cell lines: cytotoxic and cytokinetic effects. *Cancer Res* 1990; **50**: 5735–9.

77. Mutti L, Valle MT, Balbi B, *et al*. Primary human mesothelioma cells express class II MHC, ICAM-1 and B7-2 and can present recall antigens to autologous blood lymphocytes. *Int J Cancer* 1998; **78**: 740–9.

78. Leong CC, Robinson BW, Garlepp MJ. Generation of an antitumour immune response to a murine mesothelioma cell line by the transfection of allogeneic MHC genes. *Int J Cancer* 1994; **59**: 212–16.

79. Bevan M. Cross-priming for a secondary cytotoxic response to minor H antigens with H-2 congenic cells which do not cross-react in the cytotoxic assay. *J Exp Med* 1976; **143**: 1283–8.

80. Huang A, Golumbek P, Ahmadzadeh M, Jaffee E, Pardoll D, Levitsky H. Bone marrow-derived cells present MHC class I-restricted tumour antigens in priming of antitumour immune responses. *Ciba Found Symp* 1994; **187**: 229–44.

81. Robinson BW, Lake RA, Nelson DJ, Scott BA, Marzo AL. Cross-presentation of tumour antigens: evaluation of threshold, duration, distribution and regulation. *Immunol Cell Biol* 1999; **77**: 552–8.

82. Kurts C, Heath W, Carbone F, Kosaka H, Miller J. Cross-presentation of self antigens to CD8[+] T cells: the balance between tolerance and autoimmunity. *Novartis Found Symp* 1998; **215**: 172–90.

83. Houde M, Bertholet S, Gagnon E, *et al*. Phagosomes are competent organelles for antigen cross-presentation. *Nature* 2003; **425**: 402–6.

84. Marzo AL, Kinnear BF, Lake RA, *et al*. Tumour-specific CD4[+] T cells have a major 'post-licensing' role in CTL mediated anti-tumour immunity. *J Immunol* 2000; **165**: 6047–55.

85. Bright RK, Kimchi ET, Shearer MH, Kennedy RC, Pass HI. SV40 Tag-specific cytotoxic T lymphocytes generated from the peripheral blood of malignant pleural mesothelioma patients. *Cancer Immunol Immunother* 2002; **50**: 682–90.

86. Goedegebuure P, Eberlein T. The role of CD4[+] tumour-infiltrating lymphocytes in human solid tumours. *Immunol Res* 1995; **14**: 119–31.

87. Fearon E, Pardoll D, Itaya T, *et al*. Interleukin-2 production by tumour cells bypasses T helper function in the generation of an antitumor response. *Cell* 1990; **60**: 397–403.

88. Ostrand-Rosenberg S, Clements V, Thakur A, Cole G. Transfection of major histocompatibility complex class I and class II genes causes tumour rejection. *J Immunogenet* 1989; **16**: 343–9.

89. Cardin R, Brooks J, Sarawar S, Doherty P. Progressive loss of CD8[+] T cell-mediated control of a gamma-herpesvirus in the absence of CD4[+] T cells. *J Exp Med* 1996; **184**: 863–71.

90. Kurts C, Carbone FR, Barnden M, *et al*. CD4+ T cell help impairs CD8+ T cell deletion induced by cross-presentation of self-antigens and favors autoimmunity. *J Exp Med* 1997; **186**: 2057–62.

91. Zajac AJ, Blattman JN, Murali-Krishna K, *et al.* Viral immune evasion due to persistence of activated T cells without effector function. *J Exp Med* 1998; **188**: 2205–13.

92. Leigh RA, Webster I. Lymphocytic infiltration of pleural mesothelioma and its significance for survival. *S Afr Med J*; **61**: 1007–9.

93. Segal A, Whitaker D, Henderson D, Shilkin K. Pathology of mesothelioma. In: Robinson BW, CA, eds. *Mesothelioma,*. London: Martin Dunitz, 2002; 143–84.

94. Coronella JA, Spier C, Welch M, *et al.* Antigen-driven oligoclonal expansion of tumour-infiltrating B cells in infiltrating ductal carcinoma of the breast. *J Immunol* 2002; **169**: 1829–36.

95. Quan N, Zhang Z-b, Demetrikopoulos MK, *et al.* Evidence for involvement of B lymphocytes in the surveillance of lung metastasis in the rat. *Cancer Res* 1999; **59**: 1080–9.

96. Qin Z, Richter G, Schuler T, Ibe S, Cao X, Blankenstein T. B cells inhibit induction of T cell-dependent tumour immunity. *Nat Med* 1998; **4**: 627–30.

97. Rolink A, ten Boekel E, Melchers F, Fearon D, Krop I, Andersson J. A subpopulation of B220+ cells in murine bone marrow does not express CD19 and contains natural killer cell progenitors. *J Exp Med* 1996; **183**: 187–94.

98. Ardavin C, Martin P, Ferrero I, *et al.* B cell response after MMTV infection: extrafollicular plasmablasts represent the main infected population and can transmit viral infection. *J Immunol* 1999; **162**: 2538–45.

99. Toraldo G, Roggia C, Qian W-P, Pacifici R, Weitzmann MN. IL-7 induces bone loss *in vivo* by induction of receptor activator of nuclear factor kappa B ligand and tumour necrosis factor alpha from T cells. *Proc Natl Acad Sci USA* 2003; **100**: 125–30.

100. Robinson C, Robinson BWS, Lake RA. Sera from patients with malignant mesothelioma can contain autoantibodies. *Lung Cancer* 1998; **20**: 175–84.

101. Robinson C, Callow M, Stevenson S, Scott B, Robinson BWS, Lake RA (2000; Serologic responses in patients with malignant mesothelioma. Evidence for both public and private specificities. *Am J Respir Cell Mol Biol* **22**: 550–6.

102. Xie Y, Hwang C, Overwijk W, *et al.* Induction of tumour antigen-specific immunity *in vivo* by a novel vaccinia vector encoding safety-modified simian virus 40 T antigen. *J Natl Cancer Inst* 1999; **91**: 169–75.

103. Nowak A, Lake R, Kindler H, Robinson B. New approaches for mesothelioma: biologics, vaccines, gene therapy, and other novel agents. *Semin Oncol* 2002; **29**: 82–96.

104. Cote R, Jhanwar S, Novick S, Pellicer A. Genetic alterations of the p53 gene are a feature of malignant mesotheliomas. *Cancer Res* 1991; **51**: 5410–16. Erratum. *Cancer Res* 1991; **51**: 6399.

105. Ni Z, Liu Y, Keshava N, Zhou G, Whong W, Ong T. Analysis of K-*ras* and p53 mutations in mesotheliomas from humans and rats exposed to asbestos. *Mutat Res* 2000; **468**: 87–92.

106. Mayall F, Jacobson G, Wilkins R. Mutations of p53 gene and SV40 sequences in asbestos associated and non-asbestos-associated mesotheliomas. *J Clin Pathol* 1999; **52**: 291–3.

107. Mor O, Yaron P, Huszar M, *et al.* Absence of p53 mutations in malignant mesotheliomas. *Am J Respir Cell Mol Biol* 1997; **16**: 9–13.

108. Creaney J, McLaren BM, Stevenson S, *et al.* p53 autoantibodies in patients with malignant mesothelioma: stability through disease progression. *Br J Cancer* 2001; **84**: 52–6.

109. Robinson BWS, Creaney J, Lake R, *et al.* Mesothelin-family proteins and diagnosis of mesothelioma. *Lancet* 2003; **362**: 1612–16.

110. Bielefeldt-Ohmann H, Jarnicki AG, Fitzpatrick DR. Molecular pathobiology and immunology of malignant mesothelioma. *J Pathol* 1996; **178**: 369–78.

111. Restifo N, Kawakami Y, Marincola F, *et al.* Molecular mechanisms used by tumours to escape immune recognition: immunogenetherapy and the cell biology of major histocompatibility complex class I. *J Immunother* 1993; **14**: 182–90.

112. Cohen E, Kim T Neoplastic cells that express low levels of MHC class I determinants escape host immunity. *Semin Cancer Biol* 1994; **5**: 419–28.

113. Chen L, Ashe S, Brady W, *et al.* Costimulation of antitumor immunity by the B7 counterreceptor for the T lymphocyte molecules CD28 and CTLA-4. *Cell* 1992; **71**: 1093–1102.

114. Townshend S, Allison J. Tumour rejection after direct costimulation of CD8[+] T cells by B7-transfected melanoma cells. *Science* 1993; **259**: 368–70.

115. Fitzpatrick DR, Bielefeldt-Ohmann H, Himbeck RP, Jarnicki AG, Marzo AL, Robinson BW. Transforming growth factor-beta: Antisense RNA-mediated inhibition affects anchorage-independent growth, tumorigenicity and tumour-infiltrating T-cells in malignant mesothelioma. *Growth Factors* 1994; **11**: 29–44.

116. Krishnan L, Menu E, Chaouat G, Talwar G, Raghupathy R. *In vitro* and *in vivo* immunosuppressive effects of supernatants from human choriocarcinoma cell lines. *Cell Immunol* 1991; **138**: 313–25.

117. Singh S, Ross S, Acena M, Rowley D, Schreiber H. Stroma is critical for preventing or permitting immunological destruction of antigenic cancer cells. *J Exp Med* 1992; **175**: 139–46.

118. Onrust SV, Hartl PM, Rosen SD, Hanahan D. Modulation of L-selectin ligand expression during an immune response accompanying tumorigenesis in transgenic mice. *J Clin Invest* 1996; **97**: 54–64.

119. Alleva D, Burger C, Elgert K. Tumour-induced regulation of suppressor macrophage nitric oxide and TNF- alpha production. Role of tumour-derived IL-10, TGF-beta, and prostaglandin E2. *J Immunol* 1994; **153**: 1674–86.

120. Maeda J, Ueki N, Ohkawa T, *et al.* Transforming growth-factor-beta-1 (TGF-beta-1)- and beta-2-like activities in malignant pleural effusions caused by malignant mesothelioma or primary lung-cancer. *Clin Exp Immunol* 1994; **98**: 319–22.

121. Gerwin B, Lechner J, Reddel R, *et al.* Comparison of production of transforming growth factor-beta and platelet-derived growth factor by normal human mesothelial cells and mesothelioma cell lines. *Cancer Res* 1987; **47**: 6180–4.

122. Jarnicki AG, Fitzpatrick DR, Robinson BWS, Bielefeldt-Ohmann H. Altered CD3 chain and cytokine gene expression in tumour infiltrating T lymphocytes during the development of mesothelioma. *Cancer Lett* 1996; **103**: 1–9.

123. Ashcroft GS. Bidirectional regulation of macrophage function by TGF-[beta]. *Microbes Infect* 1999; **1**: 1275–82.

124. Valle MT, Castagneto B, Procopio A, Carbone M, Giordano A, Mutti L. Immunobiology and immune defence mechanisms of mesothelioma cells. *Monaldi Arch Chest Dis* 1998; **53**: 219–27.

125. Schmitter D, Lauber B, Fagg B, Stahel R. Hematopoietic growth factors secreted by seven human pleural mesothelioma cell lines: interleukin-6 production as a common feature. *Int J Cancer* 1992; **51**: 296–301.

126. Motoyama T, Honma T, Watanabe H, Honma S, Kumanishi T, Abe S. Interleukin 6-producing malignant mesothelioma. *Virchows Arch B Cell Pathol Incl Mol Pathol* 1993; **64**: 367–72.

127. Bowman RV, Manning LS, Davis MR, Robinson BW. Capacity of tumour necrosis factor to augment lymphocyte-mediated tumour cell lysis of malignant mesothelioma. *Clin Immunol Immunopathol* 1991; **58**: 80–91.

128. Monti G, Jaurand M, Monnet I, *et al.* Intrapleural production of interleukin 6 during mesothelioma and its modulation by gamma-interferon treatment. *Cancer Res* 1994; **54**: 4419–23.

129. Bielefeldt-Ohmann H, Marzo AL, Himbeck RP, Jarnicki AG, Robinson BW, Fitzpatrick DR. Interleukin-6 involvement in mesothelioma pathobiology: inhibition by interferon alpha immunotherapy. *Cancer Immunol Immunother* 1995; **40**: 241–50.

130. McLaren BR, Robinson, BWS, Lake, RA. New chemotherapeutics in malignant mesothelioma: effects on cell growth and IL-6 production. *Cancer Chemother Pharmacol* 2000; **45**: 502–8.

Chapter 11

Cytogenetic and molecular genetic changes in malignant mesothelioma

D. A. Altomare and J. R. Testa

Introduction

Malignant mesothelioma is characterized by a long latency, typically several decades, from the time of initial asbestos exposure to diagnosis [1], suggesting that multiple somatic genetic events contribute to the tumorigenic conversion of a mesothelial cell. Karyotypic analyses, which have revealed multiple clonal chromosomal alterations in most human mesothelioma specimens, provide supporting evidence for recurrent cytogenetic abnormalities in this highly aggressive neoplasm. Most of these recurrent changes involve deletions of discrete chromosomal regions, consistent with a recessive mechanism of oncogenesis. Loss and/or inactivation of tumour suppressor genes residing at these chromosomal regions is postulated to contribute to the neoplastic transformation of a mesothelial cell [2], and recent molecular genetic studies have implicated several tumour suppressor genes that are inactivated during the development and/or progression of malignant mesothelioma.

In this chapter we summarize recurrent cytogenetic and molecular genetic alterations that have been identified in malignant mesothelioma, and we suggest mechanisms by which asbestos and other aetiological factors such as simian virus 40 (SV40) contribute to a multistep tumorigenic process. Potential therapeutic approaches that target genetic alterations found in this disease will also be briefly discussed. A comprehensive review of the role of SV40 in malignant mesothelioma is presented in Chapter 8 and will not be discussed in detail here.

Mechanisms of asbestos carcinogenicity

The mechanism whereby asbestos fibres are carcinogenic to mesothelial cells may be direct or indirect via the formation of reactive oxygen species and the induction of growth factor receptors [3,4]. Asbestos fibres have been shown to associate physically with the mitotic spindle apparatus in dividing cells to prevent the proper segregation of chromosomes, potentially resulting in aneuploidy and other forms of chromosome damage [5]. Moreover, iron-rich crocidolite asbestos fibres may catalyse the generation of reactive oxygen species when hydrogen peroxide and superoxide react to form hydroxyl radicals. Reactive oxygen species may also be produced by alveolar macrophages during the phagocytosis of asbestos fibres [6]. The expression and activation of apurinic/apyrimidinic endonuclease, a mammalian DNA repair enzyme, has been linked to DNA damage caused by reactive oxygen species generated by asbestos [7]. Recent evidence indicates that the most prevalent mutations are G–T transversions in transgenic rats exposed to crocidolite asbestos fibres [8]. The inflammatory response to asbestos may induce cytokines responsible for local and systemic immunosuppressive activity [9]. In addition, asbestos activates epidermal growth factor receptor and mitogen-activated protein kinase (MAPK) signalling, and thereby increases expression of nuclear factor κB and activator protein 1 transcription factors [10,11].

Activation of transcription factors may increase early response proto-oncogenes such as *jun* and *fos* [12], leading to increased cellular proliferation and susceptibility to subsequent mutations in tumour suppressor genes. The enhanced expression of proto-oncogenes and inactivation of tumour suppressor genes may cooperate in a multistep process that contributes to the development and/or progression of mesothelioma as discussed in detail in Chapter 6.

Recurrent chromosome changes

Chromosome banding analyses of malignant mesothelioma specimens, effusions, and cell lines has revealed the complexity of genetic changes involved in this malignancy [13,14]. All but one of the 20 mesothelioma cases karyotyped by our laboratory exhibited more than 10 clonal chromosomal alterations [2]. Frequent deletions of specific chromosomal regions were observed in the short (p) arms of chromosomes 1, 3, and 9 and the long (q) arm of chromosome 6. Overlapping losses, including numerical alterations, deletions, and unbalanced rearrangements of chromosome region 1p21-22 were documented in 17 of 20 cases. Thirteen cases (65 per cent) had interstitial deletions or other rearrangements resulting in losses from 3p21. Ten cases (50 per cent) showed losses from 6q, with the shortest region of overlap being 6q15-21. Sixteen cases (80 per cent) had losses involving 9p, with the shortest region of overlap being 9p21-22. Moreover, monosomy 22 was observed in 13 cases (65 per cent) and was the single most consistent numerical change. These recurrent losses of 1p, 3p, 6q, 9p, and 22 frequently occurred in combination in a given tumour, with five of 20 cases exhibiting all of these aberrations. Various combinations of three or more of these abnormalities were observed in another 10 cases. Overall, the accumulated loss and/or inactivation of multiple genes from chromosomes 1p, 3p, 6q, 9p, and 22 appear to play a fundamental role in the pathogenesis of malignant mesothelioma.

Comparative genomic hybridization (CGH) analysis, a molecular cytogenetic technique that employs fluorescence *in situ* hybridization to identify chromosome gains and losses across an entire tumour genome, has been used to further elucidate recurrent chromosome changes in malignant mesothelioma. Analyses have revealed multiple (6–25) genomic imbalances in each of a series of 24 malignant mesothelioma cell lines derived from American patients [15], and confirmed earlier karyotypic findings by revealing recurrent losses of 1p, 3p, 6q, and 9p in 30–40 per cent of the cell lines. Losses of 22q were observed in 14 of 24 cell lines(58 per cent). Importantly, CGH analysis detected other recurrent chromosome losses not recognized by conventional cytogenetic analyses. Thirteen of 24 cell lines (54 per cent) showed losses of part or all of 15q, with the shortest region of overlap being 15q11.1-21. Furthermore, losses of 14q24.2-qter and 13q12-14 were each observed in 42 per cent of the cell lines, and loss of 8p21-pter was detected in 33 per cent of cases. Thirteen cell lines (54 per cent) also displayed a gain of chromosomal arm 5p, suggesting the involvement of a putative oncogene(s) in this region.

Similar recurrent genomic alterations were identified in malignant mesothelioma specimens from Finland [16]. However, three frequently deleted chromosome regions that were reported in the American series (i.e. losses of 15q11.1-21, 8p21-pter, and 3p21) were each observed in only one of 42 Finnish cases. Discrepancies between the studies may reflect differences in the type of asbestos exposure or genetic variations in the study populations. Alternatively, these studies may suggest the possible involvement of a cofactor (e.g. SV40) in the USA that is not associated with malignant mesothelioma in Finland [17].

Loss of heterozygosity analyses

The configuration of recurrent genomic losses in malignant mesothelioma suggests a recessive mechanism of oncogenesis, with common sites of chromosomal loss representing the locations of putative tumour suppressor genes that contribute to the development and/or progression of this malignancy. As an initial approach to isolating the putative tumour suppressor genes that may play a role in malignant mesothelioma, loss of heterozygosity (LOH) analyses using polymorphic DNA markers were used to obtain molecular maps of frequently deleted regions that were previously identified by cytogenetic studies. These investigations have been reviewed in detail elsewhere [13,14] and are briefly summarized below.

Loss of 1p22

To define the commonly deleted region of 1p genetically, 50 malignant mesotheliomas were analysed for LOH using a large panel of DNA markers distributed along the short arm of chromosome 1 [18]. Allelic losses at 1p21-22 were observed in 36 cases (72 per cent), and the shortest region of overlap was localized to a 4 centiMorgan (cM) region in 1p22. *BCL10*, which is located in 1p22 and encodes a protein motif found in several regulatory and effector apoptotic molecules, was discounted as a candidate tumour suppressor gene in malignant mesothelioma because *BCL10* mutations were not identified and transcript levels were not downregulated in mesothelioma cells compared twith normal mesothelial cells [19]. Currently, other candidate tumour suppressor genes in this region are being examined for potential involvement in malignant mesothelioma.

Loss of 3p21

It has been demonstrated by two independent research groups that 3p is a common site of allelic loss in malignant mesothelioma [20,21]. In our laboratory, 3p LOH was observed in 15 of 24 mesotheliomas (63 per cent), with the highest frequency of allelic loss at 3p21.3. Since losses from this region have been reported in other cancers, particularly lung tumours, perturbation of a tumour suppressor gene(s) at this site may contribute to the development of multiple tumour types. A homozygous deletion of the β-catenin gene (*CTNNB1*), located at 3p21.3, has been reported in one malignant mesothelioma cell line [22]. However, none of the remaining nine malignant mesothelioma cell lines or tumour specimens examined showed deletions or aberrant expression of *CTNNB1*, suggesting that this is not the critical 3p21 tumour suppressor gene.

Loss of 6q14-25

A complex pattern of allelic loss has been reported for chromosome 6q [23]. Loss of heterozygosity at 6q occurred in approximately 60 per cent of the malignant mesothelioma cases we evaluated, and deletions segregated into several discrete regions including 6q14-21, 6q16.3-21, 6q21-23.2, and 6q25. Similarly, three or four non-overlapping regions of 6q loss have been reported in breast cancer [24], ovarian cancer [25], and non-Hodgkin's lymphoma [26].

Loss of 9p21

Gene dosage analysis was performed on a series of 23 malignant mesothelioma cell lines, 83 per cent of which showed homozygous or hemizygous deletions involving a segment of size ~1 Mb located between the interferon gene cluster and the *D9S171* locus in 9p21 [27]. The *CDKN2A/ARF* locus, which encodes the alternatively transcribed tumour suppressor gene products *p16INK4a* and *p14ARF*, is located in this region. The tumour suppressor function of *p16INK4a* and *p14ARF* and their potential role in malignant mesothelioma are discussed below.

Loss of 13q13.3-14.2

Since CGH analysis previously revealed recurrent losses of 13q and 14q in malignant mesothelioma cell lines [15], LOH analyses were performed on 30 malignant mesothelioma cases using numerous microsatellite markers in 13q and 14q to identify the shortest region of overlap of deletions from these chromosomes [28]. Twenty of 30 cases (67 per cent) showed allelic loss of at least one marker in 13q, and an ~7 cM region located at 13q13.3-14.2 was designated as the shortest region of overlap. Thirteen of 30 (43 per cent) cases exhibited allelic losses from 14q, and deletions localized to at least three distinct regions of LOH at segments 14q11.2-13.2, 14q22.3-24.3, and 14q32.12. In contrast to the single region of chromosomal loss in 13q, the lower frequency and diffuse pattern of allelic losses in 14q suggest that several potential tumour suppressor genes may reside in this chromosome arm and contribute to the tumorigenic progression of a subset of mesotheliomas.

Loss of 15q15

CGH analysis was used to document losses from 15q in 13 of 24 mesothelioma cell lines, and LOH studies demonstrated that 10 of these 13 cases had allelic losses from one or more 15q loci, with the shortest region of overlap being 15q11.1-15 [15]. Other types of cancer, including metastatic tumours of the breast, lung and colon [29], display losses in this same region, suggesting that it harbours a tumour suppressor gene that may contribute to the progression of a variety of cancer types. More recently, high-density LOH analysis of 46 malignant mesotheliomas was used to define a minimally deleted region of ~3 cM at 15q15 [30].

Gene expression profiling of malignant mesothelioma

Comprehensive gene expression profiling using cDNA microarrays allows the simultaneous investigation of thousands of individual genes in a single experiment. Significant progress has been made with this technology in the assessment of global alterations in gene expression levels in mesothelioma, utilizing both clinical and research samples. An early study of four mesothelioma cell lines compared with two normal mesothelial cell cultures revealed a number of genes that are differentially expressed in tumour cells compared with normal cells, and these expression changes may effect a wide variety of cell processes such as cell cycle, cell growth, and cell motility [31]. More recently, a large cDNA microarray study of 181 pleural mesothelioma and lung adenocarcinoma specimens demonstrated that expression profiling has significant diagnostic utility and can be used to distinguish these two pathologically similar diseases [32].

Involvement of tumour suppressor genes

p16^{INK4a}

The p16^{INK4a} product of the *CDKN2A/ARF* locus is capable of binding and inhibiting cyclin-dependent kinase 4, which induces cell cycle arrest at the G_1 phase by inhibiting the phosphorylation of the retinoblastoma protein pRb [33]. The *p16^{INK4a}* gene was identified as the 9p21 tumour suppressor gene shortly after it was cloned, and homozygous deletions of *p16^{INK4a}* were detected at high frequencies in cell lines derived from various tumours [34].

Deletion mapping studies have demonstrated that 34 of 40 mesothelioma cell lines (85 per cent) had homozygous deletions of one or more *p16^{INK4a}* exons, and another had a point mutation in *p16^{INK4a}* [35]. Downregulation of *p16^{INK4a}* was observed in four of the remaining cell lines. Moreover, homozygous deletions of *p16^{INK4a}* were identified in five of 23 matched mesothelioma specimens (22 per cent). The higher frequency of *p16^{INK4a}* alterations in mesothelioma cell lines compared with tumour tissues may be attributed to a potential growth advantage provided by *p16^{INK4a}* loss during cell culture. Alternatively, malignant mesothelioma specimens often contain significant amounts of contaminating normal stroma, which may create difficulties in detecting a homozygous deletion in the malignant cell population. Downregulation of $p16^{INK4a}$ in mesothelioma cells may result from promoter hypermethylation, as has been observed in other types of cancer [36]. Abnormal $p16^{INK4a}$ protein expression has been reported in 12 of 12 malignant mesothelioma specimens and 15 of 15 tumour-derived cell lines examined by immunohistochemistry [37].

$p14^{ARF}$

The tumour suppressor gene $p14^{ARF}$ shares exons 2 and 3 with $p16^{INK4a}$, although the reading frames differ, and homozygous deletions of the CDKN2A/ARF locus often lead to inactivation of both gene products. The p14^{ARF} protein is essential for the activation of p53 in response to certain oncogene products such as Ras or Myc [38]. Therefore homozygous losses of both $p14^{ARF}$ and $p16^{INK4a}$ would affect p53- and pRb-dependent growth regulatory pathways, respectively.

NF2

Numerical loss of a copy of chromosome 22 has been consistently shown to be a frequent event in malignant mesothelioma. The neurofibromatosis type 2 (NF2) tumour suppressor gene resides at chromosome 22q12. Although dominantly inherited mutations in NF2 predispose individuals to tumours primarily of neuroectodermal origin, somatic mutations of NF2 have been identified in unrelated malignancies [39]. To determine its role in malignant mesothelioma, mutation studies of the NF2 gene were performed and demonstrated nucleotide alterations in eight of 15 mesothelioma cell lines (53 per cent) [40]. The mutations, which included deletions and insertions and one nonsense mutation, were predicted to truncate and inactivate the NF2 protein, known as merlin or schwannomin. Mutations were confirmed in the genomic DNA from six matched primary tumour specimens, and the two other alterations that could not be confirmed by genomic analysis may affect gene splicing: i.e. deletion of exon 10 in one cell line and a 43 bp insertion between exons 13 and 14 in the other. In addition, somatic mutations in one malignant mesothelioma specimen and in seven of 17 mesothelioma cell lines (41 per cent) were documented in an independent study [41].

More recently, mutations were detected in the NF2 coding region of 12 of 23 additional mesothelioma cell lines (52 per cent) [42]. Loss of merlin expression was detected in each of the 12 cell lines with NF2 gene alterations. Another two cell lines with NF2 mutations in the previous study were also found to lack NF2 expression. LOH analyses using two polymorphic DNA markers residing at or near the NF2 locus revealed that 18 of all 25 mesothelioma cell lines (72 per cent) had losses at one or both loci. LOH was evident in all cases exhibiting mutation and aberrant expression of NF2, consistent with biallelic inactivation of NF2 in malignant mesothelioma. It is also noteworthy that a malignant mesothelioma was recently reported in an NF2 patient who had been exposed to asbestos occupationally [43]. The relatively early age of onset of mesothelioma in this individual raises the intriguing possibility that patients with this rare disorder could be particularly prone to the development of this malignancy if exposed to asbestos.

Merlin has significant homology to members of the ezrin–radixin–moesin (ERM) family of proteins [44]. However, the cellular function and regulation of merlin is not well defined, and the mechanism by which merlin exerts its tumour suppressor activity is unknown. Because Rho GTPase-mediated signalling phosphorylates other ERM proteins, further studies have investigated whether merlin is regulated by a similar mechanism. These revealed that merlin is phosphorylated in response to activated Rac and activated Cdc42 [45,46]. Furthermore, merlin phosphorylation is mediated by p21-activated kinase (Pak), a downstream target of both Rac and Cdc42 [46]. Kinase assays demonstrated that Pak is capable of directly phosphorylating merlin at serine 518, a site that affects merlin activity and localization. Importantly, Pak has been shown to regulate motility in mammalian cells [47], and thus loss of merlin function may contribute to invasiveness and/or tumour spread in malignant mesothelioma.

GPC3

GPC3 is another putative tumour suppressor gene that is frequently downregulated in mesothelioma. Located at chromosome Xq26, the *GPC3* gene has been implicated as a tumour suppressor gene in ovarian cancer [48]. Using differential mRNA display, *GPC3* transcript levels have been shown to be abundant in normal rat mesothelial cells but markedly diminished in rat mesothelioma cells [49]. Northern blot analysis confirmed that *GPC3* was consistently silenced in each of 10 rat mesothelioma cell lines and two primary tumours. Human *GPC3* transcript levels were downregulated in 16 of 18 mesothelioma specimens (89 per cent) and 17 of 22 mesothelioma cell lines (77 per cent), most of which displayed aberrant methylation of the *GPC3* promoter region. Allelic loss at the *GPC3* locus was observed in only two of 31 mesothelioma cell lines (6 per cent), and no mutations were detected, contrary to a recent report of somatic *GPC3* mutations in two of 41 Wilms tumours (5 per cent) [50]. We also demonstrated that ectopic expression of *GPC3* inhibits *in vitro* colony formation of human mesothelioma cells lacking detectable endogenous expression of this gene [49]. Collectively, these data suggest that downregulation of *GPC3* frequently occurs in malignant mesothelioma and that *GPC3* may encode a negative regulator of mesothelial cell growth.

The functional significance of *GPC3* expression in tumorigenesis is not known. *GPC3* is mutated in patients diagnosed with Simpson–Golabi–Behmel syndrome (SGBS), an X-chromosome-linked congenital overgrowth disorder characterized by morphological abnormalities and increased risk of embryonal tumours of mesodermal origins [51]. The association between *GPC3* loss-of-function mutations and SGBS suggests that this gene plays a potentially critical role in maintaining homeostasis between cell growth and growth inhibition, which is disrupted in tumorigenesis. The *GPC3* gene encodes glypican-3, a heparan sulphate proteoglycan that is bound to the cell surface via a glycosyl-phosphatidylinositol anchor, and induces programmed cell death in a cell-line-specific manner [52]. Human GPC3 was initially proposed to be a negative regulator of insulin-like growth factor 2 (IGF-2) [51], but convincing biochemical evidence is still lacking. GPC3-deficient mice exhibit several of the clinical features observed in SGBS patients [53] and have been used to demonstrate that GPC3 expression is independent of IGF signalling, although the two pathways may converge downstream [54]. Other recent studies with GPC3-deficient mice have shown that glypican-3 controls response to bone morphogenetic protein 4 (BMP4) in limb patterning and skeletal development [55], and modulates BMP and fibroblast growth factor (FGF) signalling during renal branching [56].

Possible genetic predisposition to mesothelioma in Turkish villagers exposed to erionite

Volcanic tuffs and natural caves containing asbestos and zeolite fibres are indigenous to the small villages of Karain and Tuzkoy in Cappadocia, Central Anatolia, Turkey, and nearly 50 per cent of the inhabitants succumb to malignant mesothelioma [57,58]. The mineral fibre erionite, a type of zeolite, is associated with this extremely high incidence of malignant mesothelioma, and erionite has been shown to cause mesothelioma in rodents [59,60]. Cancer in these villages has occurred in clusters (referred to by villagers as 'houses of death'), such that many members of the same household developed malignant mesothelioma. However, buildings in the nearby village of Karlik were constructed with the same materials containing comparable amounts of erionite, but

(a)

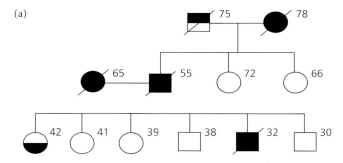

(b)

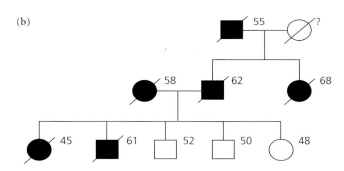

Figure 11.1 Genetic mapping study of malignant pleural mesothelioma in Cappadocia. Analysis of a six-generation extended pedigree of 526 individuals showed that it was genetically transmitted. It was suggested that vertical transmission of malignant pleural mesothelioma probably occurs in an autosomal dominant fashion. (Reproduced from I. Roushdy-Hammady *et al.* Genetic-susceptibility factor and malignant mesothelioma in the Cappadocian region of Turkey. *Lancet* 2001; 357, 444–5.)

no mesotheliomas are observed. Pedigree analysis of extended families in Karain and Tuzkoy have suggested that malignant mesothelioma is genetically transmitted, possibly as an autosomal dominant disease, and that erionite is a cofactor (Fig. 11.1) [61]. SV40 was determined not to be a cofactor in the pathogenesis of pleural malignant mesothelioma in Turkey [58,62]. Isolation of the putative malignant mesothelioma susceptibility gene could lead to the development of therapeutic approaches for members of these families and may enhance our understanding of molecular mechanisms involved in the pathogenesis of malignant mesothelioma generally.

Tumour suppressor genes and SV40 Tag as potential therapeutic targets

Information about the recurrent genetic alterations associated with various cancers has led to the realization that intrinsic molecular changes connected with the pathogenesis of a particular cancer may also be useful markers of disease susceptibility, initiation, and progression. In addition, some alterations may provide a genetic basis for targeted therapeutics in cancers such as malignant mesothelioma that are refractory to conventional therapy [63].

Clinical presentation of mesothelioma is generally localized to the pleural or peritoneal cavity [64], but there is a lack of any effective treatment for this lethal disease. Gene replacement therapy in malignant mesothelioma may be an attractive option, although obstacles such as toxicity and delivery must be effectively addressed for molecularly based therapies to become practical

[65]. As an initial approach to developing a molecularly targeted therapy, malignant mesothelioma cells with loss of a functional tumour suppressor gene were infected with virus containing a normal gene copy, and the cells were evaluated for physiological endpoints such as inhibited cell proliferation or increased apoptosis. Adenovirus-mediated gene transfer of *p16^INK4a* in mesothelioma cells lacking the endogenous gene was shown to induce cell cycle arrest and cell death, as well as tumour suppression and regression [66], and *p16^INK4a* adenovirus treatment of mice with established human mesothelioma xenografts prolonged survival [67]. Similarly, adenovirus-mediated replacement of *p14^ARF* in mesothelioma cells was shown to restore p53 function, arrest cells in the G_1 phase, and induce cell death [68]. In addition, transfection of antisense SV40 has been shown to inhibit large T antigen (Tag) expression, restore the p53 pathway, and induce growth arrest and apoptosis of SV40-positive human mesothelioma cells [69]. These findings have led some investigators to suggest that antisense SV40 strategies may be efficacious for patients with SV40-positive malignant mesothelioma [69].

Summary and conclusions

Asbestos fibres, particularly short amphibole types such as crocidolite, are associated with the induction of malignant mesothelioma, although the actual carcinogenic mechanism is unknown. Asbestos affects mesothelial cells either directly or indirectly by inducing reactive oxygen species that can damage DNA. Most somatic genetic changes are likely to be of minimal significance or alternatively lead to cell death, although a few may perturb key cell cycle regulatory genes, leading to immortalization and tumorigenesis [13].

A subset of genetic alterations (e.g. homozygous 9p21 deletions encompassing the *CDKN2A/ARF* locus encoding both the p16^Ink4a^ and p14^ARF^ tumour suppressor proteins) or the expression of SV40 Tag can disrupt Rb- and p53-dependent growth control and thereby provide cells with a proliferative advantage. Mesothelioma cells positive for SV40 exhibit Tag-mediated inhibition of p53 [70]. Recent studies have demonstrated that human mesothelial cells are susceptible to SV40-mediated transformation and that asbestos complements SV40 in this process [71]. Moreover, p53-deficient mice are more susceptible to asbestos-induced mesothelioma than wild-type mice [72]. Collectively, the data suggest that asbestos and SV40 act as cofactors to overwhelm cell cycle regulatory mechanisms, result in unchecked cell division, and permit cellular transformation that may ultimately lead to the development of mesothelioma.

Generally, to genetically inactivate a tumour suppressor gene, both copies of the gene must be lost and/or inactivated by mutation or epigenetic mechanisms. Loss of a tumour suppressor gene may occur by deletions or by asbestos-mediated chromosome mis-segregation. In many mesotheliomas, a non-disjunction event that involves chromosome 22 causes loss of one *NF2* allele, while a point mutation in the other copy produces a truncated functionally inactive product. Cytogenetic and molecular genetic studies indicate that malignant mesothelioma results from the accumulation of multiple somatic genetic events, mainly deletions, suggesting a multistep cascade that involves the inactivation of several tumour suppressor genes. It has not been possible to determine a temporal sequence of genetic events because of a lack of data from early stage disease. However, the identification and characterization of all of the putative tumour suppressor genes targeted by recurrent deletions, as well as any mesothelioma susceptibility loci, will elucidate how each component contributes to the pathogenesis of mesothelioma. Ultimately, this information will aid in the design of more effective therapeutic strategies.

Acknowledgments

Data obtained by the authors and summarized here were supported by grants from the National Cancer Institute (CA45745 and CA06927) and the Mesothelioma Applied Research Foundation, and by a gift from the Local 14 Mesothelioma Fund of the International Association of Heat and Frost Insulators & Asbestos Workers, in memory of Hank Vaughan and Alice Haas.

References

1. Selikoff IJ, Hammond EC, Seidman H. Latency of asbestos disease among insulation workers in the United States and Canada. *Cancer* 1980; **46**: 2736–40.

2. Taguchi T, Jhanwar SC, Siegfried JM, Keller SM, Testa JR. Recurrent deletions of specific chromosomal sites in 1p, 3p, 6q, and 9p in human malignant mesothelioma. *Cancer Res* 1993; **53**: 4349–55.

3. Mossman BT, Kamp DW, Weitzman SA. Mechanisms of carcinogenesis and clinical features of asbestos-associated cancers. *Cancer Invest* 1996; **14**: 466–80.

4. Pache JC, Janssen YM, Walsh ES, *et al.* Increased epidermal growth factor-receptor protein in a human mesothelial cell line in response to long asbestos fibers. *Am J Pathol* 1998;**152**: 333–40.

5. Ault JG, Cole RW, Jensen CG, Jensen LC, Bachert LA, Rieder CL. Behavior of crocidolite asbestos during mitosis in living vertebrate lung epithelial cells. *Cancer Res* 1995; **55**: 792–8.

6. Hansen K, Mossman BT. Generation of superoxide (O^{2-}.) from alveolar macrophages exposed to asbestiform and nonfibrous particles. *Cancer Res* 1987; **47**: 1681–6.

7. Fung H, Kow YW, Van Houten B, *et al.* Asbestos increases mammalian AP-endonuclease gene expression, protein levels, and enzyme activity in mesothelial cells. *Cancer Res* 1998; **58**: 189–94.

8. Unfried K, Schurkes C, Abel J. Distinct spectrum of mutations induced by crocidolite asbestos: clue for 8-hydroxydeoxyguanosine-dependent mutagenesis in vivo. *Cancer Res* 2002; **62**: 99–104.

9. Rosenthal GJ, Simeonova P, Corsini E. Asbestos toxicity: an immunologic perspective. *Rev Environ Health* 1999; **14**: 11–20.

10. Buder-Hoffmann S, Palmer C, Vacek P, Taatjes DJ, Mossman B. Different accumulation of activated extracellular signal-regulated kinases (ERK 1/2) and role in cell-cycle alterations by epidermal growth factor, hydrogen peroxide, or asbestos in pulmonary epithelial cells. *Am J Respir Cell Mol Biol* 2001; **24**: 405–13.

11. Ramos-Nino ME, Haegens A, Shukla A, Mossman BT. Role of mitogen-activated protein kinases (MAPK) in cell injury and proliferation by environmental particulates. *Mol Cell Biochem* 2002; **234–235**: 111–18.

12. Robledo R, Mossman B. Cellular and molecular mechanisms of asbestos-induced fibrosis. *J Cell Physiol* 1999; **180**: 158–66.

13. Murthy SS, Testa JR. Asbestos, chromosomal deletions, and tumor suppressor gene alterations in human malignant mesothelioma. *J Cell Physiol* 1999; **180**: 150–7.

14. Testa JR, Pass HI, Carbone M. Molecular biology of mesothelioma. In: DeVita VT Jr, Hellman S, Rosenberg SA, eds. *Principles and Practice of Oncology*, 6th edn. Philadelphia, PA: Lippincott–Williams & Wilkins, 2001; 1937–43.

15. Balsara BR, Bell DW, Sonoda G, *et al.* Comparative genomic hybridization and loss of heterozygosity analyses identify a common region of deletion at 15q11.1–15 in human malignant mesothelioma. *Cancer Res* 1999; **59**: 450–4.

16. Bjorkqvist AM, Tammilehto L, Anttila S, Mattson K, Knuutila S Recurrent DNA copy number changes in 1q, 4q, 6q, 9p, 13q, 14q and 22q detected by comparative genomic hybridization in malignant mesothelioma. *Br J Cancer* 1997; **75**: 523–7.

17. Hirvonen A, Mattson K, Karjalainen A, *et al.* SV40-like DNA sequences not detectable in Finnish mesothelioma patients not exposed to SV40 contaminated poliovaccines. *Mol Carcinog* 1999; **26**: 93–9.

18. Lee W-C, Balsara B, Liu Z, Jhanwar SC, Testa JR. Loss of heterozygosity analysis defines a critical region in chromosome 1p22 commonly deleted in human malignant mesothelioma. *Cancer Res* 1996; **56**: 4297–301.

19. Apostolou S, De Rienzo A, Murthy SS, Jhanwar SC, Testa JR. Absence of *BCL10* mutations in human malignant mesothelioma. *Cell* 1999; **97**: 684–6.

20. Lu YY, Jhanwar SC, Cheng JQ, Testa JR. Deletion mapping of the short arm of chromosome 3 in human malignant mesothelioma. *Genes Chromosomes Cancer* 1994; **9**: 76–80.

21. Zeiger MA, Gnarra JR, Zbar B, Linehan WM, Pass HI. Loss of heterozygosity on the short arm of chromosome 3 in mesothelioma cell lines and solid tumors. *Genes Chromosomes Cancer* 1994; **11**: 15–20.

22. Shigemitsu K, Sekido Y, Usami N, *et al.* Genetic alteration of the beta-catenin gene (*CTNNB1*) in human lung cancer and malignant mesothelioma and identification of a new 3p21.3 homozygous deletion. *Oncogene* 2001; **20**: 4249–57.

23. Bell DW, Jhanwar SC, Testa JR. Multiple regions of allelic loss from chromosome arm 6q in malignant mesothelioma. *Cancer Res* 1997; **57**: 4057–62.

24. Sheng ZM, Marchetti A, Buttitta F, *et al.* Multiple regions of chromosome 6q affected by loss of heterozygosity in primary human breast carcinomas. *Br J Cancer* 1996; **73**: 144–7.

25. Orphanos V, McGown G, Hey Y, *et al.* Allelic imbalance of chromosome 6q in ovarian tumours. *Br J Cancer* 1995; **71**: 666–9.

26. Offit K, Parsa NZ, Gaidano G, *et al.* 6q deletions define distinct clinico-pathologic subsets of non-Hodgkin's lymphoma. *Blood* 1993; **82**: 2157–62.

27. Cheng JQ, Jhanwar SC, Lu YY, Testa JR. Homozygous deletions within 9p21-p22 identify a small critical region of chromosomal loss in human malignant mesothelioma. *Cancer Res* 1993; **53**: 4761–3.

28. De Rienzo A, Jhanwar SC, Testa JR. Loss of heterozygosity analysis of 13q and 14q in human malignant mesothelioma. *Genes Chromosomes Cancer* 2000; **28**: 337–41.

29. Wick W, Petersen I, Schmutzler RK, *et al.* Evidence for a novel tumor suppressor gene on chromosome 15 associated with progression to a metastatic stage in breast cancer. *Oncogene* 1996; **12**: 973–8.

30. De Rienzo A, Balsara BR, Apostolou S, Jhanwar SC, Testa JR. Loss of heterozygosity analysis defines a 3-cM region of 15q commonly deleted in human malignant mesothelioma. *Oncogene* 2001; **20**: 6245–9.

31. Kettunen E, Nissen AM, Ollikainen T, *et al.* Gene expression profiling of malignant mesothelioma cell lines: cDNA array study. *Int J Cancer* 2001; **91**: 492–6.

32. Gordon GJ, Jensen. RV, Hsiao LL, *et al.* Translation of microarray data into clinically relevant cancer diagnostic tests using gene expression ratios in lung cancer and mesothelioma. *Cancer Res* 2002; **62**: 4963–7.

33. Serrano M, Hannon GJ, Beach D. A new regulatory motif in cell-cycle control causing specific inhibition of cyclin D/CDK4. *Nature* 1993; **366**: 704–7.

34. Kamb A, Gruis NA, Weaver-Feldhaus J, *et al.* A cell cycle regulator potentially involved in genesis of many tumor types. *Science* 1994; **264**: 436–40.

35. Cheng JQ, Jhanwar SC, Klein WM, *et al.* p16 alterations and deletion mapping of 9p21-p22 in malignant mesothelioma. *Cancer Res* 1994; **54**: 5547–51.

36. Merlo A, Herman JG, Mao L, *et al.* 5' CpG island methylation is associated with transcriptional silencing of the tumour suppressor p16/CDKN2/MTS1 in human cancers. *Nat Med* 1995; **1**: 686–92.

37. Kratzke RA, Otterson GA, Lincoln CE, *et al.* Immunohistochemical analysis of the p16INK4 cyclin-dependent kinase inhibitor in malignant mesothelioma. *J Natl Cancer Inst* 1995; **87**: 1870–5.

38. Palmero I, Pantoja C, Serrano M. p19ARF links the tumour suppressor p53 to Ras. *Nature* 1998; **395**: 125–6.

39. Bianchi AB, Hara T, Ramesh V, *et al.* Mutations in transcript isoforms of the neurofibromatosis 2 gene in multiple human tumour types. *Nat Genet* 1994; **6**: 185–92.

40. Bianchi AB, Mitsunaga S-I, Cheng JQ, *et al.* High frequency of inactivating mutations in the neurofibromatosis type 2 gene (*NF2*) in primary malignant mesotheliomas. *Proc Natl Acad Sci USA* 1995; **92**: 10854–8.

41. Sekido Y, Pass HI, Bader S, *et al* Neurofibromatosis type 2 (*NF2*) gene is somatically mutated in mesothelioma but not in lung cancer. *Cancer Res* 1995; **55**: 1227–31.

42. Cheng JQ, Lee W-C, Klein MA, Cheng GZ, Jhanwar SC, Testa JR. Frequent alterations of *NF2* and allelic loss from chromosome band 22q12 in malignant mesothelioma: evidence for a two-hit mechanism of *NF2* inactivation. *Genes Chromosomes Cancer* 1999; **24**: 238–42.

43. Baser ME, De Rienzo A, Altomare D, *et al.* Neurofibromatosis 2 and malignant mesothelioma. *Neurology* 2002; **59**: 290–1.

44. Gusella JF, Ramesh V, MacCollin M, Jacoby LB. Merlin: the neurofibromatosis 2 tumor suppressor. *Biochim Biophys Acta* 1999; **1423**: M29–36.

45. Shaw RJ, Paez JG, Curto M, *et al.* The NF2 tumor suppressor, merlin, functions in Rac-dependent signaling. *Dev Cell* 2001; **1**: 63–72.

46. Xiao GH, Beeser A, Chernoff J, Testa JR. p21-activated kinase links Rac/Cdc42 signaling to merlin. *J Biol Chem* 2002; **277**: 883–6.

47. Sells MA, Boyd JT, Chernoff J. p21-activated kinase 1 (Pak1) regulates cell motility in mammalian fibroblasts. *J Cell Biol* 1999; **145**: 837–49.

48. Lin H, Huber R, Schlessinger D, Morin PJ. Frequent silencing of the GPC3 gene in ovarian cancer cell lines. *Cancer Res* 1999; **59**: 807–10.

49. Murthy SS, Shen T, De Rienzo A, *et al.* Expression of *GPC3*, an X-linked recessive overgrowth gene, is silenced in malignant mesotheliomas. *Oncogene* 2000; **19**: 410–16.

50. White GR, Kelsey AM, Varley JM, Birch JM. Somatic glypican 3 (GPC3) mutations in Wilms' tumour. *Br J Cancer* 2002; **86**: 1920–2.

51. Pilia G, Hughes-Benzie RM, MacKenzie A, *et al.* Mutations in GPC3, a glypican gene, cause the Simpson–Golabi–Behmel overgrowth syndrome. *Nat Genet* 1996; **12**: 241–7.

52. Gonzalez AD, Kaya M, Shi W, *et al.* OCI-5/GPC3, a glypican encoded by a gene that is mutated in the Simpson–Golabi–Behmel overgrowth syndrome, induces apoptosis in a cell line-specific manner. *J Cell Biol* 1998; **141**: 1407–14.

53. Cano-Gauci DF, Song HH, Yang H, *et al.* Glypican-3-deficient mice exhibit developmental overgrowth and some of the abnormalities typical of Simpson–Golabi–Behmel syndrome. *J Cell Biol* 1999; **146**: 255–64.

54. Chiao E, Fisher P, Crisponi L, *et al.* Overgrowth of a mouse model of the Simpson–Golabi–Behmel syndrome is independent of IGF signaling. *Dev Biol* 2002; **243**: 185–206.

55. Paine-Saunders S, Viviano BL, Zupicich J, Skarnes WC, Saunders S. Glypican-3 controls cellular responses to Bmp4 in limb patterning and skeletal development. *Dev Biol* 2000; **225**: 179–87.

56. Grisaru S, Cano-Gauci D, Tee J, Filmus J, Rosenblum ND. Glypican-3 modulates BMP- and FGF-mediated effects during renal branching morphogenesis. *Dev Biol* 2001; **231**: 31–46.

57. Carbone M, Kratzke RA, Testa JR. The pathogenesis of mesothelioma. *Semin Oncol* 2002; **29**: 2–17.

58. Emri S, Demir A, Dogan M, *et al.* Lung diseases due to environmental exposures to erionite and asbestos in Turkey. *Toxicol Lett* 2002; **127**: 251–7.

59. Fraire AE, Greenberg SD, Spjut HJ, *et al.* Effect of erionite on the pleural mesothelium of the Fischer 344 rat. *Chest* 1997; **111**: 1375–80.

60. Kleymenova EV, Horesovsky G, Pylev LN, Everitt J. Mesotheliomas induced in rats by the fibrous mineral erionite are independent from p53 alterations. *Cancer Lett* 1999; **147**: 55–61.

61. Roushdy-Hammady I, Siegel J, Emri S, Testa JR, Carbone M. Genetic-susceptibility factor and malignant mesothelioma in the Cappadocian region of Turkey. *Lancet* 2001; **357**: 444–5.

62. De Rienzo A, Tor M, Sterman DH, Aksoy F, Albelda SM, Testa JR. Detection of SV40 DNA sequences in malignant mesothelioma specimens from the United States, but not from Turkey. *J Cell Biochem* 2002; **84**: 455–9.

63. Nowak AK, Lake RA, Kindler HL, Robinson BWS. New approaches for mesothelioma: biologics, vaccines, gene therapy, and other novel agents. *Semin Oncol* 2002; **29**: 82–96.

64. Antman KH, Pass HI, Schiff PB. Management of mesothelioma. In: DeVita VT, Jr., Hellman S, Rosenberg SA, eds. *Principles and Practice of Oncology*, 6th edn. Philadelphia, PA: Lippincott–Williams & Wilkins, 2001; 1943–69.

65. Blaese RM. Gene therapy for cancer. *Sci Am* 1997; **276**: 111–15.

66. Frizelle SP, Grim J, Zhou J, *et al*. Re-expression of p16INK4a in mesothelioma cells results in cell cycle arrest, cell death, tumor suppression and tumor regression. *Oncogene* 1998; **16**: 3087–95.

67. Frizelle SP, Rubins JB, Zhou JX, Curiel DT, Kratzke RA. Gene therapy of established mesothelioma xenografts with recombinant p16INK4a adenovirus. *Cancer Gene Ther* 2000; 7: 1421–5.

68. Yang CT, You L, Yeh CC, *et al*. Adenovirus-mediated p14(ARF) gene transfer in human mesothelioma cells. *J Natl Cancer Inst* 2000; **92**: 636–41.

69. Waheed I, Guo ZS, Chen GA, Weiser TS, Nguyen DM, Schrump DS. Antisense to SV40 early gene region induces growth arrest and apoptosis in T-antigen-positive human pleural mesothelioma cells. *Cancer Res* 1999; **59**: 6068–73.

70. Carbone M, Rizzo P, Grimley PM, *et al*. Simian virus-40 large-T antigen binds p53 in human mesotheliomas. *Nat Med* 1997; **3**: 908–12.

71. Bocchetta M, Di Resta I, Powers A, *et al*. Human mesothelial cells are unusually susceptible to simian virus 40-mediated transformation and asbestos cocarcinogenicity. *Proc Natl Acad Sci USA* 2000; **97**: 10214–19.

72. Marsella JM, Liu BL, Vaslet CA, Kane AB. Susceptibility of p53-deficient mice to induction of mesothelioma by crocidolite asbestos fibers. *Environ Health Perspect* 1997; **105**: 1069–72.

Chapter 12

The role of surgery for diagnosis, staging, and symptom control in malignant pleural mesothelioma

A. E. Martin-Ucar and D. A. Waller

Introduction

Surgery in the management of malignant pleural mesothelioma (MPM) has largely been confined to obtaining tissue diagnosis or to effect symptom control by pleurodesis. Non-invasive image-guided methods of obtaining pleural tissues are reducing the need for surgical biopsy, and the increasing use of thoracoscopy under sedation by an interventional pulmonologist may also reduce surgical involvement. However, the increasing incidence of the disease together with reports of long-term survivors has resulted in a more aggressive surgical approach towards therapy. Palliative surgical debulking may have a role in symptom control beyond that of chemical pleurodesis in patients not suitable for radical therapy because their tumour is unresectable or they are inoperable and not fit for the procedure. In this chapter we focus on the reported experiences of authors in the use of surgery for the diagnosis, staging and symptomatic control in MPM.

Invasive diagnostic procedures

Clinical suspicion of MPM can be difficult to confirm. The most common feature in chest radiographs in patients with MPM is pleural effusion. Therefore aspiration cytology is one of the most common first-line attempts to obtain confirmation of the diagnosis. However, cytological examination of pleural fluid in malignant mesothelioma is only positive in around 30 per cent of cases [1]. At the same time it is justified to perform a closed-needle pleural biopsy (using either the Cope or Abrams needle). Unfortunately, it is clear that the effectiveness of 'blind' pleural biopsy is operator dependent. If sufficient operator experience exists, the closed 'blind' pleural biopsy is still justified as a first attempt to obtain a tissue diagnosis at the time of pleural aspiration or drain insertion [2].

In most cases the sensitivity of pleural fluid cytology and 'blind' percutaneous biopsy remain comparatively low, whilst thoracoscopic biopsy is relatively expensive and invasive. The sensitivity of percutaneous biopsy may be enhanced by image guidance. Adams et al. [3] analysed the use of percutaneous image-guided cutting-needle biopsy (CNB) in the diagnosis of mesothelioma. Over a 7 year period a single radiologist (Gleeson) performed percutaneous CNB under local anaesthesia on 53 consecutive patients with pleural thickening on contrast-enhanced CT. There were only two minor complications with no mortality. Mesothelioma was correctly diagnosed in 18 of 21 cases (86 per cent sensitivity; 100 per cent specificity). Fine-needle aspiration cytology was diagnostic in only two of 17 patients and pleural fluid cytology was non-diagnostic in all patients with pleural effusion. The median pleural thickness at the site of biopsy was 1.5 cm but non-uniformity of pleural thickness emphasizes the benefits of image guidance. All patients were offered prophylactic irradiation to the biopsy site. Whilst the results are impressive, they represent the learning experience of an enthusiastic specialist and therefore must be viewed in the context of 'operator dependence'. This technique is attractive if further radical surgery is planned for MPM as it reduces the potential for wound implantation and is non-invasive. However, its efficacy in early disease with patchy slight pleural involvement remains to be established, and in these patients thoracoscopy remains the diagnostic tool of choice.

Thoracoscopy for the diagnosis of mesothelioma is increasingly being performed using a rigid scope under local or regional anaesthesia in a spontaneously ventilating patient often in a bronchoscopy suite by a non-surgeon, so-called 'medical thoracoscopy'. Boutin and Rey [4] described their experience with diagnostic thoracoscopy under local anaesthesia in 188 patients achieving diagnosis in 185 out of 188 patients (98 per cent), while fluid cytology was diagnostic in 26 per cent only. Blanc *et al.* [5] have recently reported a series of 168 medical thoracoscopies in which the diagnosis from closed biopsy was changed in 43 of 96 cases; mesothelioma was found in 16 of 66 cases erroneously diagnosed as inflammation. In four cases the diagnosis of mesothelioma on closed biopsy was corrected after thoracoscopy. Medical thoracoscopy was inaccurate in 10 of 149 cases where either the diagnosis of MPM was missed or misinterpreted as adenocarcinoma because of insufficient pleural material in the biopsy or where pleural adhesions necessitated thoracotomy. Despite these limitations and the fact that it is more expensive than percutaneous biopsy, medical or surgical thoracoscopy plays a valuable role in the majority of those with mesothelioma who are unfit for radical treatment. It can offer a one-stop diagnosis and therapeutic intervention with the administration of talc pleurodesis as described by Cardillo *et al.* [6] who performed thoracoscopy and talc pleurodesis on 611 patients with malignant pleural effusions with a postoperative mortality of 0.8 per cent and a complication rate of 3.1 per cent, and achieved 100 per cent histological diagnosis and 93 per cent control of effusion at follow-up [6].

If the patient is suitable for radical surgery, a definitive tissue type is required, i.e. epithelial vs. sarcomatoid, as cell type may influence selection and at least would define prognosis after surgery [7]. Surgical thoracoscopy is normally performed via two or three port incisions to obtain diagnosis and perform chemical pleurodesis [8]. However, if radical surgery is contemplated, it is important that the number and location of biopsy sites should be limited to a minimum. We favour a single 3–5 cm microthoracotomy in the line of a future incision to minimize the risk of biopsy site implantation. Video-assisted thoracoscopy (VATS) via this incision may direct the biopsy. Additional talc pleurodesis may facilitate subsequent pleuropneumonectomy but theoretically could interfere with pathological interpretation of the resected specimen. When biopsy is performed with the use of VATS the accuracy universally approaches 100 per cent (Table 12.1).

Table 12.1 Results of video-assisted thoracoscopic biopsy in malignant pleural mesothelioma

	Year	Number	Diagnosis obtained
Menzies and Charbonneau [9]	1991	102	96%
Boutin and Rey [4]	1993	188	98%
Waller *et al.* [8]	1994	20	100%
Canto *et al.* [10]	1997	46	100%
Grossebner *et al.* [11]	1999	23	100%
Cardillo *et al.* [6]	2002	611	100%

In any case, regardless of the method of biopsy, tumour growth along the biopsy sites is a recognized event with an incidence of around 20 per cent, although large series estimated incidences of up to 50 per cent. In a prospective randomized trial, Boutin *et al.* [12] reported complete absence of subcutaneous nodules in 20 patients after local radiotherapy in contrast with an incidence of 40 per cent in patients who were not treated with radiotherapy. Therefore local irradiation to biopsy sites should be recommended once wounds have healed.

Invasive staging procedures

Different therapeutic approaches can only be adequately assessed with adequate staging. The traditional imaging techniques such as CT and MRI scans are helpful for determining local extension of the disease, but may not accurately assess mediastinal or distant disease. The use of positron-emission tomography (PET) scanning has helped with the staging of distant metastases, but to date it has proved ineffective in the staging of mediastinal disease. The most common surgical procedures employed to stage MPM are thoracoscopy, cervical mediastinoscopy, and to a lesser extent laparoscopy.

Video-assisted thoracoscopy

At the time of surgical diagnosis exploration of the pleural cavity via thoracoscopy can aid in determining the extent of local disease in cases with suspected early stage mesothelioma. The main benefit is obtained by determining involvement of the visceral pleura by tumour. As reported by Bergonzini *et al.* [13], it appears mandatory to sample both pleural surfaces when dealing with early stages of MPM. In more advanced stages of the disease the role of thoracoscopy for staging is more limited. Confirmation of extrapleural mediastinal lymphatic involvement via VATS can be achieved for the staging of lung cancer [14] but has not been extensively employed in MPM. Technical barriers exist such as thickened mediastinal pleura.

Cervical mediastinoscopy

Involvement of extrapleural lymph nodes by tumour is a recurrent prognostic factor in most series. Some surgeons advocate not doing radical surgery in the presence of mediastinal lymph node metastases. Certainly, lymph node involvement should prompt consideration of initial treatment with chemotherapy [7,15,16]. Imaging techniques have consistently been inaccurate in providing adequate mediastinal staging. Rusch and Venkatraman [17] and Schouwink *et al.* [18] reported accuracies of mediastinal staging of 75 per cent and 67 per cent, respectively, with the use of CT scanning. In our experience contrast-enhanced MRI scanning, with a sensitivity of 66 per cent and a specificity of 73 per cent, has proved of no additional benefit to CT scanning in mediastinal staging [19]. There has been recent interest in the use of PET scanning to stage MPM. Recent reports have shown the effectiveness of PET scanning to determine the presence of distant metastases in MPM, but mediastinal staging remains inaccurate. In the largest study to date, Flores *et al.* [20] showed that nine of 31 surgically staged patients who underwent preoperative PET scanning had mediastinal nodal involvement and PET could only identify one of these. Bernard *et al.* [21] reported similar findings regarding the inaccuracy of PET scanning to stage the mediastinum. Furthermore, we have recently reported our findings in our own experience with radical surgery for MPM describing no correlation between pathological size of lymph nodes and presence of malignant involvement [16]. The inaccuracies of imaging methods to stage the mediastinum has led to high rates of extrapleural node involvement in the largest series that involve radical surgery (Table 12.2).

Table 12.2 Incidence of extrapleural lymph node metastasis (N2 disease) found in series of radical surgery for malignant pleural mesothelioma

	Year	Total number of patients	Incidence of N2 disease
Maggi et al. [15]	2001	32	9 (28%)
Schouwink et al. [18]	2003	24	4 (17%)*
Rusch and Venkatraman [17]	1999	157	82 (52%)
Sugarbaker et al. [7]	1999	176	40 (23%)
Aziz et al. [22]	2002	64	14 (22%)
Pilling et al. [16]	2003	55	17 (31%)

*After routine cervical mediastinoscopy to exclude N2 disease.

Cervical mediastinoscopy has been shown to be accurate in staging the mediastinum in MPM, thus potentially avoiding radical surgery in advanced stages of the disease. The diagnostic accuracy was 93 per cent in a recent study involving 43 patients with MPM conducted by Schouwink et al. [18]. The procedure is performed under a general anaesthesia via a 3–5 cm transverse suprasternal incision for the insertion of a mediastinoscope through the pretracheal fascia enabling inspection and biopsies of Naruke's stations 2, 3, 4, and 7 [23] (Fig. 12.1), and is associated with extremely low morbidity [24]. There are shortcomings, as mediastinoscopy does not reach lymph node stations 6, 8, or 9 or other areas such as the internal mammary or peridiaphragmatic regions where lymph nodes are frequently involved. Therefore complete lymph node staging in MPM is not possible via mediastinoscopy. The development of video-assisted techniques aid in the training and supervision of the procedure [25], and the ability to use two instruments simultaneously can increase the size of the biopsy specimens [26]. These advances have permitted us to experiment with entering the pleural cavity during cervical mediastinoscopy to perform pleural biopsy and talc pleurodesis in addition to mediastinal lymph node staging via a single mediastinoscopy incision in patients with MPM considered for radical surgery (Fig. 12.2).

At present, staging cervical mediastinoscopy is favoured as routine prior to radical surgery in mesothelioma, although not all surgeons concur with this opinion.

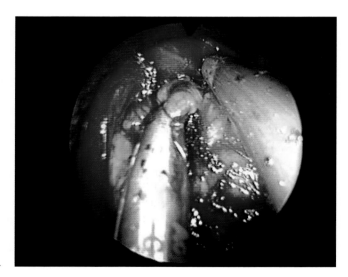

Figure 12.1 Video-assisted cervical mediastinoscopy in the staging of malignant mesothelioma. The 'bimanual' exploration facilitates sampling.

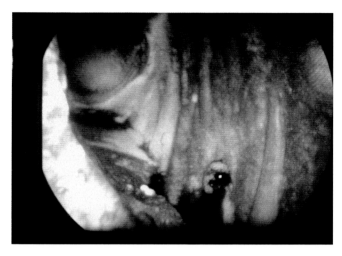

Figure 12.2 Inspection of the right pleural cavity via video-assisted cervical thoracoscopy. The procedure permits biopsy, pleurodesis, and nodal staging via single cervical incision.

Laparoscopy

Laparoscopy does not form part of routine staging of MPM. Its use has been reported in cases where imaging techniques revealed doubts about transdiaphragmatic spread of the disease, thus making it potentially non-resectable. In this subgroup of patients Conlon *et al.* [27] recommend its use following their 100 per cent staging accuracy in 12 patients with MPM who were considered for radical surgery and CT scanning was equivocal in assessing transdiaphragmatic spread of the tumour [27]. They reported no complications and a median hospital stay of 1 day, and concluded that laparoscopy should be used prior to radical surgery in cases where transdiaphragmatic spread cannot be excluded with radiology. However, there is no evidence to suggest any benefit in the routine use of laparoscopy for staging of MPM in the presence of an unequivocal CT scan.

An important example of the need for surgical staging prior to radical surgery for mesothelioma was the work by Maggi *et al.* [15] who, in a series of 32 patients, attempted to repeat the treatment regimen of Sugarbaker *et al.* [7] with extrapleural pneumonectomy followed by adjuvant chemotherapy and hemithoracic radiation. The results were encouraging, with only 6.25 per cent operative mortality. However, 50 per cent of the patients were found to be in stage III after surgery, which is reflected in the rather disappointing median survival of 9.5 months after operation. The authors confirmed that preoperative staging with CT or MRI was inaccurate in detecting mediastinal lymph node involvement or transdiaphragmatic tumour spread. Therefore they suggest transbronchial subcarinal lymph node biospy, routine cervical mediastinoscopy and laparoscopy prior to radical surgery for MPM.

Further advances are also required to determine T3 pericardial involvement prior to radical surgery as at present no staging modalities have proved accurate.

Palliative therapeutic procedures

Whilst radical surgery remains controversial, an accepted role for surgery in MPM has been to palliate its symptoms. Although clinical presentation can vary according to the stage of the disease, dyspnoea due to pleural effusion (80–100 per cent), chest pain (40–72 per cent), cough (15–60 per cent), and weight loss are the most commonly reported symptoms in surgical series [28–31]. Different surgical procedures have been advocated for symptom control in selected patients not considered for radical surgery; pleurodesis and parietal pleurectomy have been clearly shown to provide lasting symptom relief when the lung expands to occupy the pleural cavity. A more difficult decision is faced when the underlying lung fails to re-expand after drainage of the effusion due to encasement by diseased visceral pleura; this is known as 'trapped-lung syndrome'.

Chemical pleurodesis

The most common indication for intervention in malignant mesothelioma is for control of pleural effusion. Although thoracocentesis can prove effective initially, most malignant effusions will recur rapidly within 1–3 days [32]. Repeated pleural aspirations should be the very last resort reserved for terminally ill patients, but otherwise avoided at all costs because of the risks of iatrogenic pleural sepsis and malignant empyema. Effective control of the effusion is usually accomplished by chemical pleurodesis, and the outcomes appear better when performed via VATS at the time of biopsy rather than through an intercostal drain [33]. Most reports based on randomized trials and reviews conclude that sterile iodized talc is superior to other agents and should be the agent of choice for chemical pleurodesis [34,35]. Although side effects such as pain, respiratory failure, and acute pneumonitis have been reported following instillation of talc in the pleural cavity [36], their incidence is very low and normally related to administration of large doses of talc (10 g).

Success of the pleurodesis is dependent on expansion of the underlying lung to facilitate apposition of the visceral and parietal pleurae. Cardillo et al. [6] reported 93 per cent control of recurrent effusions with videothoracosocpic insufflation of 5g of sterile purified talc in this situation. Operative mortality was less than 1 per cent and there was no documented acute respiratory distress syndrome. Schulze et al. [37] reported similar results in 101 patients with malignant pleural effusion with relief of dyspnoea in 92 per cent of cases. In an institutional review of 88 patients with symptomatic mesothelioma undergoing medical or surgical thoracoscopy with insufflation of talc, Viallat et al. [38] reported initial success within 1 month of 90 per cent and life-lasting resolution of the effusion in almost 80 per cent of cases. Unfortunately, as outlined in a recent review of conservative measures, subsequent survival is limited at around 7 months although those with an epitheloid tumour survived longer [42] (Table 12.3).

Debulking pleurectomy

Debulking parietal pleurectomy may be considered as an addition to talc pleurodesis. It has shown benefits in terms of providing a lasting and effective pleurodesis, giving the opportunity

Table 12.3 Summary of reports using VATS talc pleurodesis for malignant pleural effusion

	Year	Number	Mortality	Success rate
Ohri et al. [39]	1992	100	5%	95%
LoCicero [33]	1993	40	NS	100%
Bal and Hasan [41]	1993	213	2.3%	93%
Hartman [40]	1993	39	–	95%
Viallat et al. [38]	1996	88	1%	90%
Schulze et al. [37]	2001	105	2.8%	92%
Cardillo et al. [6]	2002	611	0.8%	93%

NS, not stated.

to obtain large volumes of tissue in cases of difficult histological diagnosis, and symptomatic benefit of both dyspnoea and chest wall pain together with the potential therapeutic benefits of cytoreduction. Before the development of VATS, the role of pleurectomy for mesothelioma was explored via thoracotomy. There is controversy regarding whether the risk of surgery outweighs the benefits when thoracotomy is performed for palliation in patients whose survival is limited.

Thoracotomy

Unfortunately, pleurectomy performed through a thoracotomy has been linked in the past with high morbidity and is therefore generally avoided, although there are exceptions such as the report by Martini *et al.* [43] with an operative mortality of 10 per cent.

In the largest series to date, Achatzy *et al.* [44] reviewed their experience with 245 patients with MPM of whom 118 were treated with pleurectomy. The operative mortality and morbidity were lower (6 per cent and 8 per cent, respectively). Of note is their finding that median survival was better in patients treated surgically than in the non-operative cases (10 months vs. 6 months).

More recent studies [22,45,46] have reported success in the use of pleurectomy with lower mortality rates (ranging from zero to 2 per cent), although morbidity rates approach 20 per cent.

In some of the reports pleurectomy has been employed as part of multimodality regimes. A variety of intrapleural therapies have been attempted in this setting, aiming to enhance local control of the disease. Sauter *et al.* [47] reported a lack of benefit of intrapleural chemotherapy at the time of pleurectomy. Indeed, survival and disease progression were worse in patients who underwent intrapleural cytarabine and cisplatin therapy in addition to adjuvant systemic chemotherapy after pleurectomy than patients who did not receive pleural chemotherapy.

Takita *et al.* [48] and Pass *et al.* [45] reported protocols that incorporated intrapleural photodynamic therapy with pleurectomy. Although mortality rates were acceptable, the protocols did not improve local control of the disease or survival significantly, and the complication rates were excessive (up to 50 per cent). Overall, intrapleural therapies in addition to pleurectomy cannot be routinely recommended at present because of failure to enhance local control of the disease and the increased morbidity rates of these approaches (Table 12.4).

Table 12.4 Reports incorporating debulking pleurectomy for malignant pleural mesothelioma using thoracotomy.

	Number	Procedure	Multimodality	Mortality	Survival (months)
Martini *et al.* [43]	14	Pleurectomy	–	10%	–
McCormack *et al.* [49]	64	Pleurectomy	Variable	1.5%	12.6
Hilaris *et al.* [50]	41	Pleurectomy	Radiotherapy	0%	21
Chahinian *et al.* [29]	30	Pleurectomy	Variable	0%	13
Achatzy *et al.* [44]	118	Pleurectomy	Variable	6%	9
Brancatisano *et al.* [46]	50	Pleurectomy	–	2%	16
Rusch *et al.* [65]	28	Pleurectomy	Pleural chemotherapy	3.6%	17
Takita and Dougherty [48]	22	Pleurectomy	Pleural phototherapy	4.5%	12
Soysal *et al.* [64]	100	Pleurectomy	Variable	1%	17
Pass *et al.* [45]	39	Pleurectomy	Pleural phototherapy	2%	14
Aziz *et al.* [22]	47	Pleurectomy	Chemotherapy	0%	14
De Vries and Long [51]	29	Pleurectomy	Variable	3.8%	9

Table 12.5 Reports incorporating VATS techniques in palliative debulking surgical practice for malignant mesothelioma

	Number	Procedure	Mortality	Success
Waller *et al.* [52]	13	Pleurectomy	0	100% (13/13)
Grossebner *et al.* [11]	21	Pleurectomy and mobilization	0	71% (15/21)
Martin-Ucar *et al.* [28]	17	Pleurectomy	0	100% (17/17)
Ceresoli *et al.* [53]	54	Pleurectomy	NS	NS
Cardillo *et al.* [6]	29	Decortication	0	97% (28/29)
Atkins *et al.* [54]	7	Decortication	0	100% (7/7)

NS, not stated.

Video-assisted thoracoscopic pleurectomy

With increasing expertise and expansion in the use of VATS techniques, subtotal debulking parietal pleurectomy can be carried out effectively with minimal morbidity and over 90 per cent effusion control at 12 months [52]. The procedure is traditionally performed via three port incisions, and after division of loculations and adhesions the effusion is drained. Once lung expansion is tested with positive pressure ventilation, the pleurectomy is carried out in a similar manner to the more universal procedure for recurrent pneumothorax. In malignant cases, the parietal pleurectomy is not restricted to the apical part of the pleural cavity but extended as far as possible towards the diaphragm. The fear of postoperative haemorrhage after the procedure has not been confirmed; it is possibly prevented by lung expansion and rapid apposition onto the chest wall. In a retrospective study of 121 patients, Ceresoli *et al.* [53] found that debulking pleurectomy resulted in better survival than supportive care only, with a median survival of 12.5 months. In our own series of debulking surgery for mesothelioma, VATS pleurectomy was possible in 17 cases not suitable for radical surgery in which the lung re-expanded after the effusion was drained. In this subgroup of patients no mortality or major morbidity was encountered and a lifelong resolution of the effusion was obtained with the addition of maintained symptomatic benefit until disease progression [28]. Grossebner *et al.* [11] described the benefits of VATS pleurectomy by obtaining confirmation of diagnosis, resolution of effusion, and partial debulking in a one-stage procedure with low mortality and morbidity rates (Table 12.5).

Trapped-lung syndrome

The development of a pleural effusion causes collapse of the underlying lung parenchyma, and the disease involving the visceral pleura may lead to the development of a cortex entrapping the collapsed lung tissue in the same manner as observed during chronic empyemas, i.e. trapped-lung syndrome. By definition, because of the cortex the lung will not re-expand even after drainage of the effusion (Fig. 12.3). The management of trapped lung due to MPM remains difficult and clinicians have advocated very different strategies.

Long-term drainage

Long-term indwelling pleural drainage catheters have been employed in the management of malignant pleural effusions. The advantages include a low level of immediate complications, patients are not required to undergo a general anaesthesia, and it can even be performed as an outpatient procedure with resource implications. In these terms, Putnam *et al.* [55] described their experience of managing 100 patients with malignant pleural effusions of diverse origin (60 per cent as outpatients) with chronic indwelling pleural catheters. In their experience the compli-

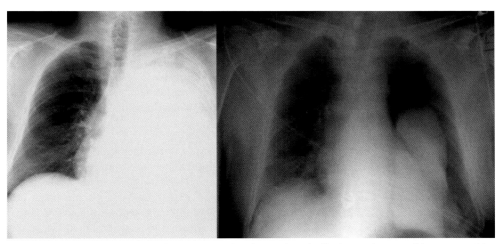

Figure 12.3 *Chest* radiographs of a patient with a large pleural effusion and trapped lung caused by mesothelioma after drainage of the effusion.

cation rate approaches 20 per cent. Pien *et al.* [56] described their experience with 11 cases (six of them with MPM) and reported a 50 per cent treatment-specific complication rate. In addition to the complications of long-term drainage, re-expansion of the lung does not occur if the lung is encased by thick tumour cortex, and this approach condemns patients to months of permanent drainage with consequences for the quality of life and the need of continuous nursing support.

Although the principle of a relatively low-invasive procedure for palliation of symptoms is very attractive, the available data suggest that the use of lifelong pleural catheters should be reserved for cases unfit to undergo any surgical procedure and with a very short life expectancy.

Pleuroperitoneal shunt

Pleuroperitoneal shunts have been described in the management of malignant pleural effusions since 1982 [57]. The device consists of a pump chamber, inserted subcutaneously, with two connected limbs with one-way valves that communicate with the pleural and peritoneal cavities. It is inserted via a limited thoracotomy or VATS with the addition of a small incision to enter the peritoneal cavity. It requires lifelong manual pumping of the device by the patient to drain the fluid from the pleural to the peritoneal cavity. Schulze *et al.* [37] has recently reported a small series of cases with malignant pleural effusion where the lung would not re-expand after effusion drainage. VATS was used to place a shunt between pleural and peritoneal cavities under vision. Although the authors reported improvement of dyspnoea in 73 per cent of cases, 30-day mortality was 21 per cent and surgical re-intervention for shunt dysfunction was required in two of 14 cases. Genc *et al.* [58] from the Royal Brompton Hospital reported similar results in their larger series where shunt specific complications requiring re-intervention occurred in 15 per cent of cases. With a hospital mortality of less than 2 per cent, median survival of patients with MPM was 10 months. Unfortunately, the authors did not include data regarding any symptomatic improvement of pain or dyspnoea following surgery. The rate of shunt complications is consistent with other reports such as that of Lee *et al.* [59] who described an incidence of shunt blockage of up to 25 per cent, or the earlier report from Tsang *et al.* [60] in 1990 who described insertion of pleuroperitoneal shunts in 16 patients with one postoperative mortality and two blocked shunts. Other complications have been described such as pneumoperitoneum and peritonitis caused by air pumping from a pneumothorax [61]. An important contraindication for insertion of shunts is the presence of pleural sepsis, which is more likely to happen if patients have undergone multiple diagnostic or palliative procedures. Despite control of the effusion by drainage into the peritoneal cavity, the relief of dyspnoea is far from universal after pleuroperitoneal shunting, reflecting the persistent problem of underlying pulmonary collapse. This problem can only really be addressed by decortication of the lung. Finally, pleuroperitoneal shunts place MPM patients at risk for tumour implantation in the peritoneum and subsequent symptomatic ascites. All in all, pleuroperitoneal shunts are not recommended for the palliative management of MPM.

Thoracotomy for decortication (Table 12.6)

The rationale for visceral decortication of trapped lung was described by Ryzman *et al.* [62] when they reported the physiological benefits of lung re-expansion following chronic empyemas. Their results after decortication concur with those of other authors with improvement of vital capacity and forced expiratory volume in 1 s (FEV_1), correction of ventilation–perfusion mismatch, and recovery of oxygenation [63]. In a retrospective review of our experience [28], we found that decortication was required in 66 per cent of a series of 51 consecutive patients with MPM; 30-day mortality was 7.8 per cent and significant morbidity was encountered in seven further patients. A significant improvement in dyspnoea and chest pain was obtained until disease progression. However, the symptomatic improvement was outweighed by the increasing mortality more than 3 months post-surgery. One year survival was only 31 per cent, but was significantly higher in those with epithelial cell type and without weight loss prior to surgery. Brancatisano *et al.* [46] reported the need to decorticate a trapped lung in 28 of 50 consecutive patients (56 per cent) surgically debulked for MPM. Soysal *et al.* [64] reviewed their experience, also reporting a 56 per cent need for decortication due to trapped lung in their series of 100 cytoreductive procedures in consecutive patients with MPM, again with a very low mortality of 1 per cent.

Thoracotomy with pleurectomy–decortication for MPM has also been reported in combination with other modalities of treatment. In 1994, Rusch *et al.* [65] reported their experience with the use of intrapleural mitomycin and cisplatin immediately after pleurectomy–decortication. This protocol resulted in a median survival of 17 months, with a mortality of 3.6 per cent and significant morbidity in over 25 per cent of cases. Unfortunately, 80 per cent of patients present-

Table 12.6 Experiences reported with the use of debulking decortication due to malignant mesothelioma via thoracotomy

	Number	Procedure	Multimodality	Mortality	Survival (months)
Rusch et al. [65]	28	Pleurectomy–decortication	Pleural chemotherapy	3.6%	17
Brancatisano et al. [46]	50	Pleurectomy–decortication		2%	16
Rice et al. [68]	19	Decortication	Pleural chemotherapy	5%	13
Soysal et al. [64]	100	Pleurectomy–decortication	Variable	1%	17
Pass et al. [69]	23	Decortication	Pleural phototherapy	–	22
Martin-Ucar et al. [28]	34	Decortication	–	11%	7
Takagi et al. [67]	73	Decortication	variable	6%	12
Aziz et al. [22]	47	Decortication	variable	0%	14
De Bree et al. [66]	11	Decortication	Pleural chemotherapy	0%	NS

NS, not stated.

ed with locoregional progression of the disease. De Bree *et al.* [66] reported open cytoreductive surgery and intraoperative chemotherapy in 11 patients with MPM with no mortality. The short follow-up at the time of their report did not permit any conclusions regarding survival benefit. Aziz *et al.* [22] performed palliative debulking via thoracotomy over 10 years on 47 patients with MPM who were not suitable for radical surgery because of advanced stage or unfitness for the procedure. They reported no mortality and the survival equalled that of extrapleural pneumonectomy as the single modality of treatment. The same conclusion was obtained from a multicentre survey in Japan [67] which included 73 patients with a 6 per cent postoperative mortality and a median survival of 12 months, similar to the results for patients who underwent radical surgery as a single modality of treatment. A similar median survival (13 months) was reported by Rice *et al.* [68] on 19 patients with MPM who underwent pleurectomy–decortication followed by intrapleural chemotherapy. They reported a 5 per cent postoperative death rate. Pass *et al.* [69] also reported their experience with pleurectomy–decortication in 39 patients and observed a median survival of 14.5 months with low postoperative morbidity. However, they were unable to debulk 17 patients because of large tumour volumes, and the median survival in this group was only 5 months (Table 12.6).

Video-assisted thoracoscopic decortication

As the use of VATS increases, new indications have been described for the technique in the belief that the perioperative complications inherent to open surgery may be ameliorated by the avoidance of muscle division and rib spreading. Cytoreductive surgery via VATS has rarely been reported, and there have been very few reports of adding visceral decortication of tumour to pleurectomy. Grossebner *et al.* [11] al reported a series of cases with MPM where a combination of VATS cytoreductive pleurectomy and lung mobilization was found to obliterate the pleural space effectively in nearly 75 per cent of cases. The use of VATS to achieve visceral decortication has been reported in postpneumonic empyema, even in chronic cases [69], and Cardillo *et al.* [6] recently reported the use of VATS to remove the visceral pleural tumour in 29 patients with an entrapped lung after effusion drainage. They achieved significantly better effusion control than with talc poudrage alone. The procedure is performed via three port incisions and, after evacuation of the effusion, the affected lung is subjected to positive ventilation of up to 40 cmH$_2$O to attempt expansion. We have found that, despite the appearance of a visceral layer encasing the affected lung, with this manoeuvre and debridement the lung achieves satisfactory expansion so that chemical or surgical pleurodesis can be performed. VATS has recently been successful in decorticating trapped lungs in seven patients with MPM in whom the lung would not re-expand after the previously reported measures [54]. By using a combination of sharp and blunt dissection the visceral cortex can be 'peeled' from the lung in a similar manner as with traditional open decortication (Figs 12.4 and 12.5). Lung expansion was achieved in all patients (Fig. 12.6). The median drainage time was 8 days and length of stay was 7 days. No postoperative mortality, major morbidity, or recurrence of effusions at follow-up occurred. Although this is a technique that requires expertise in VATS, it offers a favourable alternative to lifelong drainage or pleuroperitoneal shunts, and it can be performed in patients not fit enough to undergo open decortication.

Summary

There is a well-established role for surgery in determining diagnosis and achieving chemical pleurodesis in MPM. With more centres offering aggressive therapies that involve radical surgery, the value of surgery in improvement of staging of the disease is gaining importance. However,

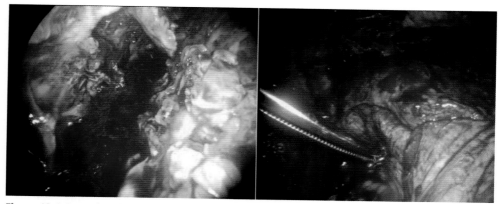

Figure 12.4 Operative view of trapped lung caused by mesothelioma treated by video-assisted thoracoscopic decortication.

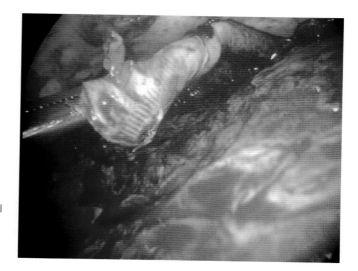

Figure 12.5 The visceral pleural peel can be removed in the same manner as for a chronic empyema.

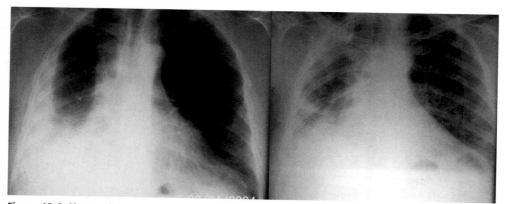

Figure 12.6 *Chest* radiographs of a trapped lung before and after video-assisted thoracoscopic decortication.

many patients with MPM will not be fit or suitable for radical surgery. Aziz *et al.* [22] assessed 302 patients in their dedicated surgical unit over 10 years, and only 64 of them (21 per cent) underwent extrapleural pneumonectomy. As the incidence of the disease increases [71] and more diagnostic operations are being performed because of the introduction of VATS [72], palliative surgical procedures for symptom control have to be considered. Improvements in perioperative care have now made more extensive surgery feasible, even in conjunction with other modalities of treatment. However, the morbidity and mortality of palliative procedures have to be justified not only by an increased survival, but also by improved quality of life. These aspects should be addressed in future prospective studies.

References

1. Renshaw AA, Dean BR, Antman KH, Sugarbaker DJ, Cibas ES. The role of cytologic evaluation of pleural fluid in the diagnosis of malignant mesothelioma. *Chest* 1997; **111**: 106–9.
2. Baumann M. Closed pleural biopsy: a necessary tool? *Pulm Perspect* 2000; **17**: 1–3
3. Adams RF, Gray W, Davies RJO, Gleeson FV. Percutaneous image-cutting needle biopsy of the pleura in the diagnosis of malignant mesothelioma. *Chest* 2001; **120**: 1798–1802.
4. Boutin C, Rey F. Thoracoscopy in pleural malignant mesothelioma: a prospective study of 188 consecutive patients.*Cancer* 1993; **72**: 389–93
5. Blanc F-X, Atassi K, Bignon J, Housset B. Diagnostic value of medical thoracoscopy in pleural disease. A 6 year retrospective review. *Chest* 2002; **121**: 1677–83.
6. Cardillo G, Facciolo F, Carbone FL, *et al.* Long-term follow-up of video-assisted talc pleurodesis in malignant recurrent pleural effusions. *Eur J Cardiothorac Surg* 2002; **21**: 302–6.
7. Sugarbaker DJ, Flores RM, Jaklitsch MT, *et al.* Resection margins, extrapleural nodal status and cell type determine postoperative long-term survival in trimodality therapy of malignant pleural mesothelioma. *J Thorac Cardiovasc Surg* 1999; **117**: 54–65.
8. Waller DA, Hasan A, Forty J, Morritt GN. Videothoracoscopy in the diagnosis of intrathoracic pathology: early experience. *Ann R Coll Surg Engl* 1994; **76**: 123–6.
9. Menzies R, Charbonneau M. Thoracoscopy for the diagnosis of pleural disease. *Ann Intern Med* 1991; **114**: 271–6.
10. Canto A, Guijarro R, Arnau A, Galbis J, Martorell M, Garcia Aguado R. Videothoracoscopy in the diagnosis and tratment of malignant pleural mesothelioma with associated pleural effusions. *Thorac Cardiovasc Surg* 1997; **45**: 16–19.
11. Grossebner MW, Arifi AA, Goddard M, Ritchie AJ. Mesothelioma—VATS biopsy and lung mobilization improves diagnosis and palliation. *Eur J Cardiothorac Surg* 1999; **16**: 619–23.
12. Boutin C, Rey F, Viallat JR. Prevention of malignant seeding after invasive diagnostic procedures in patients with pleural mesothelioma. A randomized trial of local radiotherapy. *Chest* 1995; **108**: 754–58.
13. Bergonzini R, Olivetti L, Tassi GF, Chiodera PL. Malignant mesothelioma of the pleura: correlations between thoracoscopy and radiology. *Radiol Med* 1996; **92**: 52–7.
14. Hoffmann H. Invasive staging of lung cancer by mediastinoscopy and video-assisted thoracoscopy. *Lung Cancer* 2001; **34** (Suppl 30): S3–5.
15. Maggi G, Casadio C, Cianci R, Rena O, Ruffini E. Trimodality management of malignant pleural mesothelioma. *Eur J Cardiothorac Surg* 2001; **19**: 346–50.
16. Pilling JE, Stewart DJ, Martin-Ucar AE, Muller S, O'Byrne KJ, Waller DA. The case for routine cervical mediastinoscopy prior to radical surgery for malignant pleural mesothelioma. *Eur J Cardiothorac Surg* 2004; **25**: 497–501.
17. Rusch VW, Venkatraman E. Important prognostic factors in patients with malignant pleural mesothelioma managed surgically. *Ann Thorac Surg* 1999; **68**: 1799–1804.
18. Schouwink JH, Kool LS, Rutgers EJ, *et al. Ann Thorac Surg* 2003; **75**: 1715–18.

19. Stewart D, Waller DA, Edwards JG, Jeyapalan K, Entwisle J. Is there a role for pre-operative contrast-enhanced magnetic resonance imaging for radical surgery in malignant pleural mesothelioma? *Eur J Cardiothorac Surg* 2003; **24**: 1019–24.

20. Flores RM, Akhurst T, Gonen M, Larson SM, Rusch VW. Positron emission tomography defines metastatic disease but not locoregional disease in patients with malignant pleural mesothelioma. *J Thorac Cardiovasc Surg.* 2003; **126**: 11–16

21. Bernard F, Sterman D, Smith R, Kaiser L, Albelda S, Alavi A. Metabolic imaging of malignant pleural mesothelioma with fluorodeoxyglucose positron emission tomography. *Chest* 1998; **114**: 713–22.

22. Aziz T, Jilaihawi A, Prakash D. The management of malignant pleural mesothelioma: single centre experience in 10 years. *Eur J Cardiothorac Surg* 2002; **22**: 298–305.

23. Naruke T, Suemasu K, Ishikawa S. Lymph node mapping and curability at various levels of metastasis in resected lung cancer. *J Thorac Cardiovasc Surg* 1978; **79**: 832–9.

24. Venissac N, Alifano M, Mouroux J. Video-assisted mediastinoscopy: experience from 240 consecutive cases. *Ann Thorac Surg* 2003; **76**: 208–12.

25. Martin-Ucar AE, Chetty GK, Vaughan R, Waller DA. A prospective audit of video assisted mediastinoscopy as a training tool. *Eur J Cardiothorac Surg* 2003; **26** 393–5.

26. Hurtgen M, Friedel G, Toomes H, Fritz P. Radical video-assisted mediastinoscopic lymphadenectomy (VAMLA)—technique and first results. *Eur J Cardiothorac Surg.* 2002; **21**: 348–51.

27. Conlon KC, Rusch VW, Gillern S. Laparoscopy: an important tool in the staging of malignant pleural mesothelioma. *Ann Surg Oncol* 1996; **3**: 489–94 .

28. Martin-Ucar AE, Edwards JG, Rengajaran A, Muller S, Waller DA. Palliative surgical debulking in malignant mesothelioma. Predictors of survival and symptom control. *Eur J Cardiothorac Surg* 2001; **20**: 1117–21.

29. Chaninian AP, Pajak TF, Holland JF, Norton L, Ambinder MR, Mandel EM. Diffuse malignant mesothelioma. Prospective evaluation of 69 patients. *Ann Intern Med* 1982; **96**: 746–55.

30. Sugarbaker DJ, Norberto JJ. Multimodality management of malignant pleural mesothelioma. *Chest* 1998; **113**: 61–5S.

31. Edwards JG, Abrams KR, Leverment JN, Spyt TJ, Waller DA, O'Byrne KJ. Prognostic factors for malignant mesothelioma in 142 patients: validation of CALGB and EORTC prognostic scoring systems. *Thorax* 2000; **55**: 731–5.

32. Anderson CB, Philpott GW, Ferguson TB. The treatment of malignant pleural effusions. *Cancer* 1974; **33**: 916–22.

33. LoCicero J. Thoracoscopic management of malignant pleural effusion.*Ann Thorac Surg* 1993; **56**: 641–3.

34. Keller SM. Current and future therapy for malignant pleural mesothelioma. *Chest* 1993; **103**: 63S–7S.

35. Walker-Renard PB, Vaughan LM, Sahn SA. Chemical pleurodesis in malignant pleural effusions. *Ann Intern Med* 1994; **120**: 56–64.

36. Bouchama A, Chastre J, Gaudichet A, Soler P, Gibert C. Acute pneumonitis with bilateral pleural effusion after talc pleurodesis. *Chest* 1984; **86**: 795–7.

37. Schulze M, Boehle AS, Kurdow R, Dohrmann P, Henne- Bruns D. Effective treatment of malignant pleural effusion by minimal invasive thoracic surgery : thoracoscopic talc pleurodesis and pleuroperitoneal shunts in 101 patients. *Ann Thorac Surg* 2001; **71**: 1809–12.

38. Viallat JR, Rey F, Astoul P, Boutin C. Thoracoscopic talc poudrage pleurodesis for malignant effusions. A review of 360 cases. *Chest* 1996; **110**: 1387–93.

39. Ohri SK, Oswal SK, Townsend ER, Fountain SW. (1992) Early and late outcome after diagnostic thoracoscopy and talc pleurodesis. *Ann Thorac Surg* 53: 1038–41.

40. Hartman DL, Gaither JM, Kesler KA, Mylet DM, Brown JW, Mathur PN. Comparison of insufflated talc under thoracoscopic guidance with standard tetracycline and bleomycin pleurodesis for control of malignant pleural effusions. *J Thorac Cardiovasc Surg* 1993; **105**: 743–7.

41. Bal S, Hasan SS. Thoracoscopic management of malignant pleural effusion. *Int Surg* 1993; **78**: 324–7.

42. Merritt N, Blewett CJ, Miller JD, Bennett WF, Young JEM, Urschel JD. Survival after conservative (palliative) management of pleural malignant mesothelioma. *J Surg Oncol* 2001; **78**: 171–4.

43. Martini N, Bains MS, Beattie EJ. Indications for pleurectomy in malignant effusion. *Cancer* 1975; **35**: 734–8.

44. Achatzy R, Beba W, Ritschler R, *et al*. The diagnosis, therapy and prognosis of diffuse malignant mesothelioma. *Eur J Cardiothorac Surg* 1989; **3**: 445–8.

45. Pass HI, Temeck BK, Kranda K, *et al*. Phase III randomized trial of surgery with or without intraoperative photodynamic therapy and postoperative immunochemotherapy for malignant pleural mesothelioma. *Ann Surg Oncol* 1997; **4**: 628–33.

46. Brancatisano RP, Joseph MG, McCaughan BC. Pleurectomy for mesothelioma. *Med J Aust* 1991; **154**: 455–7, 460.

47. Sauter ER, Langer C, Coia LR, Goldberg M, Keller SM. Optimal management of malignant mesothelioma after subtotal pleurectomy: revisiting the role of intrapleural chemotherapy and postoperative radiation. *J Surg Oncol*. 1995; **60**: 100–5

48. Takita II, Dougherty TJ. Intracavitary photodynamic therapy for malignant pleural mesothelioma. *Semin Surg Oncol* 1995; **11**: 368–71.

49. McCormack PM, Nagasaki F, Hilaris BS, Martini N. Surgical treatment of mesothelioma. *J Thorac Cardiovasc Surg* 1982; **84**: 834–42.

50. Hilaris BS, Nori D, Kwong E, Kutcher GJ, Martini N. Pleurectomy and intraoperative brachytherapy and postoperative radiation in the treatment of malignant pleural mesothelioma. *Int J Radiat Oncol Biol Phys* 1984; **10**: 325–31.

51. de Vries WJ, Long MA. Treatment of mesothelioma in Bloemfontein, South Africa. *Eur J Cardiothorac Surg* 2003; **24**: 434–40.

52. Waller DA, Morritt GN, Forty J. Video-assisted thoracoscopic pleurectomy in the management of malignant pleural effusion. *Chest* 1995; **107**: 1454–6.

53. Ceresoli GL, Locati LD, Ferreri AJM, *et al*. Therapeutic outcome according to histological subtype in 121 patients with malignant pleural mesothelioma. *Lung Cancer* 2001; **34**: 279–87.

54. Atkins JL, Khan OA, Martin-Ucar AE, Waller DA. An audit of thoracoscopic decortication as the treatment of choice for 'trapped lung' of unknown aetiology. *Thorax* 2003; **58** (Suppl III): iii26

55. Putnam JB Jr, Walsh GL, Swisher SG, *et al*. Outpatient management of malignant pleural effusion by a chronic indwelling pleural catheter. *Ann Thorac Surg* 2000; **69**: 369–75.

56. Pien GW, Gant MJ, Washam CL, Sterman DH. Use of an implantable pleural catheter for trapped lung syndrome in patients with malignant pleural effusion. *Chest* 2001; **119**: 1641–6.

57. Weese JL, Schouten JT. Pleural peritoneal shunts for the treatment of malignant pleural effusions. *Surg Gynecol Obstet* 1982; **154**: 391–2.

58. Genc O, Petrou M, Ladas G, Goldstraw P. The long-term morbidity of pleuroperitoneal shunts in the management of recurrent malignant effusions *Eur J Cardiothorac Surg* 2000; **18**: 143–6.

59. Lee KA, Harvey JC, Reich H, Beattie EJ. Management of malignant pleural effusions with pleuroperitoneal shunting. *J Am Coll Surg* 1994; **178**: 586–8.

60. Tsang V, Fernando HC, Goldstraw P. Pleuroperitoneal shunts for recurrent malignant pleural effusions. *Thorax* 1990; **45**: 369–72.

61. Lopez-Viego MA, Cornell JM. Pneumoperitoneum and signs of peritonitis from a pleuroperitoneal shunt. *Surgery* 1992; **111**: 228–9.

62. Ryzman W, Skokowski J, Romaniwicz G, Lass P, Dziadziuszko R. Decortication in chronic pleural empyema—effect on lung function. *Eur J Cardiothorac Surg* 2002; **21**: 502–7.

63. Swoboda L, Laule K, Blattmann H, Hasse J. Decortication in chronic pleural empyema. Investigation of lung function based on perfusion scintigraphy. *Thorac Cardiovasc Surgeon*. 1990; **38**: 359–61.

64. Soysal O, Karaoglanoglu N, Demiracan S, *et al*. Pleurectomy/decortication for palliation in malignant pleural mesothelioma: results of surgery. *Eur J Cardiothorac Surg*. 1997; **11**: 210–13.

65. Rusch VW, Saltz L, Venkatraman E, *et al.* A phase II trial of pleurectomy/decortication followed by intrapleural and systemic chemotherapy for malignant pleural mesothelioma. *J Clin Oncol* 1994; **12:** 1156–63.

66. De Bree E, van Ruth S, Baas P, *et al.* Cytoreductive surgery and intraoperative hyperthermic intrathoracic chemotherapy in patients with malignant pleural mesothelioma or pleural metastases of thymoma. *Chest* 2002; **121:** 480–7.

67. Takagi K, Tsuchiya R, Watanabe Y. Surgical approach to pleural diffuse mesothelioma in Japan. *Lung Cancer* 2001; **31:** 57–65.

68. Rice TW, Adelstein DJ, Kirby TJ, *et al.* Aggressive multimodality therapy for malignant pleural mesothelioma. *Ann Thorac Surg* 1994; **58:** 24–9.

69. Pass HI, Temeck BK, Kranda K, Steinberg SM, Feuerstein IR. Preoperative tumour volume is associated with outcome in malignant pleural mesothelioma. *J Thorac Cardiovasc Surg* 1998; **115:** 310–17.

70. Waller DA, Rengarajan A. Thoracoscopic decortication: a role for video-assisted surgery in chronic postpneumonic pleural empyema. *Ann Thorac Surg* 2001; **71:** 1813–16.

71. Peto J, Decarli A, La Vecchia C, Levi F, Negri E. The European Mesothelioma epidemic. *Br J Cancer* 1999; **79:** 666–72.

72. Atkins JL, Martin-Ucar AE, Waller DA. The impact of 10 years of video assisted thoracic surgery on respiratory practice in the UK. *Thorax* 2001; **56** (Suppl III): iii67–8.

Chapter 13

Surgical and multimodality approaches to the management of operable malignant mesothelioma

D. J. Boffa and V. W. Rusch

Introduction

Historically, malignant pleural mesothelioma (MPM) was considered to be a rapidly and universally fatal disease. Most patients were thought to die within 2 years of diagnosis, and this nihilism led to insufficient attention being given to the staging and treatment of MPM. However, during the past two decades, a few investigators have carefully defined the natural history and studied the treatment of MPM. These studies established that patients with stage Ia tumours can be expected to live for up to 2 years without treatment, and patients who undergo surgical resection for stage I and II disease usually live more than 3 years. Effective surgical and multimodality treatments are now available. The surgical mortality of 31 per cent reported by Butchart *et al.* [1] in 1976 for extrapleural pneumonectomy has decreased to 4–5 per cent, becoming similar to the mortality of standard pneumonectomy and making is possible to offer surgery as a routine part of treatment for MPM [2]. Adjuvant radiotherapy after extrapleural pneumonectomy is now an accepted means of controlling locoregional disease (Chapter 15). Newer chemotherapeutic regimens, including gemcitabine–cisplatin and pemetrexed–cisplatin, have shown encouraging response rates [3,4] In this chapter we address the staging of MPM and the surgical and multimodality treatment of this disease.

Staging: historical perspective

Prior to the present decade, it was difficult to diagnose and stage MPM accurately. MPM was frequently misclassified pathologically as metastatic adenocarcinoma, a diagnostic problem which has now been solved by the routine use of a panel of immunohistochemical stains on pleural biopsies. Chest radiography rather than computed tomography (CT) was used as the primary imaging modality, leading to inaccuracies in clinical stage classification. In addition, there was no widely accepted staging system, making it difficult to assess the natural history and to compare treatment outcomes.

Butchart *et al.* [1] proposed the first staging system in 1976 (Table 13.1), based on their experience with 29 patients who underwent extrapleural pneumonectomy. However, this study was performed before the advent of CT and the extent of disease preoperatively was assessed very crudely. Consequently, this study did not permit accurate correlations of stage and survival. Several staging systems were proposed over the next 25 years, but each faced limitations similar to the Butchart system and none was well validated or universally accepted. In 1982, Mattson [5] developed a staging system which was a variation on the Butchart system and Chahinian *et al.* [6] proposed the first TNM-based system. In 1993, the UICC proposed another TNM staging

Table 13.1 Staging proposed by Butchart *et al.* [1]

Stage I	Tumour confined within the 'capsule' of the parietal pleura, i.e. involving only ipsilateral pleura, lung, pericardium, and diaphragm
Stage II	Tumour invading chest wall or involving mediastinal structures (e.g. oesophagus, heart, opposite pleura) Lymph node involvement within the chest
Stage III	Tumour penetrating diaphragm to involve peritoneum; involvement of opposite pleura Lymph node involvement outside chest
Stage IV	Distant blood-borne metastases

Reproduced with permission from Butchart EG, Ashcroft T, Barnsley WC, Holden MP. Pleuropneumonectomy in the management of diffuse malignant mesothelioma of the pleura: experience with 29 patients. *Thorax* 1976; 31: 15–24.

system. In 1999, Sugarbaker and colleagues [7,8] published a revised staging system based solely upon patients undergoing extrapleural pneumonectomy. Because of the lack of a universally accepted staging system, the International Mesothelioma Interest Group (IMIG) developed a staging system that would be universally accepted and would be applicable to both clinical and surgical/pathological staging [9]. This system was accepted by the AJCC and the UICC and was recently published in the sixth editions of their staging manuals [10,11].

The current UICC and AJCC staging system for malignant pleural mesothelioma

T status

The current UICC–AJCC staging system groups TNM descriptors into a stage I to stage IV classification (Table 13.2) [9]. T1 is divided into 1a and 1b, where 1a describes tumour that involves only the parietal pleura of one hemithorax without mediastinal or diaphragmatic involvement (thus sparing the visceral pleura) and 1b describes a slightly more advanced tumour that involves both pleural surfaces. T1 tumours are usually associated with a free pleural space and a large effusion (Fig. 13.1).

With tumour growth the visceral and parietal pleural surfaces fuse, and the effusion may resolve or become loculated. This confluence of pleural surfaces or involvement of the underly-

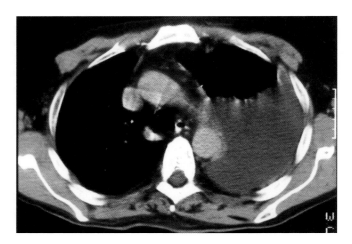

Figure 13.1 Example of stage I MPM with a large left pleural effusion and minimal parietal and mediastinal pleural thickening.

Table 13.2 AJCC–UICC Staging System

Primary tumour (T)	
TX	Primary tumour cannot be assessed
T0	No evidence of primary tumour
T1	Tumour involves ipsilateral parietal pleura, with or without focal involvement of visceral pleura
T1a	Tumour involves ipsilateral parietal (mediastinal, diaphragmatic) pleura; no involvement of the visceral pleura
T1b	Tumour involves ipsilateral parietal (mediastinal, diaphragmatic) pleura with focal involvement of visceral pleura
T2	Tumour involves any of the ipsilateral pleural surfaces with at least one of the following: confluent visceral pleural tumour (including fissure) invasion of diaphragmatic muscle invasion of lung parenchyma
T3	Describes locally advanced *but potentially resectable* tumour
	Tumour involves any of the ipsilateral pleural surfaces with at least one of the following: invasion of the endothoracic fascia invasion into mediastinal fat solitary focus of tumour invading the soft tissues of the chest wall non-transmural involvement of the pericardium
T4	Describes locally advanced *technically unresectable* tumour
	Tumour involves any of the ipsilateral pleural surfaces with at least one of the following: diffuse or multifocal invasion of soft tissues of the chest wall any involvement of rib invasion through the diaphragm to the peritoneum direct extension of any mediastinal organ direct extension to the contralateral pleura invasion into the spine extension to the internal surface of the pericardium pericardial effusion with positive cytology invasion of the myocardium invasion of the brachial plexus
Regional lymph nodes (N)	
NX	Regional lymph nodes cannot be assessed
N0	No regional lymph node metastases
N1	Metastases in the ipsilateral bronchopulmonary and/or hilar lymph nodes
N2	Metastases in the subcarinal lymph nodes and/or ipsilateral internal mammary or mediastinal lymph nodes
N3	Metastases in the contralateral mediastinal, contralateral internal mammary, or hilar lymph nodes and/or the ipsilateral or contralateral supraclavicular or scalene lymph nodes
Distant metastases (M)	
MX	Distant metastases cannot be assessed
M0	No distant metastases
M1	Distant metastases present

Table 13.2 Contd.

Stage grouping			
Stage I	T1	N0	M0
Stage IA	T1a	N0	M0
Stage IB	T1b	N0	M0
Stage II	T2	N0	M0
Stage III	T1, T2	N1	M0
	T1, T2	N2	
	T3	N0, N1, N2	
Stage IV	T4	Any N	M0
	Any T	N3	M0
	Any T	Any N	M1

Reproduced with permission from: American Joint Commission on Cancer. *Cancer Staging Manual*, 6th edn. New York: Springer Verlag, 2002; 180–1.

ing lung parenchyma designates a tumour as T2. Usually, this stage of tumour cannot be completely removed without removal of the underlying lung and diaphragmatic muscle. At this stage, only extrapleural pneumonectomy will rid the patient of all gross disease; pleurectomy–decortication will not.

T3 describes a locally advanced tumour but one that is still amenable to surgical resection by extrapleural pneumonectomy. There is involvement of all pleural surfaces (including diaphragm and pericardium) with areas of tumour invasion into the endothoracic fascia or mediastinal fat (Fig. 13.2). A solitary completely resectable focus of tumour extending directly into the chest wall, usually occurring at previous incision or chest tube sites, is also considered T3. The concept is similar to that for non-small-cell lung cancer; a single focus of tumour invading the chest wall by direct extension is removed *en bloc* with the entire specimen. This is a very different finding

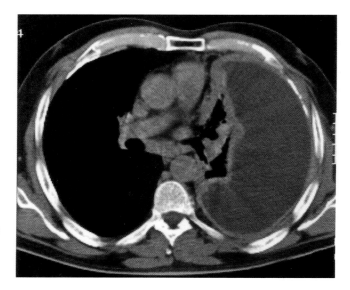

Figure 13.2 Example of more locally advanced MPM, at least T2 and possibly T3 (along anterolateral chest wall) by CT scan.

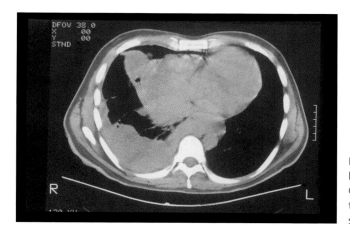

Figure 13.3 Example of a very locally advanced MPM, T4 by CT scan. There is a massive tumour extending into and shifting the mediastinum.

when compared with the locally advanced tumour that is technically unresectable because it diffusely invades the intercostal and chest wall muscles.

T4 indicates a very locally advanced and technically unresectable tumour (Fig. 13.3). It is characterized by diffuse chest wall invasion, direct extension through the diaphragm to the underlying peritoneum, direct extension to the contralateral pleura, mediastinal organs, spine, myocardium, or internal surface of the pericardium. The differences between T3 and T4 tumours have obvious implications with regard to resectability as well as survival [12,13].

N status

The N descriptors are identical to those used in the International Lung Cancer Staging System [14]. N1 indicates involvement of the ipsilateral lymph nodes from the bronchopulmonary and hilar regions; N2 includes lymph nodes from the ipsilateral mediastinal, internal mammary and subcarinal regions, and N3 describes supraclavicular, contralateral mediastinal, or contralateral hemithoracic nodal involvement.

Because of current uncertainty about the prognostic difference between N1 and N2 disease, both of these are grouped into stage III disease. Sugarbaker *et al.* [8] identified a significant difference in survival between patients with negative and positive N2 nodes. Among 176 patients surviving extrapleural pneumonectomy, 136 patients with negative N2 nodes had a significantly better survival than 40 patients with positive nodes. The adverse influence of nodal involvement was not evident in earlier surgical series [15], but analysis of this variable was confounded by the small numbers of patients in most reports, a lack of routine complete nodal sampling, and the retrospective nature of many analyses. The true incidence of nodal involvement and the routes of lymphatic spread are also poorly understood. It is possible that the N2 nodes and the internal mammary nodes may become involved before N1 nodes because of the anatomical extent of MPM and the fact that it apparently arises in the parietal pleura rather than in the parenchyma of the lung. Analysis of our series at Memorial Sloan-Kettering Cancer Center (MSKCC) [16] showed that the frequency of nodal metastasis was significantly higher (50 per cent) than in Sugarbaker's experience (23 per cent) and emphasizes the importance of systematic nodal dissection for staging. In our experience, both the presence of nodal metastases (N1 and N2) and the number of involved lymph nodes had a prognostic impact on overall survival after surgical resection. As more data become available, new analyses of the patterns of nodal metastasis and of the impact of N1 versus N2 or N3 disease should be performed. Such analyses may lead to future revisions of the UICC–AJCC staging system.

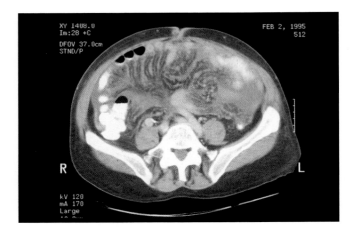

Figure 13.4 Example of MPM metastatic to the omentum and bowel mesentery, M1 by CT scan.

M status

Although mesothelioma is usually known as a disease that progresses and invades locally, a small but significant number of patients present with extrathoracic disease. Autopsy series also show that at least half of all patients have widely disseminated disease at the time of death [17]. Because of the potential magnitude of surgical procedures such as extrapleural pneumonectomy, it is important to recognize these patients and spare them an inappropriate operation.

M0 designates no evidence of metastatic disease and M1 describes distant metastasis. In MPM, metastases are often widespread but the most common sites of disease progression include the peritoneum, contralateral pleura, and contralateral lung (Fig. 13.4). These may develop by direct extension of tumour through the diaphragm (T4 tumour) or as a result of lymphatic or haematogenous dissemination. However, the prognosis is similar no matter what the route of tumour spread.

AJCC stage groupings

The TNM descriptors are used to characterize four stages of the disease. Stages I and II include node negative tumours. Stage I is subdivided into 1a and 1b, and stage II includes T2N0 tumours. Stage III includes any T3, any N1, or any N2, M0 tumour, and stage IV includes any T4, N3, or M1 tumour. Survival at 3 and 5 years for stages I, II, and III is 46 per cent and 28 per cent, 32 per cent and 15 per cent, and 15 per cent and 0 per cent, respectively (Fig. 13.5) [16].

Clinical staging in mesothelioma

Computed tomography and magnetic resonance imaging

There is some controversy over which imaging study is best and whether MRI adds to CT. In 1992, prior to the advent of helical CT scanning, Patz *et al.* [18] from the Brigham and Women's Hospital reviewed 34 consecutive MPM patients who had CT scanning and MRI prior to surgery. The radiological review focused on diaphragmatic involvement, chest wall invasion, and mediastinal invasion. The sensitivity was high (>90 per cent) for both CT and MRI in each region. The unresectability rate of patients undergoing thoracotomy was 30 per cent. CT and MRI provided similar information on resectability in most cases. Although they state that important anatomical information can be derived from MR images obtained prior to surgical intervention, this information will rarely preclude patients from surgical exploration. More recent studies have also

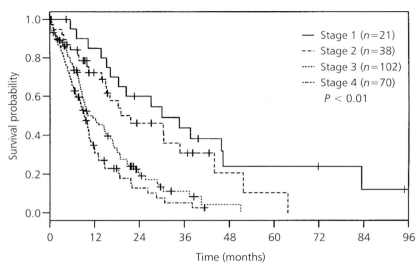

Figure 13.5 Overall survival of 231 patients by stage. When analysed across all four categories, stage had a highly significant effect on survival ($P < 0.01$). (Reproduced with permission from Rusch V, Venkatraman E. Important prognostic factors in patients with malignant pleural mesothelioma, managed surgically. *Ann Thorac Surg* 1999; 68: 1799–1804.)

claimed a slight advantage of MRI over CT. However, there is little evidence that these findings translate into clinically relevant information [19,20].

At MSKCC, we enrolled 95 patients in a prospective staging protocol. Sixty-five patients underwent CT and MRI followed by surgical resection. CT and MRI scans were interpreted by independent observers in a blinded fashion and imaging findings were then compared with surgical–pathological staging. MRI was slightly more accurate at identifying diaphragmatic invasion, invasion of endothoracic fascia, and solitary resectable foci of chest wall invasion. However, these findings were not significant enough to alter surgical treatment in these patients. Therefore we consider CT of the chest and upper abdomen to be the standard staging study before therapy [21]. However, CT does not reliably identify either N1 or N2 nodal disease and often fails to diagnose chest wall invasion. Consequently, approximately 20–25 per cent of patients who undergo surgical exploration are found to have unresectable tumour [22].

Pass *et al.* [23] conducted a study using CT to evaluate the impact of preoperative tumour volume on outcome in patients undergoing resection for pleural mesothelioma. Forty-eight patients had three-dimensional CT reconstructions of pre- and post-resection solid tumour volume, and were staged according to the AJCC staging system for mesothelioma prior to surgical resection with either extrapleural pneumonectomy or pleurectomy–decortication. The median survival for preoperative tumour volume less than 100 cm^3 was 22 months compared with 11 months for tumour volume greater than 100 cm^3 ($P = 0.03$). Progressively higher stage was associated with higher median preoperative volume: stage I, 4 cm^3; stage II, 94 cm^3; stage III, 143 cm^3; stage IV, 505 cm^3 ($P = 0.007$). Higher tumour volumes were also associated with a greater likelihood of lymph node metastasis. This study showed that preoperative tumour volume assessed by volumetric CT tumour measurement is representative of T status in malignant pleural mesothelioma and can predict survival. (See also Chapter 3).

Positron emission tomography

At MSKCC, we explored the utility of PET scanning in the preoperative staging of MPM. We reviewed 63 patients who underwent PET scans at our institution during their initial evaluation prior to surgical resection. 2-Fluoro-2-deoxyglucose (FDG) uptake was present in all except one patient with stage Ia disease (Figs 13.6 and 13.7). We did not find that PET scanning added to the assessment of locoregional disease, especially the determination of T status; neither did PET accurately diagnose lymph node involvement. However, a high standard uptake value (SUV) was associated with a greater likelihood of N2 nodal metastases. More importantly, PET was useful in identifying 10 per cent of the patients as having distant disease undetected by CT scan, thereby preventing inappropriate surgical intervention [24].

In addition, PET scan findings may have prognostic significance. Recently, we evaluated 85 MPM patients who underwent PET scanning at diagnosis and found that there was a linear relationship between increasing SUV and decreasing median survival. The relative risk of death in patients with SUV > 4 compared with patients with SUV < 4 was 3.3 ($P = 0.03$). In both univariate and multivariable analyses, SUV significantly predicted overall survival. These findings suggest that PET may assist in selecting patients for treatment [25].

Distant metastases in sites not evaluated by PET or by CT of the chest and upper abdomen, principally the central nervous system (CNS), are rare in patients with early stage MPM. CNS metastases occur rarely in patients with advanced disease. Therefore routine preoperative brain imaging is not indicated in MPM. (See also Chapter 3).

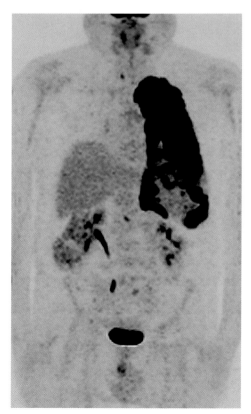

Figure 13.6 PET scan demonstrating a high SUV in a patient with a left-sided mesothelioma. The tumour involves all pleural and diaphragmatic surfaces.

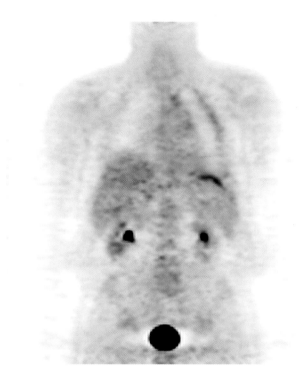

Figure 13.7 PET scan demonstrating a low SUV in a patient with a left-sided mesothelioma. The tumour involves the left lower pleural and diaphragmatic areas.

Video-assisted thoracic surgery

Video-assisted thoracic surgery (VATS) is principally used to diagnose MPM. Cytological yield is low and tissue is frequently necessary to perform immunohistochemistry and electron microscopy in order to establish a definitive diagnosis. In addition, the identification of histological subtype is useful in selecting patients for treatment protocols.

With respect to staging, the distinction between T1a and T1b tumours is best made by VATS. In 66 patients undergoing thoracoscopy, Boutin and colleagues [12,26] found subtle differences in the extent of pleural disease that are impossible to identify radiographically and that account for differences in survival found in patients believed to have similar stage early disease. In this series, 23 patients with stage Ia (parietal pleura only) disease had a median survival of 32.7 months compared with the 43 patients with stage Ib (parietal and visceral pleura) disease who had a median survival of 7 months. (See also Chapter 12).

Laparoscopy

At MSKCC we conducted a study to determine the utility of laparoscopy in detecting transdiaphragmatic tumour extension when CT findings were equivocal [27]. During a 1 year period, 12 of 36 patients considered for possible thoracotomy and surgical resection had equivocal CT findings of diaphragmatic invasion. All underwent laparoscopy with diaphragmatic and peritoneal biopsies. There were no perioperative complications and the median hospital stay was 1 day. Six patients had biopsy-proven transdiaphragmatic extension or peritoneal studding of tumour. The other six patients subsequently underwent thoracotomy: three had a complete resection, and three had unresectable tumour due to chest wall ($n = 2$) or mediastinal ($n = 1$) invasion. In no case was transdiaphragmatic extension of a tumour seen. This experience demonstrated that laparoscopy is a safe and accurate method for detecting transdiaphragmatic tumour extension when CT fails to do so and should be considered a standard part of pre-thoracotomy staging in this subset of patients. (See also Chapter 12).

Mediastinoscopy

The role of mediastinoscopy in the management of malignant pleural mesothelioma is still unclear. Schouwink et al. [28] examined the usefulness of cervical mediastinoscopy in 43 patients. Only 24 of these patients went on to thoracotomy for pathological confirmation, and therefore data were not available on the patients with potentially false-negative mediastinoscopy results. Of the 17 patients with enlarged nodes detected by CT scan, only six were confirmed to be positive by cervical mediastinoscopy, emphasizing the fact that lymph nodes that are enlarged on CT are not necessarily malignant. In addition, mediastinoscopy cannot diagnose lymph node metastases that occur frequently in MPM but are in anatomical locations inaccessible to this procedure, including the posterior mediastinal, internal mammary, and peridiaphragmatic regions. Although mediastinoscopy will clearly identify some patients with N2 disease, its role in staging MPM requires further study. Finally, while the presence of N2 disease is generally associated with a worse prognosis, it is not clear that all such patients should be denied surgical resection given current treatment options. (See also Chapter 12).

Summary

In summary, CT and PET scanning currently provide the most accurate clinical staging. MRI does not appear to add consistently to CT and PET and should be used selectively. VATS and laparoscopy can provide some additional information about T status, transdiaphragmatic tumour invasion, or peritoneal metastases. Although the current UICC–AJCC staging system and the methods available for clinical staging represent advances made in the management of MPM during the past decade, they are imperfect. Further studies to improve the accuracy of staging in MPM are warranted.

Preoperative physiological evaluation

Thorough evaluation of cardiac and pulmonary function is essential in selecting MPM patients for surgical resection, especially extrapleural pneumonectomy. Because of prior asbestos exposure, and frequently a past smoking history, many MPM patients have both obstructive and interstitial lung disease. Therefore pulmonary function is assessed through complete pulmonary function testing, including lung volumes, spirometry, diffusion capacity, and rest and exercise arterial blood gases. Quantitative ventilation–perfusion lung scanning is essential for determining where patients have sufficient pulmonary reserve to allow extrapleural pneumonectomy. In general, the calculated values of the postoperative FEV_1 (forced expiratory volume in 1 s) and the DLCO (diffusion capacity) should be 40 per cent of predicted in order to consider performing an extrapleural pneumonectomy.

Relatively advanced age and, often, a past smoking history place MPM patients at risk for coronary artery disease, which may or may not be clinically evident. Routine radionuclide stress testing in all MPM patients is indicated preoperatively as extrapleural pneumonectomy poses a significant myocardial stress, because of both the pneumonectomy and haemodynamic changes associated with blood loss intraoperatively and with fluid shifts immediately postoperatively. We would not usually consider performing an extrapleural pneumonectomy in patients whose radionuclide stress test shows a major area of myocardial ischemia. Such patients would be evaluated further by cardiac catheterization before considering surgical resection of the MPM.

Surgical resection

The two operations performed for MPM with curative intent are extrapleural pneumonectomy and pleurectomy–decortication. The surgical techniques for these two operations are described below.

Surgical techniques

Extrapleural pneumonectomy is an *en bloc* resection of the pleura, the lung, the ipsilateral hemidiaphragm, and the pericardium. It is performed via an extended S-shaped posterolateral thoracotomy incision that extends to the costal margin (Fig. 13.8). The sixth rib is excised to facilitate exposure to the extrapleural plane (Fig. 13.8). This approach is slightly lower than for a standard pulmonary resection because the greatest bulk of tumour is usually in the lower half of the hemithorax. Blunt dissection is started in the extrapleural plane between the parietal pleura and the endothoracic fascia and is continued with a sweeping motion of the hand up to the apex of the chest (Fig. 13.8). A similar dissection is then performed inferiorly from the intercostal incision down to the diaphragm. The dissection is carried anteriorly to the pericardium and posteriorly to the spine. It is important to pack each section of the chest sequentially as this dissection is performed as otherwise there can be a substantial blood loss. The Argon Beam Electrocoagulator (ConMed Corporation, Utica, New York) is very helpful in controlling this diffuse chest wall bleeding. When the parietal pleura has been mobilized away from the chest wall, a chest retractor is inserted. Dissection is continued under direct vision, mobilizing the pleura away from the mediastinum superiorly, anteriorly, and posteriorly (Fig. 13.9). On the left side, care must be taken to identify the oesophagus, the plane between the adventitia of the aorta and the tumour,

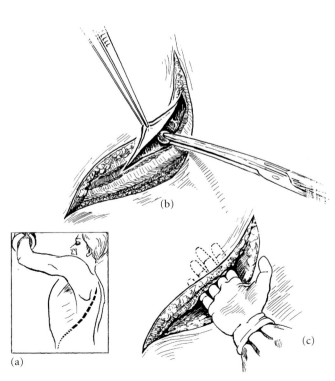

Figure 13.8 (a) Initial approach for a pleurectomy or an extrapleural pneumonectomy. An extended posterolateral thoracotomy or thoracoabdominal incision is performed. (b) A parallel counter-incision in the 10th intercostal space, with or without a separate skin incision, can be added to improve exposure to the diaphragm. (c) The extrapleural plane is opened after resection of the sixth rib, and the parietal pleura is bluntly dissected away from the endothoracic fascia. (Reproduced with permission from Rusch VW. Mesothelioma and less common pleural tumours. In Pearson FG, Cooper JD, Deslauriers J, *et al.*, eds. *Thoracic Surgery*, 2nd edn. Philadelphia, PA: Churchill Livingstone, 2002; 1253–7.)

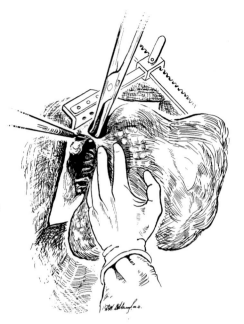

Figure 13.9 After the parietal pleura has been mobilized from the chest wall, a chest retractor is inserted and the mediastinal pleura is freed from the mediastinal structures under direct vision using a combination of sharp and blunt dissection. (Reproduced with permission from Rusch VW. Mesothelioma and less common pleural tumours. In Pearson FG, Cooper JD, Deslauriers J, *et al*., eds. *Thoracic Surgery*, 2nd edn. Philadelphia, PA: Churchill Livingstone, 2002; 1253–7.)

and the origins of the intercostal vessels. On the right side, dissection along the superior vena cava must be performed very gently. After this portion of the dissection, the pleura and lung will have been completely mobilized in the upper half of the chest, exposing the superior and posterior aspects of the hilum. A standard *en bloc* dissection of the subcarinal lymph nodes is performed for staging purposes and to expose the mainstem bronchus. The lymph nodes are submitted separately, appropriately labelled, to the pathologist. In some patients, there is a clean plane of dissection between the mediastinal pleura and the pericardium, also allowing exposure of the anterior aspect of the hilum. In other patients, this plane is obliterated and the anterior mediastinal pleura has to be resected *en bloc* with the pericardium later in the operation.

Attention is then turned to resection of the diaphragm. There is always a palpable 'edge' or cleavage plane between the tumour and the uninvolved portion of the diaphragmatic muscle or peritoneum. This plane can be entered and the tumour mobilized along the diaphragmatic surface by blunt dissection in much the way that one would perform a Kocher manoeuvre. Once the tumour is mobilized from the posterior costophrenic angle, it is rotated up into the thoracotomy incision, rolling it back upon itself and placing strong traction on the diaphragm. The plane of dissection varies from patient to patient. If the involvement of the diaphragm is extensive, the entire thickness of the diaphragmatic muscle will be removed, peeling this away from the peritoneum. If the involvement of the diaphragm is superficial, dissection can be carried through the diaphragmatic muscle using electrocautery (Fig. 13.10). Every effort is made not to enter the peritoneum because of the propensity of MPM to produce tumour implants. The most difficult area to avoid entering the abdomen is at the level at the central tendon, and often a small opening in the peritoneum is unavoidable but should be immediately reclosed. The diaphragmatic portion of the tumour is completely mobilized back to the pericardium medially. If resection of the pericardium is required, it is entered only when the tumour has been mobilized as fully as possible from all other directions because traction on the pericardium causes arrhythmias and haemodynamic instability (Fig. 13.11). The hilar structures are divided in whatever sequence is technically

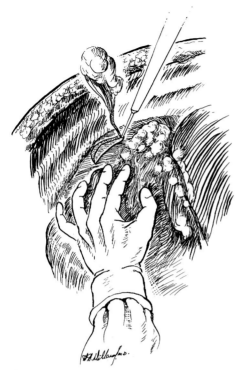

Figure 13.10 The tumour has been bluntly mobilized out of the costophrenic sulcus. Strong traction is placed on the pleural tumour and underlying lung, and cautery is used to dissect the diaphragmatic surface of the tumour away from the diaphragmatic muscle or peritoneum. (Reproduced with permission from Rusch VW. Mesothelioma and less common pleural tumours. In Pearson FG, Cooper JD, Deslauriers J, *et al.*, eds. *Thoracic Surgery*, 2nd edn. Philadelphia, PA: Churchill Livingstone, 2002; 1253–7.)

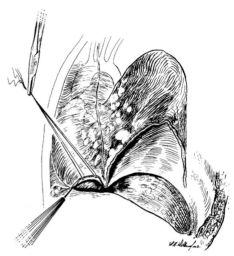

Figure 13.11 The pericardium is opened after the tumour has been completely mobilized from all other directions, including the diaphragm. (Reproduced with permission from Rusch VW. Mesothelioma and less common pleural tumours. In Pearson FG, Cooper JD, Deslauriers J, *et al.*, eds. *Thoracic Surgery*, 2nd edn. Philadelphia, PA: Churchill Livingstone, 2002; 1253–7.)

easiest and requires the least manipulation of the large tumour mass. Usually, this means dividing the mainstem bronchus first, then the inferior pulmonary vein, the superior pulmonary vein, and finally the main pulmonary artery. If the pericardium is being resected, it is gradually opened as this portion of the dissection is carried out. Traction sutures are placed on the pericardium to prevent it from retracting towards the opposite hemithorax. The traction sutures minimize changes in the position of the heart and reduce haemodynamic instability (Fig. 13.12). The specimen consisting of pleura, lung, and diaphragm, with or without pericardium, is removed *en bloc*. Sampling or dissection of the paratracheal lymph nodes if the operation is on the right, or of the aortopulmonary window nodes if the operation is on the left, is performed for staging purposes. Again, these nodes are submitted separately, appropriately labelled, to the pathologist.

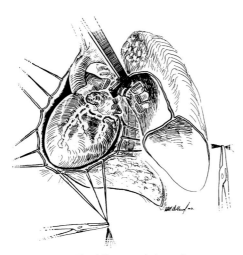

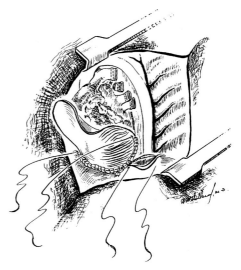

Figure 13.12 The hilar vessels have been divided intrapericardially. Traction sutures have been placed on the edge of the pericardium as it was opened to prevent it from retracting into the contralateral hemithorax. (Reproduced with permission from Rusch VW. Mesothelioma and less common pleural tumours. In Pearson FG, Cooper JD, Deslauriers J, *et al.*, eds. *Thoracic Surgery*, 2nd edn. Philadelphia, PA: Churchill Livingstone, 2002; 1253–7.)

Figure 13.13 The pericardial and diaphragmatic defects are reconstructed with prosthetic material. Reconstruction of the diaphragm is not always necessary, especially on the right side. (Reproduced with permission from Rusch VW. Mesothelioma and less common pleural tumours. In Pearson FG, Cooper JD, Deslauriers J, *et al.*, eds. *Thoracic Surgery*, 2nd edn. Philadelphia, PA: Churchill Livingstone, 2002; 1253–7.)

Reconstruction of the diaphragm is then performed (Fig. 13.13). On the right side Dexon mesh is used because the underlying liver assists in preventing herniation of the intra-abdominal contents. On the left side, Gore-Tex is used because a heavier non-absorbable material is required to prevent herniation. If the diaphragmatic muscle has been completely resected back to its costal insertion, the prosthesis is secured by placing sutures around the ribs laterally (Fig. 13.14). Posteriorly, it is sutured to the crus or gently tacked with fine sutures to the wall of the oesophagus. Medially it is sewn to the edge of the pericardium. If the pericardium has been resected, it is reconstructed with Dexon mesh. This prevents cardiac herniation into the empty hemithorax, and facilitates postoperative radiation to the hemithorax by maintaining the heart in a central position. Meticulous attention is given to obtaining haemostasis throughout the operation and particularly prior to closure of the chest. The thoracotomy incision is closed in the usual manner.

A similar approach is used for the initial portion of the operation for a pleurectomy–decortication. As for an extrapleural pneumonectomy, the intention of a pleurectomy–decortication is to remove all gross tumour; the only difference is that the lung is left in place [29] Mobilization of the parietal and mediastinal pleura and of the diaphragmatic surface is the same as for an extrapleural pneumonectomy. If the pericardium cannot be easily separated from the pleura, it is also resected and reconstructed as previously described. When all this dissection has been completed, the parietal pleura is opened and the decortication begun (Fig. 13.15). The degree to which the parietal and visceral pleura are separable, and to which the visceral pleural tumour can be peeled cleanly away from the lung, is extremely variable. Sometimes it is necessary to remove

rence [30]. Therefore most treatment regimens have focused on combined modality treatment, but it has been difficult to evaluate the results of such treatments because most series report small numbers of patients treated in a highly individualized manner over long periods of time [6,37,38]. The approaches to combined modality treatment can be categorized into those designed to enhance only local control, and those aimed at preventing both local and systemic relapse.

Approaches to enhancing local control

One way of circumventing these problems is to administer radiation therapy as adjuvant treatment after surgical resection of gross tumour. A variety of techniques can be used to minimize the radiation dose to the lung. The largest and most consistent experience with this approach was reported from the MSKCC [39,40]. After subtotal resection of gross tumour by pleurectomy–decortication, any residual tumour was implanted intraoperatively with ^{125}I or ^{192}Ir implants. Patients then received external beam irradiation to the entire hemithorax using a mixed photon-electron beam technique to a total dose of 4500 cGy, attempting to spare the underlying lung. In an updated report by Mychalczak et al. [41], 105 patients treated in this manner at MSKCC between 1976 and 1988 experienced a median survival of 12.6 months with 1 and 2 year actuarial survivals of 52 per cent and 23 per cent, respectively. However, the 27 patients who had pure epithelioid histology and minimal gross residual disease requiring only external beam irradiation without brachytherapy had a median survival of 15 months, and 1 and 2 year survivals of 68 per cent and 35 per cent, respectively. There were 19 complications, including 12 cases of radiation pneumonitis and eight patients with pericarditis and tamponade. The most common site of relapse was local, with ipsilateral recurrent pleural tumour seen in 64 of the 105 patients (63 per cent). Both this experience and experimental work by Soubra et al. [42] indicate that a low-dose mixed photon-electron beam, although theoretically attractive, does not spare the pulmonary parenchyma, does not provide long-term local control for most patients, and after pleurectomy–decortication is associated with an unacceptable risk of complications.

A very successful use of radiation is as an adjuvant therapy to prevent tumour implantation in the chest wall after thoracoscopy. In a small randomized study, Boutin et al. [43] reported that eight of 20 (40 per cent) patients who did not receive radiation therapy to the chest wall after thoracoscopy developed tumour implantation compared with none of the 20 patients who received radiation . Because the radiation regimen was a short course (700 cGy daily for 3 days), this treatment is worth considering in patients for whom no further surgical intervention is planned. Low et al. [44] confirmed the experience, using this radiation regimen in 20 patients. They found no evidence of local recurrence in irradiated sites.

In addition to the MSKCC experience with pleurectomy–decortication and radiation therapy described above, another large and relatively uniform experience with combined adjuvant radiation and chemotherapy treatment has been reported by the Dana Farber Cancer Center. Between 1980 and 1997, Sugarbaker and colleagues performed an extrapleural pneumonectomy in 183 patients, followed by CAP (cyclophosphamide–doxorubicin–cisplatin) chemotherapy or carboplatin and paclitaxel and subsequent hemithoracic irradiation at a median dose of 30.6 Gy [8]. The overall survival was 38 per cent at 2 years and 15 per cent at 5 years. The 2 and 5 year survivals were 52 per cent and 21 per cent, respectively, for patients with epithelioid cell type, and 16 per cent and zero for patients with sarcomatous or mixed histology tumours. Nodal metastases were a significant adverse prognostic factor. It is difficult to assess how much the radiation and chemotherapy each contribute to overall survival rates because these have not been tested individually as adjuvant treatment. The major problem with this modality, as reported by Baldini et al. [45], was a 35 per cent local recurrence rate most likely related to the low total dose of radiation administered.

At MSKCC we performed a phase II trial of high-dose hemithoracic radiation after complete resection to determine feasibility and to estimate rates of local recurrence and survival. After complete resection, patients received hemithoracic radiation (54 Gy) and were then followed up with serial CT scans. During a 3 year period, 88 patients were entered into the study. The operations performed included 62 extrapleural pneumonectomies (70 per cent) and five pleurectomy–decortications; procedures for exploration only were performed in 21 patients. Adjuvant radiation, administered to 57 patients (54 undergoing extrapleural pneumonectomy and three undergoing pleurectomy–decortication) at a median dose of 54 Gy, was well tolerated (grade 0–2 fatigue, oesophagitis), except for one late oesophageal fistula. The median survival was 33.8 months for stage I and II tumours but only 10 months for stage III and IV tumours ($P = 0.04$). For the patients undergoing extrapleural pneumonectomy, the sites of recurrence were locoregional in two cases, locoregional and distant in five, and distant only in 30. This study demonstrated the feasibility of administering adjuvant hemithoracic radiation at a dose not previously reported and a dramatic reduction in local recurrence rate to 8.7 per cent [22]. Since the major sites of failure were distant, we have now focused our efforts on adding systemic therapy, usually administered preoperatively as induction treatment. Adjuvant radiotherapy is discussed further in Chapter 15.

Other novel local treatment strategies have also been investigated. Photodynamic therapy (PDT) seeks to improve local control by eliminating microscopic residual disease immediately after surgical resection. This approach is based on experimental data with MPM cell lines as reported by Keller et al. [46], as well as a previous small clinical trial reported by Ris et al. [47], which suggested the feasibility of this approach. Pass et al. [48] reported that 42 patients received PDT after maximal surgical tumour debulking using escalating light doses of 15–35 J/cm^2. There was one mortality and three serious complications. Overall, this trial demonstrated the feasibility and safety of combined surgical resection and PDT.

Therefore Pass et al. [49] conducted a phase III trial comparing maximum debulking surgery and postoperative cisplatin, interferon α-2b, and tamoxifen (CIT) immunochemotherapy with and without intraoperative PDT to determine the impact on local recurrence and survival. Sixty-three patients with localized MPM were randomized to either PDT or no PDT over a 3 year period. The tumours of 15 patients could not be debulked. Patients assigned to PDT ($n = 25$) and no PDT ($n = 23$) were similar with respect to age, sex, tumour volume, and histology. The type of resection included 11 pleurectomies and 14 pneumonectomies for the PDT group compared with 12 pleurectomies and 11 pneumonectomies for the group without PDT. There was one operative death (haemorrhage), and each group had two bronchopleural fistulas. In addition, postoperative staging was equivalent and comparable numbers of CIT cycles were delivered. Median survival for the 15 non-debulked patients was 7.2 months compared with 14 months for the 48 patients on protocol. There were no major differences in median survival (14.4 vs. 14.1 months) or median progression-free time (8.5 vs. 7.7 months), and sites of first recurrence were similar. These results demonstrate that PDT does not prolong survival or increase local control for MPM.

More recently, Sterman et al. [50] explored the feasibility of treating early-stage MPM with intrapleural gene therapy. Using human MPM tumours growing in the peritoneal cavities of severe combined immunodeficient mice, Hwang et al. [51] found that the herpes simplex virus thymidine kinase (HSVtk) gene could be successfully transferred to tumour via an adenovirus. Administration of the antiviral drug ganciclovir then led to selective tumour cell death. This treatment approach has been evaluated in a phase I clinical trial [50]. However, adenovirus-mediated intrapleural gene therapy remains investigational.

Approaches to enhancing control of systemic disease

Numerous phase II studies of chemotherapeutic agents have been performed in MPM, testing virtually all the currently available drugs. These have been recently reviewed in detail by Krarup-Hansen and Hansen [52], Ong and Vogelzang [53], and Tomek *et al.* [54] (Table 13.4). Response rates as high as 30–40 per cent have been reported for either single or multiple agents in small single-institution studies, but in pooled data from multiple studies response rates are generally in the 20 per cent range. The results of these studies are influenced by the inclusion of patients with varying stages of disease and different MPM cell types, as well as by the lack of use of CT scanning to assess response. Agents reported to have activity in MPM include doxorubicin, ifosfamide, cisplatin, carboplatin, mitomycin, methotrexate, edatrexate, 5-azacitidine, and 5-fluorouracil [55–59] In the past, combination treatment has not shown clear superiority over single agents (Table 13.5). However, the response rates for newer chemotherapy drugs in MPM are more encouraging.

Byrne *et al.* [3] conducted a phase II study of combined cisplatin and gemcitabine for patients with advanced measurable MPM. Of the 21 patients treated, 62 per cent had epithelioid tumours and 18 were classified as AJCC stage III or IV. There was a 47.6 per cent (95 per cent confidence interval 26.2–69.0 per cent) response rate with symptom improvement in responding patients. Toxicity was mainly gastroenterological and haematological. This study has demonstrated the best response rate to date.

The feasibility of cisplatin and gemcitabine was confirmed in a multicentre study by Nowak *et al.* [60], but the overall response rates were lower than in the initial single-institution study. Quality of life and pulmonary function were assessed at each cycle. In 52 evaluable patients, partial response was seen in 17 patients (33 per cent), stable disease in 31 (60 per cent), and progressive disease in four (8 per cent). The median time to disease progression was 6.4 months, the median survival from start of treatment was 11.2 months, and the median survival from diagnosis was 17.3 months. Vital capacity and the global quality of life improved significantly in responding patients.

A phase III international trial comparing cisplatin with cisplatin and pemetrexed (a new multi-targeted antifolate) has recently been reported [4] During a 2 year period, 448 patients were enrolled and randomized. Overall survival was significantly better in the pemetrexed–cisplatin arm (12.1 versus 9.3 months), and the overall response rate was 41 per cent versus 17 per cent for the cisplatin-only arm. An unexpected finding was that folic acid and vitamin B12 supplements improved drug tolerance, thus leading to higher response rates. Pulmonary function tests and quality of life were also better in the cisplatin–pemetrexed arm.

Attempts to combine surgery and chemotherapy include a phase II trial at MSKCC [61]. Patients received a single dose of intrapleural cisplatin 75 mg/m^2 and mitomycin 8 mg/m^2 after complete resection of all gross tumour by pleurectomy–decortication. Additional chemotherapy was administered systemically, starting 1 month postoperatively, using two cycles of cisplatin 50 mg/m^2 per week and mitomycin 8 mg/m^2. This approach of surgical resection and short intensive chemotherapy tried to address the problems of both local control and potential distant metastases. It was based on the established use of intraperitoneal chemotherapy in ovarian cancer and on a smaller but successful experience with intracavitary chemotherapy in both pleural and peritoneal MPM reported by several authors [62–64].

A total of 23 patients received the entire treatment of pleurectomy–decortication and adjuvant chemotherapy. Although the treatment was tolerable it was associated with a high risk of local recurrence (16 of 20 patients). The overall survival was favourable (median survival of 18

Table 13.4 Examples of combination chemotherapy

Agent	Reference	No. of patients	Responders		95% CI (%)	Median survival
			Number	Percentage		
Doxorubicin-containing combinations						
Doxorubicin + cisplatin + mitomycin	Pennucci (1997) [69]	23	5	21	7–42	11
Doxorubicin + cisplatin + mitomycin + bleomycin	Breau (1991) [70]	25	11	44	27–63	NA
Cisplatin-containing combinations						
Cisplatin + DHAC	Samuels (1998) [71]	29	5	17	5–30	6.4
Cisplatin + etoposide	Eisenhauer (1988) [72]	26	3	12	4–30	NA
Cisplatin + gemcitabine	Byrne (1999) [3]	21	10	48	26–69	10.3
Cisplatin + gemcitabine	Novak (2002) [60]	52	17	33	20–46	11.2
Cisplatin + gemcitabine	Van Haarst (2000) [73]	22	4	15	NA	10
Cisplatin + irinotecan	Nakano (1999) [74]	15	4	27	8–55	7.1
Cisplatin + mitomycin + vinblastine	Middleton (1998) [75]	39	8	20	NA	6
Cisplatin + pemetrexed (phase I)	Thodtman (1999) [76]	11	5	45	NA	NA
Cisplatin + paclitaxel	Fizazi (2000) [77]	18	1	6	0–24	12
Other combinations						
Methotrexate + mitoxantrone + mitomycin	Pinto (2001) [78]	22	6	32	12–51	13.5
Carboplatin + gemcitabine	Aversa (1999) [79]	18	3	16	NA	8.6
Carboplatin + pemetrexed (phase I)	Hughes (2002) [80]	25	8	32	NA	15
Oxaliplatin + raltitrexed	Fizazi (2000) [81]	30	9	30	15–49	NA
Oxaliplatin + vinorelbine	Steele (2001) [82]	17	2	12	NA	NA
Doxetaxel + irinotecan	Knuuttila (2000) [83]	15	0	0	2–45	8.8

NA, not available.

Reproduced with permission from Tomek S, Emri S, Krejcy K, Manegold C. Chemotherapy for malignant pleural mesothelioma: past results and recent developments. *Br J Cancer* 2003; 88: 167–74.

Table 13.5 Single-agent chemotherapy since 1995

Single agent	Reference	No. of patients	Responders		95% CI (%)	Median survival (months)
			Number	Percentage		
Anthracyclines and related compounds						
Liposomal doxorubicin	Baas (2000) [84]	32	2	6	V	13
Liposomal doxorubicin	Oh (2000) [85]	24	0	0	NA	9.3
Liposomal daunorubicin	Steele (2001) [86]	11	0	0	NA	6.1
Alkylating agents						
Ifosfamide	Andersen (1999) [88]	26	1	4	0–11	10
ZD0473	Giaccone (2001) [87]	10	Two regressions of evaluable disease		NA	NA
Topoisomerase interactive agents						
Etoposide i.v.	Sahmoud (1997) [89]	49	2	4	1–15	7.3
Etoposide oral	Sahmoud (1997) [89]	45	3	7	2–20	9.5
Campthotecin analogues						
Irinotecan	Kindler (2000) [90]	28	0	0	10–55	7.9
Topotecan	Maksymiuk (1998) [91]	22	0	0	NA	8
Antimicrotubule agents						
Vinca alkaloids						
Vinorelbine	Steele (2000) [92]	64	12	21	10–44	13.4
Vincristine	Martensson (1989) [93]	23	0	0	0–14	7
Vinblastine	Cowan (1988) [94]	20	0	0	0–16	3

290

Table 13.5 Contd.

Single agent	Reference	No. of patients	Responders Number	Percentage	95% CI (%)	Median survival (months)
Taxanes						
Docetaxel	Belani (1999) [95]	19	1	5	0–26	NA
Docetaxel	Vorobiof (2000) [96]	22	3	14	7–46	12
Paclitaxel	van Meerbeck (1996) [97]	25	0	0	0–15	9.8
Paclitaxel	Vogelzang (1999) [98]	35	Three regressions of evaluable disease		2–10	5
Antimetabolites						
Edatrexate	Kindler (1999) [99]	20	5	25	9–49	9.6
Edatrexate + LV-rescue	Kindler (1999) [99]	38	6	16	6–31	6.6
Gemcitabine	Kindler (2001) [100]	17	0	0	3–13	4.1
Gemcitabine	van Meerbeck (1999) [101]	27	2	7	1–24	8
Gemcitabine	Bischoff (1998) [102]	16	5	31	NA	NA
Pemetrexed	Scagliotti (2001) [103]	62	9	6	NA	10.7

Reproduced with permission from Tomek S, Emri S, Krejcy K, Manegold C. Chemotherapy for malignant pleural mesothelioma: past results and recent developments. *Br J Cancer* 2003; 88: 167–74.

months; 40 per cent at 2 years), but the high rate of local relapse after intensive chemotherapy was believed not to warrant further trials of incorporating this approach into treatment.

The development of better-tolerated more effective chemotherapy regimens, and the establishment of extrapleural pneumonectomy and adjuvant hemithoracic radiation as a sound approach to local control, has led to new combined modality trials. At MSKCC, we are completing a phase II trial of induction cisplatin and gemcitabine (as reported by Byrne *et al.* [3]) followed by extrapleural pneumonectomy and adjuvant hemithoracic radiation (total dose 54 Gy). Pilot experience at MSKCC with this combined modality approach suggested that it was feasible. This treatment regimen has also been tested in single and multicentre phase II trials in Switzerland and is reported to be feasible [65,66]. Long-term follow-up data are awaited.

Most recently, the development of the cisplatin and pemetrexed regimen has led to a multicentre trial in the USA. Patients with clinical stages I–III MPM are eligible if their cardiopulmonary function indicates that extrapleural pneumonectomy can be tolerated. Induction therapy with cisplatin and pemetrexed [4] is followed by extrapleural pneumonectomy and 54 Gy of adjuvant hemithoracic radiation as described at MSKCC [22]. This clinical trial represents the logical summation of previous trials discussed above, which established the most effective current approaches to systemic therapy and locoregional disease control.

Summary

MPM is an uncommon and usually fatal malignancy. Much about MPM tumour biology and clinical behaviour remains poorly understood. However, during the past 20 years the diagnosis, staging, and treatment of MPM have improved significantly. Continued study of this disease is needed, but effective multimodality treatment regimens for MPM are now available.

References

1. Butchart EG, Ashcroft T, Barnsley WC, Holden MP. Pleuropneumonectomy in the management of diffuse malignant mesothelioma of the pleura. Experience with 29 patients. *Thorax* 1976; **31**: 15–24.

2. Rusch VW (1999) Indications for Pneumonectomy. Extrapleural pneumonectomy. *Chest Surg Clin N Am* 1999; **9**: 327–38.

3. Byrne MJ, Davidson JA, Musk AW, *et al.* Cisplatin and gemcitabine treatment for malignant mesothelioma: a phase II study. *J Clin Oncol* 1999; **17**: 25–30.

4. Vogelzang NJ, Rusthoven J, Symanowski J, *et al.* Phase III study of pemetrexed in combination with cisplatin versus cisplatin alone in patients with malignant pleural mesothelioma. *J Clin Oncol* 2003; **21**: 2636–44.

5. Mattson K. Natural history and clinical staging of malignant mesothelioma. *Eur J Respir Dis*1982; **63** (Suppl 124): 87.

6. Chahinian AP, Pajak TF, Holland JF, Norton L, Ambinder RM, Mandel EM. Diffuse malignant mesothelioma. Prospective evaluation of 69 patients. *Ann Int Med* 1982; **96**: 746–55

7. Sugarbaker DJ, Strauss GM, Lynch TJ, *et al.* Node status has prognostic significance in the multimodality therapy of diffuse, malignant mesothelioma. *J Clin Oncol* 1993; **11**: 1172–8.

8. Sugarbaker DJ, Flores RM, Jaklitsch MT, *et al.* Resection margins, extrapleural nodal status, and cell type determine postoperative long-term survival in trimodality therapy of malignant pleural mesothelioma: Results of 183 patients. *J Thorac Cardiovasc Surg* 1999; **117**: 54–65.

9. Rusch VW, International Mesothelioma Interest Group. A proposed new international TNM staging system for malignant pleural mesothelioma. *Chest* 1995; **108**: 1122–8.

10. Union Internationale Contre le Cancer. *TNM Classification of Malignant Tumours.* New York: Wiley–Liss, 2002.

11. American Joint Committee on Cancer. *AJCC Cancer Staging Handbook*. New York: Springer-Verlag, 2002

12. Boutin C, Rey F. Thoracoscopy in pleural malignant mesothelioma: a prospective study of 188 consecutive patients. Part 1: Diagnosis. *Cancer* 1993; **72**: 389–393

13. Tammilehto L. Malignant mesothelioma: prognostic factors in a prospective study of 98 patients. *Lung Cancer* 1992; **8**: 175–84.

14. Mountain CF. Revisions in the International System for Staging Lung Cancer. *Chest* 1997; **111**: 1710–17.

15. Allen KB, Faber LP, Warren WH. Malignant pleural mesothelioma. Extrapleural pneumonectomy and pleurectomy. *Chest Surg Clin N Am* 1994; **4**: 113–26.

16. Rusch VW, Venkatraman ES. Important prognostic factors in patients with malignant pleural mesothelioma, managed surgically. *Ann Thorac Surg* 1999; **68**: 1799–1804.

17. Ruffie P, Feld R, Minkin S, *et al.* Diffuse malignant mesothelioma of the pleura in Ontario and Quebec: a retrospective study of 332 patients. *J Clin Oncol* 1989; 7: 1157–68.

18. Patz EF, Jr., Shaffer K, Piwnica-Worms DR, *et al.* Malignant pleural mesothelioma: value of CT and MR imaging in predicting resectability. *Am J Roentgenol* 1992; **159**: 961–6.

19. Knuuttila A, Halme M, Kivisaari L, Kivisaari A, Salo J, Mattson K. The clinical importance of magnetic resonance imaging versus computed tomography in malignant pleural mesothelioma. *Lung Cancer* 1998; **22**: 215–25.

20. Stewart D, Waller D, Edwards J, Jeyapalan K, Entwisle J. Is there a role for pre-operative contrast-enhanced magnetic resonance imaging for radical surgery in malignant pleural mesothelioma? *Eur J Cardiothorac Surg* 2003; **24**: 1019–24.

21. Heelan RT, Rusch VW, Begg CB, Panicek DM, Caravelli JF, Eisen C (1999) Staging of malignant pleural mesothelioma: comparison of CT and MR imaging. *Am J Radiol* 1999; **172**: 1039–47.

22. Rusch VW, Rosenzweig K, Venkatraman E, *et al.* A phase II trial of surgical resection and adjuvant high dose hemithoracic radiation for malignant pleural mesothelioma. *J Thorac Cardiovasc Surg* 2001; **122**: 788–95.

23. Pass HI, Temeck BK, Kranda K, Steinberg SM, Feuerstein IR. Preoperative tumor volume is associated with outcome in malignant pleural mesothelioma. *J Thorac Cardiovasc Surg* 1998; **115**: 310–18.

24. Flores R, Akhurst T, Gonen M, Larson S, Rusch V. Positron emission tomography (PET) defines metastatic disease but not locoregional disease in patients with malignant pleural mesothelioma. *J Thorac Cardiovasc Surg* 2003; **126**: 11–16.

25. Flores RM, Akhurst T, Gonen M, Larson S, Rusch VW (2003) FDG-PET predicts survival in patients with malignant pleural mesothelioma. *Proc Am Soc Clin Oncol* 22: 620 (abstr 2495).

26. Boutin C, Rey F, Gouvernet J, Viallat J-R, Astoul P, Ledoray V. Thoracoscopy in pleural malignant mesothelioma: a prospective study of 188 consecutive patients. Part 2: Prognosis and staging. *Cancer* 1993; **72**: 394–404.

27. Conlon KC, Rusch VW, Gillern S. Laparoscopy: an important tool in the staging of malignant pleural mesothelioma. *Ann Surg Oncol* 1996; **3**: 489–94.

28. Schouwink JH, Kool LS, Rutgers EJ, *et al.* The value of chest computer tomography and cervical mediastinoscopy in the preoperative assessment of patients with malignant pleural mesothelioma. *Ann Thorac Surg* 2003; **75**: 1715–19.

29. Rusch VW. Pleurectomy/decortication and adjuvant therapy for malignant mesothelioma. *Chest* 1993; **103** (Suppl): 382S–4S

30. Rusch VW, Piantadosi S, Holmes EC. The role of extrapleural pneumonectomy in malignant pleural mesothelioma. *J Thorac Cardiovasc Surg* 1991; **102**: 1–9.

31. DeLaria GA, Jensik R, Faber LP, Kittle CF. Surgical management of malignant mesothelioma. *Ann Thorac Surg* 1978; **26**: 375–82.

32. Sugarbaker DJ, Heher EC, Lee TH, *et al.* Extrapleural pneumonectomy, chemotherapy, and radiotherapy in the treatment of diffuse malignant pleural mesothelioma. *J Thorac Cardiovasc Surg* 1991; **102**: 10–15.

33. Sugarbaker DJ, Garcia JP, Richards WG, *et al.* Extrapleural pneumonectomy in the multimodality therapy of malignant pleural mesothelioma. Results in 120 consecutive patients. *Ann Surg* 1996; **224**: 288–96.

34. DeValle MJ, Faber LP, Kittle CF, Jensik RJ Extrapleural pneumonectomy for diffuse, malignant mesothelioma. *Ann Thorac Surg* 1986; **42**: 612–18.

35. Rusch VW, Venkatraman E. The importance of surgical staging in the treatment of malignant pleural mesothelioma. *J Thorac Cardiovasc Surg* 1996; **111**: 815–26.

36. McCormack PM, Nagasaki F, Hilaris BS, Martini N (1982) Surgical treatment of pleural mesothelioma. *J Thorac Cardiovasc Surg* 1982; **84**: 834–42.

37. Achatzy R, Beba W, Ritschler R, *et al.* The diagnosis, therapy and prognosis of diffuse malignant mesothelioma. *Eur J Cardiothorac Surg* 1989; **3**: 445–8.

38. Alberts AS, Falkson G, Goedhals L, Vorobiof DA, Van Der Merwe CA. Malignant pleural mesothelioma: a disease unaffected by current therapeutic maneuvers. *J Clin Oncol* 1988; **6**: 527–35

39. Hilaris BS, Dattatreyudu N, Kwong E, Kutcher GJ, Martini N. Pleurectomy and intraoperative brachytherapy and postoperative radiation in the treatment of malignant pleural mesothelioma. *Int J Radiat Oncol Biol Phys* 1984; **10**: 325–31.

40. Kutcher GJ, Kestler C, Greenblatt D, Brenner H, Hilaris BS, Nori D. Technique for external beam treatment for mesothelioma. *Int J Radiat Oncol Biol Phys* 1987; **13**: 1747–52.

41. Mychalczak BR, Nori D, Armstrong JG, Martini N, Harrison LB (1989) Results of treatment of malignant pleural mesothelioma with surgery, brachytherapy, and external beam irradiation. *Endocurie Hypertherm Oncol* 1989; **5**: 245.

42. Soubra M, Dunscombe PB, Hodson DI, Wong G. Physical aspects of external beam radiotherapy for the treatment of malignant pleural mesothelioma. *Int J Radiat Oncol Biol Phys* 1990; **18**: 1521–7.

43. Boutin C, Rey F, Viallat J-R. Prevention of malignant seeding after invasive diagnostic procedures in patients with pleural mesothelioma. A randomized trial of local radiotherapy. *Chest* 1995; **108**: 754–8.

44. Low EM, Khoury GG, Matthews AW, Neville E. Prevention of tumour seeding following thoracoscopy in mesothelioma by prophylactic radiotherapy. *Clin Oncol* 1995; **7**: 317–18.

45. Baldini EH, Recht A, Strauss GM, *et al.* Patterns of failure after trimodality therapy for malignant pleural mesothelioma. *Ann Thorac Surg* 1997; **63**: 334–8.

46. Keller SM, Taylor DD, Weese JL. *In vitro* killing of human malignant mesothelioma by photodynamic therapy. *J Surg Res* 1990; **48**: 337–40.

47. Ris H-B, Altermatt JH, Inderbitzi R, *et al.* Photodynamic therapy with chlorins for diffuse malignant mesothelioma: initial clinical results. *Br J Cancer* 1991; **64**: 1116–20.

48. Pass HI, DeLaney TF, Tochner Z, *et al.* Intrapleural photodynamic therapy: results of a phase I trial. *Ann Surg Oncol* 1994; **1**: 28–37.

49. Pass HI, Temeck BK, Kranda K, *et al.* Phase III randomized trial of surgery with or without intraoperative photodynamic therapy and postoperative immunochemotherapy for malignant pleural mesothelioma. *Ann Surg Oncol* 1997; **4**: 628–33.

50. Sterman DH, Treat J, Litzky LA, *et al.* Adenovirus-mediated herpes simplex virus thymidine kinase/ganciclovir gene therapy in patients with localized malignancy: Results of a phase I clinical trial in malignant mesothelioma. *Hum Gene Ther* 1998; **9**: 1083–92.

51. Hwang HC, Smythe WR, Elshami AA, *et al.* Gene therapy using adenovirus carrying the herpes simplex-thymidine kinase gene to treat *in vivo* models of human malignant mesothelioma and lung cancer. *Am J Resp Cell Mol Biol* 1995; **13**: 7–16.

52. Krarup-Hansen A, Hansen HH. Chemotherapy in malignant mesothelioma: a review. *Cancer Chemother Pharmacol* 1991; **28**: 319–30.

53. Ong ST, Vogelzang NJ. Chemotherapy in malignant pleural mesothelioma: a review. *J Clin Oncol* 1996; **14**: 1007–17.

54. Tomek S, Emri S, Krejcy K, Manegold C. Chemotherapy for malignant pleural mesothelioma: past results and recent developments. *Br J Cancer* 2003; **88**: 167–74.

55. Dimitrov NV, Egner J, Balcueva E, Suhrland LG. High-dose methotrexate with citrovorum factor and vincristine in the treatment of malignant mesothelioma. *Cancer* 1982; **50**: 1245–7.

56. Chahinian AP, Holland JF, Mandel EM. Chemotherapy for malignant mesothelioma with adriamycin and continuous infusion of 5-azacytidine. *Cancer Treat Rep* 1978; **62**: 1108–9.

57. Dabouis G, LeMevel B, Corroller J. Treatment of diffuse pleural malignant mesothelioma by *cis* dichloro diammine platinum (C.D.D.P.) in nine patients. *Cancer Chemother Pharmacol* 1981; **5**: 209–10.

58. Raghavan D, Gianoutsos P, Bishop J, *et al.* Phase II trial of carboplatin in the management of malignant mesothelioma. *J Clin Oncol* 1990; **8**: 151–4.

59. Umsawasdi T, Dhingra HM, Charnsangavej C, Luna MA. A case report of malignant pleural mesothelioma with long-term disease control after chemotherapy. *Cancer* 1991; **67**: 48–54.

60. Nowak AK, Byrne MJ, Williamson R, *et al.* A multicentre phase II study of cisplatin and gemcitabine for malignant mesothelioma. *Br J Cancer* 2002; **87**: 491–6.

61. Rusch VW, Saltz L, Venkatraman E, *et al.* A phase II trial of pleurectomy/decortication followed by intrapleural and systemic chemotherapy for malignant pleural mesothelioma. *J Clin Oncol* 1994; **12**: 1156–63.

62. Lederman GS, Recht A, Herman T, Osteen R, Corson J, Antman KH (1987) Long-term survival in peritoneal mesothelioma. The role of radiotherapy and combined modality treatment. *Cancer* 1987; **59**: 1882–6.

63. Markman M. Response of paraneoplastic syndromes to antineoplastic therapy. *West J Med* 1986; **144**: 580–5.

64. Mintzer DM, Kelsen D, Frimmer D, Heelan R, Gralla R. Phase II trial of high-dose cisplatin in patients with malignant mesothelioma. *Cancer Treat Rep* 1985; **69**: 711–12.

65. Stahel RA, Weder W, Ballabeni P, *et al.* (2003) Neoadjuvant chemotherapy followed by pleuropneumonectomy for pleural mesothelioma: a multicenter phase II trial of the SAKK. *Lung Cancer* 2003; **41** (Suppl 2): S59 (abstr O-200).

66. Weder W, Kestenholz P, Taverna C, Bodis S, Lardinois D, Jerman M *et al.* Neoadjuvant chemotherapy followed by extrapleural pneumonectomy in malignant pleural mesothelioma. *J Clin Oncol* 2004; **22**: 3451–3457.

67. Worn H. Moglichkeiten und ergebnisse der chirurgischen behandlung des malignen pleuramesothelioms. *Thoraxchirurgie Vaskulare Chirurgie* 1974; **22**: 391.

68. Vogt-Moykopf I, Etspüler W, Bülzebruck H. Des diffuse maligne Pleuramesotheliom: Diagnostick, Therapie und Prognose. *Z Herz Thorax Gefässchir* 1987; **1**: 67.

69. Pennucci MC, Ardizzoni A, Pronzato P, Fioretti M, Lanfranco C, Verna A *et al.* Combined cisplatin, doxorubicin, and mitomycin for the treatment of advanced pleural mesothelioma. A phase II FONICAP trial. *Cancer* 1997; **79**: 1897–1902.

70. Breau J-L, Boaziz C, Morere JJF. Combination therapy with cisplatinum, adriamycin, bleomycin and mitomycin C plus systemic and intra-pleural hyaluronidase in 25 consecutive cases of stages II, II pleural mesothelioma. Presented at the first International Mesothelioma Conference Paris, France. 1991. (Unpublished Work ?)

71. Samuels BL, Herndon JE, II, Harmon DC, Carey R, Aisner J, Corson JM *et al.* Dihydro-5-azacytidine and cisplatin in the treatment of malignant mesothelioma. A phase II study of the Cancer and Leukemia Group B. *Cancer* 1998; **82**: 1578–1584.

72. Eisenhauer EA, Evans WK, Murray N, Kocha W, Wierzbicki R, Wilson K. A phase II study of VP-16 and cisplatin in patients with unresectable malignant mesothelioma. An NCI Canada Clinical Trial. *Invest New Drugs* 1988; **6**: 327–329.

73. Van Haarst JW, Burgers JA, Manegold CH. Multicenter phase II study of gemcitabine and cisplatin in malignant pleural mesothelioma. Program and Abstracts of the 9th World Conference on Lung Cancer, Tokyo, Japan September 11–15, Abstract 56. 2000. (Unpublished?)

74. Nakano T, Chahinian AP, Shinjo M, Togawa N, Tonomura A, Miyake M *et al.* Cisplatin in combination with irinotecan in the treatment of patients with malignant pleural mesothelioma. A pilot Phase II clinical trial and pharmacokinetic profile. *Cancer* 1999; **85**: 2375–2384.

75. Middleton GW, Smith IE, O'Brien MER, Norton A, Hickish T, Priest K *et al.* Good symptom relief with palliative MVP (mitomycin-C, vinblastine and cisplatin) chemotherapy in malignant mesothelioma. *Ann Oncol* 1998; **9**: 269–273.

76. Thodtmann R, Depenbrock H, Blatter J, Johnson RD, van Oosterom A, Hanauske A-R. Preliminary results of a phase I study with MTA (LY231514) in combination with cisplatin in patients with solid tumors. *Semin Oncol* 1999; **26**: 89–93.

77. Fizazi K, Caliandro R, Soulié P, Fandi A, Daniel C, Bedin A *et al.* Combination raltitrexed (Tomudex(R)-oxaliplatin: A step forward in the struggle against mesothelioma? The Institut Gustave Roussy experience with chemotherapy and chemo-immunotherapy in mesothelioma. *Eur J Cancer* 2000; **36**: 1514–1521.

78. Pinto C, Marino A, Guaraldi M, Melotti B, Piana E, Martoni A *et al.* Combination chemotherapy with mitoxantrone, methotrexate, and mitomycin in malignant pleural mesothelioma: A Phase II study. *Am J Clin Oncol* 2001; **24**: 143–147.

79. Aversa SL, Crcuri C, DePangher V. Carboplatin and gemcitabine chemotherapy for malignant pleural mesothelioma: A Phase II study of the GSTPV. *Clin Lung Cancer* 1999; **1**: 73–5.

80. Hughes A, Calvert P, Azzabi A, Plummer A, Johnsons R, Rusthoven R *et al.* Phase I clinical and pharmacokinetic study of pemetrexed and carboplatin in patients with malignant pleural mesothelioma. *J Clin Oncol* 2002; **20**: 3533–3544.

81. Fizazi K, Doubre H, Le Chevalier T, Riviere A, Viala J, Daniel C *et al.* Combination of raltitrexed and oxaliplatin is an active regimen in malignant mesothelioma: results of a phase II study. *J Clin Oncol* 2003; **21**: 349–354.

82. Steele JPC, Shamash J, Evans MT, Goonewardene TI, Nystrom ML, Gower NH *et al.* Phase II trial of vinorelbine and oxaliplatin in malignant pleural mesothelioma. *Proc ASCO* 2001; **20**: 335, abstr 1335.

83. Knuuttila A, Ollikainen T, Halme M, Mali P, Kivisaari L, Linnainmaa K *et al.* Doxetaxel and irinotecan (CPT-11) in the treatment of malignant pleural mesothelioma – a feasibility study. *Anticancer Drugs* 2000; **11**: 257–261.

84. Baas P, van Meerbeeck J, Groen H, Schouwink H, Burgers S, Daamen S *et al.* CaelyxTM in malignant mesothelioma: A Phase II EORTC study. *Ann Oncol* 2000; **11**: 697–700.

85. Oh Y, Perez-Soler R, Fossella FV, Glisson BS, Kurie J, Walsh GL *et al.* Phase II study of intravenous Doxil in malignant pleural mesothelioma. *Invest New Drugs* 2000; **18**: 243–245.

86. Steele JPC, O'Doherty CA, Shamash J, Evans MT, Gower NH, Tischkowitz MD *et al.* Phase II trial of liposomal daunorubicin in malignant pleural mesothelioma. *Ann Oncol* 2001; **12**: 497–499.

87. Giaccone G, O'Brien M, Byrne MJ, Van Steenkiste J, Cosaert J. Phase Ii trial of ZD0473 in patients with mesothelioma relapsing after one prior chemotherapy regimen. *Proc ASCO* 2001; **20**: 257b, Abs A2781.

88. Andersen MK, Krarup-Hansen A, Martensson G, Winther-Nielsen H, Thylen A, Damgaard K *et al.* Ifosfamide in malignant mesothelioma: A Phase II study. *Lung Cancer* 1999; **24**: 39–43.

89. Sahmoud T, Postmus PE, van Pottelsberghe C, Mattson K, Tammilehto L, Splinter TAW *et al.* Etoposide in malignant pleural mesothelioma: Two phase II trials of the EORTC Lung Cancer Cooperative Group. *Eur J Cancer* 1997; **33**: 2211–2215.

90. Kindler HL, Herndon JE, Vogelzang NJ, Green MR, The Cancer and Leukemia Group B. CPT-11 in malignant mesothelioma: A Phase II trial by the Cancer and Leukemia Group B (CALGB 9733). *Proc ASCO* 2000; **19**: 505 – abstr 1978.

91. Maksymiuk AW, Marschke RFJr, Tazelaar HD, Grill J, Nair S, Marks RS *et al.* Phase II trial of topotecan for the treatment of mesothelioma. *Am J Clin Oncol* 1998; **21**: 610–613.

92. Steele JPC, Shamash J, Evans MT, Gower NH, Tischkowitz MD, Rudd RM. Phase II study of vinorelbine in patients with malignant pleural mesothelioma. *J Clin Oncol* 2000; **18**: 3912–3917.

93. Martensson G, Sorenson S. A phase II study of vincristine in malignant mesothelioma – a negative report. *Cancer Chemother Pharmacol* 1989; **24**: 133–134.

94. Cowan JD, Green S, Lucas J, Weick JK, Balcerzak SP, Rivkin SE *et al*. Phase II trial of five day intravenous infusion vinblastine sulfate in patients with diffuse malignant mesothelioma: a Southwest Oncology Group study. *Invest New Drugs* 1988; **6**: 247–248.

95. Belani CP, Adak S, Aisner S, Stella PJ, Levitan N, Johnson DH *et al*. Docetaxel for malignant mesothelioma: Phase II study of the Eastern Cooperative Oncology Group (ECOG 2595). *Proc ASCO* 1999; **18**: 474 – abstr 1829.

96. Vorobiof DA, Chasen MR, Abratt RP, Rapoport BL, Cronje N, Fourie LS *et al*. Phase II trial of single agent taxotere in malignant pleural mesothelioma. *Proc ASCO* 2000; **19**: 578a, abstr 2277.

97. van Meerbeeck J, Debruyne C, Van Zandwijk N, Postmus PE, Pennucci MC, van Breukelen F *et al*. Paclitaxel for malignant pleural mesothelioma: A phase II study of the EORTC Lung Cancer Cooperative Group. *Br J Cancer* 1996; **74**: 961–963.

98. Vogelzang NJ, Herndon JE, II, Miller A, Strauss G, Clamon G, Stewart FM *et al*. High-dose paclitaxel plus G-CSF for malignant mesothelioma: CALGBN phase II study 9234. *Ann Oncol* 1999; **10**: 597–600.

99. Kindler HL, Belani CP, Herndon JE, II, Vogelzang NJ, Suzuki Y, Green MR. Edatrexate (10-ethyl-deaza-aminopterin) (NSC# 626715) with or without leucovorin rescue for malignant mesothelioma. Sequential Phase II trials by the Cancer and Leukemia Group B. *Cancer* 1999; **86**: 1985–1991.

100. Kindler HL, Millard F, Herndon JE, II, Vogelzang NJ, Suzuki Y, Green MR. Gemcitabine for malignant mesothelioma: A Phase II trial by the Cancer and Leukemia Group B. *Lung Cancer* 2001; **31**: 311–317.

101. van Meerbeeck J, Baas P, Debruyne C, Groen HJ, Manegold C, Ardizzoni A *et al*. A Phase II study of gemcitabine in patients with malignant pleural mesothelioma. *Cancer* 1999; **85**: 2577–2582.

102. Bischoff HG, Manegold C, Knopp M, Blatter J, Drings P. Gemcitabine may reduce tumor load and tumor associated symptoms in malignant pleural mesothelioma. *Proc ASCO* 1998; **17**: A1784.

103. Scagliotti G, Shin D, Kindler H, Keppler U. Phase II study of ALIMTA (pemetrexed disodium, MTA) single agent in patients with malignant pleural mesothelioma. *European Journal of Cancer* 2001; **37** (Suppl 6): S20–S21.

Chapter 14

Systemic chemotherapy for malignant pleural mesothelioma

J. P. C. Steele and R. M. Rudd

Introduction

Chemotherapy can be an effective treatment for patients with malignant pleural mesothelioma (MPM). It is arguably the most important of current treatment approaches because few patients are suitable for radical surgery. Palliative surgery is of considerable value but it must be performed by specialist surgeons for optimum benefit [1]. Radiotherapy can control symptoms but does not improve survival [2–4]. For the majority of mesothelioma patients, who generally have International Mesothelioma Interest Group (IMIG) stage III or IV disease, the major treatment decision is whether or not to opt for a course of chemotherapy. In our experience patients often hold strong views for or against chemotherapy. Some patients in the UK will not accept chemotherapy at any stage of their disease. Alternatively, other patients are determined to proceed with chemotherapy or other drug therapy 'whatever the side effects'.

The responsibility rests with the mesothelioma physician who must give the patient the best and most relevant advice as to the choice of drugs and the likely benefits and toxicities. The decision is not difficult if the patient presents with advanced disease: cachexia, anorexia, and overwhelming debility eventually occur in the majority of patients with MPM and, once established, are unlikely to be reversed by chemotherapy. Patients who present in very good condition with minimal symptoms also pose a dilemma because chemotherapy may worsen their quality of life for uncertain benefit.

Until recently the data supporting the use of chemotherapy were lacking [5,6], but we now know that it can be beneficial when used judiciously in appropriate patients [7,8]. Chemotherapy offers patients the chance of symptom palliation, improved quality of life, and prolonged survival. Although chemotherapy has been used for over two decades, it is only in the last 4 years, with the publication of important phase II and III trial data, that clinicians have been able to recommend chemotherapy with confidence. Recently, results were published from the first large randomized, international phase III trials comparing combination chemotherapy with single-agent chemotherapy [7,8]. The importance of this interesting new data is less to do with the actual drugs chosen than with the fact that large randomized trials are being conducted in this once neglected disease. The evidence for improvement in survival with effective palliative treatment is also interesting.

Clinical trials of chemotherapy in MPM

To date the majority of clinical studies reported have been phase II trials (see Chapter 13). Generally patients with unresectable MPM and of good performance status (normally Eastern Cooperative Oncology Group (ECOG) score 0–1 or equivalent) have been entered [9]. Patients are usually heterogeneous between studies with regard to stage and prognostic factors. This makes comparisons between studies difficult and potentially misleading [10,11]. Two prognostic scoring systems, those of the Cancer and Leukemia Group B (CALGB) and the European Organization for Research and Treatment of Cancer (EORTC), have been described for malignant pleural mesothelioma based on data collected from patients entered into cooperative group trials [12,13]. At our centre 134 patients treated in phase II trials were retrospectively stratified by the EORTC system. The data show that the EORTC system is able to identify different prognostic groups robustly [14].

Tumour response can be very difficult to measure by conventional radiology in patients with MPM. Standardized criteria for response evaluation by CT scan improved the consistency of reported response rates compared with older studies based on chest radiographs, but until recently conventional criteria required the presence of bidimensionally measurable tumour, even though MPM is usually only measurable in one dimension because it grows contiguously along the pleural surface.

Adoption of the unidimensional measurement standards as outlined by the Response Evaluation Criteria In Solid Tumors (RECIST) guidelines should make tumour response in

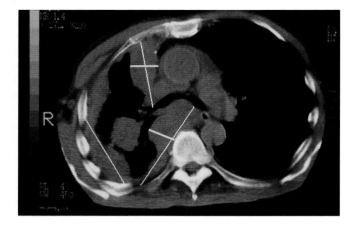

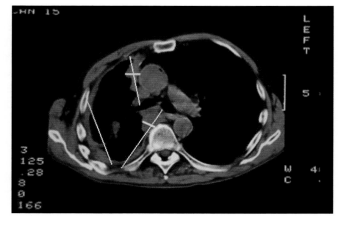

Figure 14.1 RECIST criteria and modified RECIST criteria. Right-sided mesothelioma (a) before and (b) after chemotherapy with transthoracic thickness estimated by RECIST method (white lines) and Byrne and Nowak's method (yellow lines). These images show that the method proposed by Byrne and Nowak offers a simpler technique for response assessment.

MPM studies more meaningful [15]. Byrne and Nowak [16] described a similar method of response evaluation using unidimensional measurement of the tumour at three separate levels on cross-sectional CT scan. This method incorporates measurements taken perpendicular to vital structures such as the vertebral column and the chest wall, and it may be simpler and more reproducible than the RECIST approach. This technique is illustrated in Figure 14.1.

Staging of MPM is another complex issue. In chemotherapy studies stage is often unstated or estimated according to the IMIG system [17]. The difficulty is that staging can only be defined accurately following cytoreductive surgery, a procedure performed on a minority of patients [18,19]. In future, combination of the IMIG staging system, validated prognostic scoring systems, and robust imaging techniques and protocols should allow accurate selection of patients for clinical trials, reproducible response assessment, and comparison of different patient populations between trials [10].

Most chemotherapy agents have been tested in MPM as single agents. In general, single-agent response rates are under 20 per cent. To date no clinical trial has shown a survival advantage for single-agent chemotherapy compared with best supportive care alone, but an ongoing trial in the UK [20] is attempting to address this issue (discussed below). The majority of combination chemotherapy regimens that have been studied for malignant pleural mesothelioma have been anthracycline or platinum based. These regimens generally have response rates of 20 per cent or less, with median survivals in the range of 6–12 months [9]. In the last few years, newer agents have been tested in combination regimens with more encouraging results (Table 14.1). The evidence for and against the available chemotherapy drugs is reviewed in this chapter, with an emphasis on recent data. The role of chemotherapy used prior to cytoreductive surgery is also discussed briefly. (See also Chapter 13).

Anthracyclines and anthracycline combinations

Doxorubicin was once thought to be one of the most active drugs for MPM. However, in a large retrospective series by ECOG, the response rate to single-agent doxorubicin was reported to be only 14 per cent, with a median survival of 7.3 months [21]. Epirubicin has been evaluated in two phase II trials and has a response rate of 15 per cent or less [22,23]. Other anthracycline analogues and formulations, including liposomal doxorubicin, have been tested and dose escalations have been studied. Liposomal doxorubicin has been shown to be ineffective in three phase II trials, none of which produced response rates greater than 10 per cent [24–26]. Steele *et al.* [27] treated 14 patients with liposomal daunorubicin with a median survival of 6.1 months and no responses. Severe myelosuppression occurred in most patients on at least one occasion [27]. The conclusion is that the anthracyclines currently available have no value as single agents in mesothelioma and should not be used.

Similarly, anthracyclines used in combination appear to offer little clinical benefit. Perhaps the most persuasive data in this regard are the results of two trials from over 10 years ago. In 1987, Samson *et al.* [28] compared doxorubicin, cyclophosphamide, and imidazole carboxamide with doxorubicin and cyclophosphamide. The partial response rates were 13 per cent for the three-drug combination and 11 per cent for doxorubicin with cyclophosphamide. The median survivals were 6.3 months and 7.5 months, respectively. Chahinian *et al.* [29] tested cisplatin and doxorubicin (CD) against cisplatin and mitomycin (CM). The response rates were 14 per cent for CD and 26 per cent for CM, with median survivals of 8.8 months and 7.7 months, respectively. One can conclude from these data that doxorubicin in combination with either cisplatin or cyclophosphamide is unlikely to have useful activity in mesothelioma.

Table 14.1 Selected single-agent and combination regimens for MPM[a]

Regimen	Response rate (% patients)	Median survival (months)
Non-randomized trials		
Capecitabine [55]	4	4.9
Daunorubicin (liposomal) [27]	0	6.1
Doxorubicin (liposomal) [24–26]	0–6	9.3–13.0
Gemcitabine [36–38]	0–7	4.1–8
Gemcitabine + cisplatin [39–41]	16–48	9.6–11.2
Gemcitabine + carboplatin [42]	26	15
Irinotecan [66]	0	7.9
Irinotecan + docetaxel [67]	0	8.5
Irinotecan + cisplatin [69]	27	7.1
Irinotecan + cisplatin + mitomycin [70]	43	10.1
Mitomycin + cisplatin + vinblastine [44]	15	7.0
Oxaliplatin + raltitrexed [46]	20	7.1
Oxaliplatin + gemcitabine [47]	40	13.0
Pemetrexed [58]	14	10.7
Pemetrexed + carboplatin [57]	32	14.8
Vinorelbine [63]	21	13.4
Randomized trials		
Cisplatin + mitomycin vs. cisplatin + doxorubicin [29]	26 /14	7.7/8.8
Doxorubicin + cyclophosphamide vs. doxorubicin + cyclophosphamide + DTIC [28]	11 /13	7.5/6.3
Pemetrexed + cisplatin vs. cisplatin [7]	41 /17	12.1/9.3
Raltitrexed + cisplatin vs. cisplatin [8]	23 /14	11.2/8.8
Ranparnase vs. doxorubicin [82]	NA	7.7/8.2

[a] Trials that quote response rates and median survival are included.

Platinum agents

Cisplatin

Platinum analogues have been studied both as single agents and in combined regimens for MPM. Cisplatin 100 mg/m^2 given every 21 days gave a response rate of 14 per cent in patients with diffuse malignant mesothelioma [30]. In a phase II trial reported by Planting *et al.* [31], cisplatin 80 mg/m^2 weekly produced a partial response rate of 36 per cent; however, there were a significant number of discontinuations (34 per cent) due to toxicities. Mintzer *et al.* [32] reported a 13 per cent response rate in 24 patients treated with cisplatin 120 mg/m^2 every 4 weeks.

Carboplatin

Carboplatin, an analogue of cisplatin that is better tolerated and easier to deliver, has been evaluated in three trials containing at least 14 patents. The response rates reported were similar to those with conventional doses of cisplatin (8–16 per cent) in phase II studies [33–35]. In practice, a conventional platinum agent used alone is unlikely to have meaningful clinical benefit for MPM patients.

Platinum agents in combination with gemcitabine

Gemcitabine is a nucleoside analogue drug that has proved valuable since its introduction into clinical practice over the last 10 years. There have been three phase II trials of single-agent gemcitabine in MPM, but unfortunately there is little evidence of significant activity. van Meerbeeck *et al.* [36] treated 27 patients with histologically-confirmed mesothelioma with gemcitabine 1250 mg/m^2 on days 1, 8, and 15 of a 28-day cycle. Two responses were seen, giving a response rate of only 7 per cent. The median survival was 8 months. The only major toxicity was grade 3–4 neutropenia which occurred in 30 per cent of patients. Kindler *et al.* [37] treated patients with 1500 mg/m^2 of gemcitabine on a similar 3 out of 4 weeks schedule. There were no recorded responses and the median survival was a disappointing 4.7 months. The one positive study of gemcitabine is a phase II trial by Bischoff *et al.* [38] in Germany, who used a similar schedule to the EORTC. This group reported a response rate of 31 per cent in five of 16 evaluable patients. In fact, 23 patients were entered on trial, so that the response rate by intention-to-treat analysis was five of 23 patients (i.e. 22 per cent). There appeared to be a clinical benefit even in patients without evidence of response. Therefore gemcitabine used as a single agent may occasionally provide clinical benefit for MPM patients and, despite the generally discouraging phase II data, there may be scope for further trials with the drug.

Although gemcitabine appears to have limited activity as a single agent, it has shown activity in MPM when combined with cisplatin. In the original trial reported in 1999 by Byrne and colleagues from Western Australia [39], a response rate of 48 per cent was reported in MPM patients, with symptom improvement in 90 per cent of responding and 33 per cent of non-responding patients. Grade 3 leucopenia was recorded in 38 per cent of patients and the median overall survival was 9.5 months. Unusually, a cytological diagnosis of MPM was considered sufficient for enrolment in this trial. When the same investigators used the schedule in a multi-institutional study the results remained impressive. Of the 53 patients recruited to the study, 52 had evaluable disease. The best response achieved was a partial response in 33 per cent (95 per cent confidence interval (CI) 20–46 per cent), stable disease in 60 per cent, and progressive disease in only 8 per cent. The median time to disease progression was 6.4 months, the median survival from the start of treatment was 11.2 months, and the median survival from diagnosis was 17.3 months. Vital capacity and global quality of life remained stable in all patients and improved significantly in responding patients [40]. van Haarst *et al.* [41] reported a response rate of 16 per cent for a three-weekly cycle of gemcitabine and cisplatin. Carboplatin is also effective in combination with gemcitabine, with a partial response rate of 26 per cent and median survival of 15 months [42].

Mitomycin, vinblastine, and cisplatin

A study of the combination of mitomycin, vinblastine, and cisplatin administered three-weekly, a well-known regimen in non-small-cell lung cancer, was reported by Middleton *et al.* [43] from the Royal Marsden Hospital, London. Eight out of 39 patients responded, giving a 20 per cent response rate. Sixty-two percent of patients were recorded as having symptom relief. In an extended series of 150 patients from the same institution the response rate was lower at 15 per cent, with 69 per cent having stable disease. The median survival was 7 months with 1 and 2 year survival rates of 31 per cent and 11 per cent, respectively. Median survival was 10 months for patients with ECOG performance status 0–1 and 6 months for patients with performance status 2–3 [44]. This schedule is included in the UK randomized trial in MPM [20].

Oxaliplatin combinations

New platinum agents are good candidates for investigation because of previous experience with this drug class. Oxaliplatin is a platinum analogue that has been studied in several combination regimens for MPM and is approved by the Food and Drug Administration and European Medicine Evaluation Agency for colon cancer. The combination of oxaliplatin and raltitrexed was evaluated by Fizazi *et al.* [45]. The response rate was 35 per cent, with a favourable toxicity profile in a phase I study in patients previously identified as platinum refractory. The same authors reported a phase II study in which both chemo-naive and previously treated patients were enrolled [46]. The overall response rate was 20 per cent, and median survival from start of treatment for the chemo-naive and previously treated groups was 31 weeks and 44 weeks, respectively.

Oxaliplatin is also active when combined with gemcitabine, with a response rate of 40 per cent and a median survival of 13 months reported by Schuette *et al.* [47]. However, when combined with vinorelbine in a phase II trial, oxaliplatin significantly increased the overall toxicity and did not appear to offer any advantage over vinorelbine alone [48]. The patients entered into this trial had a preponderance of poor prognosis features (such as stage 4 disease, unfavourable histology, and poor performance status) which may have adversely affected the results.

Antifolate agents

Antifolate chemotherapy drugs have modest activity as single agents in malignant pleural mesothelioma. This activity may be explained by the fact that the α-folate receptor gene is over-expressed in up to 72 per cent of MPM tumours [49].

Methotrexate and edatrexate

In a phase II trial of 60 MPM patients, high-dose methotrexate produced a partial response rate of 37 per cent and median survival of 11 months [50]. The treatment was well tolerated in light of the known effects of pleural fluid collections on methotrexate pharmacokinetics. A study of high-dose methotrexate (with leucovorin rescue) in combination with interferon-α and interferon-γ in 26 patients with localized MPM demonstrated a response rate of 29 per cent and a median survival of 17 months [51]. Survival rates at 1 year and 2 years were 62 per cent and 31 per cent, respectively. The treatment was surprisingly well tolerated, with only two patients requiring dose reductions and one patient discontinuing treatment secondary to toxicity. In a CALGB phase II study of 58 patients, weekly edatrexate with or without leucovorin demonstrated an objective response rate of 15 per cent. Toxicity was unacceptably high [52].

Fluorouracil and capecitabine

Unlike most newer antifolates tested in MPM, fluorouracil (5-FU) only exhibits minimal activity [53,54]. Capecitabine is an orally available antifolate which is widely used in place of 5-FU in patients with colorectal cancer. Disappointingly, in view of the convenience of this drug, a phase

II trial recently reported by Otterson *et al.* [55] did not show useful activity in patients with MPM. The partial response rate was 4 per cent and the median survival under 5 months.

Pemetrexed and pemetrexed combinations

Pemetrexed is a multitargeted antifolate drug that has excited considerable interest in MPM. The manufacturer of pemetrexed took the decision to test this new agent in MPM patients before more common cancers. This is an unusual and bold approach that most MPM specialists would support. During the pemetrexed phase I and II development programme [56,57] severe toxicities were observed, including grade 4 neutropenia with infection, grade 3–4 diarrhea, grade 4 thrombocytopenia, grade 3–4 mucositis, and treatment-related deaths. Analysis of patient characteristics and toxicities showed a significant association between elevated homocysteine (a marker of folate status) and increased risk of toxicities.

Because of these observations, supplemental folic acid and vitamin B12 were administered and reduced the incidence and severity of haematological and non-haematological toxicities, without apparently worsening efficacy. Sixty-four patients with MPM entered a phase II single-agent trial of pemetrexed [58]. Sixteen patients completed treatment before vitamin supplementation was required, five started taking vitamin supplementation during the treatment, and 43 received vitamins throughout their pemetrexed treatment. Nine of 64 patients (14 per cent) had a partial response, with seven of the nine responses seen in vitamin-supplemented patients. Median survival was 10.7 months, 13.0 months, and 8.0 months for all patients, supplemented patients, and non-supplemented patients, respectively. Myelosuppression was the most common toxicity. Grade 3–4 neutropenia occurred in 52 per cent of patients not receiving supplementation and 9 per cent of supplemented patients. Patients supplemented with vitamins tolerated treatment better and received a median of six cycles of treatment, while non-supplemented patients received a median of two cycles.

A large randomized phase III trial of pemetrexed–cisplatin versus single-agent cisplatin has been reported recently and has generated much interest [7,59]. A total of 456 chemo-naive patients with MPM were randomized, 448 of whom received chemotherapy and were analysed for survival (226 received pemetrexed–cisplatin, and 222 received cisplatin). Patients treated with pemetrexed–cisplatin received six cycles of treatment, while cisplatin-treated patients received four cycles. Because of early evidence of severe toxicity, possibly related to reduced folic acid and vitamin B12, all patients treated with pemetrexed subsequently received oral folic acid and intramuscular vitamin B12 supplementation. This resulted in three patient subgroups: not supplemented (completed treatment before the protocol change), partially supplemented (started treatment before the change and completed treatment after the change), and fully supplemented (began treatment after the change). The results showed that the pemetrexed–cisplatin combination was more effective than the cisplatin treatment in terms of median survival (12.1 months vs. 9.3 months, $P = 0.020$), median time to progressive disease (5.7 months vs. 3.9 months, $P = 0.001$), and response rate (41 per cent vs. 17 per cent, $P = 0.0001$) using criteria that allowed for both bidimensional and unidimensional disease.

Pemetrexed–cisplatin also appeared to be more effective than cisplatin alone in the subgroup of fully supplemented patients, although the median overall survival times (13.3 vs. 10.0 months) were not clearly statistically significant ($P = 0.051$). These data are illustrated in Figure 14.2. Time to progressive disease was 6.1 months vs. 3.9 months ($P = 0.008$), and the response rate was 45.4 per cent vs. 19.6 per cent ($P < 0.001$). A similar treatment effect was seen when the fully and partially supplemented subgroups were combined. Toxicity was more common in the pemetrexed–cisplatin arm, with grade 3–4 neutropenia (28 per cent) and leucopenia (18 per cent)

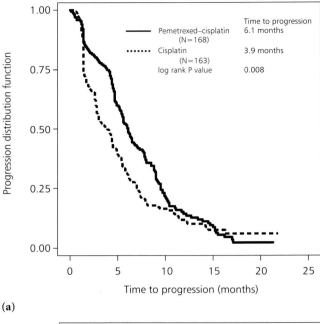

(a)

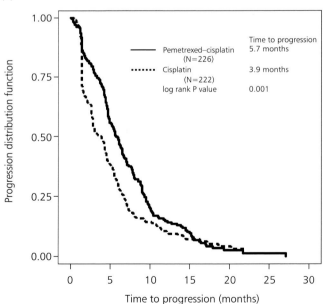

Figure 14.2 Time to tumour progression in (a) patients receiving supplementation with vitamin B12 and folate, and (b) all patients treated in the study.

(b)

being the most common toxicities. Vitamin-supplemented patients did consistently better in terms of efficacy and toxicity than non-supplemented patients. Pulmonary function tests (PFTs) and clinical benefit measures were also collected in this study. Pemetrexed–cisplatin showed significant improvement in both PFT and major disease-related symptoms such as dyspnoea and pain.

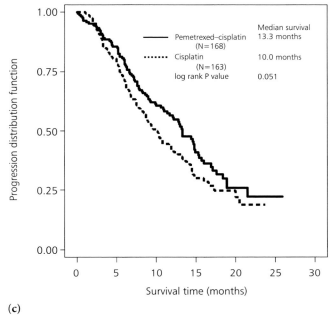

(c)

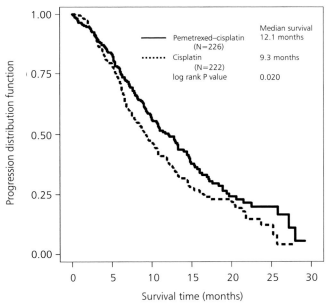

Figure 14.2 Contd. Median survival in (c) patients receiving supplementation with vitamin B12 and folate, and (d) all patients treated in the study.

(d)

This is an important study, not least because it has brought publicity for MPM. The result in terms of improved survival, response rate, and clinical benefits is also highly provocative. However, a degree of caution must be exercised [59]. First, the control arm must be considered. Who would use single-agent cisplatin as treatment for mesothelioma? Most recent trials have tested combinations of a platinum drug with a newer agent or, indeed, newer agents used singly.

This new trial has shown that pemetrexed–cisplatin is more effective than therapy that is inappropriate. Indeed, the quality-of-life analysis showed that the cisplatin control arm was essentially detrimental to symptoms. The authors of this study recommend pemetrexed–cisplatin with full vitamin supplementation as the treatment of choice for MPM, even though this precise combination was not clearly significantly better at prolonging survival than treatment with single-agent cisplatin and vitamins. Despite these reservations about the data from this trial, one can say that pemetrexed and cisplatin is an active regimen which should be compared with other doublet or sequential regimens or regimens containing biological agents in future randomized studies.

Raltitrexed

Raltitrexed, a thymidylate synthase inhibitor, produced a response rate of 21 per cent in a multicentre phase II trial including 24 patients [60] and has subsequently entered trials in Europe in combination with other agents including cisplatin. Raltitrexed has recently been studied in a phase III trial by EORTC [8]. As with the pemetrexed–cisplatin trial discussed above, the comparator arm consisted of cisplatin administered three-weekly. Two hundred and fifty patients were randomized to receive either raltitrexed 3 mg/m^2 with cisplatin 80 mg/m^2 or cisplatin 80 mg/m^2 as a single agent. All treatment was given three-weekly. This was a multicentre international trial. RECIST criteria were used for response assessment. Sixty-eight percent of patients had epithelioid histology. The median age was 58 years (range 19–80 years). There were no toxic deaths and other toxicities were manageable. In the combination chemotherapy group, 16 per cent of patients experienced grade 3 or 4 neutropenia. The figure was 8 per cent for the cisplatin-only group. Other toxicities included fatigue (12 per cent/6 per cent), nausea (14 per cent/10 per cent), emesis (13 per cent/7 per cent), pleuritic pain (6 per cent/10 per cent); and dyspnoea (10 per cent/8 per cent). The overall toxicity of the raltitrexed–cisplatin combination was comparable to that reported in the pemetrexed–cisplatin trial. No harmful effects in health related quality of life were seen in both arms. The treatment led to improvement over time in dyspnoea. This effect was considered clinically meaningful in the cisplatin–raltitrexed arm [61].

How should one interpret this result, especially in relation to the previous data for the pemetrexed–cisplatin combination which had appeared to set a new standard? The response rates and median overall survival figures reported for the raltitrexed–cisplatin combination were inferior to those reported for pemetrexed–cisplatin. These data are presented in Table 14.2. However, this must be seen in the context of slightly different patient populations. Specifically, the EORTC trial included 13 per cent of patients of performance status 2, whereas the pemetrexed investigators excluded such patients. It is possible that even this relatively small proportion of poor-condition

Table 14.2 Comparison of results of randomized trials of antifolate agents in combination with cisplatin

	Pemetrexed–cisplatin trial [7]	Raltitrexed–cisplatin trial [8]
Total number of patients randomized	448	250
ECOG performance score 0–1 (%)	100	87
Overall response rate for antifolate–cisplatin group (%)	41	24
Overall survival for antifolate–cisplatin group (months)	12.1	11.4
Overall survival for cisplatin group (months)	9.3	8.8
P-value for overall survival for log-rank test	0.02	0.048

patients made the results for survival and response worse. Our view is that the EORTC trial result tells us two things: (1) an antifolate (pemetrexed or raltitrexed) in combination with cisplatin is a reasonable first-choice chemotherapy regimen for fit patients with MPM; (2) pemetrexed may or may not offer a new level of activity in the treatment of the disease but is certainly as good a combination as is available. Raltitrexed might prove to be a good alternative drug if economic considerations preclude the use of pemetrexed. The manufacturer of raltitrexed is not pursuing a product license for raltitrexed in MPM which might limit its availability.

Vinca alkaloid agents

Vincristine, vinblastine, and vindesine do not have useful activity against MPM [9]. Vinorelbine is a newer vinca alkaloid agent which has a rather different spectrum of activity from the other drugs in the class being active as a single agent in solid tumours (e.g. breast cancer [62]) and has been evaluated in patients with MPM. Steele *et al.* [63] treated 29 patients with evaluable histogically confirmed MPM (performance status 0, 1, or 2) with weekly vinorelbine 30 mg/m². The response rate was 24 per cent, and an improvement in general physical symptoms was recorded in 41 per cent of patients. Stable disease was seen in 55 per cent of patients and median survival was an encouraging 10.6 months. Serious toxicity was low. In an extended series of 64 MPM patients treated at the mesothelioma unit of St Bartholomew's Hospital, London, a median overall survival of 11.8 months was recorded [64]. Although the response rate with this vinorelbine schedule is modest, the acceptability and ease of administration have led to its acceptance as a possible treatment for patients unable to enter a clinical trial or tolerate combination chemotherapy with a platinum-based regimen. This schedule is under further evaluation in a randomized phase III trial in the UK [20].

Camptothecin agents

Topotecan and irinotecan

Irinotecan and topotecan are topoisomerase I inhibitors with activity in several tumour types including colon cancer, lung cancer, and cervical cancer. They have been evaluated in MPM in several trials. Maksymiuk *et al.* [65] conducted a phase II trial of topotecan; the median survival in 19 patients was 7.6 months and there were no partial responses in the full cohort of 22 patients. The schedule used was 1.5 mg/m² on days 1–5 of a 3 week cycle. Toxicity was substantial, with the majority of patients experiencing grade 3 or 4 myelosuppression. There were no responses with single-agent irinotecan in a phase II trial of the CALGB [66]. Again, toxicity was notable.

When used in combination with docetaxel in 15 patients with IMIG stage III–IV MPM, it failed to produce an objective response, with 15 per cent of the patients exhibiting minor responses [67]. Toxicity was severe, with almost 50 per cent of patients developing neutropenic fever and 40 per cent developing grade 3–4 diarrhoea. Irinotecan may be more effective in combination with at least one other drug. Irinotecan (three-weekly) with gemcitabine (days 1 and 8 every 3 weeks) was evaluated by Ferrari *et al.* [68]. They reported a 14 per cent response rate in 15 patients with MPM. Toxicity was reasonable. Irinotecan with cisplatin may also be an effective combination as it produced a response rate of 27 per cent, with tolerable toxicities, in a 15 patient phase II trial coordinated by Nakano *et al.* [69].

Fennell *et al.* [70] used a combination of irinotecan, cisplatin, and mitomycin C in a 28-day cycle in patients with previously untreated MPM. This trial had previously shown activity in advanced cytokine-resistant kidney cancer [71]. Partial responses were seen in 35 per cent of patients with progression-free survival and overall survival of 6.5 months and 10.1 months, respectively. The most common toxicities were haematological, with 25 patients experiencing grade 3 or 4 neutropenia. Of note, when the same regimen was tested in a group of previously treated patients with MPM, partial responses were seen in three of 13 patients. Vinorelbine was the most commonly used therapy in the first-line setting in these patients [72].

Other agents

Etoposide appears to be inactive in MPM, whether administered orally or intravenously [72]. Taxanes have activity in non-small-cell lung cancer and many other tumours but they are not effective as single agents in MPM. Paclitaxel has been evaluated in two phase II studies, neither of which produced response rates greater than 10 per cent [74,75]. The data for docetaxel are similar with two reported trials, both with low response rates [76,77]. As previously discussed, docetaxel proved very toxic when administered with irinotecan [67]. Other agents, including mitomycin, temozolomide, and ifosfamide, have also been studied as single agents in MPM with poor results [78–80]. Ranpirnase, a ribonuclease extracted from leopard frog eggs, has been studied in mesothelioma. In a phase II trial of 105 patients with unresectable MPM, ranpirnase demonstrated a response rate of only 5 per cent, but it produced stable disease in 43 per cent of patients [81]. Overall survival was 6 months in the intent-to-treat population but 8.3 months in a subset of patients with a good prognosis defined by CALGB criteria. In a randomized phase III trial, ranpirnase showed an improvement in survival by 2 months over doxorubicin (11.3 months vs. 9.1 months) in patients with a CALGB prognostic score of 1–4 [82]. However, overall quality of life in the ranpirnase-treated group was inferior to that of patients treated with doxorubicin, and survival analysis in the intent-to-treat population was hampered by an imbalance between groups of patients with a poor prognosis.

The palliative benefit of chemotherapy

What is the palliative gain for patients from chemotherapy? The pemetrexed–cisplatin trial showed that patients treated with this combination lived longer than those treated with cisplatin alone. But how much longer do patients treated with chemotherapy live than those not treated with any chemotherapy? These questions are being addressed in a randomized study (designated MS01) organized by the British Thoracic Society, the Medical Research Council, and Cancer Research UK [20]. This study, which aims to recruit 840 patients, is in progress in the UK. Patients are randomized between three arms: weekly vinorelbine, the MVP combination (mitomycin, vinblastine, and cisplatin), and an active symptom control (ASC) arm. The ASC arm includes regular review by oncologists, palliative care physicians, and specialist nurses. The feasibility study that preceded the full trial showed that ASC alone is capable of producing substantial symptom relief, confirming the importance of this trial [83].

A recent small randomized trial from O'Brien *et al.* [84] compared the palliative and survival benefits of early versus late use of chemotherapy. Forty-three patients were randomized to receive early treatment with chemotherapy or delayed chemotherapy treatment (DT) commenced at the time of symptomatic progression. The chemotherapy used was mitomycin C, vinblastine, and cisplatin/carboplatin. Twenty-one patients received immediate chemotherapy and 17 of the 22 patients in the delayed treatment group received chemotherapy at symptomatic progression. The median time to progression was 25 weeks in the immediate arm and 11 weeks in the DT group ($P = 0.01$). The median overall survival was 14 months in the immediate arm and 10 months in the DT group ($P = 0.01$). The groups were well matched for clinical features. This study result is very interesting, especially the clear suggestion of a benefit for the early use of palliative chemotherapy. The assumption could be that a large-scale phase III trial with a similar design would convincingly show the benefit of early chemotherapy. This is the question that the UK MS01 trial, due to be completed by Summer 2006, should answer. For fit patients agreeable to chemotherapy, the data of O'Brien *et al.* [84] add weight to the argument for chemotherapy to be given before the onset of severe symptoms.

Neoadjuvant chemotherapy

Chemotherapy given prior to cytoreductive surgery ('neoadjuvant' or 'primary' chemotherapy) is under investigation (see also Chapter 13). The theoretical advantages are that disease may be shrunk prior to surgery and that metastases may be eliminated. The approach is entirely investigational at present, but the recent encouraging data from chemotherapy trials in unresectable patients gives cause for optimism. A recent report presented preliminary data from a feasibility study of neoadjuvant therapy followed by surgery from the Swiss Group for Clinical Cancer Research [85]. Patients with potentially resectable malignant mesothelioma underwent preoperative mediastinoscopy to rule out N2 disease, and were then treated with three cycles of cisplatin (80 mg/m^2 on day 1) and gemcitabine (1000 mg/m^2 on days 1, 8, and 15) in a 28-day cycle. The response rate to neoadjuvant chemotherapy was 32 per cent. Of the 19 patients studied, 16 subsequently underwent extrapleural pneumonectomy with no perioperative mortality. All major postoperative complications, which occurred in six patients, were treated successfully. Postoperative radiotherapy was administered to 13 patients. The overall median survival time was 23 months. The investigators concluded that neoadjuvant chemotherapy was well tolerated in patients with potentially resectable MPM and that the resection rate was encouraging.

Conclusions

Chemotherapy for MPM is starting to have clinical impact. The first two large international randomized trails in MPM have recently been reported and show a survival advantage for cisplatin combined with either pemetrexed or raltitrexed compared with cisplatin alone. The control arms of these trials were not optimal and may have exaggerated the clinical benefit of pemetrexed in combination with cisplatin, although the response rates for single-agent cisplatin were similar to those reported in earlier studies [59].

Other schedules such as gemcitabine and cisplatin may also produce clinical benefit in a proportion of patients. Single-agent protocols may also produce modest clinical benefits; for example, weekly vinorelbine offers useful palliation with low toxicity. Questions remain as to which patients to treat and whether patients with poor performance status should be offered chemotherapy. Other issues to be resolved concern fit patients who are enjoying excellent quality of life. Should chemotherapy be withheld from such patients for a period of time until symptoms appear? The place of chemotherapy before and after surgery is unknown.

Certainly there are more questions than answers, but at least MPM specialists can feel more confident when advising chemotherapy treatment. With the data gained in the last 5 years and the promise of better drugs we can be optimistic that real progress will be achieved. Well-designed randomized trials are needed to achieve this aim.

References

1. Rusch VW, Piantadosi S, Holmes EC. The role of extrapleural pneumonectomy in malignant pleural mesothelioma: a Lung Cancer Study Group trial. *J Thorac Cardiovasc Surg* 1991; **102**: 1–9.

2. Ball DL, Cruickshank DG. The treatment of malignant mesothelioma of the pleura: review of a 5-yr experience, with special reference to radiotherapy. *Am J Clin Oncol* 1990; **13**: 4–9.

3. Bissett D, Macbeth FR, Cram I. The role of palliative radiotherapy in malignant mesothelioma. *Clin Oncol (R Coll Radiol)* 1991; **3**: 315–17.

4. Davis SR, Tan L, Ball DL. Radiotherapy in the treatment of malignant mesothelioma of the pleura, with special reference to its use in palliation. *Australas Radiol* 1994; **38**: 212–14.

5. Chahinian AP, Pajak TF, Holland JF, *et al.* Diffuse malignant mesothelioma. Prospective evaluation of 69 patients. *Ann Intern Med* 1982; **96**: 746–55.

6. Alberts AS, Falkson G, Goedhals L, *et al.* Malignant pleural mesothelioma: a disease unaffected by current therapeutic maneuvers. *J Clin Oncol* 1988; **6**: 527–35.

7. Vogelzang NJ, Rusthoven JJ, Symanowski J, *et al.* Phase III study of pemetrexed in combination with cisplatin versus cisplatin alone in patients with malignant pleural mesothelioma. *J Clin Oncol* 2003; **21**: 2636–44.

8. van Meerbeeck JP, Gaafar R, Manegold C, *et al.* Randomized phase III study of cisplatin with or without raltitrexed in patients with malignant pleural mesothelioma: an intergroup study of the European Organisation for Research and Treatment of Cancer Lung Cancer Group and the National Cancer Institute of Canada. *J Clin Oncol* 2005; **23**: 6881–6889.

9. Baas P. Chemotherapy for malignant mesothelioma: from doxorubicin to vinorelbine. *Semin Oncol* 2002; **29**: 62–9.

10. Steele JP, Rudd RM. Malignant mesothelioma: predictors of prognosis and clinical trials. *Thorax* 2000; **55**, 725–6.

11. Steele JP. Prognostic factors in mesothelioma. *Semin Oncol* 2002; **29**: 36–40.

12. Curran D, Sahmoud T, Therasse P, *et al.* Prognostic factors in patients with pleural mesothelioma: the European Organization for Research and Treatment of Cancer experience. *J Clin Oncol* 1998; **16**: 145–52.

13. Herndon JE, Green MR, Chahinian AP, *et al.* Factors predictive of survival among 337 patients with mesothelioma treated between 1984 and 1994 by the Cancer and Leukemia Group B. *Chest* 1998; **113**: 723–31.

14. Fennell DA, Parmar A, Shamash J, *et al.* Statistical validation of the EORTC prognostic model for malignant pleural mesothelioma based on three consecutive phase II trials. *J Clin Oncol* 2005; **23**: 184–9.

15. Therasse P, Arbuck SG, Eisenhauer EA, *et al.* New guidelines to evaluate the response to treatment in solid tumors. *J Natl Cancer Inst* 2000; **92**: 205–16.

16. Byrne MJ, Nowak AK. Modified RECIST criteria for assessment of response in malignant pleural mesothelioma. *Ann Oncol* 2004; **15**: 257–60.

17. International Mesothelioma Interest Group. A proposed new international TNM staging system for malignant pleural mesothelioma. *Chest* 1995; **108**: 1122–8.

18. Rusch VW. A proposed new international TNM staging system for malignant pleural mesothelioma from the International Mesothelioma Interest Group. *Lung Cancer* 1996; **14**: 1–12.

19. Sugarbaker DJ, Flores RM, Jaklitsch MT, *et al.* Resection margins, extrapleural nodal status, and cell type determine postoperative long-term survival in trimodality therapy of malignant pleural mesothelioma: results in 183 patients. *J Thorac Cardiovasc Surg* 1999; **117**: 54–63.

20. Girling DJ, Muers MF, Qian W, Lobban D. Multicenter randomized controlled trial of the management of unresectable malignant mesothelioma proposed by the British Thoracic Society and the British Medical Research Council. *Semin Oncol* 2002; **29**: 97–101.

21. Lerner HJ, Schoenfeld DA, Martin A, *et al.* Malignant mesothelioma: the Eastern Cooperative Oncology Group (ECOG) experience. *Cancer* 1983; **52**: 1981–5.

22. Magri MD, Veronesi A, Foladore, *et al.* Epirubicin treatment of malignant mesothelioma: a phase II cooperative study. *Tumori* 1991; **77**: 49–51.

23. Mattson K, Giaccone G, Kirkpatrick A, *et al.* Epirubicin in malignant mesothelioma: A phase II study of the EORTC Lung Cancer Cooperative Group. *J Clin Oncol* 1992; **10**: 824–8.

24. Baas P, van Meerbeeck J, Groen H, *et al.* Caelyx in malignant mesothelioma: a phase II EORTC study. *Ann Oncol* 2000; **11**: 697–700.

25. Hillerdal G, Brodin O, Hjerpe A, *et al.* Malignant pleural mesothelioma: treatment with liposomized doxorubicin: a phase II Scandinavian study. *Eur J Cancer* 2001; **37**: s44.

26. Oh Y, Perez-Soler R, Fossella FV, *et al.* Phase II study of intravenous Doxil in malignant pleural mesothelioma. *Invest New Drugs* 2000; **18**: 243–5.

27. Steele JP, O'Doherty CA, Shamash J, *et al.* Phase II trial of liposomal daunorubicin in malignant pleural mesothelioma. *Ann Oncol* 2001; **12**: 497–9.

28. Samson MK, Wasser LP, Borden EC, *et al.* Randomized comparison of cyclophosphamide, imidazole carboxamide, and adriamycin versus cyclophosphamide and adriamycin in patients with advanced stage malignant mesothelioma: a Sarcoma Intergroup Study. *J Clin Oncol* 1987; **5**: 86–91.

29. Chahinian AP, Antman K, Goutsou M, *et al.* Randomized phase II trial of cisplatin with mitomycin or doxorubicin for malignant mesothelioma by the Cancer and Leukemia Group B. *J Clin Oncol* 1993; **11**, 1559–65.

30. Zidar BL, Green S, Pierce HI, Roach RW, Balcerzak SP, Militello L. A phase II evaluation of cisplatin in unresectable diffuse malignant mesothelioma: a Southwest Oncology Group Study. *Invest New Drugs* 1988; **6**: 223–6.

31. Planting AS, Schellens JH, Goey SH, *et al.* Weekly high-dose cisplatin in malignant pleural mesothelioma. *Ann Oncol* 1994; **5**: 373–4.

32. Mintzer DM, Kelsen D, Frimmer D, Kheelan R, Gralla R. Phase II trial of high-dose cisplatin in patients with malignant mesothelioma. *Cancer Treat Rep*1985; **69**: 711–12.

33. Vogelzang NJ, Goutsou M, Corson JM, *et al.* Carboplatin in malignant mesothelioma: a phase II study of the Cancer and Leukemia Group B. *Cancer Chemother Pharmacol* 1990; **27**: 239–42.

34. Raghavan D, Gianoutsos P, Bishop J, *et al.* Phase II trial of carboplatin in the management of malignant mesothelioma. *J Clin Oncol* 1990; **8**: 151–4.

35. Mbidde EK, Harland SJ, Calvert AH, Smith IE. Phase II trial of carboplatin (JM8) in treatment of patients with malignant mesothelioma. *Cancer Chemother Pharmacol* 1986; **18**: 284–5.

36. van Meerbeeck JP, Baas P, Debruyne C, *et al.* A phase II study of gemcitabine in patients with malignant pleural mesothelioma. European Organization for Research and Treatment of Cancer: Lung Cancer Cooperative Group. *Cancer* 1999; **85**: 2577–82.

37. Kindler HL, Millard F, Herndon JE 2nd, *et al.* Gemcitabine for malignant mesothelioma: a phase II trial by the Cancer and Leukemia Group B. *Lung Cancer* 2001; **31**: 311–17.

38. Bischoff HG, Manegold C, Knopp M, *et al.* Gemcitabine (Gemzar) may reduce tumour load and tumour associated symptoms I malignant pleural mesothelioma. *Proc Am Soc Clin Oncol* 1998; **17**: 464.

39. Byrne MJ, Davidson JA, Musk AW, *et al.* Cisplatin and gemcitabine treatment for malignant pleural mesothelioma: a phase II study. *J Clin Oncol* 1999; **17**: 25–30.

40. Nowak AK, Byrne MJ, Williamson R, *et al.* A multicentre phase II study of cisplatin and gemcitabine for malignant mesothelioma. *Br J Cancer* 2002; **87**: 491–6.

41. van Haarst JM, Baas P, Manegold Ch, *et al.* Multicentre phase II study of gemcitabine and cisplatin in malignant pleural mesothelioma. *Br J Cancer* 2003; **86**: 342–5.

42. Favaretto AG, Aversa SM, Paccagnella A, *et al..* Gemcitabine combined to carboplatin in malignant pleural mesothelioma: a multicentric phase II study. *Lung Cancer* 2003; **41** (Suppl 2): 218.

43. Middleton GW, Smith IE, O'Brien ME, *et al.* Good symptom relief with palliative MVP (mitomycin-C, vinblastine and cisplatin) chemotherapy in malignant mesothelioma. *Ann Oncol* 1998; **9**: 269–73.

44. Andreopoulou E, Ross PJ, O'Brien ME, *et al.* The palliative benefits of MVP (mitomycin C, vinblastine and cisplatin) chemotherapy in patients with malignant mesothelioma. *Ann Oncol* 2004; **15**: 1406–12.

45. Fizazi K, Caliandro R, Soulié P, *et al.* Combination raltitrexed (Tomudex®)–oxaliplatin: a step forward in the struggle against mesothelioma? The Institut Gustave Roussy experience with chemotherapy and chemo-immunotherapy in mesothelioma. *Eur J Cancer* 2000; **36**: 1514–21.

46. Fizazi K, Doubre H, Le Chevalier T, *et al.* Combination of raltitrexed and oxaliplatin is an active regimen in malignant mesothelioma: results of a phase II study. *J Clin Oncol* 2003; **21**: 349–54.

47. Schuette W, Blankenburg T, Lauerwald, *et al.* A multicenter phase II study of gemcitabine and oxaliplatin for malignant pleural mesothelioma. *Clin Lung Cancer* 2003; **4**, 294–7.

48. Fennell DA, Steele JP, Shamash J, *et al.* Phase II trial of vinorelbine and oxaliplatin as first-line therapy in malignant pleural mesothelioma. *Lung Cancer* 2005; **47**: 277–81.

49. Bueno R, Appasani K, Mercer H, *et al.* The alpha folate receptor is highly activated in malignant pleural mesothelioma. *J Thorac Cardiovasc Surg* 2001; **121**: 225–33.

50. Solheim OP, Saeter G, Finnanger AM, Stenwig AE. High-dose methotrexate in the treatment of malignant mesothelioma of the pleura. A phase II study. *Br J Cancer* 1992; **65**: 956–60.

51. Halme M, Knuuttila A, Vehmas T, *et al.* High-dose methotrexate in combination with interferons in the treatment of malignant pleural mesothelioma. *Br J Cancer* 1999; **80**: 1781–5.

52. Kindler HL, Belani CP, Herndon JE II, *et al.* Edatrexate (10-ethyl-deaza-aminopterin) (NSC #626715) with or without leucovorin rescue for malignant mesothelioma. Sequential phase II trials by the Cancer and Leukemia Group B. *Cancer* 1999; **86**: 1985–91.

53. Baas P, Ardizzoni A, Grossi F, *et al..* The activity of raltitrexed (Tomudex) in malignant pleural mesothelioma: an EORTC phase II study. *Eur J Cancer* 2003; **39**: 353–7.

54. Harvey VJ, Slevin ML, Ponder BA, *et al.* Chemotherapy of diffuse malignant mesothelioma. Phase II trials of single-agent 5-fluorouracil and adriamycin. *Cancer* 1984; **54**: 961–64.

55. Otterson GA, Herndon JE 2nd, Watson D, *et al.* Capecitabine in malignant mesothelioma: a phase II trial by the Cancer and Leukemia Group B (39807). *Lung Cancer* 2004; **44**, 251–9.

56. Takimoto CH, Baker SD, Sweeney CJ, *et al.* Phase I and pharmacokinetic study of pemetrexed disodium (LY231514, MTA, Alimta) in patients (pts) with impaired renal function. *Proc Am Soc Clin Oncol* 2001; **20**: 93.

57. Hughes A, Calvert P, Azzabi A, *et al.* Phase I clinical and pharmacokinetic study of pemetrexed and carboplatin in patients with malignant pleural mesothelioma. *J Clin Oncol* 2002; **20**, 3533–44.

58. Scagliotti GV, Shin DM, Kindler HL, *et al.* Phase II study of pemetrexed with and without folic acid and vitamin B_{12} as front-line therapy in malignant pleural mesothelioma. *J Clin Oncol* 2003; **21**: 1556–61.

59. Steele JP. The new front line treatment for malignant pleural mesothelioma? *Thorax* 2003; **58**: 96–7.

60. Baas P, Ardizzoni A, Grossi F, *et al.* The activity of raltitrexed (Tomudex) in malignant pleural mesothelioma: an EORTC phase II study (08992). *Eur J Cancer* 2003; **39**: 353–7.

61. Bottomley A, Gaafur R, Manegold C *et al.* Short-term treatment-related symptoms and quality of life: results from an international randomized phase II study of cisplatin with or without raltitrexed in patients with malignant pleural mesothelioma: an EORTC Lung-Cancer Group and National Cancer Institute, Canada, Intergroup Study. *J Clin Oncol* 2006; **24**: 1435–1442.

62. Rossi A, Gridelli C, Gebbia V, *et al.* Single agent vinorelbine as first-line chemotherapy in elderly patients with advanced breast cancer. *Anticancer Res* 2003; **23**, 1657–64.

63. Steele JP, Shamash J, Evans MT, *et al.* Phase II study of vinorelbine in patients with malignant pleural mesothelioma. *J Clin Oncol* 2000; **18**, 3912–17.

64. Steele JP, Shamash J, Gower NH, *et al.* Vinorelbine (Navelbine) given as a single agent for malignant pleural mesothelioma. Results from 65 patients at a single centre. *Lung Cancer* 2000; **29** (Suppl 1):18.

65. Maksymiuk AW, Marschke RF Jr, Tazelaar HD, *et al.* Phase II trial of topotecan for the treatment of mesothelioma. *Am J Clin Oncol* 1998; **21**: 610–13.

66. Kindler HL, Herndon JE, Zhang C, Green MR. Cancer and Leukemia Group B. Irinotecan for malignant mesothelioma. A phase II trial by the Cancer and Leukemia Group B. *Lung Cancer* 2005; **48**: 423–428.

67. Knuuttila A, Ollikainen T, Halme M, *et al*. Docetaxel and irinotecan (CPT-11) in the treatment of malignant pleural mesothelioma—a feasibility study. *Anti-Cancer Drugs* 2000; **11**: 257–61.

68. Ferrari VD, Simoncini E, Marini G, *et al*. Gemcitabine (GEM) plus irinotecan (CPT11) in malignant mesothelioma (MM): a phase II study. Preliminary report. *Proc Am Soc Clin Oncol* 2002; **21**: 2755.

69. Nakano T, Chahinian AP, Shinjo M, *et al*. Cisplatin in combination with irinotecan in the treatment of patients with malignant pleural mesothelioma: a pilot phase II clinical trial and pharmacokinetic profile. *Cancer* 1999; **85**: 2375–84.

70. Fennell DA, Steele JP, Shamash J, *et al*. A phase II study of irinotecan, cisplatin, and mitomycin C (IPM) in malignant pleural mesothelioma. *Lung Cancer* 2003; **41** (Suppl 2), S221b.

71. Shamash J, Steele JP, Wilson P, *et al*. IPM chemotherapy in cytokine refractory renal cell cancer. *Br J Cancer* 2003; **19**: 1516–21.

72. Fennell DA, Steele JP, Shamash J, *et al*. Second line therapy of malignant pleural mesothelioma with irinotecan, cisplatin, and mitomycin C (IPM): a phase II study. *Lung Cancer* 2003; **41** (Suppl 2): S221c.

73. Sahmoud T, Postmus PE, van Pottelsberghe C, *et al*. Etoposide in malignant pleural mesothelioma: two phase II trials of the EORTC Lung Cancer Cooperative Group. *Eur J Cancer* 1997; **33**: 2211–15.

74. Vogelzang NJ, Herndon JE 2nd, Miller A, *et al*. High-dose paclitaxel plus G-CSF for malignant mesothelioma: CALGB phase II study 9234. *Ann Oncol* 1999; **10**: 597–600.

75. van Meerbeeck J, Debruyne C, van Zandwijk N, *et al*. Paclitaxel for malignant pleural mesothelioma: a phase II study of the EORTC Lung Cancer Cooperative Group. *Br J Cancer* 1996; **74**: 961–3.

76. Belani CP, Adak S, Aisner S, *et al*. Docetaxel for malignant mesothelioma: phase II study of the Eastern Cooperative Oncology Group. *Clin Lung Cancer* 2004; **6**: 43–7.

77. Vorobiof DA, Rapoport BL, Chasen MR, *et al*. Malignant pleural mesothelioma: a phase II trial with docetaxel. *Eur J Cancer* 2002; **33**: 2211–15.

78. Bajorin D, Kelsen D, Mintzer DM. Phase II trial of mitomycin in malignant mesothelioma. *Cancer Treat Rep* 1987; **71**: 857–8.

79. van Meerbeeck JP, Baas P, Debruyne C, *et al*. A phase II EORTC study of temozolomide in patients with malignant pleural mesothelioma. *Eur J Cancer* 2002; **38**, 779–83.

80. Andersen MK, Krarup-Hansen A, Martensson G, *et al*. Ifosfamide in malignant mesothelioma: a phase II study. *Lung Cancer* 1999; **24**: 39–43.

81. Mikulski SM, Costanzi JJ, Vogelzang NJ, *et al*. Phase II trial of a single weekly intravenous dose of ranpirnase in patients with unresectable malignant mesothelioma. *J Clin Oncol* 2002; **20**: 274–81.

82. Vogelzang N, Taub R, Shin D, *et al*. Phase III randomized trial of onconase (ONC) vs. doxorubicin (DOX) in patients (pts) with unresectable malignant mesothelioma (UMM): analysis of survival. *Proc Am Soc Clin Oncol* 2000; **19**: 577.

83. Muers MF, Rudd RM, O'Brien ME, *et al*. BTS randomised feasibility study of active symptom control with or without chemotherapy in malignant pleural mesothelioma: ISRCTN 54469112. *Thorax* 2004; **59**: 144–8.

84. O'Brien ME, Watkins D, Ryan C *et al*. A randomised trial in malignant mesothelioma (M) of early (E) versus delayed (D) chemotherapy in symptomatically stable patients: the MED trial. *Ann Oncol* 2006; **17**: 270–275.

85. Weder W, Kestenholz P, Taverna C, *et al*. Neoadjuvant chemotherapy followed by extrapleural pneumonectomy in malignant pleural mesothelioma. *J Clin Oncol* 2004; **22**: 3451–7.

Chapter 15

Radiotherapy for mesothelioma

C. W. Stevens, K. M. Forster, and W. R. Smythe

Rationale for radiation

Malignant pleural mesotheliomas (MPMs) are almost impossible to cure with radiotherapy as a single modality. The tumours are large, so that potential cure requires commensurately large radiation doses. The treatment volumes are also very large, extending from the supraclavicular fossa to the insertion of the diaphragm, because the entire pleural space, even the intrapulmonary fissures, is at risk for recurrence. The treatment volumes are also very close to radiosensitive structures such as the lung, kidney, liver, oesophagus and heart. These issues challenge the radiation oncologist at many levels.

Although these technical challenges remain, several lines of evidence suggest that radiotherapy should be effective in treating mesothelioma. First, mesothelioma cell lines are not particularly radioresistant *in vitro* and have radiosensitivities similar to non-small-cell lung cancer [1,2]. While *in vitro* and *in vivo* results do not always correlate, the reported radiosensitivities do not preclude the use of radiotherapy in the control of microscopic disease. Secondly, there is a clinically meaningful dose response for symptom palliation, such that doses greater than 40 Gy appear to be more effective than lower doses [3]. This dose response suggests that clinically significant cell killing results from modest radiation doses. Thirdly, modest radiation doses can dramatically reduce the local MPM failure rate at thoracotomy or other instrumentation sites. This demonstrates that radiation can effectively kill mesothelioma cells in regions where the tumour burden is low. Since MPM is moderately radiosensitive, it follows that postoperative radiotherapy should be effective in preventing loco-regional recurrence and potentially improve survival.

In this chapter we first describe the use of radiation in the palliative setting. This provides the background for the important combined modality approaches that will be described later, and also suggest therapeutic approaches for those patients for whom cure is not yet possible. Then several approaches to potentially curative therapy are described in detail. Finally, the future role of radiotherapy in trimodality therapy is discussed.

Palliative radiotherapy

Pain control

It has long been known that radiation can provide effective palliation for patients with MPM. A radiation dose response has been reported following the review of outcomes of 29 courses of palliative external beam radiotherapy delivered to 17 patients with MPM [3]. Four of six patients treated with more than 40 Gy achieved significant relief of symptoms. All four with a good outcome were treated for thoracic pain, while those with a poor outcome were treated for superior vena cava obstruction and dyspnoea. Only one patient treated with lower doses achieved significant palliation of any symptom, and this was for a painful chest wall mass.

In another study [4], 26 radiotherapy courses were reviewed for any symptomatic improvement. Pain was improved in 13 of 18 cases, and the response was similar irrespective of dose and fractionation (20 Gy in five fractions, or 30 Gy in 10 fractions). Palliative treatment was also delivered for 'mass', Pancoast's syndrome, and superior vena cava obstruction. Although the sample size is small, palliation was achieved in approximately 50 per cent of cases in this heterogeneous patient group. The duration of response was not assessed in either study. These data suggest that symptoms from mesothelioma can usually be palliated effectively with brief courses of radiotherapy.

Drain sites

Unlike most malignancies, MPM has a tendency to recur along tracks of previous chest wall instrumentation [5]. One group has hypothesized that local radiotherapy might prevent this type of painful tumour growth pattern [6]. Forty consecutive patients with pathologically proven MPM were randomized to immediate prophylactic radiotherapy to each site of instrumentation or to observation. Prophylactic treatment was 21 Gy in 3 fractions delivered using *en face* electron fields. Tissue-equivalent bolus material overlay each target to improve dose delivery to the skin. The prescription point was not further described. The authors found no subcutaneous MPM progression in the irradiated patients, whereas such nodules developed in eight of the 20 untreated patients (40 per cent) with a median time to recurrence of 6 months. Subcutaneous recurrence was not correlated with a positive cytological study, histological type, disease stage, subsequent treatment, or size of tracts. They concluded that, since such recurrences are typically painful, prophylactic irradiation was a safe and effective means of maintaining patient quality of life.

Summary

Palliative therapy must be individualized. Pain is fairly well controlled with radiotherapy doses above 40 Gy, and prophylactic treatment can work well with 21 Gy delivered in three fractions. Our approach has been to use 45 Gy in 15 fractions for patients with good performance status, since this has shown better palliative effects for patients with other thoracic malignancies [7]. This approach also combines a relatively short treatment course with a dose above 40 Gy. Superior vena cava obstruction, dyspnoea, and Pancoast's syndrome are more difficult to palliate, with only about 50 per cent of patients demonstrating benefit. Investigation to determine the role of prophylactic radiotherapy to the mediastinum as well as drain sites is warranted.

Curative radiotherapy

Radiotherapy alone

Radiotherapy alone is clearly not the treatment of choice for this disease. The lung is very sensitive to radiotherapy, and the volume of lung irradiated above 20 Gy (V_{20}) has been linked to pulmonary toxicity. A 41 per cent rate of pneumonitis has been reported for $V_{20} > 40$ per cent, with more than half of these being severe (grade >3) [8]. Delivery of a potentially curative dose (e.g. >60 Gy) would irradiate the entire ipsilateral lung (or 50 per cent of the total lung volume) above 20 Gy unless parts of the lung can be spared.

Such sparing is difficult if the lung and diaphragm remain in place because of two problems with the target volumes. The first problem is the intrapulmonary fissures. The fissures are bathed in pleural fluid, and therefore with mesothelioma cells. Thus the fissures should be included as part of the target volume. Unfortunately, the intrapulmonary fissures are complex three-dimensional structures surrounded by lung (Fig. 15.1). Three-dimensional conformal radiotherapy (3D-CRT) cannot irradiate the fissures and spare any significant lung volume.

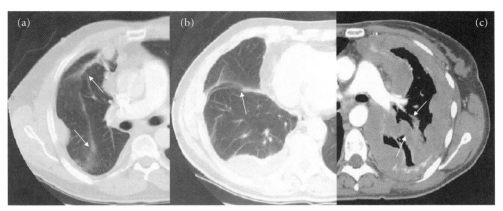

Figure 15.1 The interlobar fissures are complex three-dimensional structures. They are bathed in pleural fluid which often contains mesothelioma cells (arrows). Without pneumonectomy, irradiation of the fissures would therefore be desirable. Unfortunately, the fissures between (a) the right upper and middle lobes, (b) the right middle and lower lobes, and (c) the left upper and lower lobes are very complex structures. These cannot be irradiated to tumoricidal doses and spare adjacent uninvolved lung.

Intensity-modulated radiotherapy (IMRT) also cannot treat these structures because they move with respiration if the diaphragm is intact.

Respiratory motion is the second, and most important, problem for radiotherapy as a sole modality. When the diaphragm is in place, there can be 2–3 cm of superior–inferior motion, 1–2 cm of mediolateral motion along the mediastinum, and 1–1.5 cm of anterior chest wall motion. Expanding the pulmonary target volume (PTV) to account for this motion will result in destruction of the liver in right-sided MPM, the most common side, and deliver very high cardiac and bowel doses in left-sided MPM. Thus radiotherapy without surgery is best considered as a palliative treatment, with doses and volumes appropriately limited.

These concerns have led to rather limited data from small studies. In one of the largest, 12 patients were irradiated with curative intent at the Peter MacCallum Cancer Institute between 1981 and 1985. These results were described as part of a larger retrospective study [4]. Patients were treated with AP–PA beam geometry, including the mediastinum, to 40 Gy. The mediastinum/spinal cord was then shielded and an additional 10 Gy delivered. No attempt was made to shield the lung or the liver. The target volume included any surgical scars, but the inferior borders were not described. The median survival time for those 12 patients was 17 months, compared with 7 months for 20 patients treated palliatively, but both curves converged by 24 months. Two patients died from treatment. The first patient died from liver failure 7 weeks after completing treatment because the entire liver was irradiated to 50 Gy. The second patient died from progressive neurological deterioration about 11 months after irradiation. Autopsy revealed radiation myelopathy despite spinal cord shielding after 40 Gy.

Radiotherapy combined with surgery

Several groups have recently reported promising outcomes for MPM patients treated with surgery and radiotherapy, with or without chemotherapy. Operative approaches have used either pleurectomy–decortication or extrapleural pneumonectomy (EPP).

Radiotherapy after pleurectomy–decortication

Thirty-four patients with pathologically proven MPM were treated between 1982 and 1988 at the Helsinki University Central Hospital [9,10]. Twenty nine patients had partial pleurectomy, while the others had only biopsy. Patients were irradiated with one of three schedules that delivered between 55 and 70 Gy to the hemithorax. The extent of disease and the field borders were not described, but no lung or liver shielding was employed. The median survival was approximately 12 months [11], with about a third having in-field progression and the remainder 'stable' disease. This approach also led to progressive deterioration of pulmonary function. Within 12 months, all patients showed complete destruction of all visible alveoli. This paralleled a decrease in diffusion capacity (DLCO) that was consistent with complete pneumonectomy. Forced vital capacity (FVC) also decreased, which is consistent with the complete pulmonary fibrosis described. Interestingly, PaO_2 decreased transiently 2–4 months after irradiation but then returned to baseline, suggesting that there is minimal left–right 'shunting' after whole-lung irradiation for MPM. The authors did not describe any effects on renal or hepatic function.

A similar study was performed at the Memorial Sloan-Kettering Cancer Centre. The authors reported the results for 41 patients treated with parietal pleurectomy. Measurable gross residual disease was treated with permanent 125I implantation where feasible. Residual diffuse disease was treated with a temporary 192Ir implant or post-operative instillation of 32P. External radiation therapy was given 4–6 weeks post-operatively to the involved hemi-thorax, utilising a combination of photon and electron fields so as to treat the superficial chest wall and spare the underlying lung. Radiation doses were 45 Gy to the pleural surface, while keeping 'most of the lung' below 20 Gy. Local recurrence developed in 29 of the 41 patients, with 22 having distant failure. Median survival was 21 months with 1- and 2-year survivals of 65 per cent and 40 per cent respectively. The median disease-free survival was 11 months and the 1- and 2-year disease free survival rates were 44 per cent and 13 per cent respectively. Complications developed in 6 patients including radiation pneumonitis, pulmonary fibrosis, pericardial effusion and oesophagitis.

These data were subsequently updated [14,15]. In all 105 patients were treated with the protocol from 1976 to 1988 with a median survival of 12.6 months with 1- and 2-year actuarial survivals of 52 and 23 per cent, respectively. Subset analysis revealed that the 27 patients with epithelioid histology and minimal gross residual disease, treated with external beam irradiation alone had a median survival of 15 months, and 1- and 2-year survivals of 68 and 35 per cent, respectively. Twelve patients developed radiation pneumonitis and a further eight, pericarditis. Ipsilateral recurrent pleural tumour occurred in 64 of the 105 patients (63%). These results indicate that low-dose mixed photon-electron beam radiotherapy does not provide long-term local control for most patients. Furthermore the cardio-pulmonary toxicities indicate that the technique does not spare the pulmonary parenchyma.

A recent retrospective review of the efficacy and morbidity of radical pleurectomy-decortication and intraoperative radiotherapy (IORT) followed by external beam radiation therapy with or without chemotherapy for diffuse malignant pleural mesothelioma was performed in 26 patients [16]. Surgical staging demonstrated AJCC T1, T2 and T3 tumours in one, 18 and seven patients, respectively. Three patients also had known lymph node metastases. Of these 24 received IORT targeted mainly to the intrapulmonary fissures, pericardium, and diaphragm, with doses ranging from 5 to 15 Gy. External beam radiation therapy was generally started 1 to 2 months after resection. Fourteen patients were irradiated using 3-dimensional conformal radiation therapy (3D-CRT) and 10 with intensity-modulated radiation therapy (IMRT). The target volumes for the external beam treatments were not described, but the doses ranged from 30.1 to 48.8 Gy (median 41.4 Gy). Twelve patients also received 2 to 3 cycles of chemotherapy (cyclophosphamide, doxorubicin and cisplatin – CAP) initiated 1 to 2 months after completion of radiation at the discretion of the treating physician. Despite the early stage of the disease, the median overall and progression-free survivals from the time of the operation were relatively poor at 18.1 and 12.2 months, respectively. Although the site of failure was mostly locoregional there were 4 abdominal and 1 contralateral lung relapses. Major complications included radiation pneumonitis in four patients, pericarditis in one patient, and oesophageal stricture in one patient who had received previous radiotherapy to the oesophagus. Only the oesophageal stricture required more than conservative management (balloon dilation for the oesophageal stricture). There was no difference in the toxicity between 3D CRT and IMRT, although the patient numbers were quite small. Tumour recurrence was 'mostly locoregional' at sites of previous gross tumour. Only the number of IORT sites was predictive of overall survival, suggesting that higher external beam doses might be required for this approach to be widely used.

Pleurectomy–decortication followed by radiotherapy can reduce loco-regional failure compared with historical controls. However, local failure is common, and survival is disappointing even when modern IMRT techniques are applied. Furthermore, there are no prospective randomized trials to guide therapy.

Radiotherapy after extrpleural pneumonectomy

The first large report of combined modality therapy including EPP was described in 1997 [18]. In this series, 49 patients underwent EPP. Four to six cycles of chemotherapy were given postoperatively, followed by radiation in 35 patients. The target volumes, stage, and technique were not described. The prescribed dose was 30.6 Gy to the 'hemithorax' followed by a boost to bring the dose to about 50 Gy. The boost criteria, the locations, the volumes, and the techniques were not described. Sixteen irradiated patients had a 'local' recurrence. However, of those patients with 'abdominal' failure, five had a chest mass extending into the abdomen, two had ascites, and four had a 'retroperitoneal mass'. This last is potentially important because the diaphragm is reconstructed much higher than its insertion, thus 'abdominalizing' the retroperitoneal posterior chest wall (Fig. 15.2). Failure to irradiate this region, which can be below the ipsilateral kidney, can result in apparent retroperitoneal recurrences. Thus the true rate of loco-regional failure was at least 21/49, and possibly as high as 25/49. Despite this, the 3 year overall survival was 34 per cent. Radiation morbidity was tolerable, and included oesophagitis (one patient) and thrombocytopenia (three patients). No radiation pneumonitis was described, but five patients experienced 'respiratory compromise', one of whom died of pneumonia. These data suggest that postoperative radiotherapy can reduce local recurrence and result in long-term survival in well-selected patients.

The same Dana Farber Cancer Institute group subsequently reported their overall results from patients treated with multi-modal therapy between 1980 to 1997. An extrapleural pneumonectomy was performed in 183 patients, followed by CAP or carboplatin and paclitaxel chemotherapy and subsequent hemithoracic irradiation at a median dose of 30.6 Gy [17]. The overall median survival was 19 months, the 2- and 5-year survival rates being 38 per cent and 15 per cent, respectively. The outcome at 52% and 21% for 2- and 5-year survival, respectively, was better for patients with epithelioid mesothelioma than those with mixed or sarcomatoid tumours with no patients surviving 5 years. Again the major problem with the regimen was a 35% local recurrence rate most likely related to the low total dose of radiation administered. The impact of chemotherapy on outcome is difficult to assess emphasising the need for randomised controlled studies in this area.

Encouraging results have also been reported from the Memorial Sloan-Kettering Cancer Center. Between 1995 and 1998, 54 patients underwent EPP followed by radiotherapy using previously published techniques [19]. Two-thirds of the patients were stage III. The target volume was described as the 'hemithorax' and drain sites, and the inferior field edge 'rarely' included the ipsilateral kidney. The treatment technique, which is described in more detail below, involved

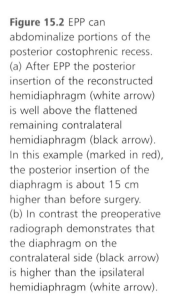

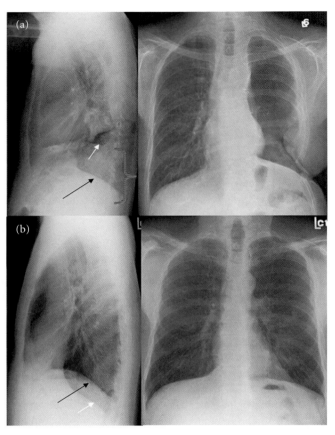

Figure 15.2 EPP can abdominalize portions of the posterior costophrenic recess. (a) After EPP the posterior insertion of the reconstructed hemidiaphragm (white arrow) is well above the flattened remaining contralateral hemidiaphragm (black arrow). In this example (marked in red), the posterior insertion of the diaphragm is about 15 cm higher than before surgery. (b) In contrast the preoperative radiograph demonstrates that the diaphragm on the contralateral side (black arrow) is higher than the ipsilateral hemidiaphragm (white arrow).

photon radiation to a dose of 54 Gy in 30 fractions. The spinal cord was shielded after 41.4 Gy, and the liver, heart, and stomach were appropriately shielded. The chest wall dose in the shielded regions were irradiated with matched electron fields so that the target dose of 54 Gy could be more safely achieved. The median survival was approximately 18 months. Only seven patients had local recurrence (two local only). Another 22 patients had 'peritoneal' or 'ipsilateral visceral' recurrence. It is not clear whether any of these were in the radiation fields, or whether some might have been marginal misses.

The results for 28 patients treated with EPP followed by IMRT have recently been reported [20–22]. Twenty-six were stage III, most had involved lymph nodes, and all required partial chest wall resection. During the EPP, radio-opaque surgical clips were placed at the insertion of the diaphragm, including the crus and the anterior-medial pleural extension which often crosses the midline over the heart. The target volume included the entire hemithorax and all surgical clips, all sites of instrumentation, and the ipsilateral mediastinum. Boosts were given to any close or positive resection margins. All volumes were reviewed with the surgeon. The target dose was 45–50 Gy to the hemithorax and 60 Gy to the boost volume. All irradiation was completed in 25 fractions. The 2 year overall survival was 62 per cent and there were no in-field failures. Two marginal misses occurred, one near the crus and one across midline anterior to the heart. Major toxicities include nausea and vomiting, fatigue, and skin irritation (see below). This series has now been extended to 45 patients with EPP followed by IMRT to 45 or 50 Gy. There have been no in-field failures and only two marginal misses. One fatal case of radiation pneumonitis occurred several weeks after completion of IMRT (unpublished data).

A very recent update of the Memorial Sloan-Kettering Cancer Center experience regarding their radiotherapy technique and outcome has been published [23]. Thirty-five patients underwent radiotherapy after EPP, with the goal of delivering 54 Gy in 30 fractions. The target volume was the ipsilateral hemithorax from the top of T1, ideally the bottom of L2, and laterally to flash the skin. All drain sites were included. The medial field edge was the contralateral edge of the vertebral bodies if mediastinal lymph nodes were negative; otherwise, the field was extended 1.5–2 cm beyond the contralateral edge of the vertebral bodies. For right-sided lesions, the liver and ipsilateral kidney were blocked. For left-sided lesions, the heart was blocked after 19.8 Gy. The blocked regions were boosted to the target dose with electrons. After 41.4 cGy, the medial field edge was moved to the ipsilateral edge of the vertebral bodies. Patients tolerate this therapy well, with the main toxicities being nausea, vomiting and dysphagia.

However, the results of this study were difficult to interpret. Local failure was documented in 13 of 35 patients, but in-field failures were not separated from marginal misses. Thus it is not clear whether the pattern of failure results from inadequate margins or inadequate dose. However, only five of the remaining 22 patients with local control are disease free. Clearly, better systemic therapy is needed.

These data demonstrate several important points (Table 15.1). First, high-dose postoperative radiotherapy can dramatically reduce ipsilateral thoracic failures. This is consistent with the radiosensitivity of MPM cell lines and suggests that postoperative radiotherapy should be a component of all future trials. Secondly, radiotherapy after pleural decortication results in a much higher rate of loco-regional failure than does radiotherapy after EPP. It is not clear whether this is due to lower radiation doses, motion of the target volume, or inadequate delineation of target volumes. Thus EPP with postoperative radiotherapy seems preferable to less morbid but much less effective approaches. Thirdly, a detailed description of the target volumes has been published

Table 15.1 Large studies combining surgery with postoperative radiotherapy.

Reference	Surgery	No. of patients	Radiotherapy dose	Local failure	Survival
Maasilta [10]	Pleurectomy	34	55–70 Gy	33% progression, but remainder 'stable'	Median 12 months
Hilaris et al. [12]	Pleurectomy	41	45 Gy + implant	29/41	Median 12.6 months
Lee et al. [16]	Pleurectomy	24	Median 41.4 Gy IORT 5–15 Gy	'Most'	Median 18 months
Baldini et al. [17]	EPP	49	30.6 Gy ~20 Gy boost	21/49	22 months
Rusch et al. [19]	EPP	55	54 Gy	7/55	Stage I–II, 34 months Stage III–IV, 10 months
Ahamad et al. [21]	EPP	28	45–50 Gy	0 2 marginal miss	Not yet reached (2 year OS 62%)
Yajnik et al. [23]	EPP	35	54 Gy	13/35	Not reported

EPP, extrapleural pneumonectomy; IORT, intraoperative radiotherapy; OS, overall survival.

[20]. Because earlier reports did not precisely define the target, it is difficult to distinguish a local failure from a marginal miss. True in-field failure needs to be well documented so that it can be explained. Fourthly, postoperative radiotherapy is well tolerated. Finally, postoperative radiotherapy changes the pattern of relapse so that distant metastases become more prevalent. This indicates the need for systemic therapy. These observations are critical to the development of future clinical MPM trials.

Radiotherapy technique

Patient immobilization and setup

The IMRT techniques for the postoperative treatment of MPM have recently been described [20,22]. This level of detail is required to ensure that the very complex target volumes can be identified and reproducibly treated for 5 weeks.

CT simulation
Because of the propensity of MPM to recur at sites of previous instrumentation, all incision/drain sites should be included in the clinical target volume (CTV). Any chest tube or thoracotomy site should be included. We have not included laparoscopy or mediastinoscopy sites provided that the mediastinoscopy was pathologically negative. To accomplish this, each site can be marked with radio-opaque wire on the skin. The wire should be covered with a tissue-equivalent bolus of thickness 0.5 cm at the time of CT simulation to facilitate treatment planning. The tissue-equivalent bolus should extend to 3.5 cm on each side of the wire and 4 cm beyond each end. This bolus material helps to increase the skin dose near surgically disrupted skin and allows better radiation dose distributions.

The patients are then immobilized supine on the CT simulator using a combination of a vacuum bag and an 'extended wing board with T-bar handgrip' immobilization device used in conjunction with a headrest, since this reduces daily setup variation compared with a vacuum bag alone. The standard deviation for setup uncertainty falls from 5 to 3.5 mm when this approach is used. Once the patient is properly aligned and immobilized, three radio-opaque markers should be placed on the patient to define a CT reference point, and all should be in a single axial plane. One marker can be placed at a point on the sternum at which the motion associated with respiration is negligible. The contralateral marker should be placed at the isocentre at exhalation, since this point is more reproducible than any other during quiet respiration. Because patients have a minimal respiratory motion, because of the surgically reconstructed diaphragm on the ipsilateral side, no adjustment for motion is needed. The positions of the markers are then tattooed on the patient's skin. The markers give a visible means of verifying the CT reference point in the inverse treatment planning system.

The scanning parameters should be selected to minimize the number of slices required for this treatment to help speed scan acquisition, volume delineation, and dose calculation, while not compromising the accuracy of the treatment and volume definition. CT slice thickness and spacing of 4–5 mm is optimal in this regard. Intravenous contrast is not needed. The patient should be scanned from the mid-neck to the anterior superior iliac spine. This low inferior border allows complete definition of both kidneys, which is important for proper dose–volume histogram evaluation.

One of the consequences of EPP is that shoulder pain is often experienced. The simulation process typically takes 60–90 min, and for a significant portion of this time the patients' hands are positioned over their heads as they hold onto a T-bar immobilization device. Because of postoperative shoulder pain, most patients require presimulation narcotic analgesia and such medication should be available.

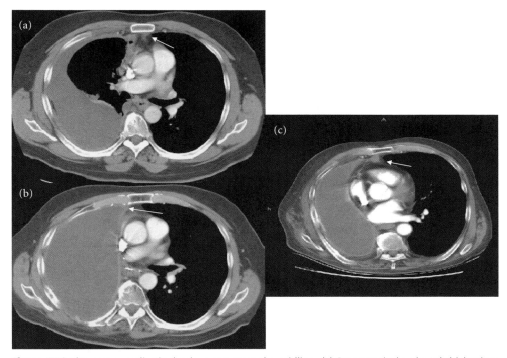

Figure 15.3 The costo-mediastinal sulcus can cross the midline. (a) Preoperatively, pleural thickening can be appreciated to cross the midline anteriorly (arrow). (b) This involvement is obliterated by EPP, and the medial edge of the CTV was placed at the insertion of the rib (arrow). (c) Unfortunately, the tumour recurred immediately adjacent to the CTV in a region that received less than 40 Gy.

Target volume delineation

There is general consensus that the ipsilateral mediastinum should be included in the target volume [13,18,20,23]. The superior border is at the thoracic inlet. The medial border includes the ipsilateral nodal regions, the trachea, and the subcarinal regions[22] or the vertebral body [23]. The posterior mediastinal structures behind the heart need not be included, and no failures in this region have been recorded as a result [20; unpublished data].

The anterior-medial pleural reflection is also a potential problem for target volume delineation. As shown in Fig. 15.3a, the medial pleural space can sometimes cross the midline, and this anatomical relationship can be lost after surgery (Fig. 15.3b). When possible, this region should be marked intraoperatively with radio-opaque clips. Alternatively, the medial extent of the pleura could be identified on preoperative CT scans, and this extent estimated on the treatment planning CT. This has been the site of a marginal miss in the M. D. Anderson Cancer Centre series (Fig. 15.3c, arrow).

The inferior border should be the insertion of the diaphragm. The location of this is quite variable, ranging from L1 to L4. Because of this variability, the diaphragm insertion should be marked either by intraoperative placement of radio-opaque clips [21] or by suturing the neodiaphragm in this location [23]. When the border of intrathoracic contents and abdominal contents is well marked, the radiotherapy margins can be maximally reduced. Figure 15.4 shows the lowest clips in two cases in which the clips are at the bottom of L2 (note the proximity of the rib; Fig. 15.4a) or at the bottom of L3 (no ribs; Fig. 15.4b). The change in chest shape and the level at

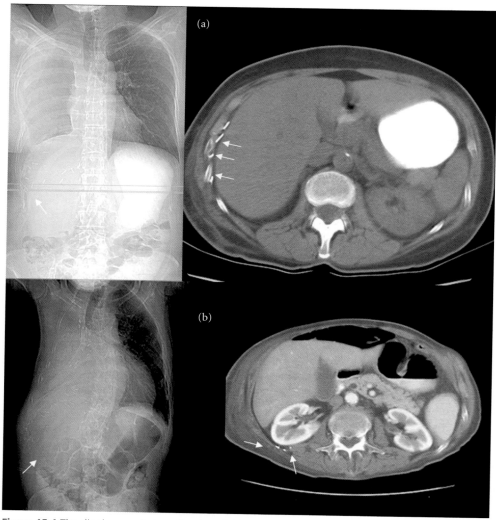

Figure 15.4 The diaphragmatic insertion is variable. The lowest point of the diaphragm is identified in two cases in which radio-opaque clips were placed at the time of EPP. The lowest insertion point in patient (a) was above the lowest ribs (arrow), while in patient (b) it was well below the ribs. Note also that the neodiaphragm was reconstructed much lower in patient (a) than in patient (b), which helped to keep the ipsilateral kidney far from the CTV.

which the diaphragm is reconstructed (higher in Fig. 15.4a) can have a profound effect on the proximity of the radiation field to organs at risk. Also, the placement of a radio-opaque neodiaphram is quite helpful in differentiating thoracic fluid from liver. The Gore-Tex neodiaphragm is quite apparent on CT scan (Fig. 15.5). In this case, there was a partial dehiscence of the posterior insertion with partial herniation of the abdominal contents. It can be very difficult to differentiate between liver and thoracic fluid, shown with the arrows on both projections. The transverse section was obtained at the level of the yellow arrows in the sagittal section. The treatment-planning CTs were obtained without intravenous contrast. Differentiation between liver and thoracic fluid is easier when contrast is used.

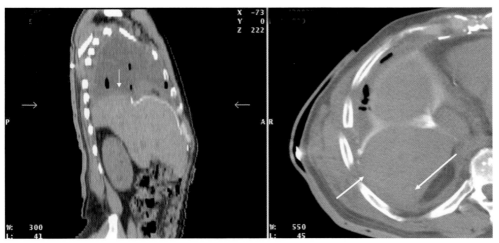

Figure 15.5 Contouring is easier with a radio-opaque neodiaphragm. This example demonstrates a case in which the posterior insertion of the neodiaphragm has dehisced. Regions bounded by the Gore-Tex neodiaphragm are easily identified, but the extent of the liver is more difficult to identify. In such cases, generous margins are needed to ensure that the regions at risk are within the CTV. This approach tends to irradiate more liver than would be necessary if the interface was more clearly seen.

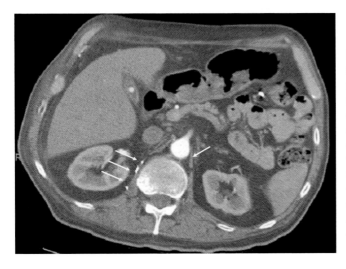

Figure 15.6 The crus can be difficult to identify without clips. After the crus (the inferior medial extent of the diaphragm) is resected as low as possible, radio-opaque clips are placed intraoperatively (yellow arrows). This region would be much more difficult to identify than the unresected crus (white arrow). The clips also determine the medial extent of the diaphragm resection.

Another potential source of contouring error is the medial extent of the crus of the diaphragm, especially at its most inferior extent (Fig. 15.6). Compare the remnants of the crus on the right (yellow arrows) with the contralateral crus (white arrow). The ipsilateral crus would be difficult to identify without clips. The best way to individualize the inferior edge of the target volume is with extensive intraoperative placement of radio-opaque clips, paying particular attention to the crus.

All chest tube or biopsy sites are also included because of the risk of tumour tracking along the instrumentation track. These should be contoured to the skin, as should any regions of subcutaneous tissue disruption. Typically, the skin incision does not directly overlie the regions where

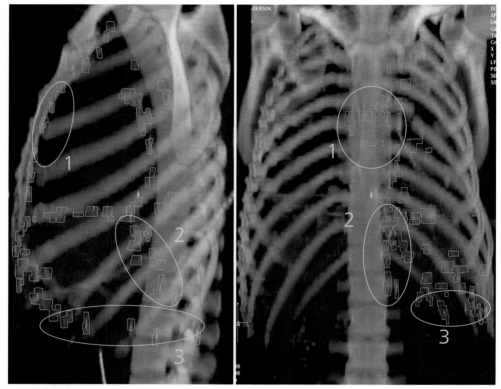

Figure 15.7 Potential problem areas for CTV determination. Three parts of the CTV are potentially difficult to appreciate without great care. These are (1) the anterior-medial pleural reflection of the sterno-pericardial recess, (2) the inferior and medial extents of the crus of the diaphragm, and (3) the inferior insertion of the diaphragm.

the ribs are entered. Since there is tunnelling under the subcutaneous fat, the entire disturbed region should be irradiated. This often includes the subscapular tissues. Disrupted tissue planes can often be identified at postoperative CT simulation and should be included in the CTV.

When the entire region is extensively clipped, a pattern such as that seen in Figure 15.7 emerges, with regions of potential pitfall highlighted. These potential problem areas include the anterior medial pleural reflection, the crus of the diaphragm, and the inferior aspect of the diaphragmatic insertion.

Ideally, the surgeon, radiation oncologist, and radiation-treatment-planning physicist should discuss the target volumes at the planning workstation. This allows for unambiguous target volume identification and helps the radiation oncologist to understand better the anatomy and extent of disease. Likewise, the surgeon gains an appreciation of the limits of target volume identification/clipping. Furthermore the treatment planner gains insight into which regions of this very large CTV are critical, and the physicist, into the planning constraints for each case.

Treatment planning

Three dimensional conformal radiotherapy (3D-CRT) The 3D-CRT approach has been best described in two reports from the Memorial Sloan-Kettering Cancer Center [13,23]. The technique applies AP–PA beam geometry to the hemithorax using the volumes described above as

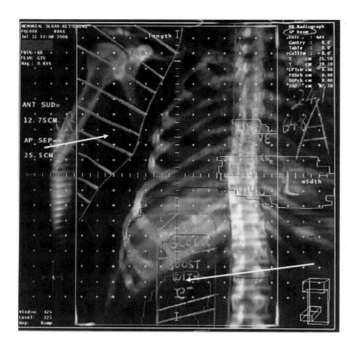

Figure 15.8 Diagram of the AP/PA fields used for traditional irradiation of MPM. After contouring normal structures, field borders are placed at the contralateral edge of the vertebral bodies. Blocks are placed to protect the shoulder and kidney (arrows). The kidney block is expanded to cover the liver. (Reprinted from Yajnick et al., 23).

CTV (Fig. 15.8). For right-sided cases, an abdominal block is present throughout treatment and the region is boosted with electrons at 1.53 Gy/day, which accounts for scatter under the block. For left-sided cases, the kidney and heart are blocked. The kidney block is present throughout treatment and the heart block is added after 19.8 Gy. The spinal cord is shielded after 41.4 Gy in all cases. The target dose to the target volume is 54 Gy in 30 fractions, with dose calculated at midplane with equally weighted beams. Patients are treated with arms akimbo.

Treatment by this simple approach results in good coverage of the vast majority of the volumes at risk (Fig. 15.9) to the target dose of 54 Gy. Doses are very homogeneous within the regions at risk, although some regions (Fig. 15.9, arrows), such as the crus, the pericardium, and the neodiaphragm, may be difficult to treat. The radiosensitive structures such as the liver and heart can be spared quite well. Protection of the ipsilateral kidney is clearly better than with IMRT (see below).

Intensity modulated radiotherapy (IMRT) First, minimal motion of the target volume is determined. This is important because respiratory motion can be significant in the chest, and such motion would be a contraindication to IMRT. This is a problem partly because of the unknown heterogeneity of dose that might occur within the target volume, but is most worrisome because of the potential for normal tissues to move into the field during treatment. Fortunately, there is little motion of the involved hemithorax (Fig. 15.10a) compared with the contralateral hemithorax (Fig. 15.10b).

The target doses and the dose–volume limits for the critical structures are given in Table 15.2. Treatment is delivered with 13–27 intensity-modulated fields using 8–11 gantry angles, typically with 100 segments per intensity-modulated field. The dose limits for critical structures are the standard values used in clinical practice at the M. D. Anderson Cancer Center, with the exception of the contralateral lung dose. Because patients have only one lung after EPP, the volumes of contralateral lung irradiated should be limited such that the mean lung dose is less than 9.5 Gy. This is consistent with results of whole-lung irradiation [24]. All patients can be set up and treated within a 45 min period.

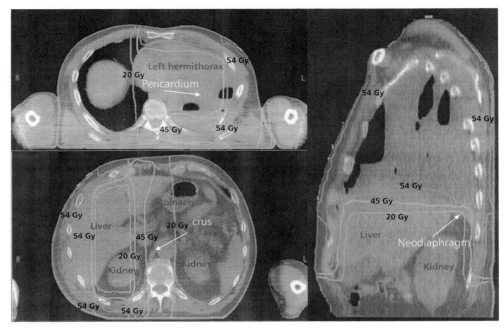

Figure 15.9 Dose distributions from traditional MPM treatment. The dose distribution from traditional radiation covers the target fairly well. Regions which may be more difficult to irradiate with this technique include the pericardium, crus, and diaphragm (arrows). (Reprinted from Yajnick et al., 23).

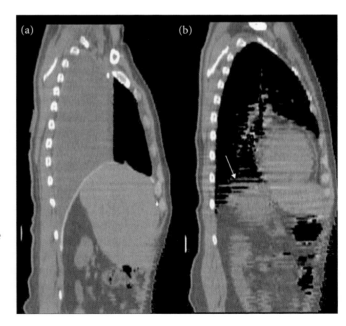

Figure 15.10 There is little motion of the involved hemithorax after EPP. (a) A postoperative treatment-planning CT scan revealed little motion artefact on the operated side. (b) In contrast, there is significant respiratory-driven motion artefact on the contralateral side (arrow).

Table 15.2 Target doses to the targets and dose–volume constraints of the organs at risk

Target or organ	Target dose or constraint dose
CTV	50 Gy in 25 fractions
bCTV	60 Gy in 25 fractions
Lung	<20% to receive >20 Gy
	Mean <9.5 Gy
Liver	<30% to receive >30 Gy
Contralateral kidney	<20% to receive >15 Gy
Heart	<50% to receive >45 Gy
Spinal cord	<10% to receive >45 Gy
	No portion to receive >50 Gy
Oesophagus	<30% to receive >55 Gy

CTV, clinical target volume.

The verification process has four components: delivered dose, relative dose distributions, leaf sequences, and patient position. Measurements to verify all four components are acquired for each patient using a variety of standard techniques customized for these unusual cases.

Ion chamber measurements are used to verify the absolute dose for each patient. Before making these measurements, the dose distribution resulting from delivering the intensity-modulated beams from the patient's treatment plan to a phantom is calculated. Initially, three ion chamber measurements are made, one near the apex of the field, one near the centre, and one corresponding to a point roughly at the centre of the liver. The measurement points are selected in regions of relatively uniform doses. The phantom, ion chamber, and electrometer are appropriately calibrated for each set of measurements. The IMRT phantom is appropriately positioned, and the entire treatment is delivered for each measurement point. Because the phantom is only 25 cm long, an additional 6 cm of Lucite blocks is stacked on its inferior and superior borders to generate the scatter from the large fields.

Initially, intensity maps for each intensity-modulated field are verified by film measurement. For each field, an *en-face* (gantry at 0°) film showing the leaf sequence is generated by exposing a film (Kodak V, Eastman Kodak, Rochester, NY) with the field's intensity-modulated field at a source–axis distance of 100 cm without build-up. Each film is qualitatively compared with the corresponding intensity maps calculated by the treatment-planning system.

At the M. D. Anderson Cancer Centre a phantom was constructed for assessing the relative dose distribution. The phantom holds a 14–17 inch film (Kodak XV) with three slabs of 2-cm-thick polystyrene on either side of the film. The film is oriented in a sagittal plane and irradiated. Because the prescription dose is 2 Gy/fraction, monitor units are adjusted to deliver 80 cGy to the film. The film is scanned on a film scanner (Lumisys Lumiscan 75, Humboldt, CT) and the scanned image is converted to a two-dimensional dose distribution. On the treatment-planning system, a dose calculation is performed using the calculated beam configuration with the phantom. The absolute isodose lines are printed out from both the treatment-planning system and the film scanning software (Wellhoffer, Schwarzenbruck, Germany) and compared visually.

On the first day of treatment, a dry run is performed in which AP and lateral isocentre verification films are acquired. The isocentre verification films are compared with the AP and lateral digitally reconstructed radiographs generated from the treatment plan. During the first week of treatment, two sets of isocentre verification films are acquired on consecutive days. Subsequently, additional portal images are acquired twice weekly.

Clearly, IMRT is more complicated to deliver than 3D-CRT. However, very good coverage of the target can be achieved. As shown in Figure 15.11, the 50 Gy isodose line encompasses most of the CTV. Review of the dose–volume histogram for this case (Fig. 15.12) demonstrates that the target volume is well covered and the normal tissue constraints are met. The liver and contralateral lung are spared with this technique. In this patient it was possible to spare the ipsilateral kidney because the organ was particularly low. This is unusual. The ipsilateral kidney usually receives a high dose because the CTV typically abuts its posterior edge. Adequate contralateral renal function is ensured by pretreatment renal assessment. For left-sided lesions, the spleen is also likely to receive a high radiation dose (Fig. 15.13). Therefore pneumococcal prophylaxis is recommended.

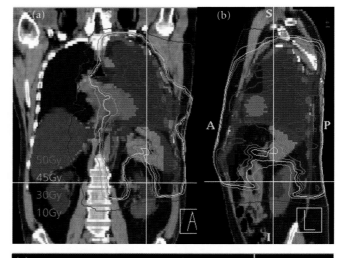

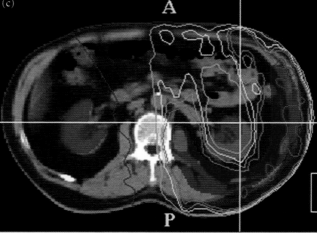

Figure 15.11 Dose distributions from IMRT. The dose distribution demonstrates good coverage of the CTV and the high dose gradients achievable with this technique. The target was 50 Gy to the CTV. The 50 Gy, 45 Gy, 30 Gy, and 10 Gy isodose lines are shown in magenta, orange, green, and blue, respectively.

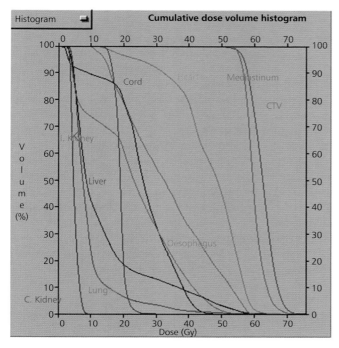

Figure 15.12 Dose volume histogram for the case shown in Fig. 15.11. Coverage of the target volumes is adequate. The contralateral kidney (C. kidney) was well below the target dose, as was about 25 per cent of the ipsilateral kidney (I. kidney). The mean lung dose was about 9.5 Gy. In this left-sided case, the heart dose was slightly higher than the target dose (60 per cent to 45 Gy, rather than 50 per cent).

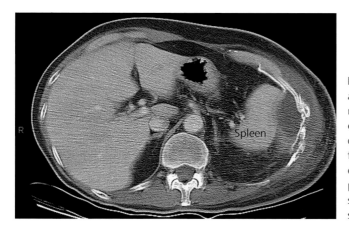

Figure 15.13 The spleen closely approximates the neodiaphragm in left-sided cases. There are no good dose–response data for splenic function. Therefore we electively provide pneumococcal vaccine before starting radiation therapy in such cases.

Summary

A review of the limited patient studies (Table 15.1) in MPM suggests that EPP followed by irradiation gives better local control than pleurectomy followed by radiation. Postoperative radiotherapy should include the entire volume immediately adjacent to the pleural space that is at highest risk for microscopic residual disease. This volume should include all sites of pleural reflection, the ipsilateral mediastinum, and the insertion of the diaphragm. The technique by which radiation is delivered (traditional vs. IMRT) is probably not as important as the target volume delineation and coverage.

Future directions

From a radiation oncology point of view, the most important aspect of future trials will be firm documentation of sites of regional relapse. True in-field failures need to be documented and explained. This will help to determine the adequacy of target volume delineation, and to determine if more, or possibly less, dose is needed to prevent recurrence.

EPP followed by radiation changes the pattern of recurrence such that distant metastases are the most common cause of death. This has several implications. First, it will be important to include systemic therapy in the treatment programme. The optimal sequencing of systemic therapy is unclear at present. However, unlike non-small-cell lung cancer, concurrent chemoradiotherapy does not seem necessary at this time because of excellent loco-regional control. One currently planned trial will use induction cisplatin–pemetrexed followed by EPP followed by radiation. Secondly, the current staging system may need modification, since it was designed at a time when loco-regional recurrence was the most common cause of death. Now, survival is more dependent on distant metastases. While some risk factors for metastases, perhaps nodal metastases, will probably continue to be important predictors, others such as parietal vs. visceral pleural involvement might become less important. Thirdly, now that loco-regional failure can be dramatically reduced, more emphasis should be placed on screening programs to identify patients with earlier disease. In summary, this is a time for cautious optimism in MPM.

References

1. Hakkinen AM, Laasonen A, Linnainmaa K, Mattson K, Pyrhonen S. Radiosensitivity of mesothelioma cell lines. *Acta Oncol* 1996; **35**: 451–6.
2. Carmichael J, Degraff WG, Gamson J, *et al.* Radiation sensitivity of human lung cancer cell lines. *Eur J Cancer Clin Oncol* 1989; **25**: 527–34.
3. Gordon W Jr, Antman KH, Greenberger JS, Weichselbaum RR, Chaffey JT. Radiation therapy in the management of patients with mesothelioma. *Int J Radiat Oncol Biol Phys* 1982; **8**: 19–25.
4. Ball DL, Cruickshank DG. The treatment of malignant mesothelioma of the pleura: review of a 5-year experience, with special reference to radiotherapy. *Am J Clin Oncol* 1990; **13**: 4–9.
5. Van Ooijen B, Eggermont AMM, Wiggers T. Subcutaneous tumor growth complicating the positioning of Denver shunt and intrapleural Port-A-Cath in mesothelioma patients. *Eur J Surg Oncol* 1992; **18**: 638–40 .
6. Boutin C, Rey F, Viallat JR. Prevention of malignant seeding after invasive diagnostic procedures in patients with pleural mesothelioma. A randomized trial of local radiotherapy. *Chest* 1995; **108**: 754–75.
7. Nguyen LN, Komaki R, Allen P, Schea RA, Milas L. Effectiveness of accelerated radiotherapy for patients with inoperable nonsmall cell lung cancer (NSCLC) and borderline prognostic factors without distant metastasis: a retrospective review. *Int J Radiat Oncol Biol Phys* 1999; **44**: 1053–6.
8. Graham MV. Purdy JA. Emami B. Harms W. Bosch W. Lockett MA. Perez CA. Clinical dose–volume histogram analysis for pneumonitis after 3D treatment for non-small cell lung cancer (NSCLC) *Int J Radiat Oncol Biol Phys* 1999; **45**: 323–9.
9. Maasilta P. Deterioration in lung function following hemithorax irradiation for pleural mesothelioma. *Int J Radiat Oncol Biol Phys* 1991; **20**: 433–8.
10. Maasilta P, Kivisaari L, Holsti LR, Tammilehto L, Mattson K. Radiographic chest assessment of lung injury following hemithorax irradiation for pleural mesothelioma. *Eur Respir J* 1991; **4**: 76–83.
11. Mattson K, Holsti LR, Tammilehto L, *et al.* 1992; Multimodality treatment programs for malignant pleural mesothelioma using high-dose hemithorax irradiation. *Int J Radiat Oncol Biol Phys* **24**: 643–50.
12. Hilaris BS, Nori D, Kwong E, Kutcher GJ, Martini N. Pleurectomy and intraoperative brachytherapy and postoperative radiation in the treatment of malignant pleural mesothelioma. *Int J Radiat Oncol Biol Phys* 1984; **10**: 325–31.

13. Kutcher GJ, Kestler C, Greenblatt D, Brenner H, Hilaris BS, Nori D. Technique for external beam treatment for mesothelioma. *Int J Radiat Oncol Biol Phys* 1987; **13**: 1747–52.

14. Mychalczak BR, Nori D, Armstrong JG, Martini N, and Harrison LB. Results of treatment of malignant pleural mesothelioma with surgery, brachytherapy, and external beam irradiation. *Endocurie Hypertherm Oncol* 1989; **5**: 245.

15. Rusch VW. Pleurectomy/decortication and adjuvant therapy for malignant mesothelioma. *Chest* 1993; **103** (Suppl): 382S–4S.

16. Lee TT, Everett DL, Shu H-KG, *et al*. Radical pleurectomy/decortication and intraoperative radiotherapy followed by conformal radiation with or without chemotherapy for malignant pleural mesothelioma. *J Thorac Cardiovasc Surg* 2002; **124**: 1183–9.

17. Baldini EH, Recht A, Strauss GM, *et al*. Patterns of failure after trimodality therapy for malignant pleural mesothelioma. *Ann Thorac Surg* 1997; **63**: 334–8.

18. Sugarbaker DJ, Flores RM, Jaklitsch MT, *et al*. Resection margins, extrapleural nodal status, and cell type determine postoperative long-term survival in trimodality therapy of malignant pleural mesothelioma: results in 183 patients. *J Thorac Cardiovasc Surg* 1999; **117**: 54–63.

19. Rusch VW, Rosenzweig K, Venkatraman E, *et al*. A phase II trial of surgical resection and adjuvant high-dose hemithoracic radiation for malignant plural mesothelioma. *J Thorac Cardiovasc Surg* 2001; **122**: 788–95.

20. Ahamad A, Stevens CW, Smythe WR, *et al*. Intensity-modulated radiation therapy: a novel approach to the management of malignant pleural mesothelioma. *Int J Radiat Oncol Biol Phys* 2003; **55**: 768–75.

21. Ahamad A, Stevens CW, Smythe WR, *et al*. Promising early local control of malignant pleural mesothelioma following postoperative intensity modulated radiotherapy (IMRT) to the chest. *Cancer J* 2004; **9**: 476–84.

22. Forster KM, Smythe WR, Starkschall G, *et al*. Intensity-modulated radiotherapy following extrapleural pneumonectomy for the treatment of malignant mesothelioma: clinical implementation. *Int J Radiat Oncol Biol Phys* 2003; **55**: 606–16.

23. Yajnik S, Rosenzweig KE, Mychalczak B, *et al*. Hemithoracic radiation after extrapleural pneumonectomy for malignant pleural mesothelioma. *Int J Radiat Oncol Biol Phys* 2003; **56**: 1319–26.

24. Della Volpe A, Ferreri AJ, Annaloro C, *et al*. Lethal pulmonary complications significantly correlate with individually assessed mean lung dose in patients with hematologic malignancies treated with total body irradiation. *Int J Radiat Oncol Biol Phys* 2002; **52**: 483–8.

Chapter 16

Immunotherapy for malignant mesothelioma

M. E. R. O'Brien, A. U. Ribate, and B. Souberbielle

Introduction

As with most other solid tumours, there is a need for new therapeutic approaches in the treatment of malignant mesothelioma (MM) because of its increasing incidence and the lack of effective options that significantly improve outcome. Although chemotherapy continues to be used [1] and new drugs are showing additional efficacy in this disease [2], a detailed knowledge of the molecular events responsible for MM, as well as the molecular profile of established MM, is limited. Consequently potential molecular targets for developing new drugs against MM have been scant until recently. Alternative and novel therapies, such as immunotherapy, have been explored to treat MM. There have been reports and discussions suggesting that the immune response may influence or even control the growth of some cases of MM, adding some weight to the potential use of immunotherapy in this disease [3–8].

Immunotherapy can be classified into two main approaches with some overlap, i.e. specific (or targeted) immunotherapy and non-specific immunotherapy. Specific immunotherapy targets particular antigens on the tumour, either through the active response of the patient to tumour vaccines, or passively by the administration of tumour-specific antibodies or lymphocytes. The definition of non-specific tumour immunotherapy is somewhat less precise but encompasses the use of immunomodulators which modify the immune biology of the host and/or tumour in such a way as to bring about an antitumour effect.

Active immunotherapy for MM has been so far restricted by the lack of identified MM specific antigens. Until recently MM was thought to be 'immunologically silent', unlike other tumours such as melanoma or even lung cancer [9]. The lack of specific MM antigens has also been a hindrance in the histopathological diagnosis of the disease. Panels of antibodies are necessary to help differentiate MM from other tumour types, such as adenocarcinoma, but no single antibody used in immunohistochemistry can be considered MM specific [10,11]. However, extensive work on MM has identified antigens which are useful for the diagnosis of epithelioid MM and which could be explored as potential targets for specific immunotherapy (see below).

Surface antigens are potential targets for antibody-based immunotherapy, and this approach has recently been successful in other tumour types (e.g. trastuzumab targeting HER-2/neu in breast cancer [12] and rituximab targeting CD20 in non-Hodgkin's lymphoma [13]). Similarly, nuclear antigens may provide targets for cytotoxic T lymphocytes (CTLs). Small parts of these nuclear proteins, called epitopes, can be processed and combined with HLA class I (and class II) molecules intracellularly, and then transported with these HLA molecules to the cell surface and presented with the HLA molecules to be recognized by CTLs [14,15]. This presentation is HLA specific and therefore will differ between patients. A tumour-specific HLA-A2-restricted CTL response has been the focus of intense research because the prevalence of HLA-A2 in the general Western population is about 40 per cent, making HLA-A2-based immunotherapy a reasonable approach in that part of the world.

Potential MM antigens for immunotherapy, as in any other tumour types, fall into three main categories: (a) tumour-specific antigens which are found in tumours but not in normal tissues (mutated oncogene products fall into this category); (b) tumour-associated antigens which are also found in normal cells, a good example being differentiation antigens which are found in normal tissues from which the tumour arose although over-expressed oncogene products also fall into this category; (c) oncofetal antigens which are expressed during gestation and re-expressed in tumours. These oncofoetal antigens are mainly tumour-associated antigens (as in b) as there is still a low background expression of such antigens in adult tissues. All these antigens represent potential targets for cancer vaccination [16,17].

MM-associated antigens

A study based on western blotting showed that about a third of patients suffering from MM have high titres of immunoglobin G (IgG) specific for MM antigens [8]. Some of these antigens were identified by the recombinant expression cloning technique SEREX as self-antigens such as topoisomerase IIb [18]. The fact that antibodies in these patients do not lead to tumour rejection is not a reason to dismiss antibody therapy for MM. Indeed, the humoral response to MM may be improved [19] either through modification of the antibodies (e.g. higher affinity, better specificity or complement-binding capability, or simply targeted to a different antigen) or manipulated in the test tube (e.g. by linking the antibody to a powerful toxin [20] to produce a pharmaceutical drug capable of bringing about tumour destruction).

Mesothelin is over-expressed in MM. It is a 40 kDa glycoprotein expressed on the cell surface of both normal mesothelium and MM as well as other tumour types such as squamous carcinoma of the oesophagus and lung, cervical, ovarian, and pancreatic cancer [21]. Monoclonal antibodies specific to mesothelin have been linked to immunotoxins, such as a truncated form of *Pseudomonas* exotoxin, and showed activity *in vitro* against cell lines and xenograft-implanted nude mice [20,22].

Calretinin is a 29 Kda protein expressed in neural tissue and some non-neural cells, such as mesothelium [23,24]. However, it appears that some antibody clones targeting calretinin may be relatively specific for MM [25]. Anti-calretinin specific staining in MM is nuclear and therefore it is conceivable that calretinin epitopes may act as CTL targets.

Cancer-testis antigens have restricted expression in normal tissues and may represent candidate molecules for immunotherapy of cancer as the testis is an immunologically privileged and should not suffer autoimmune reaction or attack. The cancer-testis antigens MAGE-1, MAGE-2 and MAGE-3, GAGE-1–2, GAGE-1–6, SSX-2, and SSX1–5 have recently been shown to be expressed in MM. MAGE-4 and NY-ESO-1 are detected less frequently in MM than the other antigens in this group [26]. NY-ESO-1 has been shown *in vitro* to act as a CTL antigen on cell lines raised from thoracic tumours [27] or to induce NY-ESO-1 peptide-specific CD8-positive lymphocytes, which are HLA-A2 restricted, in patients with cancer after immunization [28]. Other molecules such as the still uncharacterized glycoprotein 90K may also be of interest [29].

In relation to oncogene products, p53 over-expression in MM is common but p53 mutations are rare [30–32]. It is not known whether immune response against non-mutated p53 would be useful as a therapy but it is unlikely. Antibodies specific to p53 are detected at a low frequency (about 10 per cent) in patients with MM and do not have prognostic significance [33]. Wilms tumour susceptibility gene 1 [WT1] product is another tool for diagnosis as it is over-expressed [nuclear staining] in MM [34–38] and the gene has been found to be mutated in some reports [39]. WT1 has been explored for T-cell-mediated immunotherapy in preclinical models [40] and WT1-specific CTL can be detected and raised from human subjects [41]. There is one report of the neurofibromatosis type 2 (NF2) gene being mutated in mesothelioma [42], but to our knowledge the NF2 gene product has not been investigated as a potential target for immunotherapy. There has also been one report of over-expression of the c-*myc* gene product in MM compared with non-neoplastic mesothelium which also expresses this protein [43].

The role of simian virus 40 (SV40) in the pathogenesis of MM is beyond the scope of this chapter (see Chapter 7) [44]. However, at least 50 per cent of MM express SV40 antigens [45,46], especially the SV40 large tumour antigen (Tag) [47,48] which could be targeted by the immune system [49]. Specific HLA-A2-restricted Tag peptides have been characterized [50], and there is evidence of Tag-specific CTL, HLA-A2 restricted, and humoral IgG immune response in the peripheral blood of some patients with MM [51]. To our knowledge SV40 is not expressed in normal tissues in patients suffering from MM and therefore can be considered a truly tumour-specific antigen. As such, it is a good candidate vaccine target, both in the preventive and therapeutic settings [52]. Another potential CTL antigen in MM is telomerase [53] which has recently been the focus of intense attention [54]. SV40 infection induces telomerase activity in human mesothelial cells, adding even further interest to this field of MM [55].

Rationale of immunotherapy in MM

It is likely that for tumour immunotherapy to be successful, in addition to targeting specific tumour antigens, it may be necessary to achieve two goals, first, correcting a possible systemic immunosuppression and, secondly, changing the immunosuppressive local tumour environment to a more immune-potentiating one. The mechanism of the systemic and local immunosuppression is complex [56,57] (see Chapter 10), but correcting or overriding this defect is the basis of the use of non-specific immunotherapy in patients with cancer. MM may be even more amenable to local immunotherapy than most other tumour types because in practice it is usually confined to one organ and the pleural cavity can easily be accessed for local treatments or sampling.

Two approaches have the potential to break systemic/local immune tolerance (Fig. 16.1). The first is the exogenous enhancement of the host's immune response via a non-specific stimulation either using recombinant inflammatory or immunopotentiating cytokines (interleukin 2 (IL-2), interferon (IFN), tumour necrosis factor, colony-stimulation factor) or attenuated bacterial antigens (e.g. BCG, SRL 172). The second approach is to overcome the local immunosuppressive effects of the tumour by the injection of a non-specific immunostimulant intralesionally or intracavitarily [58]. These two approaches can also be used in combination. Furthermore, non-specific immunotherapy approaches can be used as immunological adjuvants to MM vaccines. This is where gene therapy overlaps with immunotherapy. For example, whole-cell tumour vaccines which provide tumour antigens can be genetically modified to secrete specific cytokines in order to sustain an antitumour response. The vaccines can also be modified to express co-stimulatory molecules which provide the second signal to T cells (the first signal is the tumour antigen) so that an efficient antitumour T-cell response can be generated. The other strategy is to provide the immunostimulatory signals at the level of the tumour, so that the tumour itself acts as the vaccine.

Some of these approaches have been tested in preclinical models of MM with antitumour responses. For example, both systemic and intratumoral administration of IL-12 showed anti-MM activity [59]. IFN-α showed anti-MM activity preclinically, especially when used with a

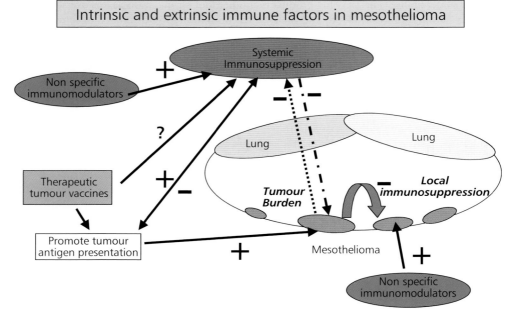

Figure 16.1 Intrinsic and extrinsic factors which may influence an immunological antitumour response: + factors have a positive antitumour effect; – factors have a negative effect on the antitumour immune mechanisms.

small tumour load and in combination with immunomodulatory and antiproliferative agents such as α-carotene or α-difluoromethylornithine [60]

Intralesional/intracavitary administration of bacterial-derived products have also been tested as MM therapy with promising results in preclinical models. Intraperitoneal administration of cationic:bacterial DNA complexes elicited strong anti-MM activity [61] due to the CpG motif of the DNA fragments [62]. It has also been reported that intrapleurally administered BCG can prevent or treat intrapleural or intraperitoneal rat sarcomas [63]. SRL-172, a heat-killed non-pathogenic mycobacterium, has been tested *in vitro* and in humans (see below).

MM cell lines genetically modified to express different cytokine/immunological signals have been shown to grow more slowly than the non-modified cell, and these effects are immunologically mediated. Examples include IL-2 secreting MM cells [64], B7–1-expressing MM cells [65], allogeneic MHC-expressing MM cells [66], IL-12 [59], and IFN-γ [67]. Furthermore, the antitumour effects of granulocyte macrophage–colony-stimulating factor (GM–CSF) and B7 gene transfection appeared to be enhanced by prior debulking surgery [68]. Viral vectors expressing particular cytokines have also been administered intralesionally so that the mesothelioma cells in the tumour secrete the cytokines of interest; this has been studied, for example, with adenoviral vectors encoding IFN-α [69].

In general, most of the immunotherapies used in preclinical models, when tested, have been shown to mediate their anti-MM activity through CD8+ lymphocytes, often with help from the CD4+ lymphocyte population [59,61,64,69,70]. To date, natural killer (NK) cells have not been shown to be involved in antitumour activity in MM. In addition, IFN and possibly IL-2 also have some antiproliferative properties on MM cells which are not immunologically mediated [4,67,71,72].

Clinical immunotherapy

The first interest in immune therapy in general, and specifically in MM, came following the encouraging results with the use of BCG in patients in the 1970s and 1980s. Thirty patients with MM were treated and survival was reported to be prolonged [73]. These results were not followed up as the appearance of recombinant molecules became the focus of clinical trials in the 1980s.

Interleukin 2 (Table 16.1)

Five studies of the use of IL-2 alone given intrapleurally have been reported. In a phase I study, Goey et al. [74] did not document any dose response but did have a response rate of 19 per cent with antitumour activity seen at all doses. Castagneto et al. [75] treated 31 patients with MM presenting with a pleural effusion with intrapleural administration of IL-2 at a dose of 9 MU twice a week, followed by subcutaneous treatment in non-progressing patients. Ninety per cent of patients had control of the pleural effusion with only one relapse. Twenty-nine patients were reported to have stage I or II disease and only two had stage IV disease. A significant rate of response was obtained, with 22 per cent (10 patients) achieving a partial response (PR) and 32 per cent stable disease (SD). The most significant toxicity was grade III fever in 19 per cent of patients and cardiac failure in one patient. The median survival was 15 months. Astoul et al. [76] also achieved an encouraging 54 per cent response rate in patients with MM also using IL-2 alone. The toxicity was acceptable, but patients were highly selected with 16 of the global 22 patients having stage II disease.

One other study used IL-2 intravenously in MM patients [77]. A dose of 18 MU was given on days 1 and 2 followed by subcutaneous IL-2 6 MU on days 5–20 every 42 days. Again, the patients had early stage I and II disease. The response was disappointing at 8 per cent, but the two patients who did respond were alive 18.1 and 18.7 months later.

IL-2 has been used with chemotherapy in the treatment of mesothelioma among other tumours. When it was given with epirubicin the response rate of the combination was 5 per cent

Table 16.1 Clinical studies using IL-2 alone and in combination

Reference	No of patients	Route	Stage	Overall response	Median survival (months)
Goey et al. [74]	23	IP	NA	19%	15.6
Castagneto et al. [75]	31	IP + SC	effusion	22%	15
Astoul et al. [76]	22 16	IP	Stage II	54% 5% CR	Resp: 28 NR: 8
Mulatero et al. [77]	29	IV + SC	Stage I/II	8%	8.6
Bretti et al. [78]	21	SC + epirubicin	NA	5%	10
Nowak et al. [3]	5	SC + LAK	NA	0	NA
Robinson et al. [81]	6	Vaccinia-IL-2	NA	0	NA

IP, intrapleural; SC, subcutaneous; IV, intravenous; LAK, lymphokine-activated killer cells; NA, not available; CR, complete response; Resp, responder; NR, non-responder

[78]. A Japanese group gave two patients with intraperitoneal MM IL-2 plus autologous tumour cells plus doxorubicin and cisplatin and they reported partial responses [79].

IL-2 has been used with lymphokine-activated killer (LAK) cells to treat five patients in Australia but no responses were seen [3]. Two patients also treated with LAK cells have been reported from Japan. One received autologous LAK cells intrapleurally and the other received allogenic cells; both received systemic IL-2 and the authors reported a reduction in pleural effusions [80]. Robinson *et al.* [81] used a gene therapy approach to expose tumours to high levels of cytokines using a vaccinia IL-2 recombinant given intrapleurally. Six patients have been treated and no responses have been seen.

Interferon (Table 16.2)

The three IFN subtypes have all been used in the treatment of MM in one way or another. IFN-γ has been given intrapleurally by continuous infusion in the largest study of this type. Boutin *et al.* [82] treated 89 patients and documented a response rate in 20 per cent of patients with a 9 per cent complete response (CR) rate overall. The response rate increased to 45 per cent in stage I disease, suggesting that a small burden of tumour may be a good predictive factor for response to local inmuno-based treatment. Recently, IFN-γ has been combined with autologous human activated macrophages and given intrapleurally in 19 patients with early stage MM [83]. The response rate was 11 per cent, and two patients had a PR with a duration of 30 and 3 months, respectively. Pleurodesis was achieved in seven of 14 patients who completed the treatment.

IFN-β used by an Italian group in 29 patients gave a response rate of 37.9 per cent with 27.6 per cent CR [84]. However, when it was used by the Southwest Oncology Group in 14 patients no activity was seen [85].

To date, IFN-α has been the most frequently used agent in studies using one of the IFNs combined with chemotherapy. Two studies described the use of IFN-α as monotherapy [86,87]. The response rate was low (of the order of 8–12 per cent), but CRs were still seen. There are three similar studies of IFN-α combined with cisplatin. Response rates to this combination can reach 40 per cent with no benefit from increasing the IFN doses [88–91]. The highest response rate was seen with weekly cisplatin 60 mg/m^2 and IFN-α. However, this combination was toxic with grade 3–4 haematological toxicities in 30 per cent, grade 3–4 emesis in 40 per cent, neuropathy in 8 per cent and a decrease in performance status in 56 per cent [88]. This combination was not improved by the addition of IL-2 [92]. One trial combining carboplatin with IFN-α in an attempt to minimize the side effects of the combination failed to show an appreciable rate of response [93]. IFN-α with doxorubicin was only modestly active, with a response rate of 16 per cent [94].

Three more studies explored the combination of subcutaneous IFN-α and doublet chemotherapy. Two groups tried adding mitomycin to cisplatin and IFN-α [95,96], and another group added doxorubicin to cisplatin and IFN-α [97]. None of them improved the response rate achieved with cisplatin and IFN-α. Metintas *et al.* [95], using IFN-α 9 MU/week, cisplatin 60 mg/m^2/4 weeks and mitomycin 8 mg/m^2/4 weeks, achieved a median survival of 11.5 months. The median survival in 19 other patients who did not receive chemotherapy was 7 months and it was 21.3 months for those patients who responded to chemotherapy. Parra *et al.* [97], using IFN-α with doxorubicin 60 mg/m^2 and the same dose of cisplatin achieved a median survival of 9.3 months but with 45 per cent alive at 1 year and 34 per cent alive at 2 years; 46 per cent had stage I disease and 38 per cent had stage III disease. Halme *et al.* [98] combined IFN-α and IFN-γ with high-dose methotrexate (3 g/m^2). Toxicity was tolerable, and both response rate (29 per cent) and median survival (17 months) make it an attractive schedule to explore further.

Table 16.2 Clinical studies using the interferons alone and in combination

Reference	No of patients	Type and route	Overall response	Median survival (months)
Boutin et al. [82]	89	IFN-γ	20% Stage I: 45% CR	
Monnet et al. [83]	19	IFN-γ + AAM	11%	PR 30, 3
Rosso et al. [84]	29	IFN-β	37.9% 27.6% CR	
Von Hoff et al. [85]	14	IFN-β	0%	
Ardizzoni et al. [86]	14	IFN-α	5%	
Christmas et al. [87]	25	IFN-α	12% 4% CR	
Soulie et al. [88]	26	IP IFN-α 3 MU + cisplatin 60 mg/m²/week	38%	12
Trandafir et al. [89]	30	SC IFN-α 6 MU + cisplatin 60 mg/m²/week	27%	NA
Purohit et al. [90]	13	SC IFN-α 6 MU + cisplatin 60 mg/m²/week	42%	NA
Pass et al. [91]	36	SC IFN-α 5 MU + tamoxifen + cisplatin 100 mg/ m²/3 weeks	19%	8.7
Caliandro et al. [92]	18	SC IFN-α 3 MU + IL-2 + cisplatin 100 mg/m2/3 weeks	15%	15
O'Reilly et al. [93]	15	SC IFN-α 3 MU + carboplatin	7%	6
Upham et al. [94]	25	SC IFN-α + doxorubicin	16%	
Metintas et al. [95]	43	SC IFN-α + cisplatin + mitomycin	23%	11.5
Rodier et al. [96]	24	SC IFN-α + cisplatin + mitomycin	21%	12
Parra et al. [97]	37	SC IFN-α 3 MU + cisplatin + doxorubicin	29%	9.3
Halme et al. [98]	26	SC IFN-α + IFN-g + methotrexate	29%	17

IP, intrapleural; SC, subcutaneous; NA, not available; CR, complete response; PR, partial response; AAM, human autologous activated macrophages.

Other immune agents and combinations

Three trials have explored GM–CSF as a therapeutic agent in MM. One trial used GM–CSF as an intrapleural agent and showed a single response out of 14 cases [99], and another demonstrated no responses in eight patients [81]. The third trial using GM–CSF with high-dose doxorubicin (120 mg/m²), given with dexrazoxane in an attempt to avoid cardiac toxicity, was suspended because of toxicity [100]. Tumour necrosis factor α (TNF-α) can induce local inflammatory responses and therefore could potentially have a local effect in the treatment of MM. A study by Stam *et al.* [101] in only five patients yielded no effect on the pleural effusions despite a high recorded level of induced IL-6 and IL-8. An anecdotal report from Japan described a patient alive 6 years after treatment with TNF and 5–fluorouracil [102]. TNF-α given intramuscularly in

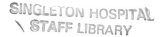

combination with IFN-γ was toxic with only a transient clearance of malignant cells in the pleural effusion of one patient with MM in a phase I study [103].

Mycobacterium vaccae

Mycobacterium vaccae SRL172 is a heat-killed non-pathogenic mycobacterium. Following on from laboratory results with SRL172 [104] which showed that it was a powerful immunological adjuvant with whole-cell vaccine, the non-specific immune stimulator was studied in patients with MM and non-small-cell lung cancer (NSCLC) (SIRON 5 series) with a separate randomization for patients with small-cell lung cancer [105]. Patients in the SIRON 5 series were divided on the basis of their symptoms into an asymptomatic and a symptomatic group. Asymptomatic patients were randomized to either a watch and wait policy or to receive intradermal four-weekly injections of SRL 172. This study recruited 14 patients to each arm from patients with NSCLC (n = 13) and MM (n = 15). Nine patients with MM were allocated to the watch and wait policy and six to SRL172. A cross-over to SRL172 was allowed at symptom progression for patients initially allocated to watch and wait. There were no objective responses to SRL172 and the median survival in both groups was 14 months with no difference between the two arms on an intention-to-treat analysis. Symptomatic patients at presentation with NSCLC and MM were randomized to chemotherapy with or without SRL172. The drug combination was mitomycin, vinblastine, and cisplatin (MVP). In each group in which mesothelioma patients were included, two out of four patients with mesothelioma had a PR with chemotherapy plus SRL172 while one out of five mesothelioma patients responded to chemotherapy alone [106]. Phase III studies were started in NSCLC (SIRON 12 series) and SCLC (Small Vac series) and have been completed.

With MM this work was expanded in an attempt to improve local disease control. A phase I study was commenced in patients with MM using SRL172 at increasing doses given intrapleurally in addition to intradermal SRL172 at standard doses and MVP chemotherapy. The results describe a bell-shaped curve in terms of activity with increasing doses of intrapleural SRL172. The overall response rate was 37.5 per cent and responses were seen at all dose levels [107]. In addition, patients showed a decreasing level of IL-4 and an increasing level of NK cells that was not predictive of objective response to treatment.

Despite the plethora of phase II studies in mesothelioma, no phase III studies comparing chemo-immunotherapy with either modality alone, or indeed with best supportive care only, have been performed. However, where these modalities have been explored in other solid tumours, either alone or in combination, the only positive clinical trials combining an immune therapy with cytotoxic drugs have been with the use of specific antibodies in combination with chemotherapy such as trastuzimab with doxorubicin and/or paclitaxel in the treatment of breast cancer or rituximab with chemotherapy for lymphoma [12,13]. These trials show an improved survival with combined antibody and chemotherapy compared with chemotherapy alone, which could be an additive rather that a synergistic effect. Trials in renal cancer and malignant melanoma with combinations of chemotherapy with IFN and interleukin show no such additive effect, but neither do they show an inhibitory effect.

With the increasing incidence of MM large trials of immunotherapy should be performed given the body of evidence suggesting that there is some activity with locally applied cytokines. However, if control of pleural effusions is all that can be achieved, a chemical pleuredesis performed medically or surgically will probably achieve the goal more rapidly and is probably less toxic overall. MM can have a long natural history. Immune function may be relatively normal when the disease is of small volume, but become progressively more impaired in the presence of bulky disease. The observation that immunosuppression tends to increase with disease progression supports an underlying hypothesis that immunotherapy will never be successful with bulky disease and should preferentially be employed after some form of debulking process (surgery, radiotherapy or chemotherapy). Chemotherapy has recently moved on and treatments with acceptable toxicities with good objective response rates are currently taking over from immune trials. This will probably continue until another immunomodulator shows promise and the cycle starts again.

References

1. Middleton GW, Smith IE, O'Brien ME, *et al.* Good symptom relief with palliative MVP (mitomycin-C, vinblastine and cisplatin) chemotherapy in malignant mesothelioma. *Ann Oncol* 1998; **9**: 269–73.

2. Vogelzang N, Rusthoven J, Paoletti P, *et al.* Phase III single-blinded study of pemetrexed + cisplatin vs cisplatin alone in chemonaive patients with malignant pleural mesothelioma. *Proc Am Soc Clin Oncol* 2002;

3. Nowak AK, Lake RA, Kindler HL, Robinson BW. New approaches for mesothelioma: biologics, vaccines, gene therapy, and other novel agents. *Semin Oncol* 2002; **29**: 82–96.

4. Porta C, Danova M, Orengo AM, *et al.* Interleukin-2 induces cell cycle perturbations leading to cell growth inhibition and death in malignant mesothelioma cells *in vitro*. *J Cell Physiol* 2000; **185**: 126–34.

5. Mutti L, Valle MT, Balbi B, *et al.* Primary human mesothelioma cells express class II MHC, ICAM-1 and B7–2 and can present recall antigens to autologous blood lymphocytes. *Int J Cancer* 1998; **78**: 740–9.

6. Valle MT, Castagneto B, Procopio A, Carbone M, Giordano A, Mutti L. Immunobiology and immune defense mechanisms of mesothelioma cells. *Monaldi Arch Chest Dis* 1998; **53**: 219–27.

7. Robinson BW, Robinson C, Lake RA. Localised spontaneous regression in mesothelioma – possible immunological mechanism. *Lung Cancer* 2001; **32**: 197–201.

8. Robinson C, Robinson BW, Lake RA. Sera from patients with malignant mesothelioma can contain autoantibodies. *Lung Cancer* 1998; **20**: 175–84.

9. Al-Moundhri M, O'Brien M, Souberbielle BE. Immunotherapy in lung cancer. *Br J Cancer* 1998; **78**: 282–8.

10. Ordonez NG. Immunohistochemical diagnosis of epithelioid mesotheliomas: a critical review of old markers, new markers. *Hum Pathol* 2002; **33**: 953–67.

11. Roberts F, Harper CM, Downie I, Burnett RA. Immunohistochemical analysis still has a limited role in the diagnosis of malignant mesothelioma. A study of thirteen antibodies. *Am J Clin Pathol* 2001; **116**: 253–62.

12. Slamon DJ, Leyland-Jones B, Shak S, *et al.* Use of chemotherapy plus a monoclonal antibody against HER2 for metastatic breast cancer that overexpresses HER2. *N Engl J Med* 2001; **344**: 783–92.

13. Coiffier B, Lepage E, Briere J, *et al.* CHOP chemotherapy plus rituximab compared with CHOP alone in elderly patients with diffuse large-B-cell lymphoma. *N Engl J Med* 2002; **346**: 235–42.

14. Van den Eynde BJ, van der Bruggen P. T cell defined tumor antigens. *Curr Opin Immunol* 1997; **9**: 684–93.

15. Robbins PF, Kawakami Y. Human tumor antigens recognized by T cells. *Curr Opin Immunol* 1996; **8**: 628–36.

16. Moingeon P. Cancer vaccines. *Vaccine* 2001; **19**: 1305–26.

17. Pardoll DM. Cancer vaccines. *Nat Med* 1998; **4** (Suppl): 525–31.

18. Robinson C, Callow M, Stevenson S, Scott B, Robinson BW, Lake RA. Serologic responses in patients with malignant mesothelioma: evidence for both public and private specificities. *Am J Respir Cell Mol Biol* 2000; **22**: 550–6.

19. Carter P. Improving the efficacy of antibody-based cancer therapies. *Nat Rev Cancer* 2001; **1**: 118–29.

20. Hassan R, Viner JL, Wang QC, Margulies I, Kreitman RJ, Pastan I. Anti-tumor activity of K1-LysPE38QQR, an immunotoxin targeting mesothelin, a cell-surface antigen overexpressed in ovarian cancer and malignant mesothelioma. *J Immunother* 2000; **23**: 473–9.

21. Argani P, Iacobuzio-Donahue C, Ryu B, *et al*. Mesothelin is overexpressed in the vast majority of ductal adenocarcinomas of the pancreas: identification of a new pancreatic cancer marker by serial analysis of gene expression (SAGE). *Clin Cancer Res* 2001; **7**: 3862–8.

22. Brinkmann U, Webber K, Di Carlo A, *et al*. Cloning and expression of the recombinant FAb fragment of monoclonal antibody K1 that reacts with mesothelin present on mesotheliomas and ovarian cancers. *Int J Cancer* 1997; **71**: 638–44.

23. Comin CE, Novelli L, Boddi V, Paglierani M, Dini S. Calretinin, thrombomodulin, CEA, and CD15: a useful combination of immunohistochemical markers for differentiating pleural epithelial mesothelioma from peripheral pulmonary adenocarcinoma. *Hum Pathol* 2001; **32**: 529–36.

24. Cury PM, Butcher DN, Fisher C, Corrin B, Nicholson AG. Value of the mesothelium-associated antibodies thrombomodulin, cytokeratin 5/6, calretinin, and CD44H in distinguishing epithelioid pleural mesothelioma from adenocarcinoma metastatic to the pleura. *Mod Pathol* 2000; **13**: 107–12.

25. Ordonez NG. Value of calretinin immunostaining in differentiating epithelial mesothelioma from lung adenocarcinoma. *Mod Pathol* 1998; **11**: 929–33.

26. Sigalotti L, Coral S, Altomonte M, *et al*. Cancer testis antigens expression in mesothelioma: role of DNA methylation and bioimmunotherapeutic implications. *Br J Cancer* 2002; **86**: 979–82.

27. Weiser TS, Guo ZS, Ohnmacht GA, *et al*. Sequential 5-aza-2 deoxycytidine-depsipeptide FR901228 treatment induces apoptosis preferentially in cancer cells and facilitates their recognition by cytolytic T lymphocytes specific for NY-ESO-1. *J Immunother* 2001; **24**: 151–61.

28. Gnjatic S, Jager E, Chen W, *et al*. CD8(+) T cell responses against a dominant cryptic HLA-A2 epitope after NY-ESO-1 peptide immunization of cancer patients. *Proc Natl Acad Sci USA* 2002; **99**: 11813–18.

29. Strizzi L, Muraro R, Vianale G, *et al*. Expression of glycoprotein 90K in human malignant pleural mesothelioma: correlation with patient survival. *J Pathol* 2002; **197**: 218–23.

30. Segers K, Backhovens H, Singh SK, *et al*. Immunoreactivity for p53 and mdm2 and the detection of p53 mutations in human malignant mesothelioma. *Virchows Arch* 1995; **427**: 431–6.

31. Mor O, Yaron P, Huszar M, *et al*. Absence of p53 mutations in malignant mesotheliomas. *Am J Respir Cell Mol Biol* 1997; **16**: 9–13.

32. Mayall FG, Jacobson G, Wilkins R. Mutations of p53 gene and SV40 sequences in asbestos associated and non-asbestos-associated mesotheliomas. *J Clin Pathol* 1999; **52**: 291–3.

33. Creaney J, McLaren BM, Stevenson S, *et al*. p53 autoantibodies in patients with malignant mesothelioma: stability through disease progression. *Br J Cancer* 2001; **84**: 52–6.

34. Hecht JL, Lee BH, Pinkus JL, Pinkus GS. The value of Wilms tumor susceptibility gene 1 in cytologic preparations as a marker for malignant mesothelioma. *Cancer* 2002; **96**: 105–9.

35. Foster MR, Johnson JE, Olson SJ, Allred DC. Immunohistochemical analysis of nuclear versus cytoplasmic staining of WT1 in malignant mesotheliomas and primary pulmonary adenocarcinomas. *Arch Pathol Lab Med* 2001; **125**: 1316–20.

36. Kumar-Singh S, Segers K, Rodeck U, *et al*. WT1 mutation in malignant mesothelioma and WT1 immunoreactivity in relation to p53 and growth factor receptor expression, cell-type transition, and prognosis. *J Pathol* 1997; **181**: 67–74.

37. Amin KM, Litzky LA, Smythe WR, *et al*. Wilms" tumor 1 susceptibility (WT1) gene products are selectively expressed in malignant mesothelioma. *Am J Pathol* 1995; **146**: 344–56.

38. Oates J, Edwards C. HBME-1, MOC-31, WT1 and calretinin: an assessment of recently described markers for mesothelioma and adenocarcinoma. *Histopathology* 2000; **36**: 341–7.

39. Park S, Schalling M, Bernard A, *et al*. The Wilms tumour gene WT1 is expressed in murine mesoderm-derived tissues and mutated in a human mesothelioma. *Nat Genet* 1993; **4**: 415–20.

Chapter 17

Intrathoracic photodynamic diagnosis and treatment of malignant mesothelioma with photodynamic therapy or hyperthermia

P. Baas

Introduction

Diagnosis of pleural malignancies such as malignant pleural mesothelioma (MPM) is sometimes difficult. Despite the relatively good diagnostic yield of cytological examination for malignancies, the differentiation between MPM and adenocarcinoma is often a problem. Histological samples are then required for a definitive diagnosis. Reports on the efficacy of thoracoscopies indicate that in 90 per cent of the cases this procedure is conclusive; however, at least 10, and preferably, 20 biopsies have to be taken during this procedure. Furthermore, adhesions and streaks of fibrosis can make it difficult to determine where the actual pathology is located. Therefore the use of a 'tumour-seeking' agent could be of value in such cases to guide biopsies and shorten the thoracoscopy procedure.

MPM is characterized by being relatively resistant to standard anticancer treatment modalities [1]. Surgery alone has little impact on survival and is associated with high local recurrence rates and significant impact on quality of life. The high rate of local recurrence is due to the microscopic nests of tumour that remain after surgery. Therefore the development of combinations of surgery with other treatments to sterilize the tumour bed has been emphasized. A number of innovative treatments have been examined, such as photodynamic therapy (PDT), a light-based cancer treatment, and hyperthermic intraoperative lavage with chemotherapy (HITHOC).

In this chapter we discuss new developments in the diagnosis of pleural malignancies and review the results of PDT and HITHOC in the management of MPM.

Photodynamic diagnosis of pleural diseases

Although at least 65 per cent of patients present with clinical signs of pleural effusion, the diagnosis of MPM often cannot be made on the basis of cytological examination alone and further invasive investigations are needed. Transthoracic pleural biopsy is diagnostic in 30–50 per cent of cases [2]. The diagnosis can best be made by invasive procedures such as thoracoscopic or open pleural biopsy. It is advisable to obtain multiple biopsies from different sites of the parietal pleura to reduce the number of false-negative results. However, it may be difficult to identify tumour lesions in early-stage MPM. Photodynamic diagnosis (PDD) is one of the new developments that can aid the physician in obtaining appropriate biopsies.

PDD can be performed as autofluorescence or photosensitizer-mediated fluorescence [3–8]. In both methods, abnormal fluorescence images are obtained when light of a specific wavelength is changed and reflected by tumour tissue. The reflected light is passed through a long bandpass filter and compared with the normal reflection spectrum. In autofluorescence, changes in vascularization are considered to be a major cause of the increased reflection of red light. In addition, changes in cell-layer thickness, tumour cell metabolism, and/or differences in the concentration of chromophores can result in a change in reflection. This approach has already led to the development of systems for the early diagnosis of oesophageal cancer [10] and lung cancer [11].

Sensitizer-mediated PDD has also been performed with 5-aminolaevulinic acid (5-ALA) [9]. This naturally occurring precursor of haemoglobin is administered in a low dose (15–30 mg/kg) orally, locally, or intravenously a few hours before the procedure. It is retained in both normal and malignant cells [6,7]. In normal cells 5-ALA is readily metabolized to protoporphorin IX (PP-IX) and subsequently to haeme. Tumour cells often lack the enzyme ferrochelatase that facilitates the metabolism of PP-IX to haeme. Therefore the concentration of PP-IX in the tumour

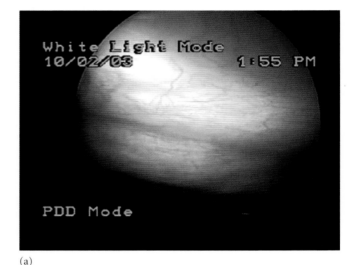

(a)

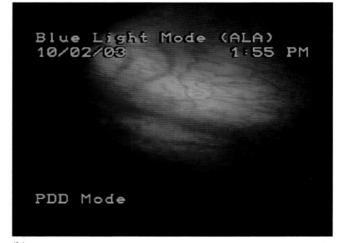

Figure 17.1 (a) Normal appearance of pleura in white light mode. (b) Same image in PDD mode. Abnormal fluorescence is now visible. Microscope examination showed malignant mesothelioma in the biopsies.

(b)

cells is increased compared with the surrounding normal cells. PP-IX fluoresces when activated by blue light and will emit red light of a specific wavelength that can be visualized in real time. PDD is now under investigation to determine whether it has any additional value compared with standard thorascopic examination.

Some examples of the application of this technology to the diagnosis of mesothelioma are shown in Figure 17.1 where images obtained using standard white light and 5-ALA PDD are compared. In these cases, white-light inspection during thoracoscopy identified tumour nodules that were highly fluorescent after the administration of 5-ALA. Tumour areas appear to be more clearly distinguished from the surrounding tissue and the extent of spread of the disease is more easily appreciated. Pathological examination of these specimens confirmed the tumour in the lesions with intense reflections and connective tissue at the control sites [9]. Currently the sensitivity and specificity of this approach is being analysed.

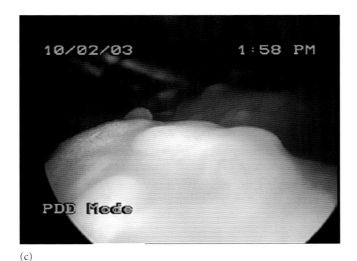

(c)

(d)

Figure 17.1 Contd.
(c) Pathological pleura with clear signs of lesions of the visceral pleura and fibrous depositions. Biopsies showed malignant mesothelioma in the white lesions (d) Same image in PDD mode. The lesions show intense fluorescence and contain tumour at biopsy.

PDT treatment of mesothelioma

Surgical debulking

Residual microscopic disease after surgical resection is considered to be one of the major problems in the surgical approach to MPM. After debulking of all gross tumour, PDT can be used to treat the residual microscopic disease. There are several surgical approaches for the treatment of pleural malignancies, and these are discussed in more detail in other chapters. In general, patients are treated under general anaesthesia in a lateral position. An endotracheal double-lumen tube is inserted and a latero-posterior thoracotomy is performed through the fifth or sixth intercostal space. An extrapleural dissection (between the chest wall, diaphragm and mediastinum) is performed until the hilar structures are reached. Resection is performed by pleurectomy–decortication alone or if necessary, by an extrapleural pneumonectomy (EPP). Care is taken not to open the diaphragm or pericardium. If this is not possible, the defect is closed by sutures or the implantation of a prosthetic mesh. It is naive to assume that no microscopic disease will remain even after complete gross resection of MPM. Although resection can be accomplished by either pleurectomy–decortication or EPP, the latter operation can have a detrimental impact on the patient's pulmonary reserve and quality of life, and can also be associated with significant mortality. As a result, many surgeons prefer to perform lung-sparing procedures whenever possible.

Photodynamic therapy

PDT utilizes a photosensitizer that is activated by light of a specific wavelength. The photosensitizer is believed to be retained in the tumour vasculature and to a lesser extent in the malignant cells after administration [12]. Direct illumination of the tumour by (laser) light results in the destruction of the endothelial cells, the vasculature, and tumour cells. The process involves the absorption of light by the sensitizer which is activated to a triplet state. In the presence of molecular oxygen the absorbed energy will be transferred, producing highly reactive singlet oxygen. Cell death occurs by vascular shutdown, apoptosis, or direct destruction of certain cellular elements [13,14]. There is also evidence that PDT can initiate a cascade of immunological effects that may enhance the host's antitumour response [15].

Photosensitizers

Only two commercially available photosensitizers have been used in patients with MPM. Photofrin® (di-haematoporphyrin derivate) was the first photosensitizer to be commercially available. It has a major excitation wavelength in the green region of visible light (530 nm) and a small peak in the red region (630 nm). Since the depth of penetration is significantly better at longer (red) wavelengths, excitation at the 630 nm peak is clinically important. Depending on the fluorophore content of the tissue, the light can penetrate to a depth of up to 1.0 cm. The absorption peak at 630 nm is relatively low and results in limited production of singlet oxygen. This indicates that the illumination time required will depend on the power of the laser and the surface treatment area [16,17]. Photofrin® is usually given in a dose of 2.0 mg/kg 2 days before the illumination to achieve good tissue concentration. Drug concentrations in tissue generally remain high for several days and the major toxicity is skin photosensitivity. Patients have to stay out of the sun or intense light for a period of 4–8 weeks after injection. The advantage of Photofrin® is that re-treatment is possible 2 or 3 days after the first illumination.

Foscan® (meta-tetrahydroxyphenylchloride) has an absorption peak in the green region of the spectrum (520 nm) and a major peak in the red region (652 nm) [12] The penetration depth of

is limited to a few hours, only drugs with a direct cytotoxic effect can be used. Drugs with these properties that have been tested are cisplatin, doxorubicin, cytosine arabinoside, and mitomycin.

Initially, this procedure was tested for diseases such as pseudomyxoma peritonei, ovarian carcinoma, and colonic carcinoma. Recently, studies have also tested hyperthermic intracavitary chemotherapy in the thoracic cavity. Lee *et al.* [33] described the use of intrapleural cisplatin and cytosine arabinoside after pleurectomy–decortication for pleural malignancies including MPM. They reported a median survival of 11.5 months. Since then, other studies have been performed in the thoracic cavity focusing on MPM and pleural metastases from thymomas [34–37].

Perfusion technique

After tumour resection, a perfusion system is set up. In general, one catheter (Tenckhof catheter) is used for inflow of the perfusion fluid and several outflow catheters are used to recycle the perfusion fluid. These are placed at strategic sites (apex of the pleural space, and anterior and posterior costophrenic sulci) to allow optimal circulation. Temperature sensors can be placed at the inflow and outflow catheters to maintain the temperature at 40–41°C. When all tubes are in place, a watertight locking suture is used to close the skin, leaving enough space for the probes and catheters. An overview of the system is presented in Figure 17.4. For the perfusion fluid, chemotherapeutic drugs are dissolved in isotonic dialysis fluid.

Drug concentrations

Several studies have addressed the issue of the optimal concentration of the cytotoxic drug. Because of differences in treatment methods (duration of perfusion, types of drugs, and perfusion concentrations) and the lack of an evaluable endpoint, these studies have only focused on toxicity and the systemic concentrations of the drugs [33,34,38–42]. Measurements of systemic drug levels in these studies indicated that cisplatin 90–200 mg/m^2 could be used with acceptable toxicity [42]. When combined with others drugs such as doxorubicin, cisplatin doses of 50–80 mg/m^2 have been tested and are considered safe as long as preoperative hydration is given. The recommended total dose for doxorubicin and its analogues is 40–60 mg/m^2 [43]. Studies of mit-

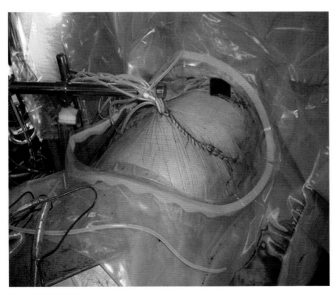

Figure 17.4 Hyperthermic intracavitary chemotherapy in a patient with a left-sided pleural mesothelioma. The chest wall is closed after tumour debulking and placement of the inflow and outflow catheters. A sterile covering is applied to prevent leakage of the heated chemotherapy solution. Three outflow catheters are placed at different sites in the cavity and one inflow catheter is placed in the middle. (Courtesy of Dr Zoetmulder and Dr Verwaal, Netherlands Cancer Institute.)

omycin suggest that doses of 13 mg/m² can be used without significant side effects, but that leukopenia occurs in 50 per cent of patients at a dose of 35 mg/m² [44,45]. Contraindications to hyperthermic intracavity chemotherapy include congestive heart failure, fibrous adhesions, and tissue necrosis of the pleura or diaphragm.

Results of hyperthermic intracavitary chemotherapy

In studies reported to date, intrathoracic chemotherapy has not been administered alone but has been combined with various amounts of postoperative radiation or systemic chemotherapy. These variations, along with the nature of the study design (phase I–II) and the differences in inclusion criteria, make it difficult to evaluate study results. The actual contribution of hyperthermic intrathoracic chemotherapy lavage cannot be estimated. In the studies to date, the patient median survival ranges from 9 to 18 months with acceptable mortality and a maximum 2 years survival rate of 40 per cent. Reported toxicities included nephrotoxicity and cytopenia. Ototoxicity was not a frequent problem. Longer survival was observed in cases of minimal residual disease after the pleurectomy–decortication compared with more incomplete resections. The site of recurrence in the study by Rice et al. [37] was local in 58 per cent of the cases and distant in 17 per cent. In a quarter of patients both local and distant recurrences were seen. In addition to surgery and hyperthermic intrathoracic chemotherapy, some studies have addressed a multimodality approach in which radiotherapy was given postoperatively. Ratto et al. [39] treated patients with 45 Gy of radiation to the chest wall incisions after perfusion. In a very small number of patients (10) there was no additional mortality or morbidity associated with this approach. A study combining resection and intraoperative hyperthermic intrathoracic chemotherapy in patients with early-stage MPM was performed at the Netherlands Cancer Institute [46]. Cisplatin and doxorubicin were perfused for 90 min under mild hyperthermic conditions (40–41°C). Doxorubicin was the drug of choice because it had enhanced cytotoxic activity under hyperthermic conditions despite limited depth of penetration. Postoperative irradiation was given to thoracotomy scars and drainage tracks to prevent tumour recurrence. In 11 patients this approach proved feasible with acceptable toxicity. Therefore this study was expanded for patients with stage I MPM [47]. Of the 20 patients subsequently treated, 16 had an epithelioid tumour histology and four a biphasic type. Surgical resection with optimal debulking was performed in 15 of the 20 patients, including pneumonectomy in eight patients. Tumour involving the diaphragm or pericardium was seen in 13 and 15 patients, respectively. The median duration of the entire procedure (resection plus perfusion) was 7 h (range 5–8.5 h), the median hospital stay was 17 days (range 11–77 days), and the median intensive care unit stay was 4 days (range 1–7 days). There was no perioperative mortality, but significant morbidity occurred in 13 of the 20 patients, including bronchopleural fistulas (four patients) and diaphragmatic ruptures, persistent parenchymal air leak, pulmonary emboli, and persistent chylothorax (two patients each). The bronchopleural fistulas were treated with reoperation using a pectoral muscle flap and, in two patients, a Clagget procedure. In one patient only palliative care was given. The diaphragmatic ruptures were reconstructed with prosthetic mesh. Persistent parenchymal air leaks led to subsequent pneumonectomy in both patients. Nineteen of 20 patients received additional radiation to the surgical scars which was well tolerated. The median survival was 11 months (range 3–19 months) and the 1 year survival was 42 per cent. Fourteen patients developed recurrent disease after a median period of 8 months (range 2–14 months). Recurrences in the abdomen were observed in four patients, in 3 of whom the diaphragm had been opened during surgery. Ten of a total of 16 patients who did not develop abdominal recurrences had small openings made in the diaphragm during the procedure. Opening of the pericardium did not result in a pericardial localization of the mesothelioma. It is clear from the studies reported that the median survival in the American series is superior to that in the Dutch study. An explanation for this difference could be that mesothelioma cells are relatively insensitive to the cisplatin and doxorubicin or that the approach described by van Ruth *et al.* [47] fails to reach all tumour cells. Perhaps the addition of systemic chemotherapy or hemithoracic irradiation should be considered as additional treatment. Currently, hyperthermic intrathoracic chemotherapy alone or in combination with surgical resection cannot be recommended as standard treatment in patients with MPM.

Conclusions

The initial results of photodynamic diagnosis with 5-ALA in pleural malignancies seems promising, but additional studies are required to determine the exact place and indication of this approach.

Although many physicians believe that the role of surgery in MPM is controversial, a subset of highly selected patients appear to benefit from combined modality therapy including resection via EPP.

The role of PDT in the treatment of MPM is controversial and this therapy is associated with significant risks. The number of centres exploring this technology is very limited because it requires both specialized equipment and a specialized multidisciplinary team. The number of patients treated in different trials is too small and no definitive conclusions can be drawn thus far. Other factors complicating the interpretation of published results are the number of variables (type of sensitizer, light dose, drug dose, drug–light interval, methods of light measurement, technique of light delivery, surgical debulking techniques) and patient selection in these single-centre studies. The only phase III study, performed with an earlier-generation photosensitizer, reported no advantage for the use of PDT in combination with surgery and immunochemotherapy.

Results of hyperthermic intrathoracic chemotherapy have also shown that this procedure is not easily combined with surgery. The best results of surgery are expected when this is combined with systemic therapy and radiation therapy in a group of highly selected patients.

We can conclude that intraoperative PDT and hyperthermic intracavitary lavage are still experimental and should only be performed in specialized centres within the context of prospective clinical trials.

References

1. van Ruth S, Baas P, Zoetmulder FA. Surgical treatment of malignant pleural mesothelioma: a review. *Chest* 2003; **123**: 551–61.
2. Canto A, Rivas J, Saumench J, Morera R, Moya J. Points to consider when choosing a biopsy method in cases of pleurisy of unknown origin. *Chest* 1983; **84**: 176–9.
3. Palcic B, Lam S, Hung J, MacAulay C. Detection and localization of early lung cancer by imaging techniques. *Chest* 1991; **99**: 742–3.
4. Alian W. Andersson-Engels S, Svanberg K, Svanberg S. Laser-induced fluorescence of meso-tetra(hydroxy)phenylchlorin in malignant and normal tissues in rats. *Br J Cancer* 1994; **70**: 880–5.
5. Hung J, Lam S, LeRiche JC, Palcic B. Autofluorescence of normal and malignant bronchial tissue. *Lasers Surg Med* 1991; **11**: 99–105.
6. Kennedy JC, Marcus SL. Photodynamic therapy (PDT) and photodiagnosis (PD) using endogenous photosensitization induced by 5-aminolevulinic acid (ALA): mechanisms and clinical results. *J Clin Laser Med Surg* 1996; **14**: 289–304.
7. Leunig A, Rick K, Steep H, *et al.* Fluorescence imaging and spectroscopy of 5-aminolevulinic acid induced protoporphyrin IX for the detection of neoplastic lesions in the oral cavity. *Am J Surg* 1996; **172**: 674–7.

8. Haringsma J. Tytgat G. Fluorescence and autofluorescence. *Baillieres Best Pract Res Clin Gastroenterol* 1999; **13**: 1–5.

9. Baas P, Triesscheijn M, Burgers S, van Pel R, Stewart F, Aalders M. Fluorescence detection of pleural malignancies using 5-aminolaevulinic acid. *Chest* 2006; **129**: 718–24.

10. Mayinger B, Neidhardt S, Reh H, Martus P, Hahn EG. Fluorescence induced with 5-aminolevulinic acid for the endoscopic detection and follow-up of esophageal lesions. *Gastrointest Endosc* 2001; **54**: 572–8.

11. Lam S, MacAulay C, le Rich JC, Palcic B. Detection and localization of early lung cancer by fluorescence bronchoscopy. *Cancer* 2000; **89**(Suppl): 2468–73.

12. Berenbaum MC, Akande SL, Bonnett R, *et al.* Mesotetra(hydroxyphenyl)porphyrins, a new class of potent tumour photosensitizer with favourable selectivity. *Br J Cancer* 1986; **54**: 717–25.

13. Oleinick NL, Evans HH. The photobiology of photodynamic therapy: cellular targets and mechanisms. *Radiat Res* 1998; **150**: 146S–56S.

14. Fingar VH. Vascular effects of photodynamic therapy. *J Clin Laser Med Surg* 1996; **14**: 323–8.

15. Korbelik M. Induction of tumor immunity by photodynamic therapy. *J Clin Laser Med Surg* 1996; **14**: 329–34.

16. Pass HI, Delaney T, Tochner Z, *et al.* Intrapleural photodynamic therapy: results of a phase I trial. *Ann Surg Oncol* 1994; **1**: 28–37.

17. Takita H, Mang TS, Loewen GM, *et al.* Operation and intracavitary photodynamic therapy for malignant mesothelioma: a phase II study. *Ann Thorac Surg* **58**: 995–8.

18. Baas P, Murrer, Zoetmulder FA, *et al.* Photodynamic therapy as adjuvant in surgically treated pleural malignancies. *Br J Cancer* 1997; **76**: 819–26.

19. Copper MP, Tan IB, Oppelaar H, Ruevekamp MC, Stewart FA. Meta-tetra(hydroxyphenyl)chlorin photodynamic therapy in early-stage squamous cell carcinoma of the head and neck. *Arch Otolaryngol Head Neck Surg* 2003; **129**: 709–11.

20. Ris HB, Altermatt HJ, Nachbur B, *et al.* Intraoperative photodynamic therapy with mTHPC for chest malignancies. *Lasers Surg Med* 1996; **18**: 39–45.

21. Pass HI, Temecj BK, Kranda K, *et al.* Phase III randomized trial of surgery with or without intraoperative photodynamic therapy, and postoperative immunochemotherapy for malignant pleural mesothelioma. *Ann Surg Oncol* 1997; **4**: 628–33.

22. Schouwink H, Rutgers ET, van der Sijp J, *et al.* Intraoperative photodynamic therapy after pleuropneumonectomy in patients with malignant pleural mesothelioma. Dose finding and toxicity results. *Chest* 2001; **120**: 1167–74.

23. Moskal TL, Dougherty TJ, Urschel JD, *et al.* Operation and photodynamic therapy for pleural mesothelioma: 6-yearfollow-up. *Ann Thorac Surg* 1998; **66**: 1128–33.

24. Vulcan TG, Zhu TC, Rodriguez CE, *et al.* Comparison between isotropic and non-isotropic dosimetry systems during intraperitoneal photodynamic therapy. *Lasers Surg Med* 2000; **26**: 292–301.

25. Ris HB, Altermatt HJ, Inderbitzi, *et al.* Photodynamic therapy with chlorins for diffuse malignant mesothelioma: initial clinical results. *Br J Cancer* 1991; **64**: 1116–20.

26. Friedberg JS, Mick R, Stevenson J, *et al.* A phase I study of Foscan-mediated photodynamic therapy and surgery in patients with mesothelioma. *Ann Thorac Surg.* 2003; **75**: 952–9.

27. Schouwink JH, Kool LS, Rutgers EJ, *et al.* The value of chest computer tomography and cervical mediastinoscopy in the preoperative assessment of patients with malignant pleural mesothelioma. *Ann Thorac Surg.* 2003; **75**: 1715–19.

28. Markman M. Intraperitoneal chemotherapy. *Semin Oncol* 1991; **18**: 248–54.

29. Storm FK. Clinical hyperthermia and chemotherapy. *Radiol Clin North Am* 1989; **27**: 621–7.

30. Barlogie B, Corry PM, Drewinko B. *In vitro* thermochemotherapy of human colon cancer cells with *cis*-dichlorodiammineplatinum (II) and mitomycin C. *Cancer Res* 1980; **40**: 1165–8.

31. Teicher BA, Kowal CD, Kennedy KA, Santorelli AC. Enhancement by hyperthermia of the in vitro cyotoxicity of mitomycin C toward hypoxic tumor cells. *Cancer Res* 1981; **41**: 1096–9.

normal mesothelial cells and express the Flt-1 and KDR receptors for VEGF. Treatment of cells in culture with recombinant human VEGF results in Flt-1 and KDR receptor activation (phosphorylation) and increased cell growth. These effects can be inhibited by antibodies against VEGF, Flt-1, or KDR [14]. The closely related molecule VEGF-C and its cognate receptor VEGFR-3 are also co-expressed in mesothelioma cell lines, and cellular proliferation can be inhibited using antisense oligonucleotide complementary to VEGF [15].

Levels of circulating serum VEGF in patients with mesothelioma are higher than in patients with other pulmonary malignancies such as small-cell and non-small-cell lung cancer. Higher VEGF levels have been detected in the pleural effusions of mesothelioma patients than in the effusions of patients with non-malignant pleural disease [16]. The expression of VEGF also correlates with microvessel density in mesothelioma biopsies [17,18], and serum VEGF levels correlate inversely with survival in patients with mesothelioma ($r = 0.72$; $P < 0.01$) [14]. Thus there is a rationale for testing VEGF inhibitors in mesothelioma, and the *in vitro* data suggest that such drugs may act by a dual mechanism with suppression of mesothelioma cell growth in addition to angiogenesis.

Relatively less data is available for other angiogenic factors that may play a role in mesothelioma. The c-Met tyrosine kinase receptor and its ligand, hepatocyte growth (or scatter) factor (HGF) have been implicated in angiogenesis, tumour invasion and metastasis. C-Met expression was increased in 82 per cent of mesothelioma biopsies compared to normal tissue. c-Met-specific small interference RNA (siRNA) blocks receptor expression. Both c-Met siRNA and the small molecule SU11274 inhibit mesothelioma cell proliferation, migration and HGF-induced Akt and erk 1/2 activation. The most significant reduction of cell growth by SU11274 was seen in 2 cell lines, H513 and H2596, with juxtamembrane domain T1010I mutations [19]. Serum concentrations of HGF are also significantly higher in patients with mesothelioma than in healthy matched controls [20]. Therefore angiogenesis is believed to be a critical process in the pathogenesis of mesothelioma and a key target for therapeutic control. A number of anti-angiogenic drugs that act via diverse mechanisms are currently in clinical development, and those that are being evaluated for the treatment of mesothelioma are discussed below.

Inhibitors of angiogenesis

SU5416

SU5416 (Semaxanib, Sugen Inc.)is a parenterally administered quinolone derivative which inhibits both VEGFR-2 (Flk-1) tyrosine kinase and c-*kit* mediated signalling [21]. In phase I trials, the most commonly encountered side effects of SU5416 were nausea, vomiting, headache, diarrhoea, pain, and fever. The dose-limiting toxicities were headache and projectile vomiting [22]. The National Cancer Institute (NCI) sponsored a phase II trial of SU5416 in 23 patients with mesothelioma who had not received more than one previous chemotherapy regimen. Patients received 145 mg/m^2 twice weekly for 8 weeks following premedication with dexamethasone, H$_1$ and H$_2$ blockers, and coumadin. Antitumour activity was observed with a partial response rate of 11 per cent and a minor response rate of 11 per cent, and stable disease was achieved in 33 per cent of patients [23]. The mechanism of tumour regression for SU5416 is more likely via VEGF inhibition than inhibition of the c-*kit* receptor because c-*kit* is infrequently expressed in mesothelioma (see later). However, the adverse toxicity profile of this drug may preclude its further development for the treatment of mesothelioma. In this study, grade 3 and 4 hyperglycaemia occurred in 19 per cent of patients, thrombosis in 14 per cent and lymphopenia in 19 per cent. Furthermore, numerous adverse events including pulmonary emboli, myocardial infarctions, cerebrovascular events, grade 4 hypoxia, and pulmonary infiltrates have occurred in trials of SU5416 in combination with gemcitabine and cisplatin, or with paclitaxel [24,25].

Bevacizumab

Bevacizumab (RhuMAb VEGF, Avastin, Genentech) is a recombinant humanized monoclonal antibody against VEGF that has been shown to inhibit the growth of a variety of human cancers *in vitro*. It may also act synergistically with chemotherapy. In a phase I trial, bevacizumab reduced serum VEGF concentrations to undetectable levels when administered at doses of 3 mg/kg/week or more, and no adverse pharmacological interactions have been identified to date for bevacizumab in combination with a variety of chemotherapeutic agents [26,27]. Promising activity of bevacuzimab in combination with chemotherapy has been demonstrated in randomised phase III studies in both non-small cell lung cancer and colorectal cancel [28,29]. The latter study was a landmark trial in that it provided the first proof of principle that inhibition of angiogenesis through the antagonism of VEGF signalling can improve on established therapy with cytotoxic chemotherapy.

In the majority of patients bevacizumab appears to be well tolerated. However, in patients with NSCLC, life-threatening haemoptysis was observed in four patients who had central tumours and squamous cell histology therefore, caution is warranted in patients with a history of haemoptysis [30]. There may also be an increased risk of hypertension [29].

The efficacy of bevacizumab as a single agent in mesothelioma has not been reported on. Preclinical studies in animal models suggest that it is highly synergistic with cisplatin [31]. This, together with the observation of responses to the anti-angiogenic SU5416 as described above, has prompted the University of Chicago to conduct a 106-patient multicentre double-blind placebo-controlled randomized phase II trial of bevacizumab or placebo given together with gemcitabine and cisplatin. In this trial, patients are stratified for performance status and histology. The primary endpoint is time to progression and secondary endpoints are objective response rate, survival, and toxicity; plasma VEGF and serum vascular cell adhesion molecule 1 (VCAM-1) levels will be correlated with response [32].

Thalidomide

Thalidomide is known to possess both immunomodulatory and anti-angiogenic properties. Its mechanism of action is not clear but it may inhibit angiogenesis induced by bFGF and VEGF, inhibit TNF-α and cyclo-oxygenase 2 (COX-2) (see later section), change intercellular adhesion molecule (ICAM) expression, and modify the extracellular matrix [33]. At doses of 100–500 mg/day, the main toxicities of thalidomide are fatigue, nausea, and vomiting constipation and peripheral neuropathy. A phase II study performed in Australia evaluated thalidomide in 16 patients with mesothelioma who had previously received chemotherapy or who were medically unfit for chemotherapy. A partial response rate of 6 per cent was observed with stable disease in 50 per cent of patients. Stable disease for more than 6 months was demonstrated in 25 per cent of patients [32]. Two further phase II trials are ongoing. In the Dutch multicentre trial the primary endpoint is time to progression using the EORTC database and prognostic groups as a reference. In the University of Maryland trial the primary endpoint is response and functional imaging using 2-fluoro-2-deoxyglucose positron-emission tomography (FDG-PET) scans, and simian virus 40 (SV40) T antigen expression will also be examined and correlated with response [32].

Thalidomide at a dose of 100–500 mg four times daily has also been evaluated in combination with gemcitabine (800 mg/m^2 on days 1, 8, and 15) and cisplatin (25 mg/m^2, days 1, 8, and 15) in 22 chemonaive patients with mesothelioma. A partial response rate of 14 per cent was observed, with stable disease in 55 per cent of patients and stable disease for more than 6 months in 32 per cent [34]. Response rates ranging from 16 to 48 per cent have been reported from phase II studies that have examined gemcitabine and cisplatin, so there is not a clear potential benefit from the addition of thalidomide [35]. If data from single-agent trials of thalidomide demonstrate activity, a sequential trial with thalidomide treatment following combination chemotherapy may be warranted.

PTK787

PTK787 (1-[4-chloroanilino]-4-[4-pyridylmethyl]phthalazine succinate) (ZK222584)is an orally bioavailable drug under codevelopment by Novartis Pharmaceuticals (East Hanover, NJ) and Schering AG (Berlin, Germany). It is a potent inhibitor of the VEGF receptor tyrosine kinases VEGFR-1 (Flt-1) and VEGFR-2 (KDR), PDGF-α tyrosine kinase (see later section on PDGF in mesothelioma), c-Kit, and c-Fms. PTK787 has demonstrated promising activity against endothelial cell growth, migration, and survival *in vitro* and in animal models [36]. Phase I studies are ongoing. A phase II trial of this agent in 40 previously untreated patients with mesothelioma is currently under way (Cancer and Leukaemia Group B (CALGB) trial 30107). The primary endpoint is time to progression, using the CALGB prognostic database as a reference. Laboratory endpoints will also be evaluated to determine whether pretreatment serum levels of PDGF/VEGF and VEGF mRNA isoforms isolated from circulating cells correlate with response.

Tetrathiomolybdate

Tetrathiomolybdate (TM) is an oral copper-depleting agent that inhibits angiogenesis and decreases levels of VEGF when ceruloplasmin is reduced to 5–15 mg/dl. Pass *et al.* [37] recently reported on a phase II trial of TM in 34 patients with mesothelioma who had undergone cytoreductive surgery. The TM dose was commenced at 180 mg/day and adjusted to maintain ceruloplasmin at 5–15 mg/dl until progression. The most common toxicity was anaemia. There was a corresponding decrease in VEGF levels when optimal suppression of ceruloplasmin to the target range was achieved. In this series of patients who had undergone surgical resection, the 2 year survival was 60 per cent for stage I–II patients (progression-free survival was 69 per cent for stage I–II patients) and 23 per cent for stage III patients. These data suggest that TM might have efficacy in mesothelioma and further studies are required for confirmation.

Epidermal growth factor receptors

Epidermal growth factor receptors (EGFRs) are widely expressed in epithelial cells and frequently expressed or overexpressed in cancer [4]. The EGFR family comprises four distinct but structurally similar tyrosine kinase receptors encoded by the proto-oncogenes c-*erbB1*/EGFR/EGFR1 (EGFR), c-*erbB2*/HER2 (HER2), c-*erbB3*/HER3 and c-*erbB4*/HER4. The principal ligands for EGFR are epidermal growth factor (EGF) and TGF-α. Upon binding of ligand, EGFR dimerizes with itself (homodimer) or with a different EGFR family member (heterodimer) and becomes activated by phosphorylation. This results in downstream signal transduction through the Ras–Raf–MAPK, PI3K-PKB/Akt, and STAT-3 pathways that regulate cellular proliferation and survival (Fig. 18.1) [38].

In experimental studies, asbestos exposure is associated with EGFR phosphorylation and MAPK signal transduction [39]. Immunohistochemical analyses of human mesothelioma biopsies have demonstrated high EGFR expression in up to 70 per cent of cases [40]. Simon *et al.* [41] noted moderate to high staining for phosphorylated (and therefore activated) EGFR in epithelial regions of mesothelioma but low staining in sarcomatous areas and sarcomatoid mesotheliomas. In a small study, Govindan *et al.* [42] also demonstrated that EGFR staining was more prevalent in epitheloid mesotheliomas (11/13) compared with mesotheliomas with biphasic histology (2/4) or sarcomatoid histology (1/7).

Betta *et al.* [43] reported that serum levels of EGF measured by an ELISA method in 20 newly diagnosed mesothelioma patients were twice those of 17 matched healthy controls, and there was a non-significant trend to inferior survival in patients with higher pretreatment levels of EGF (median survival 5.3 months vs 14 months). EGFR expression is an adverse prognostic factor for several types of cancer, but this has not yet been demonstrated in mesothelioma. Dazzi *et al.* [44] found that 68 per cent of mesotheliomas expressed EGFR, but there was no correlation with clinical outcome. Notably, EGFR expression was an independent prognostic factor for a *better* prognosis in a study of 44 patients with mesothelioma [45]. However, EGFR signal transduction is a dynamic process that may not be reflected in the 'snapshot' of expression provided by an immunohistochemical study. Also, prognostic significance may not be relevant for response to a targeted inhibitor. As a case in point EGFR is expressed in at least 80 per cent of NSCLC, yet it does not appear that expression can reliably predict for response to EGFR inhibitors in the clinical trials reported to date [4]. This, and the observation that treatment of mesothelioma cell lines from chemonaive patients with the small-molecule EGFR inhibitor gefitinib (Iressa) can suppress EGFR signalling and slow the rate of cellular proliferation [46], has prompted evaluation of EGFR inhibitors in patients with mesothelioma.

Gefitinib and erlotinib

Gefitinib (Iressa, ZD1839) and erlotinib (Tarceva, OSI774) are small-molecule inhibitors of EGFR that are now at an advanced stage in clinical development. They are orally bioavailable anilinoquinazoline-based compounds which compete with, and prevent binding of, adenosine triphosphate to the tyrosine kinase domain of EGFR. In preclinical studies these drugs were demonstrated to decrease EGFR phosphorylation and inhibit growth of tumour xenografts. Their main toxicities are diarrhoea, a maculopapular acneiform rash that is assumed to arise from blockade of EGFR-1 in keratinocytes, and, more rarely, an interstitial pneumonitis. Trials of these agents in NSCLC have been very promising, with response rates of 9–19 per cent and symptomatic benefit in approximately 40 per cent of patients in phase II studies that recruited patients who had previously received at least one chemotherapy regimen [4]. Trials of both of these drugs have been conducted in mesothelioma.

Gefitinib

The Cancer and Leukemia Group B (CALGB 30101) recently reported on a phase II study of gefitinib in 43 patients with mesothelioma [42]. Gefitinib was given orally at a dose of 500 mg/day to patients with a good performance status (PS 0–1) and previously untreated mesothelioma. The primary endpoint was 3 months failure-free survival, defined as time to disease progression or death. Secondary objectives were response rate, toxicity, overall survival, and correlation between EGFR-1 expression and clinical outcome. A total of 43 eligible patients were enrolled, of whom 79 per cent had epithelioid histology, 7 per cent sarcomatoid, 12 per cent mixed, and 2 per cent unknown. The median number of cycles administered was only 2 (range 1–8). The partial response rate was 2 per cent, stable disease occurred in 46 per cent, and progressive disease was recorded in 37 per cent.

Patients were not preselected for EGFR expression but correlative studies were performed in retrospect. The data on EGFR expression score was interesting in that high EGFR expression was associated with *longer* survival among a subset of 28 patients examined. The median survival for those with low EGFR expression was 4.5 months compared with 8.4 months for those with high EGFR expression. The finding may be explained by an association of negative or low EGFR expression with sarcomatoid histology which carries a worse prognosis.

There was no correlation between EGFR expression and failure-free survival. The median failure-free survival was 1.7 months (95 per cent confidence interval (CI) 1.5–4.0) and 66 per cent of patients had a failure-free survival of less than 3 months [43]. These data are discouraging for further trials of gefitinib in chemonaive patients with mesothelioma. It has recently been suggested that the response to gefitinib in NSCLC is dependent on the presence of activating mutations in the EGFR [46]. It is not yet known whether these mutations exist in a subset of patients with mesothelioma.

Data is also awaited from the British–Canadian study of gefitinib in which the primary endpoint is response. The secondary endpoints will include quality of life using the lung cancer symptom scale and may help to determine whether disease-related symptoms can improve in the absence of an objective response in patients who achieve stable disease.

Erlotinib

The Southwest Oncology group (SWOG SO218) [47] have examined the activity of erlotinib in mesothelioma. They evaluated erlotinib at a dose of 150 mg/day in chemonaive mesothelioma patients with PS 0–1, and correlated tumour molecular expression of the EGFR signalling pathways with clinical outcomes. Sixty-four patients were enrolled, of whom 30 had measurable disease evaluable for response. No objective responses were seen; 47 per cent had stable disease and 43 per cent had progressive disease. Using data for 63/64 patients, 6 month survival was estimated at 60 per cent (95 per cent CI 48–73 per cent); progression-free survival was estimated at 28 per cent (95 per cent CI 16 –38 per cent) at 6 months. For 60 patients, rash (82 per cent), fatigue (50 per cent), diarrhoea (53 per cent), and pruritus (30 per cent) were the most frequent toxicities, and one patient died of grade 5 respiratory failure.

This trial also included analysis of immunohistochemical correlates that may predict for response or resistance to EGFR inhibition. The majority of tumours (92 per cent of 23) were negative for phospho-Akt and PTEN (75 per cent of 55) in this study suggesting that this pathway is not active in mesothelioma. This may be a mechanism of clinical resistance to erlotinib although in other types of cancer it is *activation* of phospho-Akt with loss of PTEN that has been associated with resistance to an EGFR inhibitor [4]. These data imply a complex mechanism of resistance to erlotinib that may be cancer-type specific. A further observation was that ERK was variably activated among the tumours, particularly in the sarcomatous elements. Therefore specific inhibitors of ERK may be of value for the treatment of the more aggressive sarcomatous subtype of mesothelioma.

Platelet-derived growth factor and c-kit receptors

PDGF is a potent mitogen for mesenchymal cells which is also implicated in angiogenesis and is an autocrine growth factor for mesothelioma [48]. PDGF is composed of two polypeptide subunits, the A and B chains. Mesothelioma cell lines express PDGF-B receptors whereas normal mesothelial cells express PDGF-A receptors [49]. A common genetic abnormality in mesothelioma involves the c-*sis* proto-oncogene on 22q13 which encodes the B chain of PDGF that is co-expressed with the PDGF receptor (PDGF-R). This results in an autocrine-growth-stimulating loop. Transduction of a hammerhead ribozyme against PDGF-B mRNA into mesothelioma cells reduces PDGF-B expression and decreases cell growth [50]. To date, there have been no reports on the expression of PDGF-B and its prognostic significance in mesothelioma.

The Kit transmembrane tyrosine kinase receptor is structurally similar to the PDGF receptor and is encoded by the c-*kit* proto-oncogene. Activation of Kit tyrosine kinase by somatic mutation has been documented in mastocytosis, seminoma, acute myelogenous leukaemia, and at least 90 per cent of GISTs. Over-expression of wild-type Kit has also been demonstrated in several malignancies including small-cell lung cancer. In the absence of somatic mutation, Kit signal transduction is believed to occur via autocrine activation of the receptor due to binding of the Kit ligand stem cell factor [2]. Simon et al. [41] demonstrated expression of c-kit in sarcomatous areas of 18 mesotheliomas by immunohistochemistry with the CD117 antibody. However, in a study of 37 patients, there was no significant c-kit expression, suggesting that this oncogene is not commonly expressed in mesothelioma [51].

Imatinib

Imatinib (imatinib mesylate, Glivec, Gleevec, STI157) is an orally bioavailable tyrosine kinase inhibitor that was originally developed to inhibit the bcr-abl kinase characteristic of chronic myeloid leukaemia. Subsequently, activity against PDGF-R and the c-kit tyrosine kinase receptors was detected [52]. A role for imatinib in the treatment of GISTs is now well established. Imatinib is generally well tolerated, with gastrointestinal side effects occurring most commonly [2].

Two phase II trials of imatinib in patients with advanced pleural mesothelioma have been reported. Millward et al. [53] treated 29 patients with unresectable mesothelioma (PS 0–2) and measurable disease with a starting dose of 800 mg/day. Seven patients had received one prior chemotherapy regimen. In 25 patients evaluable for response, the best response was stable disease ($n = 11$) in which one patient had a 25 per cent reduction in pleural thickness. To determine biological activity in the absence of an objective response by tumour measurements, the authors performed functional imaging with FDG-PET scans at baseline and after 4 weeks of treatment in 13 of the patients. Mesothelioma was glucose avid in all patients and no significant reductions in FDG uptake were observed. In patients with stable disease, FDG uptake was unchanged at 4 weeks in six out of seven patients. Uptake was increased over baseline in three of five patients with progressive mesothelioma. The patient with 25 per cent reduction did not have PET scanning. Serial lung function tests were either unchanged or progressively deteriorated.

In a phase II trial performed by Villano et al. [54], 17 patients with mesothelioma (PS 0–1) were treated with 600 mg/day. Baseline expression of PDGF, PDGF-R, and KIT-R was performed and plasma levels of PDGF isoforms were assayed. The majority of patients had epitheliod histology (80 per cent) and the remainder were biphasic. There were no objective responses. Progression-free survival was 7.4 weeks. Baseline plasma levels of PDGF isoforms did not correlate with time to progression ($P = 0.4$) or thrombocytosis.

Two further studies confirmed that single agent imatinib mesylate has limited activity in mesothelioma [55,56]. Preliminary in vitro and clinical trial data, however, suggest that imatinib combined with gemcitabine mat be an active regimen in PDGF-β receptor positive tumours. Of 10 patients with treated, 2 had a partial response and the remaining 8, all with stable disease, had reduced FGD uptake on PET imaging (Luciano Mutti, personal communication).

A notable feature of the phase II trials reported for imatinib in mesothelioma is that, in contrast with experience with this drug in chronic myeloid leukaemia and patients with GISTs, imatinib appeared to be less well tolerated in the patients with mesothelioma. A significant number of patients required a dose reduction, and toxicities such as fatigue, nausea and vomiting, and anorexia were common. These findings suggest a lack of symptom control even in patients with stable disease and so there is not a strong rationale to perform any further evaluation of imatinib in mesothelioma. That said, it is intriguing that c-kit receptor expression has been noted to be more prevalent in the rarer sarcomatoid variant in one study [41]. Given that there is a particularly poor prognosis for patients with the sarcomatoid variant of mesothelioma, there may be a case for examining the efficacy of imatinib exclusively in this subset. Overall, these trials do not suggest that PDGF receptor inhibition is an effective strategy for mesothelioma either. Notably, the anti-angiogenic PTK87 also has activity against PDGF-R *in vitro* (see section on angiogenesis) and results from trials of this agent are still awaited.

Cyclo-oxygenase 2

Cyclo-oxygenases 1 and 2 (COX-1 and COX-2) catalyse the initial rate-limiting steps of prostaglandin synthesis from arachidonic acid. The COX-2 isoform leads preferentially to the formation of prostaglandins such as PGE_2 and has been implicated in carcinogenesis since it is associated with downregulation of cell-mediated immunity, promotion of angiogenesis, and the formation of carcinogenic metabolites such as malondialdehyde. Human mesothelioma samples have been noted to over-express COX-2, and growth of mesothelioma cell lines *in vitro* is suppressed by inhibition of COX-2 [57]. COX-2 appears to be expressed early in models of experimental cancer, and so its inhibition may also be an effective chemopreventive strategy [58]. Two reports have also identified COX-2 as an independent adverse prognostic factor [59,60].

A number of preclinical studies have explored the mechanism of COX-2 in the pathogenesis of mesothelioma. In animal models, exposure to asbestos is associated with activation of macrophages and other cell types that generate reactive oxygen and nitrogen species, cytokines, and growth factors [61]. A chronic inflammatory process with upregulation of COX isoforms ensues [62]. There is release of PGE_2 from alveolar macrophages and inhibition of cell-mediated cytotoxicity that can be restored by COX inhibitors such as indomethacin. DeLong *et al.* [63] reported that COX-2 inhibition by oral administration of rofecoxib significantly slowed but did not stop the growth of small tumours in mesothelioma-bearing mice; however, large tumours were not affected. This effect was dependent on the presence of CD8+ T cells and was associated with increased tumour-infiltrating lymphocytes. These data have prompted interest in combining COX-2 inhibition with immunotherapy and immunogene therapy approaches.

Catalano *et al.* [58] characterized the effects of non-steroidal anti-inflammatory drugs (NSAIDs) on experimental models of mesothelioma. The selective COX-2 inhibitor celecoxib reduced the proliferation of mesothelioma cells grown *in vitro* that had been derived from mesothelioma biopsies of previously untreated patients but did not alter the growth of normal mesothelial cells. Celecoxib inhibited mesothelioma cell colony formation in soft agar and had antitumour activity that led to long-term survival in more than 37 per cent of nude mice bearing intraperitoneal mesothelioma that were treated. Celecoxib was a more efficient inhibitor of mesothelioma cell growth than acetylsalicylic acid, indomethacin, and the COX-2 inhibitor NS-398. Its activity did not correlate with the amount of COX-2 protein present in the mesothelioma cells but did involve induction of apoptosis in a time- and dose-dependent manner through decreased Akt phosphorylation, loss of Bcl-2 and Survivin protein expression, and caspase-3 activation. VEGF is an Akt inducer that can rescue celecoxib-induced apoptosis and Akt dephosphorylation. The VEGF receptor (KDR/Flk-1) inhibitor SU-1498 in combination with celecoxib reduced the IC_{50} of celecoxib *in vitro* by 65 per cent. Thus there may be synergy between COX-2 and VEGF inhibitors. The COX-2 inhibitors celecoxib and rofecoxib are being evaluated for efficacy as single agents, and in combination with chemotherapy in NSCLC, but no trials have been reported for mesothelioma to date. The British Thoracic Oncology Group plans to study rofecoxib for chemoprevention of mesothelioma.

Induction of apoptosis

The limited effectiveness of cytotoxic drugs and radiotherapy in mesothelioma implicates an important functional defect in apoptosis signalling. Crocidolite asbestos is known to induce apoptosis via generation of free radicals that damage DNA. Mesothelioma cells have been postulated to arise from selection of cells that can survive the chronic cytotoxicity associated with exposure to asbestos fibres [64]. Improved insights into the molecular blocks in the apoptosis pathway that are present in solid tumours are providing new hypotheses for restoration/amplification of apoptosis and therapeutic control [65].

Two general pathways for apoptotic cell death have been characterized, the extrinsic and intrinsic pathways (Fig. 18.2). The extrinsic pathway is activated by ligation of plasma membrane death receptors (e.g. Fas, TRAIL) to drive the formation of a death-inducing signalling complex (DISC) that in turn activates a proteolytic caspase cascade. The intrinsic pathway is activated by drug-induced damage, among a wide range of other stimuli. Damage signals are relayed to the mitochondria where commitment to apoptosis follows increased permeability of the outer and inner mitochondrial membranes mediated by interactions between pro-apoptotic proteins (including bad, bid, bim, bak, and bax) and anti-apoptotic proteins of the bcl-2 family (including bcl-2, bcl-xl, bcl-w, and mcl-1), and the release of apoptogenic factors including cytochrome c and Smac. Cytosolic cytochrome c activates the apoptosome complex and a caspase cascade while Smac, once released into the cytosol, binds to inhibitors of apoptosis proteins (IAPs) to inactivate their restraint of caspase activity [66]. There are links between the two pathways such as the bid/t-bid proteins. In mesothelioma, mechanisms of evading apoptosis that have been identified to date include impaired permeabilization of the mitochondrial membrane due to altered bcl-2 family function and inhibition of caspase activity by upregulation of IAP family members [65]. Thus we shall focus on agents targeting these two areas, but many other com-

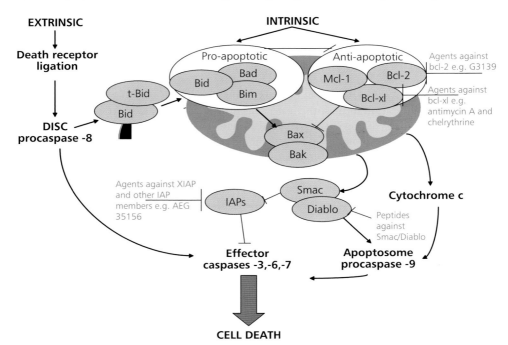

Figure 18.2 General pathways for apoptotic cell death.

pounds directed at other parts of the apoptotic pathway are being assessed at the present time. For example, TNF-related apoptosis-inducing ligand (TRAIL) has attracted interest as a target for anticancer therapy as it selectively induces apoptosis in many transformed cells but not in normal cells [67]. In mesothelioma cell lines, TRAIL plus doxorubicin resulted in more apoptosis than TRAIL or chemotherapy alone [68].

Altered bcl-2 family function

The anti-apoptotic bcl-2 family proteins bcl-xl and mcl-1 are upregulated in mesothelioma [69]. Interestingly, bcl-2, the prototype for this family that is frequently implicated in common types of cancer, does not appear to be as prevalent as bcl-xl in either mesothelioma cell lines or primary tumours.

Resistance to apoptotic stimuli *in vitro* does not appear to correlate with expression of bcl-2 [70], whereas downregulation of bcl-xl by the histone deacetylase inhibitor sodium butyrate induces apoptosis in mesothelioma cells [71]. Antisense inhibition of bcl-xl leads to apoptosis and augments response to cisplatin chemotherapy in human mesothelioma cells [72]. These data suggest that bcl-xl, rather than bcl-2, may be a critical component of apoptosis for therapeutic intervention in mesothelioma. Several small-molecule antagonists of bcl-xl interactions are now in early preclinical development [73] but have yet to be tested in patients with mesothelioma. These include BHI compounds [74], antimycin A [75], terephthalamide derivatives [76], and chelerythrine [77]. There are also bispecific antisense oligonucleotides which downregulate both bcl-2 and bcl-xl, and are more effective at inducing apoptosis in mesothelioma cells than bcl-xl alone [78].

The inhibitor of apoptosis family

Eight IAP family proteins have been found in the human genome, including X-linked inhibitor of apoptosis protein (XIAP) and survivin [79]. IAPs block execution of the final common pathway of apoptosis through inhibition of caspases. XIAP is the most potent IAP, but there is no published study yet on the expression and association of XIAP with clinical factors such as response to chemotherapy and overall survival in mesothelioma. There are limited data on other IAP proteins in mesothelioma. In one study the concentration of cIAP2 mRNA was 90 times higher in mesothelioma samples (39 primary mesothelioma and nine mesothelioma cell lines) compared with healthy pleura and expression was more abundant in the epithelioid subtype, but there was no correlation with survival [80]. Survivin is also frequently expressed (>80 per cent) in mesothelioma [81].

AEG 35156

A Cancer Research UK sponsored phase 1 trial to evaluate AEG 35156, an antisense oligonucleotide targeting XIAP, has recently been initiated in the UK. Toxicity is envisaged to be low since absence of XIAP does not significantly affect the development of normal tissues. As well as delineating the pharmacokinetics of AEG 35156, this trial incorporates the development and validation of pharmacodynamic endpoint assays to determine the biological efficacy of the antisense treatment in the target tissue. Patient tumour biopsies will be examined using western blotting and immunohistochemistry for the detection of XIAP protein knockdown and for apoptotic cells. Serum caspase cleaved cytokeratin 18 levels are also being assayed as a circulatory biomarker of tumour cell apoptosis using the M30 assay [82]. Further preclinical studies have been performed with small-molecule antagonists of XIAP that both induce apoptosis of tumour cells and sensitize these cells to anticancer drugs *in vitro*, and have antitumour effects *in vivo* [83]. These agents should enter clinical trials in the near future.

A number of inhibitors to other members of the IAP family are currently in development. Stable downregulation of cIAP2 increased spontaneous apoptosis, and was associated with a 20-fold increase in susceptibility to cisplatin-induced apoptosis in mesothelioma cell lines [80]. Spontaneous apoptosis was enhanced by antisense downregulation of survivin *in vitro* [81]. Survivin, unlike XIAP, is not thought to inhibit caspase-3, is not bound by Smac, and is associated with Aurora-B, which plays a part in chromosome segregation [84–86]. Thus agents targeting survivin may yield different results from those against XIAP. In addition, the mitochondrial protein Smac/diablo usually antagonizes the IAP family during apoptosis. Peptide agonists to Smac/diablo can inhibit the XIAP family and so induce apoptosis *in vitro* and *in vivo* [87]. The outcomes of clinical trials of apoptosis inducers in mesothelioma, particularly in combination with chemotherapy or other novel agents, are awaited with interest.

Phosphatidylinositol 3-kinase/Akt, mTOR and proteasome inhibition

The phosphatidylinositol 3-kinase (PI3K)/Akt (protein kinase B) pathway plays a central role in cancer cell survival (see Chapter 8). Phosphorylation of Akt, seen in the majority of mesothelioma samples, leads to the activation of anti-apoptotic factors such as MDM2 that inhibit p53, and inhibition of a range of pro-apoptotic factors including the forkhead receptor (FKHR) trancription factor, caspase-9 and Bad [66] (see Chapter 8; Figure 8.10). The selective PI3K inhibitor LY294002 has been demonstrated to completely block Akt phosphorylation in mesothelioma *in vitro*. This is associated with both inhibition of cell proliferation and induction of apoptosis. The combination of LY294002 with cisplatin has been shown to have greater anti-tumour efficacy than either agent alone [88] (unpublished data).

Mammalian target of rapamycin (mTOR) is a kinase that functions as a master switch between catabolic and anabolic metabolism. mTOR is downstream of, and activated by Akt. mTOR inhibition by rapamycin and its derivatives can induce long-lasting objective tumour responses in solid tumours. CCI-779, a first-in-class mTOR inhibitor, improves the survival of patients with renal cell carcinoma [89]. Treatment of mesothelioma cells with rapamycin results in growth arrest in the G1 phase of the cell cycle [88]. Several novel PI3K/Akt (PKB) and mTOR pathway inhibitors currently under development may have a role to play in the management of mesothelioma [89,90].

The proteasome plays a major role in the elimination of polyubiquitinated proteins some of which may have vital tumour suppressor activity in the cancer cell [91]. Bortezomib (velcade™, PS-341) is a dipeptidyl boronic acid proteasome inhibitor that has been shown to promote apoptosis of tumour cells through the stabilisation of p53, p21, p27 and bax. Furthermore inhibition of ubiquitination of IκBα results in inhibitory modulation of NFκB, a transcription factor involved in the upregulation of pro-inflammatory cytokines and cell survival factors (see Chapter 8). Bortezomib is approved for the management of relapsed malignant myeloma and is showing encouraging anti-tumour activity in a range of solid tumours [92].

The *Gruppo Italiano Mesotelioma* have demonstrated that Bortezomib induces mesothelioma cytotoxicity as a single agent *in vitro* and *in vivo* (manuscript in preparation). The proapoptoxic efficacy of the proteasome inhibitor PSI has also been recently reported in mesothelioma cells [93]. Bortezomib is currently being evaluated in a multicentre iternational phase II clinical trial in patients with chemonaive and relapsed mesothelioma. The EORTC will be initiating a combination phase II trial of Bortezomib with cisplatin in mesothelioma in the first line setting. Together, these trials will establish whether the proteosome is a valid target for therapeutic intervention in mesothelioma.

Future challenges

Trials of novel therapies that target critical processes involved in cancer, such as angiogenesis, growth factor receptor signalling, and apoptosis, are just beginning to be performed in patients with mesothelioma. While progress has been made in bringing a number of promising agents through to phase II evaluation in mesothelioma, it is still too early to predict which, if any, of the novel therapies that are currently available will impact on this aggressive disease. There are several difficulties that need to be addressed in trials to evaluate novel therapies for the treatment of mesothelioma. The accurate assessment of therapy, especially in relatively small phase II trials, is complicated by the variable natural history of mesothelioma and lack of an accurate staging system. Among the trials discussed in this chapter, some investigators have incorporated adjustment for known prognostic groupings such as the EORTC and CALGB groups to identify clinically homogeneous populations for comparison and provide more meaningful interpretation of the results. With greater insight into the molecular mechanisms of mesothelioma, it is becoming apparent that molecular heterogeneity may also confound the interpretation of data. In preliminary studies reported by Gordon *et al.* [94], gene expression ratios accurately predicted treatment-related patient outcome independent of the histological subtype of the mesothelioma. However, these data require validation in larger prospective series of patients before they can be incorporated into a molecular classification for routine clinical use. Mesothelioma is frequently diagnosed from small pleural biopsy specimens, and lack of adequate tissue specimens for such molecular correlative studies may be a major barrier to improving existing classification based on stage and histological subtype.

The growth pattern of malignant pleural mesothelioma also poses problems for staging and objective measurement of radiological response in patients in clinical trials [95]. The Response Evaluation Criteria in Solid Tumors (RECIST) relies on a single largest dimension of tumour rather than the product of perpendicular diameters on which the World Health Organization (WHO) response evaluation was previously based. RECIST is intended to simplify the assessment of tumour response and it is well validated for tumours with a spherical growth pattern. However, several groups have highlighted the inadequacy of RECIST for mesothelioma with a non-spherical growth pattern. It has recently been proposed that the WHO criteria should be used for bidimensional measurable lesions, RECIST should be used for unidimensional measurable lesions, and a modified RECIST response evaluation, in which the short axis perpendicular to the chest wall is measured, should be employed for accurate assessment of thickened pleural rind disease [89].

In addition to problems due to the nature of mesothelioma, a general problem in negative studies of novel agents is the difficulty in determining whether the dose of drug tested was adequate. The traditional method of dose selection based on determination of the maximum tolerated dose may not apply with targeted agents proposed to have a cytostatic rather than cytotoxic mode of action. Targets or enzymes may be saturated by drug at levels well below toxic doses, and the converse may also apply. The incorporation of novel pharmacodynamic assays to ensure that a biologically effective dose is delivered has rarely been performed in trials to date, and investigators are realizing that such assays are essential for the continued development of these drugs. Equally, early clinical trials need to incorporate molecular correlative studies to confirm expression of the target and trials may need to be designed in which patients are selected on the basis of target expression, rather than found to lack the target in retrospect. To avoid the need to obtain tissue biopsies functional imaging techniques such as PET and dynamic enhanced magnetic resonance imaging (DEMRI) have been employed with some success in the quantification of anti-angiogenesis [96]. Surrogate assays based on circulating lymphocytes or serum markers of processes such as apoptosis are also under investigation for clinical utility. It is hoped that the incorporation of techniques such as these into the design of phase I–II clinical trials will provide objective evidence of the appropriate dose to take forward into randomized trials. However, even if the desired biological effect of a novel agent is confirmed, it cannot be assumed that this will translate to a therapeutic effect and a clinically meaningful endpoint such as improvement in symptoms, tumour response, or prolonged survival. For this reason it is preferable to evaluate targeted agents alone, in the phase II setting, for therapeutic efficacy. Also, several targeted therapies such as thalidomide and bevacizumab are currently being evaluated in combination with chemotherapy in phase II trials, and the absence of single-agent data is likely to pose additional problems in the interpretation of the results. Studies in NSCLC have already provided unexpected negative results for the matrix metalloproteinases and the small-molecule EGFR-TK inhibitors erlotinib and gefitinib in combination with chemotherapy, and so caution is warranted in assuming synergy between targeted therapies and chemotherapy even if preclinical data are promising.

The clinically meaningful endpoints for mesothelioma that should be examined in early clinical trials are also a matter for debate. Overall survival is the hardest endpoint and the gold standard, but investigators frequently favour time to progression. The definition of time to progression is usually assumed to be radiological progression, which in turn is influenced by the frequency of imaging. Also, radiological progression may be asymptomatic. The point at which disease progression is associated with deterioration in symptoms and performance status may be the clinically meaningful endpoint. Mesothelioma frequently causes symptoms that are difficult to palliate such as pleuritic chest pain, sweats, fatigue, weight loss, cough, and severe dyspnoea. For example, the EGFR-TKIs improved symptoms in up to 40 per cent of patients with advanced and heavily pretreated NSCLC in contrast with response rates of 10–20 per cent [4]. If trials in mesothelioma do not include assessment of symptom control and quality of life, important benefits of targeted therapies with a cytostatic rather than a cytotoxic mechanism of action may be missed. Although the overall aim is to prolong the life expectancy of patients with mesothelioma, there are so few available options that treatments capable of improving quality of life without prolonging survival would be of benefit. Finally, compared with other types of cancer, relatively few clinical trials of novel agents have been performed to date. Given the anticipated rise in the incidence of this disease over the next few decades, there is a pressing need to prioritize patients with mesothelioma. The number of novel agents in development continues to increase and the future should witness renewed optimism for their evaluation in mesothelioma.

References

1. Hanahan D, Weinberg RA. The hallmarks of cancer. *Cell* 2000; **100**: 57–70.
2. Logrono R, Jones DV, Faruqi S, Bhutani MS. Recent advances in cell biology, diagnosis, and therapy of gastrointestinal stromal tumor (GIST). *Cancer Biol Ther* 2004; **3**: 251–8.
3. Kaklamani V, O'Regan RM. New targeted therapies in breast cancer. *Semin Oncol* 2004; **31** (Suppl 4): 20–5.
4. Ranson M. Epidermal growth factor receptor tyrosine kinase inhibitors. *Br J Cancer* 2004; **90**: 2250–5.
5. Iqbal S, Lenz HJ. Integration of novel agents in the treatment of colorectal cancer. *Cancer Chemother Pharmacol* 2004; **54** (Suppl 1): S32–9.
6. Folkman J. Tumor angiogenesis: therapeutic implications. *N Engl J Med* 1971; **285**: 1182–6.
7. Branchaud RM, MacDonald JL, Kane AB. Induction of angiogenesis by intraperitoneal injection of asbestos fibers. *FASEB J* 1989; **3**: 1747–52.
8. Kumar-Singh S, Vermeulen PB, Weyler J, *et al*. Evaluation of tumour angiogenesis as a prognostic marker in malignant mesothelioma. *J Pathol* 1997; **182**: 211–16.
9. Edwards JG, Cox G, Andi A, *et al*. Angiogenesis is an independent prognostic factor in malignant mesothelioma. *Br J Cancer* 2001; **85**: 863–8.
10. Carmeliet P, Jain RK. Angiogenesis in cancer and other disease. *Nat Med* 1995; **1**: 27–31.

11. Stamenkovic I. Extracellular matrix remodelling: the role of matrix metalloproteinases. *J Pathol* 2003; **200**: 448–64.

12. Edwards JG, McLaren J, Jones JL, Waller DA, O'Byrne KJ. Matrix metalloproteinases 2 and 9 (gelatinases A and B) expression in malignant mesothelioma and benign pleura. *Br J Cancer* 2003; **88**: 1553–9.

13. Linnekin, D. Early signaling pathways activated by c-Kit in hematopoietic cells. *Int J Biochem Cell Biol* 1999; **31**: 1053–74.

14. Strizzi L, Catalano A, Vianale G, *et al.* Vascular endothelial growth factor is an autocrine growth factor in human malignant mesothelioma. *J Pathol* 2001; **193**: 468–75.

15. Masood R, Kundra A, Zhu S, *et al.* Malignant mesothelioma growth inhibition by agents that target the VEGF and VEGF-C autocrine loops. *Int J Cancer* 2003; **104**: 603–10.

16. Linder C, Linder S, Munck-Wikland E, Strander H. Independent expression of serum vascular endothelial growth factor (VEGF) and basic fibroblast growth factor (bFGF) in patients with carcinoma and sarcoma. *Anticancer Res* 1998; **18**: 2063–8.

17. Konig JE, Tolnay E, Wiethege T, Muller KM. Expression of vascular endothelial growth factor in diffuse malignant pleural mesothelioma. *Virchows Arch* 1999; **435**: 8–12.

18. Ohta Y, Shridhar V, Kalemkerian GP, Bright RK, Watanabe Y, Pass HI. Thrombospondin-1 expression and clinical implications in malignant pleural mesothelioma. *Cancer* 1999; **85**: 2570–6.

19. Jagadeeswaran R, Ma PC, Seiwert TY, *et al.* Functional analysis of c-Met/hepatocyte growth factor pathway in malignant pleural mesothelioma. *Cancer Res* 2006; **66**: 352–361.

20. Betta P-G, Libener R, Orecchia S, *et al.* Serum hepatocyte growth factor (HGF), epidermal growth factor (EGF) and stem cell factor (SCF) in pleural malignant mesothelioma. *Proc Am Soc Clin Oncol* 2002; **21**: abstr 1773

21. Fong TA, Shawver LK, Sun L, Tang C, App H, Powell TJ. SU5416 is a potent and selective inhibitor of the vascular endothelial growth factor receptor (Flk-1/KDR) that inhibits tyrosine kinase catalysis, tumor vascularization, and growth of multiple tumor types. *Cancer Res* 1999; **591**: 99–106.

22. Stopeck A, Sheldon M, Vahedian M, Cropp G, Gosalia R, Hannah A. Results of a phase I dose-escalating study of the antiangiogenic agent, SU5416, in patients with advanced malignancies. *Clin Cancer Res* 2002; **8**: 2798–805.

23. Kindler HL, Vogelzang NJ, Chien K, *et al.* SU5416 in malignant mesothelioma: a University of Chicago phase II consortium study. *Proc Am Soc Clin Oncol* 2001; **20**: 341a (abstr).

24. Rosen L, Mulay M, Mayers A, *et al.* Phase I dose-escalating trial of SU5416, a novel angiogenesis inhibitor in patients with advanced malignancies. *Proc Am Soc Clin Oncol* 1999; **18**: 161a (abstr 618).

25. Kuenen BC, Rosen L, Smit EF, *et al.* Dose-finding and pharmacokinetic study of cisplatin, gemcitibine, and SU5416 in patients with solid tumors. *J Clin Oncol* 2002; **20**: 1657–67.

26. Gordon MS, Margolin K, Talpaz M, *et al.* Phase I safety and pharmacokinetic study of recombinant human anti-vascular endothelial growth factor in patients with advanced cancer. *J Clin Oncol* 2001; **19**: 843–50.

27. Margolin K, Gordon MS, Holmgren E, *et al.*, Phase 1b trial of intravenous recombinant humanized monoclonal antibody to vascular endothelial growth factor in combination with chemotherapy in patients with advanced cancer: pharmacologic and long-term safety data. *J Clin Oncol* 2001; **19**: 851–6.

28. Sandler AB, Gray R, Brahmer J, *et al.* Randomised phase II/III trial of paclitaxel (P) plus carboplatin (C) with or wothput bevacizumab (NSC #704865) in patients with advanced non-squamous non-small cell lung cancer (NSCLC): An Eastern Cooperative Oncology Group (ECOG) Trial – E4599. *J Clin Oncol* 2005; **23** (No 16S, Part I of II): 2s – abstract LBA4.

29. Hurwitz H, Fehrenbacher L, Novotny W, *et al.* Bevacizumab plus irinotecan, fluorouracil, and leucovorin for metastatic colorectal cancer. *N Engl J Med* 2004; **350**: 2335–42.

30. Johnson DH, Fehrenbacher L, Novotny WF, *et al.* Randomized phase II trial comparing bevacizumab plus carboplatin and paclitaxel with carboplatin and paclitaxel alone in previously untreated locally advanced or metastatic non-small-cell lung cancer. *J Clin Oncol* 2004; **22**: 2184–91.

31. Kabbinavar FF, Wong JT, Ayala RE, *et al.* The effect of antibody to vascular endothelial growth factor and cisplatin on the growth of lung tumors in nude mice. *Proc Am Assoc Cancer Res* 1995; **36**: 488 (abstr).

32. Kindler HL. Moving beyond chemotherapy: novel cytostatic agents for malignant mesothelioma. *Lung Cancer* 2004; **45** (Suppl 1): S125–7.

33. D'Amato RJ, Loughnan MS, Flynn E, Folkman J. Thalidomide is an inhibitor of angiogenesis. *Proc Natl Acad Sci USA* 1994; **91**: 4082–5.

34. Pavlakis N, Williams G, Harvey R, Aslani A, Abraham R, Wheeler H. Thalidomide alone and in combination with cisplatin/gemcitabine chemotherapy for malignant mesothelioma (MM): preliminary results from two phase II studies. *Proc Am Soc Clin Oncol* 2002; **21**: abstr 1885.

35. Kindler HL, van Meerbeeck JP. The role of gemcitabine in the treatment of malignant mesothelioma. *Semin Oncol* 2002; **29**: 70–6.

36. Wood JM, Bold G, Buchdunger E, *et al*. PTK787/ZK 222584, a novel and potent inhibitor of vascular endothelial growth factor receptor tyrosine kinases, impairs vascular endothelial growth factor-induced responses and tumor growth after oral administration. *Cancer Res* 2000; **60**: 2178–89.

37. Pass HI, Brewer G, Stevens T, *et al*. A phase II trial of tetrathiomolybdate (TM) after cytoreductive surgery for malignant pleural mesothelioma (MPM). *Proc Am Soc Clin Oncol* 2004; **23**: abstr 7051.

38. Mendelsohn J, Baselga J. The EGF receptor family as targets for cancer therapy. *Oncogene* 2000; **19**: 6550–65.

39. Zanella CL, Posada J, Tritton TR, Mossman BT Asbestos causes stimulation of the extracellular signal-regulated kinase 1 mitogen-activated protein kinase cascade after phosphorylation of the epidermal growth factor receptor. *Cancer Res* 1996; **56**: 5334–8.

40. Cai YC, Roggli V, Mark E, Cagle PT, Fraire AE. Transforming growth factor alpha and epidermal growth factor receptor in reactive and malignant mesothelial proliferations. *Arch Pathol Lab Med* 2004; **128**: 68–70.

41. Simon GR, Coppola D, Bepler G. Epidermal growth factor receptor and C-KIT expression in mesotheliomas. *Proc Am Soc Clin Oncol* 2003; **22**: 247 (abstr 991).

42. Govindan R, Kratzke RA, Herndon JE, 2nd *et al*. Gefitinib in patients with malignant mesothelioma: a phase II study by the Cancer and Leukemia Group B. *Clin Cancer Res* 2005; **11**: 2300–4.

43. Betta P-G, Libener R, Orecchia S, *et al*. Epidermal growth factor in serum from patients with malignant pleural mesothelioma. *Proc Am Soc Clin Oncol* 2004; **23**: abstr 7315.

44. Dazzi H, Hasleton PS, Thatcher N, Wilkes S, Swindell R, Chatterjee AK. Malignant pleural mesothelioma and epidermal growth factor receptor (EGF-R). Relationship of EGF-R with histology and survival using fixed paraffin embedded tissue and the F4, monoclonal antibody. *Br J Cancer* 1990; **61**: 924–6.

45. Edwards JG, Faux SP, Jones JL, Waller DA, O'Byrne KJ. Towards a biologic prognostic model for malignant mesothelioma. Preclinical studies of novel target identification. *Proc Am Soc Clin Oncol* 2002; **21**: abstr 1778.

46. Janne PA, Taffaro ML, Salgia R, Johnson BE. Inhibition of epidermal growth factor receptor signaling in malignant pleural mesothelioma. *Cancer Res* 2002; **62**: 5242–7.

47. Garland L, Rankin C, Scott K, *et al*. Molecular correlates of the EGFR signaling pathway in association with SWOG S0218: a phase II study of oral EGFR tyrosine kinase inhibitor OSI-774 (NSC-718781) in patients with malignant pleural mesothelioma (MPM). *Proc Am Soc Clin Oncol* 2004; **23**: abstr 3007.

48. Gerwin BI, Lechner JF, Reddel RR, *et al*. Comparison of production of transforming growth factor-beta and platelet-derived growth factor by normal human mesothelial cells and mesothelioma cell lines. *Cancer Res* 1987; **47**: 6180–4.

49. Versnel MA, Claesson-Welsh L, Hammacher A, *et al*. Human malignant mesothelioma cell lines express PDGF beta-receptors whereas cultured normal mesothelial cells express predominantly PDGF alpha-receptors. *Oncogene* 1991; **6**: 2005–11.

50. Dorai T, Kobayashi H, Holland JF, Ohnuma T. Modulation of platelet-derived growth factor-beta mRNA expression and cell growth in a human mesothelioma cell line by a hammerhead ribozyme. *Mol Pharmacol* 1994; **46**: 437–44.

51. Horvai AE, Li L, Xu Z, Kramer MJ, Jablons DM, Treseler PA. c-Kit is not expressed in malignant mesothelioma. *Mod Pathol* 2003; **16**: 818–22.

52. Buchdunger E, Cioffi CL, Law N, *et al*. Abl protein-tyrosine kinase inhibitor STI571 inhibits *in vitro* signal transduction mediated by *c-kit* and platelet-derived growth factor receptors. *J Pharmacol Exp Ther* 2000; **295**: 139–45.

53. M. Millward, F. Parnis, M. Byrne, *et al*. A Phase II trial of imatinib mesylate in patients with advanced pleural mesothelioma. *Proc Am Soc Clin Oncol* 2003; **22**: 228 (abstr 912).

54. Villano JL, Husain AN, Stadler WM, Hanson LL, Vogelzang NJ, Kindler HL. A phase II trial of imatinib mesylate in patients (pts) with malignant mesothelioma (MM). *Proc Am Soc Clin Oncol* 2004; **23**: abstr 7200.

55. Mathy A, Baas P, Dalesio O, van Zandwijk N. Limited efficacy of imatinib mesylate in malignant mesothelioma: a phase II trial. *Lung Cancer* 2005; **50**: 83–6.

56. Porta C, Mutti L, Tassi G. Negative results of an Italian Group for Mesothelioma (G.I.Me) pilot study of single-agent imatinib mesylate in malignant pleural mesothelioma. *Cancer Chemother Pharmacol* 2006.

57. Marrogi A, Pass HI, Khan M, Metheny-Barlow LJ, Harris CC, Gerwin BI. Human mesothelioma samples overexpress both cyclooxygenase-2 (COX-2) and inducible nitric oxide synthase (NOS2): *in vitro* antiproliferative effects of a COX-2 inhibitor. *Cancer Res* 2000; **60**: 3696–700.

58. Catalano A, Graciotti L, Rinaldi L, *et al*. Preclinical evaluation of the nonsteroidal anti-inflammatory agent celecoxib on malignant mesothelioma chemoprevention. *Int J Cancer* 2004; **109**: 322–8.

59. Edwards JG, Faux SP, Plummer SM, *et al*. Cyclooxygenase-2 expression is a novel prognostic factor in malignant mesothelioma. *Clin Cancer Res* 2002; **8**: 1857–62.

60. Baldi A, Santini D, Vasaturo F, *et al*. Prognostic significance of cyclooxygenase-2 (COX-2) and expression of cell cycle inhibitors p21 and p27 in human pleural malignant mesothelioma. *Thorax* 2004; **59**: 428–33.

61. Kamp DW, Weitzman SA. The molecular basis of asbestos induced lung injury. *Thorax* 1999; **54**: 638–52.

62. Mossman BT, Churg A. Mechanisms in the pathogenesis of asbestosis and silicosis. *Am J Respir Crit Care Med* 1998; **57**: 1666–80.

63. DeLong P, Tanaka T, Kruklitis R, *et al*. Use of cyclooxygenase-2 inhibition to enhance the efficacy of immunotherapy. *Cancer Res* 2003; **63**: 7845–52.

64. Lund LG, Aust AE. Iron-catalyzed reactions may be responsible for the biochemical and biological effects of asbestos. *Biofactors* 1991; **3**: 83–9.

65. Fennell DA, Rudd RM. Defective core-apoptosis signalling in diffuse malignant pleural mesothelioma: opportunities for effective drug development. *Lancet Oncol* 2004; **5**: 354–62.

66. Makin G, Dive C. Recent advances in understanding apoptosis: new therapeutic opportunities in cancer chemotherapy. *Trends Mol Med* 2003; **9**: 251–5.

67. Baetu TM, Hiscott J. On the TRAIL to apoptosis. *Cytokine Growth Factor Rev* 2002; **13**: 199–207.

68. Liu W, Bodle E, Chen JY, *et al*. Tumour necrosis factor-related apoptosis-inducing ligand and chemotherapy cooperate to induce apoptosis in mesothelioma cell lines. *Am J Respir Cell Mol Biol* 2001; **25**: 111–18.

69. Soini Y, Kinnula V, Kaarteenaho-Wiik R, *et al*. Apoptosis and expression of apoptosis regulating proteins bcl-2, mcl-1, bcl-X, and bax in malignant mesothelioma. *Clin Cancer Res* 1999; **5**: 3508–15.

70. Narasimhan SR, Yang L, Gerwin BI, Broaddus VC. Resistance of pleural mesothelioma cell lines to apoptosis: relation to expression of Bcl-2 and Bax. *Am J Physiol* 1998; **275**: L165–71.

71. Cao XX, Mohuiddin I, Ece F, *et al*. Histone deacetylase inhibitor downregulation of bcl-xl gene expression leads to apoptotic cell death in mesothelioma. *Am J Respir Cell Mol Biol* 2001; 25: 562–68.

72. Ozvaran MK, Cao XX, Miller SD, Monia BA, Hong WK, Smythe WR. Antisense oligonucleotides directed at the bcl-xl gene product augment chemotherapy response in mesothelioma. *Mol Cancer Ther* 2004; **3**: 545–50.

73. Wang S, Yang D, Lippman ME. Targeting Bcl-2 and Bcl-XL with nonpeptidic small-molecule antagonists. *Semin Oncol* 2003; **30** (Suppl 16): 133–42.

74. Degterev A, Lugovskoy A, Cardone M, *et al*. Identification of small-molecule inhibitors of interaction between the BH3 domain and Bcl-xL. *Nat Cell Biol* 2001; **3**: 173–82.

75. Tzung SP, Kim KM, Basanez G, *et al.* Antimycin A mimics a cell-death-inducing Bcl-2 homology domain 3. *Nat Cell Biol* 2001; **3**: 183–91.

76. Yin H, Hamilton AD. Terephthalamide derivatives as mimetics of the helical region of Bak peptide target Bcl-xL protein. *Bioorg Med Chem Lett* 2004; **14**: 1375–9.

77. Chan SL, Lee MC, Tan KO, *et al.* Identification of chelerythrine as an inhibitor of BclXL function. *J Biol Chem* 2003; **278**: 20453–6.

78. Hopkins-Donaldson S, Cathomas R, Simoes-Wust AP, *et al.* Induction of apoptosis and chemosensitisation of mesothelioma cells by bcl-2 and bcl-xl antisense treatment. *Br J Cancer* 2003; **106**: 160–6.

79. Ferreira CG, van der Valk P, Span SW, *et al.* Assessment of IAP (inhibitor of apoptosis) proteins as predictors of response to chemotherapy in advanced non-small-cell lung cancer patients. *Ann Oncol* 2001; **12**: 799–805.

80. Gordon GJ, Appasani K, Parcells JP, *et al.* Inhibitor of apoptosis protein-1 promotes tumor cell survival in mesothelioma. *Carcinogenesis* 2002; **23**: 1017–24.

81. Xia C, Xu Z, Yuan X, *et al.* Induction of apoptosis in mesothelioma cells by antisurvivin oligonucleotides. *Mol Cancer Ther* 2002; **1**: 687–94.

82. Kramer G, Erdal H, Mertens HJMM, *et al.* Differentiation between cell death modes using measurements of different soluble forms of extracellular cytokeratin 18. *Cancer Res* 2004; **64**: 1751–6.

83. Schimmer AD, Welsh K, Pinilla C, *et al.* Small-molecule antagonists of apoptosis suppressor XIAP exhibit broad antitumour activity. *Cancer Cell* 2004; **5**: 25–35.

84. Reed JC. The survivin saga goes *in vivo*. *J Clin Invest* 2001; **108**: 965–9.

85. Marusawa H, Matsuzawa S-I, Welsh K, *et al.* HBXIP functions as a cofactor of surviving in apoptosis expression. *EMBO J* 2003; **22**: 2729–40.

86. Chen J, Jin S, Tahir SK, *et al.* Survivin enhances Aurora-B kinase activity and localises Aurora-B in human cells. *J Biol Chem* 2003; **278**: 486–90.

87. Fulda S, Wick W, Weller M, *et al.* Smac agonists sensitise for Apo2L/TRAIL-or anticancer drug-induced apoptosis and induce regression of malignant glioma *in vivo*. *Nat Med* 2002; **8**: 808–15.

88. Altomore DA, You H, Xiao GH, *et al.* Human and mouse mesothelioma exhibit elevated AKT/PKB activity, which can be targeted pharmacologically to inhibit tumor cell growth. *Oncogene* 2005; **24**: 6080–9.

89. Faivre S, Kroemer D, Raymond E. Current development of mTOR inhibitors as anticancer agents. *Nat Rev Drug Discov* 2006; **5**: 671–88.

90. Collins I, Caldwell J, Fonseca T, *et al.* Structure-based design of isoquinoline-5-sulfonamide inhibitors of protein kinase B. *Bioorg Med Chem* 2006; **14**: 1255–73.

91. Adams J. The proteasome: a suitable antineoplastic target. *Nat Rev Cancer* 2004; **4**: 349–60.

92. Ludwig H, Khayat D, Giaccone G, Facon T. Proteasome inhibition and its clinical prospects in the treatment of hematologic and solid malignancies. *Cancer* 2005; **104**: 1794–807.

93. Sun X, Gulyas M, Hjerpe A, Dobra K. Proteasome inhibitor PSI induces apoptosis in human mesothelioma cells. *Cancer Lett* 2006; **232**: 161–9.

94. Gordon GJ, Jensen RV, Hsiao LL, *et al.* Using gene expression ratios to predict outcome among patients with mesothelioma. *J Natl Cancer Inst* 2003; **95**: 598–605.

95. van Klaveren RJ, Aerts JG, de Bruin H, Giaccone G, Manegold C, van Meerbeeck JP. Inadequacy of the RECIST criteria for response evaluation in patients with malignant pleural mesothelioma. *Lung Cancer* 2004; **43**: 63–9.

96. Morgan B, Thomas AL, Drevs J, *et al.* Dynamic contrast-enhanced magnetic resonance imaging as a biomarker for the pharmacological response of PTK787/ZK222584, an inhibitor of the vascular endothelial growth factor receptor tyrosine kinases, in patients with advanced colorectal cancer and liver metastases: results from two phase I studies. *J Clin Oncol* 2003; **21**: 3955–64.

Chapter 19

Gene therapy for malignant pleural mesothelioma

D. H. Sterman and P. A. DeLong

Introduction

Malignant pleural mesothelioma (MPM) is minimally responsive to most chemotherapy and radiotherapy regimens, and is almost uniformly fatal. Radiation therapy is primarily useful for palliation of localized chest wall invasion or after debulking surgery. Furthermore, radical surgical resection of all involved pleural surfaces, ipsilateral lung, pericardium, and diaphragm has not been demonstrated to prolong survival, although non-randomized large phase II studies have yielded encouraging results in highly selected groups of patients as part of multimodality treatment involving surgery, chemotherapy, and/or radiation therapy [1–5]. New chemotherapy drugs administered in combination may provide symptomatic relief and clinical/radiographic responses in a subset of patients with advanced disease, but have been shown to prolong survival at best by only a few months [6] (see Chapters 14–16 and 18). In this context new therapeutic approaches to the management of MPM are urgently needed. The genetic revolution in biology in general, and in oncology in particular, over the past 30 years has facilitated the investigation of gene therapy as a new therapeutic modality. Investigations of the role of gene therapy in cancer have involved the insertion of 'therapeutic' genes via various delivery systems ('vectors') into tumour cells for the purpose of inducing apoptosis, necrosis, and antitumour immune responses.

MPM has several characteristics that make it an attractive target for gene therapy, including the absence of standard effective therapy, accessibility of the pleural space for biopsy, local (as opposed to systemic) vector delivery, and analysis of treatment effects and morbidity and mortality related to local extension of disease, rather than distant metastases. Therefore, unlike other tumours that metastasize earlier in their course, relatively small increments of improvement in local control in MPM could result in significant symptomatic and survival benefit. In addition, gene therapy clinical trials for MPM could serve as a paradigm for treatment of malignancies localized to other body cavities such as carcinoma of the bladder or ovary.

Gene therapy: principles and vectors

Although gene therapy was originally conceived as a treatment for inherited recessive disorders in which transfer of a normal copy of a defective gene could prevent disease onset or reverse phenotypic expression [1], it soon became clear that cancer would be one of its most important targets. The concept of cancer gene therapy is defined as the transfer of genetic material, including complementary DNA (cDNA), full-length genes, RNA, or oligonucleotides into cancer or host cells. The transport mechanism for delivery and expression of this genetic material is termed the 'vector'.

Table 19.1 Characteristics of gene therapy vectors

Vector	DNA-carrying capacity (kb)	Cell range	In vivo gene delivery efficiency	Duration of expression	Co-transfer viral gene elements	Inflammatory response
Retrovirus	<8	Replicating cells only	Low	Stable	Yes	Low
Adenovirus (Ad)	7–8	Most cells	Moderate	Transient	Yes	High
Adeno-associated virus (AAV)	<5	Primarily muscle, liver, and brain	Low	Stable	Minimal	Low
Lentivirus (HIV-like)	<8	Many non-dividing cells	Low	Stable	Yes	Low
Liposome	>10	Most cells	Low	Transient	No	Moderate

Vectors used in gene therapy

A prerequisite for successful gene therapy is efficient gene transfer. A variety of viral and non-viral gene transfer vectors are currently available, which range from replicating and non-replicating viruses to bacteria and liposomes. As summarized in Table 19.1, each of these vectors has certain advantages with regard to DNA-carrying capacity, types of cells targeted, *in vivo* gene transfer efficiency, duration of expression, and induction of inflammation. It has become clear that no single gene delivery strategy is suitable for all candidate disorders.

The most widely used vector system for *in vivo* cancer gene therapy has been recombinant adenovirus (Ad). Recombinant Ad vectors have been derived by genomic deletion of early viral genes involved in replication (i.e. the E1A/B regions) and provision of these functions *in trans* via a packaging cell line [7–11]. The genomic deletion of the early viral genes renders the Ad vector's replication incompetent. The deleted gene regions can then be replaced with expression cassettes containing the desired gene under the control of general or tumour-specific promoters. Recombinant Ad vector systems offer numerous advantages including efficient transduction of a wide range of target cells, including non-dividing cells, and high expression levels of the passenger transgene [12,13]. Importantly, these vectors are stable *in vivo*, permitting direct gene delivery to many tissue sites including the bronchial epithelium and the pleural space. The two primary disadvantages of adenoviral vectors are transient gene expression and prominent local and systemic inflammatory responses elicited by the virions. The inflammatory response, including an early 'innate' immune response resulting in cytokine release and a late 'acquired' immune response resulting in the generation of neutralizing anti-adenoviral antibodies and cytotoxic T lymphocytes, has been the primary source of adenoviral vector toxicity and limited the amount of vector that can be delivered [14–19].

Gene therapy strategies in mesothelioma

Several different cancer gene therapy approaches are currently being explored for MPM including the use of so-called 'suicide genes', delivery of tumour suppressor genes, and transfer of immunomodulatory genes. Several of these have been applied in phase I clinical trials of MPM utilizing a variety of vector systems including recombinant adenovirus, vaccinia virus, and modified ovarian carcinoma cells [12,20,21]. Others remain in the preclinical stage, but with plans for clinical trials in the near future (Table 19.2).

'Suicide' gene therapy

One prominent approach in the cancer gene transfer armamentarium is so-called 'suicide' gene therapy. This method involves the transduction of tumour cells with cDNA encoding for an enzyme that converts a benign prodrug to a toxic metabolite [13]. Administration of the prodrug thus engenders selective accumulation of the toxic metabolite within the tumour cells, resulting in tumour cell death. The enzymes encoded by the suicide gene are often of non-human origin, i.e. the *Escherichia coli* cytosine deaminase (CDA) gene [14] or the herpes simplex virus-1 thymidine kinase (HSV*tk*) gene, which limits toxicity in normal tissue [15]. For instance, HSV*tk* differs enough from mammalian cellular kinases that transfect malignant cells, but not normal non-transduced cells, to convert the nucleoside analogue ganciclovir to its toxic metabolite.

The drug ganciclovir (GCV) (9-[1,3-dihydroxy-2-propoxy)methyl]-guanine) is an acyclic nucleoside that is poorly metabolized by mammalian cells and therefore is generally non-toxic. However, after enzymatic conversion to GCV-monophosphate (GCV-MP) by HSV*tk*, it is rapidly metabolized to GCV-triphosphate (GCV-TP) by endogenous mammalian kinases. Intracellular production of these GCV metabolites causes tumour cell death, or 'suicide' [13,16]. GCV-TP is

Table 19.2 Gene therapy approaches for mesothelioma

Strategy	Vector	Therapeutic gene	Molecular mechanism	Location
Suicide gene	Recombinant replication-deficient adenovirus	Herpes simplex Thymidine kinase	Delivery of enzyme capable of generating toxic metabolite after exposure to GCV	University of Pennsylvania Medical Center, Philadelphia, PA, USA 1995–1999
Genetic immunopotentiation	Replication-restricted vaccinia virus	Human IL-2	Augmentation of immune response to tumour	Queen Elizabeth II Medical Centre, Perth, Australia 1990s
	Vaccinia virus	Modified SV40 T-antigen	Stimulation of immune response against SV40+ mesothelioma cells	Wayne State University Medical Center, Detroit, IL, USA Pending
	Replication-deficient adenovirus	Interferon-β	Induction of antitumour immune response	University of Pennsylvania Medical Center, Philadelphia, PA, USA Ongoing
	Cationic liposome	Prokaryotic DNA	Non-specific induction of innate and acquired immunity	No known clinical protocols
Combined suicide gene–tumour vaccine	Irradiated allogeneic ovarian carcinoma cells	Herpes simplex Thymidine kinase	Generation of toxic metabolite and antitumour immune responses	LSU Medical Center, New Orleans, LA, USA Completed
Mutation compensation	Oligonucleotides	Anti-sense SV40 TAg	Inhibition of dominant oncogenes.	No known clinical protocols
	Adenovirus	Wild-type p14(ARF)/p16	Restoration of tumour suppressers	No known clinical protocols
	Adenovirus	Wild-type p53/Bak	Induction of apoptosis	No known clinical protocols
Replication-competent viral lytic therapy	Replication-restricted adenovirus (ONYX-015)	None	Tumour-restricted viral replication and cytotoxicity	No known clinical protocols

toxic to the cell because it is a potent inhibitor of DNA polymerase and competes with normal mammalian nucleosides for DNA replication [16]. In addition, incorporation of GCV-MP into the cellular DNA template can itself induce significant cytotoxicity [17]. This process is facilitated by the presence of the 'bystander' effect, whereby neighbouring non-transduced tumour cells also perish, achieving maximal tumour response [18].

Bystander effects of HSV*tk* suicide gene therapy

Given the limited gene transfer efficiency of adenoviral vector systems *in vivo*, direct killing of significant numbers of malignant cells within a solid tumour may be difficult to achieve. Thus the presence of a 'bystander effect', whereby non-transduced cells are killed by an indirect mechanism, is extremely important. The genesis of the bystander effect hypothesis lay in the observation that tumour regression in *in vivo* HSV*tk* experiments occurred without transgene expression in every tumour cell. This 'bystander' effect was demonstrated in *in vitro* mixing experiments using retrovirally infected tumour cells, as well as in *in vivo* experiments involving tumours with only 10–20 per cent HSV*tk* expression. Complete tumour regression was noted in tumour-bearing animals treated with HSV*tk* after GCV treatment [19,22–25]. The nature of this bystander effect is complex and appears to involve passage of toxic GCV metabolites from transduced to non-transduced cells via gap junctions or apoptotic vesicles [26,27] and induction of antitumour immune responses capable of killing tumour cells not expressing the HSV*tk* transgene ('cross tolerance') [18].

HSV*tk*–GCV gene therapy for MPM: preclinical data

Initial experiments demonstrated that replication-deficient adenoviral HSV*tk* (Ad.HSV*tk*) vectors transduced mesothelioma cells in both tissue culture and animal models and facilitated HSV*tk*–mediated killing of human mesothelioma cells in the presence of low concentrations of GCV [28,29]. Subsequently, Ad.HSV*tk*–GCV gene therapy was used to treat established intraperitoneal human mesothelioma and lung cancer xenografts in immunodeficient mice [30,31], resulting in significant tumour reduction and prolongation of survival [32]. The *in vitro* and *in vivo* sensitivities of human mesothelioma cells to HSV*tk*–GCV gene therapy have been independently confirmed by other investigators [33].

Based on this efficacy data in animals, preclinical toxicity studies designed to simulate human clinical trials were conducted. Rats were given high doses of virus intrapleurally followed by intraperitoneal administration of GCV at the same dose proposed for initial use in the clinical trial (10 mg/kg/day). Toxicity was limited to localized inflammation of the pleural and pericardial surfaces. Formal toxicology studies were also done in three non-human primates given high doses of Ad.HSV*tk* (10^{12} plaque forming units (PFU)) and GCV [34]. No adverse clinical effects or any haematological or biochemical abnormalities were documented. Necropsy findings were limited to inflammatory changes in the chest wall and intrathoracic serosa.

Phase I clinical trials

A phase I clinical trial for patients with MPM began in November 1995 at the University of Pennsylvania Medical Center in conjunction with the University of Pennsylvania Institute for Human Gene Therapy. The goals of this trial were to determine the toxicity, gene transfer efficacy, and immune responses generated in response to the intrapleural instillation of Ad.HSV*tk*. The protocol was designed as a dose escalation study, starting with a vector dose of 1×10^9 PFU and increasing in half-log increments to the maximum dose level of 1×10^{12} PFU. MPM patients who met inclusion criteria, including the presence of a patent pleural space, underwent intrapleural administration of a single dose of Ad.HSV*tk* vector followed by 2 weeks of intravenous GCV at 'standard' doses of 5 mg/kg twice daily [35,36].

Table 19.3 Results of University of Pennsylvania phase I clinical trials of Ad.tk–GCV gene therapy for mesothelioma

Patient no.	Age (years)	Sex	Stage	Cell type	Vector dose (PFU)	Post-treatment survival (months)	Gene transfer	Tumour response
1[a]	62	M	IA	E	1×10^9	111	−	SD × 2 years
2	56	M	III	E	1×10^9	8[d]	−	−
3	69	M	III	B	1×10^9	20[d]	+	−
4	66	M	II	E	3.2×10^9	11[d]	−	−
5	71	M	IA	E	3.2×10^9	58[d]	−	SD × 3 years
6	71	M	II	B	1×10^{10}	4[d]	+	−
7	70	M	II	E	1×10^{10}	6[d]	−	−
8	60	M	II	E	1×10^{10}	27[d]	+	−
9	74	M	II	B	3.2×10^{10}	2[d]	NP	−
10	60	M	III	E	3.2×10^{10}	9[d]	−	−
11	37	F	IV	E	1×10^{11}	16[d]	−	−
12	37	M	III		1×10^{11}	2[d]	−	−
13	65	F	III	E	1×10^{11}	10[d]	+	−
14	66	F	IA	E	3.2×10^{11}	50[d]	+	SD × 2 years
15	60	M	IV	B	3.2×10^{11}	5[d]	+	−
16	69	M	IB	E	3.2×10^{11}	8[d]	+	−
17	70	F	IB	E	3.2×10^{11}	15[d]	+	−
18	69	F	IB	E	3.2×10^{11}	14[d]	+	−
19[b]	75	M	II	E	3.2×10^{11}	8[d]	+	−
20[b]	68	M	IV	B	3.2×10^{11}	1[d]	+	−
21[b]	71	M	IB	E	3.2×10^{11}	41[d]	+	−
22[b]	76	M	IB	E	3.2×10^{11}	33[d]	+	−
23[b]	81	M	II	E	3.2×10^{11}	25[d]	+	−
24	71	M	II	E	1×10^{12}	21[d]	+	−
25	65	M	II	E	1×10^{12}	5[d]	+	−
26	67	M	IA	E	1×10^{12}	22[d]	+	PR (CT)
27[c]	67	M	III	B	1×10^{11}	7[d]	+	−
28[c]	53	M	III	E	1×10^{11}	13[d]	+	−
29[c]	30	F	I	E	5×10^{11}	77	+	SD
30[c]	56	F	IA	E	5×10^{11}	77	+	SD
31[c]	66	M	II	E	5×10^{11}	9[d]	+	−
32[ac]	74	M	I	E	5×10^{11}	19[d]	+	PR (PET)
33[ac]	64	M	I	E	5×10^{11}	10[d]	+	−
34[ac]	69	M	II	E	5×10^{11}	28[d]	NP	−

PFU, plaque-forming unit; E, epithelioid; B, biphasic; NP, test not performed; SD, stable disease; PR, partial response.
[a]Received GCV 15 mg/kg/day for 14 days.
[b]Received adjuvant corticosteroids.
[c]Received third-generation E1/E4-deleted adenoviiral vector.
[d]Deceased.

The adenoviral vector initially used was a so-called 'first-generation' replication-incompetent virus, deleted in the early genes E1a and E3 with the HSV*tk* gene inserted in the E1a region. Participants were evaluated for evidence of toxicity, viral shedding, immune responses to the virus, and radiographic evidence of tumour response.

Twenty-six patients (21 male, five female), ranging in age from 37 to 81 years, were enrolled in the study between November 1995 and November 1997 (Table 19.3). Intratumour HSV*tk* gene transfer was documented in 17 of 25 evaluable patients in a dose-related fashion by DNA polymerase chain reaction (PCR), reverse transcription-PCR (RT-PCR), *in situ* hybridization, and immunohistochemistry (IHC) utilizing a murine monoclonal antibody directed against HSV*tk*. All patients treated at a dose of 3.2×10^{11} PFU or greater demonstrated evidence of intratumour HSV*tk* protein expression via IHC [36]. The Ad.*tk*–GCV combination was generally well tolerated, and a maximum tolerated dose was not achieved. Toxicities included reversible liver function test abnormalities, anaemia, fever, and bullous exanthema at the instillation site. At the highest dose level of 1×10^{12} PFU, two of three patients developed transitory hypotension and hypoxaemia within hours after vector instillation that resolved with supplemental oxygen and intravenous fluids [37].

Strong anti-adenoviral humoral and cellular immune responses were noted, including generation of high serum and pleural fluid titres of anti-adenoviral neutralizing antibodies, generation of serum antibodies against adenoviral structural proteins, and increased peripheral blood mononuclear cell proliferative responses to adenoviral proteins [38].

In a small pilot study five patients (patients 19–23) received intravenous corticosteroids around the time of vector instillation. This trial was designed as a preliminary assessment of the effects of immunosuppression upon the degree of intratumour gene transfer and anti-adenoviral immune responses. Decreased fever and hypoxaemia were noted in the corticosteroid-treated cohort, but there was also an increased incidence of reversible mental status changes [38]. No diminution in anti-adenoviral immune responses was demonstrated among the patients who received corticosteroids, nor were there any appreciable differences in the degree of intratumour gene transfer.

Of the 26 patients enrolled in the initial phase I trial, 25 have since died, with a median post-treatment survival of approximately 11 months (Table 19.3). One patient (patient 20) in the corticosteroid pilot study who had stage IV MPM at the time of enrolment died from rapid progression of his mesothelioma with malignant involvement of the contralateral hemithorax 2 weeks after completion of the protocol.

Several patients with stage IA–IB epithelioid MPM had post-treatment survivals of more than 3 years, with one patient surviving over 4 years. The initial patient enrolled in the trial (patient 1) remains alive with minimal residual disease over 9 years after completion of the Ad.*tk*–GCV protocol. He did have evidence of local tumour recurrence approximately 3 years after enrolment, and subsequently underwent pleurectomy–decortication followed by intraoperative photodynamic therapy. Of the trial participants who are deceased, all had progressive MPM as their primary cause of death, typically with invasion of mediastinum, contralateral hemithorax, and transdiaphragmatic extension, as well as widespread metastatic disease. Only one of the 26 patients (patient 26) had radiographic evidence of intrathoracic tumour regression post-Ad.*tk*–GCV on follow-up chest CT scan (Fig. 19.1). This patient eventually died from intraperitoneal disease progression 26 months after completion of the protocol. At autopsy there was extensive intra-abdominal tumour, but scant disease in the treated thoracic cavity.

In summary, this phase I trial demonstrated that intrapleural Ad.HSV*tk*–GCV gene therapy carried minimal toxicity, effectively delivered transgene to superficial tumour regions, and induced significant humoral and cellular responses to the Ad vector [36,37]. Improved intratu-

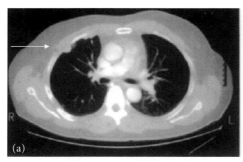 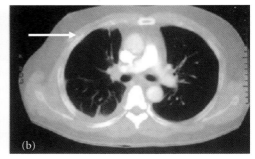

Figure 19.1 Chest CT scans (a) before and (b) 60 days after intrapleural infusion of the Ad.HSVtk vector followed by 14 days of intravenous ganciclovir (GCV) in patient 26. The pleural-based nodules seen in the anterior aspect of the right hemithorax (thin arrow in (a)) were biopsy confirmed as sarcomatoid mesothelioma prior to study entry. These nodules regressed dramatically after Ad.tk–GCV treatment (thick arrow in (b)). Patient 26 died approximately 2 years after completion of the gene therapy protocol from extensive intraperitoneal tumor, but with minimal intrathoracic disease noted on autopsy.

moral gene transfer efficacy was necessary; one option was to increase the vector dose, but doing this with the 'first generation' vector became problematic because of high levels of replication-competent adenovirus in the vector lots.

For these reasons, a phase I clinical trial employing an advanced-generation adenoviral vector containing deletions in the E1 and E4 regions with preservation of the E3 region was initiated in June 1998. The presence of an intact E4 region, unlike E3, is critical to the late phase of the viral life-cycle. E4 deletions decrease viral DNA synthesis and late gene expression. For these reason, adenoviral vectors with lethal deletions in E1 and E4 offered theoretical advantages over first-generation vectors by virtue of diminished cytopathic effects and reduced cellular immune responses [39]. In addition, since two replication-necessary genes were deleted, simple recombination could not produce replication-competent virus in the vector production process.

The primary goals of the second phase I clinical trial were to determine the toxicity, gene transfer efficiency, and immune responses associated with the intrapleural injection of high titres of the E1/E4-deleted Ad.RSV*tk* vector combined with systemic GCV. Five patients were treated under this protocol, starting at a dose 1 log lower than the highest dose used with the E1/E3-deleted Ad vector (1.5×10^{13} viral particles). There was minimal toxicity, primarily transitory fever (grade 1), in the two patients treated at this lower dose. The next three patients were treated with a dose of 5.0×10^{13} viral particles with evidence of increased, but non-dose-limiting, toxicity. All three patients experienced acute febrile responses (grade 1) after vector instillation, with rapid defervescence. One patient (patient 29) developed hypotension and hypoxaemia (grade 2) within hours of vector administration that resolved with supplemental oxygen and intravenous fluids. This patient also developed elevated serum transaminases (NCI grade 2) after vector delivery, peaking during the first week of GCV administration but returning to normal levels by completion of the protocol. The patient had no associated elevations in serum bilirubin or prothrombin time, and no clinical evidence of hepatic dysfunction. The third patient treated at the higher dose level (patient 31) developed low-grade fever (grade 1) after intrapleural vector instillation, as well as contralateral pleural inflammation. Overall, there appeared to be a trend towards lower hepatoxicity in the patients treated with the E1/E4-deleted vector than in patients treated with equivalent doses of the E1/E3-deleted adenovirus, but with a similar pattern of increased systemic side effects at higher dose levels [40].

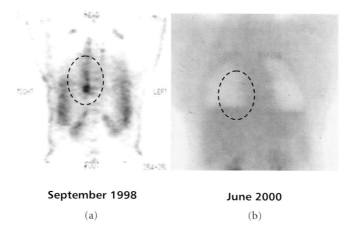

September 1998   June 2000

(a)   (b)

Figure 19.2 [18]FDG-PET scan response to Ad.RSVtk–GCV gene therapy. One of the eight patients enrolled in E1/E4-deleted vector protocols (patient 29) had objective evidence of tumour response on pre- and post-gene therapy [18]FDG-PET imaging, with almost complete absence of FDG uptake on an FDG-PET scan performed 18 months after completion of the protocol (see above). This objective metabolic response correlated with her excellent clinical status and stability on serial chest CT scans. The patient had no antineoplastic therapy other than our gene therapy protocol. A repeat PET scan performed in October 2003 showed a small area of new metabolic activity along the right hemi-diaphragm, but the patient has declined biopsy as she remains asymptomatic.

Dose-related gene transfer was detected via immunohistochemistry using an anti- HSV*tk* monoclonal antibody in all patients at both dose levels. As in the initial phase I trial, significant humoral responses to the recombinant adenoviral vector were seen in all five patients, with the development of high serum titres of total and neutralizing anti-adenoviral antibodies within 15–20 days of vector instillation [40].

Of the five patients treated in this second phase I trial, two are surviving (patients 29 and 30), both of whom were treated at the higher dose level of 5.0×10^{13} particles of Ad.HSV*tk* (Table 19.3). Each of these patients had stage I epithelioid MPM at diagnosis. Remarkably, both have clinically and radiographic evidence of minimal residual disease without other interceding antineoplastic therapy for more than 6 years after completion of the Ad.*tk*–GCV protocol. Patient 29 demonstrated diminished tumour metabolic activity on serial follow-up 18-fluordeoxyglucose positron emission tomography ([18]FDG-PET) scans (Fig. 19.2). This delayed decrease in tumour metabolic activity several months after completion of the gene therapy protocol suggests that a secondary immune bystander effect was induced by Ad.RSV*tk*–GCV [40]. Patient 29 had evidence of possible focal tumour recurrence/progression at a new anatomical location along the mid-portion of the right hemidiaphragm on repeat PET scan performed in October 2003. However, she has deferred any biopsy or resection of this lesion as she remains generally asymptomatic. Patient 30 recently had evidence of focal tumour recurrence at an old left-sided thoracostomy tube site, which was treated with excisional biopsy only. She also refused additional therapy (chemotherapy or radiation) because she was otherwise feeling well.

Based upon *in vitro* and animal experiments in mesothelioma models demonstrating a direct correlation between GCV dose and cytotoxic response after tumour transduction with HSV*tk*, a further phase I clinical trial was initiated involving gradual dose escalation of GCV in combination with intrapleural delivery of the E1/E4-deleted Ad vector [31,36,41–43]. Each of the first cohort of three patients was treated with 3.0×10^{13} particles of Ad.RSVtk (E1/E4-deleted) and 7.5 mg/kg GCV intravenously twice daily (15 mg/kg/day). All three patients tolerated the treatment well. Toxicities were non-dose-limiting, and included fever, lymphopenia, liver function test abnormalities, hyponatraemia, and hypokalaemia. No durable clinical responses were noted in any of the three patients treated with this protocol, although the initial patient treated (patient 101) demonstrated reduced ^{18}FDG uptake in the mediastinal and parietal pleural regions on his post-treatment scan. However, subsequent ^{18}FDG-PET scanning at day 170 showed significant increase in tracer uptake consistent with increased tumour metabolic activity. This correlated with the patient's increasing clinical symptoms and progressive pleural thickening and nodularity on repeat chest CT scan. Patients 102 and 103 both demonstrated increased ^{18}FDG uptake on their follow-up PET studies on day 80, and also had clear evidence of progression on chest CT.

Challenges and future directions

Based on acceptable toxicity, successful gene transfer, and anecdotal tumour responses, Ad.HSVtk–GCV 'suicide gene' therapy shows promise for future treatment of MPM as well as other localized malignancies. Unfortunately, these phase I trials were halted in midstream because of the death of a participant in an unrelated gene transfer clinical trial for ornithine transcarbamylase deficiency at the University of Pennsylvania Medical Center involving intrahepatic artery infusion of an adenoviral vector with a similar backbone [7].

The initial Ad.HSVtk–GCV strategy carried significant limitations, particularly that therapeutic efficacy could only be expected in patients with relatively small tumour burdens. An alternative approach would be to maximize the ratio of vector to tumour cell by surgical 'debulking' to minimize tumour mass, followed by adjuvant administration of Ad.HSVtk–GCV. Another method of improving efficiency of intratumour gene transfer would be repeated administration of vector and GCV (i.e. three doses over a 3 week period). Studies in immunocompetent mice with established peritoneal tumours [8,9] demonstrated marked increases in efficacy after multiple intraperitoneal injections of Ad.HSVtk, each followed by a course of GCV. Importantly, data from the initial clinical trials suggest that gene transfer is possible even in patients with titres of anti-Ad neutralizing antibodies of up to 1:500, as would be expected with repeated administration of Ad vector.

Another approach to the gene transfer problem is to maximize the efficacy of the expressed HSVtk enzyme. One intriguing aspect of the HSVtk suicide gene schema is that, compared with mammalian cellular kinases, the herpes simplex thymidine kinase 1 enzyme has a relaxed specificity that allows it to phosphorylate not only thymidine, but other nucleoside analogues such as GCV and aciclovir (ACV). Unfortunately, HSVtk has a high affinity for thymidine ($K_m = 0.5\ \mu M$), whereas the affinities for GCV ($K_m = 45\ \mu M$) and ACV ($K_m \geq 400\ \mu M$) are much lower. 'Molecular remodelling' of the HSVtk enzyme engendered increased specificity for GCV and ACV and concomitantly decreased thymidine utilization [10]. These HSVtk mutants show increased ACV- and GCV-mediated cytotoxicity, and enhanced bystander effects in mixing experiments [7,11]. Adenoviral vectors containing mutated HSVtk demonstrated enhanced cell killing and augmented bystander effect in *in vitro* and *in vivo* models of mesothelioma [44]

An additional mechanism of maximizing intratumour gene transfer would involve the use of HSVtk-bearing adenoviral vectors capable of selective replication in mesothelioma cells. In this system, tumour killing could occur via two mechanisms: direct tumour lysis due to viral replication, and HSVtk-mediated killing after administration of GCV. Widespread dissemination would be precluded by the intact host immune response [45]. Tumour-selective replicating Ad.HSVtk vectors have been developed by substituting the adenoviral E1 promoter with promoters for tumour-related proteins such as manganese superoxide dismutase (MnSOD), calretinin, and mesothelin [46]. Recent work by Kinnula's group in Finland elucidated the fact that MnSOD is highly expressed in human malignant mesothelioma explants and cell lines [47]. Calretinin is a 29 kDa calcium-binding protein that is expressed primarily in the nervous system, but high levels of expression have also been noted in cells of mesothelial origin [48,49]. Mesothelin is a 40 kDa surface protein of unknown function that is expressed only on the mesodermal-derived tissues forming the pleural, pericardial, and peritoneal membranes [50]. Other more general tumour-selective promoters, such as those responsive to the transcription factor E2F [46] or the survivin gene [51], would also be potential candidates to drive mesothelioma-selective adenoviral vectors.

Suicide gene vaccines

A growing body of evidence supports the hypothesis that treatment with HSV*tk*–GCV results in an immunological bystander effect that enhances antitumour cytotoxicity both at the site of vector delivery and at distant non-transduced tumour sites [18,25,52–54]. One example of this immune bystander effect may have been the progressive decline in tumour metabolic activity seen on the post-treatment PET scan in patient 29 in our phase I mesothelioma clinical trials. This putative antitumour immune reaction may result from non-apoptotic HSV*tk*–GCV-mediated tumour necrosis, a type of cell death that releases so-called 'danger signals' which then activate significant cellular immune responses [54,55]. Generation of these 'danger signals' may be enhanced by transduction of tumour cells with the HSV*tk* gene plus a cytokine gene such as the gene for interleukin 2 (IL-2). Augmented tumour cytotoxicty has been reported with HSV*tk* plus IL-2 in murine models of colon carcinoma, squamous cell carcinoma, and melanoma [56–59]. Current *in vivo* studies in murine mesothelioma models aim to determine the optimal combination of cytokines with HSV*tk*.

This method of destroying mesothelioma tumours via the immunological bystander effects of HSV*tk*–GCV gene therapy, a presumptive 'suicide gene vaccine', was studied in a phase I clinical trial conducted by Schwarzenberger's group at the Louisiana State University (LSU) Medical Center in New Orleans (Table 19.2). The protocol designed by the LSU investigators consisted of intrapleural instillation, via an indwelling pleural catheter, of an irradiated ovarian carcinoma cell line retrovirally transfected with HSV*tk* (PA1-STK cells), followed by systemic administration of GCV [21]. Schwarzenberger and colleagues hypothesized that the the PA-1-STK cells would migrate to areas of intrapleural tumour after instillation, undergo necrotic cell death after exposure to GCV, and generate immune responses that would facilitate killing of adjacent mesothelioma cells. The LSU group performed *in vitro* mixing experiments showing that PA-1-STK cells, in combination with GCV, killed both mouse and human mesothelioma cells in a dose-dependent manner. In syngeneic murine models of mesothelioma, administration of PA-1-STK cells with GCV prolonged survival when the percentage of transduced tumour cells was high (70 per cent), but there was no survival benefit when the percentage of PA-1-STK cells was low (30 per cent) [60].

Anti-mesothelioma immune responses in this system are related to the local generation of pro-inflammatory cytokines which, in turn, summon an influx of cytotoxic lymphocytes to the area producing haemorrhagic tumour necrosis [21,61]. Minimal side effects have been seen in patients treated to date, while preliminary findings showed significant post-treatment increases in the percentage of CD8 T lymphocytes in pleural fluid [61].

The LSU investigators have also demonstrated that PA-1-STK cells home to mesothelioma deposits in patients after intrapleural instillation. They performed a substudy in which the gene-modified ovarian cancer cells expressing the thymidine kinase gene (PA1-STK) were radiolabelled with technetium-99 and infused into the pleural space of four patients with malignant pleural mesothelioma. The patients were then scanned to determine the distribution of the cells.

PA-1-STK cells recognized and adhered preferentially to MPM lining the chest wall, confirming the feasibility of this treatment concept [62].

Cytokine gene therapy for mesothelioma

There has been significant interest in the delivery of genes encoding for pro-inflammatory cytokines to the pleural space of patients with MPM. One of the rationales for cytokine gene therapy is that exogenous cytokines are known to have direct antiproliferative effects upon mesothelioma cells, as well as the ability to activate intrapleural and intratumoral immune effector cells *in vivo*. Expression of cytokine genes by tumour cells generates a high intratumour level of cytokines in an autocrine and paracrine fashion, inducing powerful local cytokine effects without significant systemic toxicity. Prolonged local cytokine expression can induce activation of tumour-associated dendritic cells (DCs) to express MHC–tumour antigen complexes in conjunction with co-stimulatory molecules. These activated DCs can then migrate to regional lymph nodes where they stimulate proliferation of tumour-specific CD8 and CD4 lymphocytes, inducing antitumour cytotoxicity at distant tumour sites. In addition, some pro-inflammatory cytokines such as IL-2 have the capability of direct intratumour activation of CD8+ tumour infiltrating lymphocytes, overcoming tolerance signals to produce tumour-specific cytotoxic T lymphocytes. Increased intratumour IL-2 may also activate natural killer (NK) cells and lymphokine-activated killer (LAK) cells. Animal experiments have shown that injection of IL-2-transduced tumour cells increases specific antitumour activity, generates systemic responses to the parental tumour, augments the immune response against autologous tumour, and causes rejection of rechallenged tumour cells [63,64].

Several published phase I and phase II human clinical trials have documented MPM responses to intrapleural infusion of IL-2, interferon β (IFN-β), and interferon γ (IFN-γ) [65–71]. In particular, Boutin's group at the Hôpital de la Conçeption, Marseille, France, demonstrated significant response rates in MPM after intrapleural instillation of IFN-γ, including several complete pathological responses in patients with stage IA disease (tumour limited to the parietal and diaphragmatic pleura) [68,69].

The first human clinical trial of direct intratumoral delivery of cytokine genes in MPM using this method of *in vivo* genetic immunotherapy was conducted by investigators at Queen Elizabeth II Hospital, Perth, Australia, using a recombinant vaccinia virus (VV) expressing the human IL-2 gene (Table 19.2). A vaccinia vector was chosen because of its large genome and proven safety in human vaccines, and the availability of anti-VV antibodies for evaluation of vector-induced immune responses. In addition, insertion of the IL-2 gene into the thymidine kinase region of the VV rendered it partially replication restricted, allowing relatively more expression in tumour cells. The VV-IL-2 vector was serially injected at a dose of 1×10^7 PFU into palpable chest wall lesions of six patients with advanced MPM. Toxicities were minimal, and there was no clinical or serological evidence of spread of VV to patient contacts. No significant tumour regression was seen in any of the patients, and only modest intratumour T-cell infiltration was detected. VV-IL-2 mRNA was detected by RT-PCR in serial tumour biopsies for up to 6 days after injection, but declined to low levels by day 8. The prolonged nature of IL-2 gene expression in this trial was remarkable considering the fact that significant serum titres of anti-VV neutralizing antibodies were generated in all patients [72].

The use of cellular vectors to deliver the IL-2 gene in patients with pleural mesothelioma has also been studied in a phase II European clinical trial sponsored by Transgene Inc. (Strasburg, France). Mertelsmann and colleagues in Freiburg, Germany, are conducting a phase II randomized study of non-specific immunotherapy of malignant mesothelioma by repeated intratumoral injection of 'Vero cells' engineered to produce human IL-2 (Vero-IL2). Vero cells are immortalized monkey fibroblasts capable of constitutive expression of therapeutic human proteins such as inflammatory cytokines. They can be grown in culture, packaged in vials, tested for quality, stored, and administered to the patient like a standard medicinal product. Transgene Inc. has engineered Vero cells to secrete very high levels of human IL2 or other cytokines including IFN-γ. The first two MPM patients in this study were enrolled in March 1999 with a total planned enrolment of 20 patients. This phase II trial was based upon earlier animal studies demonstrating the efficacy of Vero-IL-2 therapy in the treatment of spontaneously occurring tumours, as well as two phase I clinical trials completed in France and Switzerland documenting the safety of this product in human subjects and preliminary evidence of antitumour activity [73].

The future of genetic immunotherapy for mesothelioma

Several other candidate cytokine genes are being evaluated for therapeutic effectiveness in animal models of mesothelioma. Caminschi's group at the Queen Elizabeth II Medical Center, Perth, Australia, investigated genetic alteration of murine mesothelioma cell lines with the gene for IL-12, one of the most active immunomodulatory cytokines. The same group previously demonstrated that systemic administration of exogenous IL-12 induced strong antitumour immune responses in mice bearing syngeneic mesothelioma tumours [74]. They showed that injection of murine mesothelioma cells transfected with the IL-12 gene (AB1-IL-12) did not produce tumours in immune-competent mice, but did so in athymic nude mice, implicating a T-cell-dependent mechanism of IL-12 activity. Immune competent mice challenged with AB1-IL-12 were protected from subsequent challenge with parental tumour not expressing IL-12, demonstrating induction of long-term immunity. In addition, AB1-IL-12 injection reduced the incidence of tumour development from parental cell challenge at a distant site [75].

Non-specific immune stimulation

Innate and adaptive antitumour immune responses can also be elicited by targeted expression of non-specific immunostimulatory genes. As an example of this paradigm, Lukacs et al. [76] delivered a mycobacterial heat shock protein gene (HSP-65) via cationic liposomes into the abdominal cavities of mice bearing intraperitoneal sarcomas, resulting in significant antitumour responses. The rationale for the in vivo efficacy of HSP-65 gene transfer was that heat shock proteins expressed in tumour cells could serve as 'molecular chaperones', facilitating more efficient tumour antigen presentation via MHC molecules. Lanuti et al. [77] found that the antitumour effects of HSP-65 gene transfer via cationic liposomes could be reproduced in an immunocompetent murine mesothelioma model, but appeared to be related to non-specific effects of lipid–pDNA complexes. Significant survival advantages compared with saline control were observed with plasmid delivery of HSP-65, the E.coli β-galactosidase marker gene lacZ, and a null vector. There was no survival benefit for heat shock gene transfer compared with instillation of the null vector alone. Lanuti and colleagues postulated that the unmethylated CpG motifs of the prokaryotic DNA in the null vector were sufficient to activate 'danger signals' and initiate innate and adaptive antitumour immune responses.

These findings were similar to those of Lukacs et al. [78] in their study of intraperitoneal delivery of the β-gal gene into immunocompetent mice bearing intraperitoneal mesotheliomas. Transfection of tumour cells with plasmid–liposome complexes or replication-incompetent retroviruses (with and without liposomes) encoding for β-gal engendered significant reduction in intraperitoneal mesothelioma burden in immunocompetent, but not immunodeficient, mice. Although the retrovirus–liposome constructs provided the greatest β-gal expression, there was no correlation with superior antitumour response. Lukacs and colleagues reported the generation of tumour-specific cytotoxic T lymphocytes in mice treated with intraperitoneal β-gal–plasmid–liposome complexes. Therefore the antitumour effect induced by intratumour expression of bacterial antigen is probably T-cell mediated.

Rudginsky et al. [79] further explored the potential of prokaryotic DNA induction in in vivo mesothelioma models. They conducted a series of experiments demonstrating antitumour responses and increased survival with liposomal delivery of fragments of bacterial plasmid DNA, genomic E.coli DNA, and synthetic CpG oligonucleotides. No increased survival or tumour reductions were seen with liposomal delivery of eukaryotic DNA or with methylated bacterial DNA. Therefore the unmethylated CpG motifs of prokaryotic DNA play a crucial role in the development of innate and adaptive antitumour immune responses. Intraperitoneal lavage after liposomal delivery revealed elevations in the pro-inflammatory cytokines TNF-α and IL-12 only, with those complexes inducing antitumour immunity.

Therefore, based upon the Lanuti, Lukacs, and Rudginsky experiences, there is a rationale for a phase I clinical trial of intrapleural delivery of lipid–prokaryotic DNA complexes in patients with mesothelioma (Table 19.2).

Interferon-β gene therapy

As previously mentioned, the type I (α, β) and type II (γ) interferons have demonstrable antitumour activity when administered exogenously to patients with MPM. For example, IFN-β has potent antiproliferative effects on mesothelioma cells in vitro and strong immunostimulatory actions in animal models, but is limited in clinical use by toxicity of systemic administration [80]. Therefore Odaka's group at the University of Pennsylvania Medical Center investigated the effects of IFN-β gene therapy in murine models of mesothelioma. These investigators showed that a single intraperitoneal injection of a recombinant adenovirus engineered to express the murine IFN-β gene (Ad.muIFN-β) eradicated syngeneic murine mesothelioma in the vast majority of animals tested. Intraperitoneal Ad.muIFN-β gene therapy also resulted in significant reduction in the size of distant subcutaneous tumours. Odaka et al. [81] showed that these effects of Ad.muIFN-β were mediated by CD8+ T lymphocytes.

Based on these results, investigators at the University of Pennsylvania Medical Center, in conjunction with Biogen-IDEC Corporation, recently initiated a phase I trial of Ad.huIFN-β (BG00001) in patients with MPM as well as in metastatic pleural tumours (Table 19.2). To date, nine patients have undergone intrapleural infusion of a single dose of Ad.IFN-β at two dose levels after pretreatment leucophoresis. Six patients had mesothelioma, two had metastatic non-small-cell lung cancer, and the other had metastatic ovarian cancer. The first three patients received 9×10^{11} viral particles of Ad.IFN-β. They all tolerated dosing with mild to moderate toxicities (NCI grade 1–2). None of the patients experienced a dose-limiting toxicity or a serious adverse event. Lymphopenia was the most common toxicity seen in two of three patients. The other toxicities included chest pain, coyrza, fever, anaemia, and elevated liver enzymes. Two of three patients in the first cohort are still alive up to 16 months after receiving the vector.

Four patients with MPM were enrolled at dose level 2 (3×10^{12} viral particles). One patient experienced an episode of transient hypoxia (grade 3) approximately 11 h after dosing but rapidly recovered to baseline. This patient has now completed 6 months of evaluations without any further complications. The next two patients at dose level 2 tolerated dosing well and have completed their 2 month evaluations. Both are doing well clinically but have had evidence of progressive disease. The fourth patient treated at dose level 2 developed grade 3 elevations in liver function tests (LFTs) without clinical evidence of hepatic dysfunction. These LFT elevations gradually decreased to baseline levels over a period of several months. Subsequently, as per protocol, two additional patients have been dosed at dose level 1 (9×10^{11} viral particles) without evidence of serious adverse events.

Eight of the nine patients dosed to date with IPl Ad.IFN-β have undergone repeat imaging studies 60 days after discharge. Two of three patients at dose level 1 and two of four patients at dose level 2 had interval disease progression at the 60 day time point. The other two patients in dose level 2 had stable disease on CT scan at 60 days, one of whom had evidence of a delayed partial response on ^{18}FDG-PET scan at 180 days. An additional patient with metastatic epithelial ovarian carcinoma had a complete metabolic response of her pleural malignancy at 60 days, although her abdominal tumour ultimately progressed. Repeat CT scan of the chest and abdomen at 10 months, after several months of therapy with the anti-vascular endothelial growth factor monoclonal antibody bevacizumab (Avastin®), demonstrated continued regression of the intrathoracic tumour, interim resolution of intra-abdominal ascites, and decreased size of intraperitoneal tumour nodules. A 68-year-old male with sarcomatoid mesothelioma who was treated at dose level 1 (9×10^{11} viral particles), after this was established as the maximum tolerated dose, had evidence of partial anatomical and metabolic responses on CT and PET scanning at day 60 after Ad.IFN-β infusion

Current efforts in the Thoracic Oncology Research Laboratory, University of Pennsylvania Medical Center, are focused on augmenting the response to immuno-gene therapy. Marked augmentation of efficacy has been obtained with combinations including Ad.IFN-β plus COX-2 inhibition, surgical debulking, vascular disruptive agents, and neoadjuvant chemotherapy with cisplatin and gemcitabine. These approaches will be incorporated in future human clinical trials.

Induction of apoptosis

One of the primary cancer gene therapy approaches has been mutation compensation—the replacement of absent or mutated tumour suppressor genes responsible for the malignant phenotype of the cancer cell. Intratumour delivery of the wild-type p53 gene has been the most widely utilized schema of experimental cancer gene therapy, as mutations in the p53 tumour suppressor gene account for the majority of genetic abnormalities in solid tumours. However, most MPMs contain wild-type p53 and a normal copy of the cell cycle regulator pRB. The most common molecular abnormality found in MPM is absent expression of the cyclin-dependent kinase (cdk) inhibitor, p16^{INK4a}. This mutation results in unmitigated progression through the cell cycle despite the presence of normal pRB expression and wild-type p53, and therefore can engender a neoplastic phenotype [82].

Kratzke's group at the University of Minnesota School of Medicine have demonstrated that re-expression of p16^{INK4a} in mesothelioma cells *in vitro* and *in vivo* results in cell cycle arrest, cell growth inhibition, apoptosis, and tumour reduction [83]. In addition, the Minnesota investigators have shown that repeated administration of an Ad vector expressing wild-type p16^{INK4a} into established human mesothelioma xenografts in athymic nude mice resulted in prolongation of survival compared with controls [82]. Successful application of this technology to human clinical trials is dependent upon the development of more efficient means of tumour cell transduction.

Jablons' group at the Thoracic Oncology Laboratory, University of California at San Francisco (UCSF), targeted another common MPM mutation for mutation compensation gene therapy, homozygous deletion of the INK4a/ARF locus. The p14(ARF) protein encoded by the INK4a/ARF locus promotes degradation of the MDM2 protein and thus prevents the MDM2-mediated inhibition of p53. Therefore deletion of the INK4a/ARF locus abrogates p14(ARF) protein expression, thereby inactivating p53, via MDM2, leading to unchecked progression through the cell cycle. The UCSF group transfected human mesothelioma cell lines *in vitro* with an Ad vector encoding for human p14(ARF) complementary DNA (Ad.p14). Over-expression of p14(ARF) within the mesothelioma cells led to increased intracellular levels of p53 and p21, as well as dephosphorylation of pRb. In addition, Ad.p14 inhibited mesothelioma cell growth via induction of G_1-phase cell cycle arrest and apoptotic cell death. This gene therapy approach has not yet been tested in human clinical trials [84].

Jablons and colleagues also investigated the efficacy of the ONYX-015 adenovirus in mesothelioma cells and found that the cytolytic effect of this agent in mesothelioma is dependent upon absence of p14(ARF) expression. ONYX-015 is a conditionally replication competent adenovirus lacking the E1b 55 kDa gene, the product of which can bind and inactivate wild-type p53. Therefore ONYX-015 is theoretically replication restricted to tumour cells lacking functional p53. Clinical trials of ONYX-015 in patients with head and neck cancer and lung cancer have demonstrated preliminary evidence of tumour responses with minimal toxicity. In MPM, unlike most other solid tumours, genetic alterations in p53 are uncommon, but functional inhibition of p53 can be achieved via deletions in the INK4a/ARF locus. Jablons and colleagues demonstrated *in vitro* cytotoxicity of ONYX-015 on mesothelioma cell lines lacking p14(ARF), and increased resistance of these same cell lines to ONYX-015 after transfection of the tumour cells with Ad.p14 [85].

Despite the fact that most mesotheliomas contain wild-type p53 (wt-p53), the function of p53 in mesothelioma cells may be abnormal secondary to p53 binding by inhibitor proteins such as MDM-2 and SV40 large T antigen (Tag). Therefore there may be a rationale for gene therapy of mesothelioma via overexpression of wt-p53 within the cell. Giuliano *et al.* [86] performed a series of experiments involving transfection of human mesothelioma cells with a replication-deficient Ad.wt-p53 vector. They demonstrated significant inhibition of tumour cell growth *in vitro* with documentation of apoptosis induction in the dying tumour cells. In addition, they showed that *ex vivo* transfer of the wt-p53 gene to mesothelioma cells inhibited growth of tumour implants in nude mice. Intratumoral injection of the wt-p53 gene inhibited tumour growth and prolonged survival in immunodeficient mice with established human mesothelioma xenografts. Therefore it may be reasonable to propose human clinical trials of Ad.wt-p53 gene therapy in mesothelioma akin to those conducted in lung cancer, head and neck cancer, and metastatic colon cancer (Table 19.2).

An alternative method of inhibiting mesothelioma cells is the introduction of 'downstream' promoters of apoptosis such as the pro-apoptotic Bcl-2 family member Bak. Pataer's group at the M.D. Anderson Cancer Center, Houston, co-delivered binary adenoviral-Bak/GV-16 vectors into wt-p53 positive and mutated p53 mesothelioma cell lines *in vitro*, along with binary Ad.*lacZ*/GV-16 control vectors [87]. They demonstrated marked induction of apoptosis and decreased cellular viability in both p53 'sensitive' and 'resistant' cell lines with Bak gene transfer, but not with *lacZ* delivery. Thus gene transfer *in vivo* with pro-apoptotic Bcl-2 family members would be a reasonable strategy for future mesothelioma gene therapy clinical trials, if hurdles surrounding transduction efficiency could be surmounted.

Simian virus 40: has it a role in therapy for mesothelioma?

One of the most remarkable and controversial developments in mesothelioma research in recent years has been the identification of simian virus 40 (SV40) sequences in mesothelioma tumour specimens from the USA and several European countries. SV40, a non-human polyomavirus which was a contaminant of some poliovaccines in the 1950s and 1960s, has the ability to transform normal cells via the oncogenic properties of its large T antigen (Tag), and can induce the formation of mesotheliomas in hamsters after injection into the pleural space or peritoneal cavity [88]. Laboratory analysis of a subset of human mesotheliomas has demonstrated co-immuno-precipitation of SV40 Tag with tumour suppressor gene products such as the p53 and pRB proteins [89]. The presence of SV40 Tag within tumour cells binding and inactivating wild-type p53 and pRB may explain the unusually high rate of wild-type p53 and pRb within mesotheliomas, unlike most other solid tumours.

The potential role for SV40 as a causative factor in mesothelioma carcinogenesis has elicited several new experimental gene therapy approaches. Schrump and Waheed [90], at the National Cancer Institute, demonstrated that antisense oligonucleotides directed against SV40 Tag mRNA induce apoptosis and enhance sensitivity to chemotherapeutic agents in SV40(+) mesothelioma cells *in vitro*. Imperiale *et al.* [91], at the University of Michigan and Wayne State University Medical Centers, proffered an alternative strategy involving a genetically engineered vaccine to SV40 Tag. SV40 is an ideal candidate for antigen-specific immunotherapy because Tag is a viral antigen which, unlike most other tumour-associated antigens, should not induce immune tolerance. Imperiale and colleagues devised a recombinant truncated version of Tag (mTag) modified to exclude regions with oncogenic function (the J domain and the p53–pRB binding domains). They cloned the mTag gene into a vaccinia vector (vac-mTag) and demonstrated significant antitumour immune responses in Balb/c mice bearing Tag(+) tumours. A phase I dose-escalation safety and toxicity trial in patients with Tag-expressing mesotheliomas is planned (Table 19.2).

Summary

Gene therapy for mesothelioma remains in its infancy, nonetheless, novel preclinical studies and ongoing phase I trials offer significant hope for the future. Both intrapleural and intratumoral injections of viral vectors carrying various therapeutic genes have proved safe in humans, with evidence of intratumoral gene transfer and anecdotal tumour responses. Expanding knowledge of the molecular abnormalities responsible for mesothelioma carcinogenesis facilitated the development of gene therapy modalities targeting specific oncoproteins and mutant tumour suppressor genes. Implementation of these gene therapy approaches as part of standard medical care for mesothelioma patients remains several years from actuality. Nevertheless, the marginal benefit seen from standard anticancer treatments in mesothelioma argues strongly for continued patient enrolment in clinical studies of various experimental approaches, including gene therapy trials, to determine safety, toxicity, and efficacy, as well as to guide future laboratory investigation.

Acknowledgements

The HSV TK and interferon β studies were supported by Grant P01 CA66726 from the National Cancer Institute and Grant MO1-RR00040 to the General Clinical Research Center of the University of Pennsylvania Medical Center, as well as by the BiogenIDEC Corporation, the National Gene Vector Laboratories, the Nicolette Asbestos Trust, the Benjamin Shein Foundation for Humanity, the Edward J. Walton Jr Fund, and the Samuel H. Lunenfeld Charitable Foundation. Institutional support was provided by the Abramson Cancer Center of the University of Pennsylvania.

References

1. Sterman D, Kaiser L, Albelda S. Advances in the treatment of malignant pleural mesothelioma. *Chest* 1999; **116**: 504–20.
2. Rusch V. Trials in malignant mesothelioma. LCSG 851 and 882. *Chest* 1994; **106**: 359S–62S.
3. Rusch V. Pleurectomy/decortication and adjuvant therapy for malignant mesothelioma. *Chest* 1993; **103**: 382S–4S.

4. Martini N, McCormack PM, Bains MS, Kaiser LR, Burt ME, Hilaris BS. Pleural mesothelioma. *Ann Thorac Surg* 1987; **43**: 113–20.

5. Rusch VW, Figlin R, Godwin D, Piantadosi S. Intrapleural cisplatin and cytarabine in the management of malignant pleural effusions: a Lung Cancer Study Group trial. *J Clin Oncol* 1991; **9**: 313–19.

6. Vogelzang NJ, Rusthoven JJ, Symanowski J, *et al.* Phase III study of pemetrexed in combination with cisplatin versus cisplatin alone in patients with malignant pleural mesothelioma. *J Clin Oncol.* 2003; **21**: 2636–44.

7. Carmen IH. A death in the laboratory: the politics of the Gelsinger aftermath. *Mol Ther* 2001; **3**: 425–8.

8. Lambright ES, Force SD, Lanuti ME, *et al.* Efficacy of repeated adenoviral suicide gene therapy in a localized murine tumor model. *Ann Thorac Surg.* 2000; **70**: 1865–71.

9. Al-Hendry A., Magliocco AM, Al-Tweigeri T, *et al.* Ovarian cancer gene therapy: repeated treatment with thymidine kinase in an adenovirus vector and ganciclovir improves survival in a novel immunocompetent murine model. *Am J Obstet Gynecol* 2000; **182**: 553–9.

10. Black ME, Newcomb TG, Wilson HMP, Loeb LA. Creation of drug-specific herpes simplex virus type 1 thymidine kinase mutants for gene therapy. *Proc Natl Acad Sci USA* 1996; **93**: 3525–9.

11. Qiao J, Chen SH, Pham-Nguyen KB, Mandell J, Woo SL. Construction and characterization of a recombinant adenoviral vector expressing human interleukin-12. *Cancer Gene Ther* 1999; **6**: 373–9.

12. Robinson BW, Mukherjee SA, Davidson A, *et al.* Cytokine gene therapy or infusion as treatment for solid human cancer. *J Immunother* 1998; **21**: 211–17.

13. Tiberghien P. Use of suicide genes in gene therapy. *J Leukoc Biol* 1994; **56**: 203–9.

14. Huber BE, Austin EA, Richards CA, Davis ST, Good SS. Metabolism of 5-fluorocytosine to 5-fluorouracil in human colorectal tumor cells transduced with the cytosine deaminase gene: significant antitumor effects when only a small percentage of tumor cells express cytosine deaminase. *Proc Natl Acad Sci USA* 1994; **91**: 8302–6.

15. Hoganson DK, Batra RK, Olsen JC, Boucher RC. Comparison of the effects of three different toxin genes and their levels of expression on cell growth and bystander effect in lung adenocarcinoma. *Cancer Res* 1996; **56**: 1315–23.

16. Matthews T, Boehme R. Antiviral activity and mechanism of action of ganciclovir. *Rev Infect Dis* 1988; **10**: S490–4.

17. Rubsam LZ, Davidson BL, Shewach DS. Superior cytotoxicity with ganciclovir compared with acyclovir and 1-b-D-arabinofuranosylthymine in herpes simplex virus-thymidine kinase expressing cells: a novel paradigm for cell killing. *Cancer Res* 1998; **58**: 3873–82.

18. Pope IM, Poston GJ, Kinsella AR. The role of the bystander effect in suicide gene therapy. *Eur J Cancer* 1997; **33**: 1005–16.

19. Moolten FL, Wells JM, Mroz PJ. Multiple transduction as a means of preserving ganciclovir chemosensitivity in sarcoma cells carrying retrovirally transduced herpes thymidine kinase genes. *Cancer Lett* 1992; **64**: 257–63.

20. Treat J, Kaiser LR, Sterman DH, *et al.* Treatment of advanced mesothelioma with the recombinant adenovirus H5.010RSVTK: a phase 1 trial (BB-IND 6274). *Hum Gene Ther* 1996; **7**: 2047–57.

21. Schwarzenberger P, Harrison L, Weinacker A, *et al.* Gene therapy for malignant mesothelioma: a novel approach for an incurable cancer with increased incidence in Louisiana. *J La State Med Soc* 1998; **150**: 168–74.

22. Ram Z, Culver KW, Walbridge B, Blaese RM, Oldfield EH. In situ retroviral-mediated gene transfer for the treatment of brain tumors in rats. *Cancer Res* 1993; **53**: 83–8.

23. Freeman SM, Abboud CN, Whartenby KA, *et al.* The 'bystander effect': tumor regression when a fraction of the tumor mass is genetically modified. *Cancer Res* 1993; **53**: 5274–83.

24. Hasegawa Y, Emi N, Shimokata K, *et al.* Gene transfer of herpes simplex virus type I thymidine kinase gene as a drug sensitivity gene into human lung cancer lines using retroviral vectors. *Am J Respir Cell Mol Biol* 1993; **8**: 655–61.

25. Caruso M, Panis Y, Gagandeep S, Houssin D, Salzmann JL, Klatzmann D. Regression of established macroscopic liver metastases after in situ transduction of a suicide gene. *Proc Natl Acad Sci USA* 1993; **90**: 7024–8.

26. Elshami AA, Saavedra A, Zhang HB, *et al*. Gap junctions play a role in the bystander effect of the herpes simplex virus thymidine kinase/ganciclovir system *in vitro*. *Gene Ther* 1996; **3**: 85–92.

27. Mesnil M, Yamasaki H. Bystander effect in herpes simples virus-thymidine kinase/ganciclovir cancer gene therapy: role of gap-junctional intercellular communication. *Cancer Res* 2000; **60**: 3989–99.

28. Smythe WR, Hwang HC, Amin KM, *et al*. Use of recombinant adenovirus to transfer the herpes simplex virus thymidine kinase (HSV*tk*) gene to thoracic neoplasms: an effective *in vitro* drug sensitization system. *Cancer Res* 1994; **54**: 2055–9.

29. Smythe WR, Kaiser LR, Amin KM, *et al*. Successful adenovirus-mediated gene transfer in an *in vivo* model of human malignant mesothelioma. *Ann Thorac Surg* 1994; **57**: 1395–1401.

30. Smythe WR, Hwang HC, Elshami AA, *et al*. Successful treatment of experimental human mesothelioma using adenovirus transfer of the herpes simplex-thymidine kinase gene. *Ann Surg* 1995; **222**: 78–86.

31. Hwang HC, Smythe WR, Elshami AA, *et al*. Gene therapy using adenovirus carrying the herpes simplex thymidine kinase gene to treat *in vitro* models of human malignant mesothelioma and lung cancer. *Am J Respir Cell Mol Biol* 1995; **13**: 7–16.

32. Elshami A, Kucharczuk J, Zhang H, *et al*. Treatment of pleural mesothelioma in an immunocompetent rat model utilizing adenoviral transfer of the HSV-thymidine kinase gene. *Hum Gene Ther* 1996; **7**: 141–8.

33. Esandi MC, van Someren GD, Vincent AJ, *et al*. Gene therapy of experimental malignant mesothelioma using adenovirus vectors encoding the HSV*tk* gene. *Gene Ther* 1997; **4**: 280–7.

34. Kucharczuk JC, Raper S, Elshami AA, *et al*. Safety of adenoviral-mediated transfer of the herpes simplex thymidine kinase cDNA to the pleural cavity of rats and non-human primates. *Hum Gene Ther* 1996; **7**: 2225–33.

35. Treat J, Kaiser LR, Sterman DH, *et al*. Treatment of advanced mesothelioma with the recombinant adenovirus H5.010RSV*TK*: a phase 1 trial (BB-IND 6274). *Hum Gene Ther* 1996; **7**: 2047–57.

36. Sterman DH, Treat J, Litzky LA, *et al*. Adenovirus-mediated herpes simplex virus thymidine kinase gene delivery in patients with localized malignancy: results of a phase 1 clinical trial in malignant mesothelioma. *Hum Gene Ther* 1998; **9**: 1083–92.

37. Molnar-Kimber KL, Sterman DH, Chang M, *et al*. Humoral and cellular immune responses induced by adenoviral-based gene therapy for localized malignancy: results of a phase 1 clinical trial for malignant mesothelioma. *Hum Gene Ther* 1998; **9**: 2121–33.

38. Sterman DH, Molnar-Kimber K, Iyengar T, *et al*. A pilot study of systemic corticosteroid administration in conjunction with intrapleural adenoviral vector administration in patients with malignant pleural mesothelioma. *Cancer Gene Ther* 2000; **7**: 1511–18.

39. Gao GP, Yang Y, Wilson JM. Biology of adenovirus vectors with E1 and E4 deletions for liver-directed gene therapy. *J Virol* 1996; **70**: 8934–43.

40. Sterman DH, Recio A, Molnar-Kimber K, *et al*. Herpes simplex virus thymidine kinase (HSV*tk*) gene therapy utilizing an E1/E4-deleted adenoviral vector: preliminary results of a phase I clinical trial for pleural mesothelioma. *Am J Respir Crit Care Med* 1999; **159**: A237.

41. Alavi JB, Eck SL. Gene therapy for malignant gliomas. *Hematol Oncol Clin North Am* 1998; **12**: 617–629.

42. Perez-Cruet MJ, Trask TW, Chen SH, *et al*. Adenovirus-mediated gene therapy of experimental gliomas. *J Neurosci Res* 1994; **39**: 506–11.

43. Morris JC, Ramsey WJ, Wildner O, Muslow HA, Aguilar-Cordova E, Blaese RM. A phase I study of intralesional administration of an adenovirus vector expressing the HSV-1 thymidine kinase gene (AdV.RSV-*TK*) in combination with escalating doses of ganciclovir in patients with cutaneous metastatic melanoma. *Hum Gene Ther* 2000; **11**: 487–503.

44. Wiewrodt R, Amin K, Kiefer M, et al. Adenovirus-mediated gene transfer of enhanced herpes simplex virus thymidine kinase mutants improves prodrug-mediated tumor cell killing. Cancer Gene Ther 2003; 10: 353–64.

45. Al-Hendry A., Magliocco AM, Al-Tweigeri T, et al. Ovarian cancer gene therapy: repeated treatment with thymidine kinase in an adenovirus vector and ganciclovir improves survival in a novel immunocompetent murine model. Am J Obstet Gynecol 2000; 182: 553–9.

46. Tsukuda K, Wiewrodt R, Molnar-Kimber K, Jovanovic VP, Amin KM. An E2F-responsive replication-selective adenovirus targeted to the defective cell cycle in cancer cells: potent antitumoral efficacy but no toxicity to normal cells. Cancer Res. 2002; 62: 3438–47.

47. Kahlos K, Anttila S, Asikainen T, et al. Manganese superoxide dismutase in healthy human pleural mesothelium and in malignant pleural mesothelioma. Am J Respir Cell Mol Biol 1998; 18: 579–80.

48. Doglioni C, Dei Tos AP, Laurino L, et al. Calretinin: a novel immunocytochemical marker for mesothelioma. Am J Surg Pathol 1996; 20: 1037–46.

49. Gotzos V, Vogt P, Celio M. The calcium binding protein calretinin is a selective marker for malignant pleural mesotheliomas of the epithelial type. Pathol Res Pract 1996; 192: 137–47.

50. Chang K, Pastan I. Molecular cloning of mesothelin, a differentiation antigen present on mesothelium, mesotheliomas, and ovarian cancers. Proc Natl Acad Sci USA 1996; 93: 136–40.

51. Ambrosini G, Adid C, Altieri DC. A novel anti-apoptosis gene, surviving, expressed in cancer and lymphoma. Nat Med 1997; 3: 917–21.

52. Hall SJ, Sanford MA, Atkinson G, Chen SH. Induction of potent antitumor natural killer cell activity by herpes simplex virus-thymidine kinase and ganciclovir therapy in an orthotopic mouse model of prostate cancer. Cancer Res 1998; 58: 3221–5.

53. Freeman SM, Ramesh R, Marogi AJ. Immune system in suicide gene therapy. Lancet 1997; 349: 2–3.

54. Vile RG, Castleden S, Marshall J, Camplejohn R, Upton C, Chong H. Generation of an anti-tumor immune response in a non-immunogenic tumour: HSVtk killing in vivo stimulates a mononuclear cell infiltrate and a Th1-like profile of intratumoral cytokine expression. Int J Cancer 1997; 71: 267–74.

55. Melcher A, Todryk S, Hardwick N, Ford M, Jacobson M, Vile R. Tumor immunogenicity is determined by the mechanism of cell death via induction of heat shock protein expression. Nat Med 1998; 4: 581–7.

56. Chen SH, Li Chen XH, Wang Y, et al. Combination gene therapy for liver metastasis of colon carcinoma in vivo. Proc Natl Acad Sci USA 1995; 92: 2577–81.

57. O'Malley B Jr, Cope KA, Chen SH, Li D, Schwartz M, Woo SLC. Combination gene therapy for oral cancer in a murine model. Cancer Res 1996; 56: 1737–41.

58. Castleden SA, Chong H, Garcia-Ribas I, et al. A family of bicistronic vectors to enhance both local and systemic antitumor effects of HSVtk or cytokine expression in a murine melanoma model. Hum Gene Ther 1997; 8: 2087–102.

59. Coll J, Mesnil M, Lefebvre M, Lancon A, Favrot M. Long-term survival of immunocompetent rats with intraperitoneal colon carcinoma tumors using herpes simplex thymidine kinase/ganciclovir and IL-2 treatments. Gene Ther 1997; 4: 1160–6.

60. Schwarzenberger P, Lei D, Freeman SM, et al. Antitumor activity with the HSV-tk-gene cell line PA-1-STK in malignant mesothelioma. Am J Respir Cell Mol Biol 1998; 19: 333–7.

61. Kolls J, Freeman S, Ramesh R, et al. The treatment of malignant pleural mesothelioma with gene modified cancer cells: a phase I study. Am J Respir Crit Care Med 1998; 157: A563.

62. Harrison LH Jr, Schwarzenberger PO, Byrne PS, Marrogi AJ, Kolls JK, McCarthy KE Gene-modified PA1-STK cells home to tumor sites in patients with malignant pleural mesothelioma. Ann Thorac Surg 2000; 70: 407–11.

63. Leong CC, Marley JV, Loh S, Robinson BWS, Garlepp MJ. The induction of immune responses to murine mesothelioma by IL-2 gene transfer. Immunol Cell Biol 1997; 75: 356–9.

64. Fakharai H, Shawler D, Gjerset R, et al. Cytokine gene therapy with interleukin-2-transduced fibroblasts: effects of IL-2 dose on anti-tumor immunity. Hum Gene Ther 1995; 6: 591–601.

65. Christmas T, Manning LS, Garlepp MJ, Mush AW, Robinson BW. Effect of interferon-alpha 2a on malignant mesothelioma. *Interferon Res* 1993; **13**: 9–12.

66. Astoul P, Viallat JR, Laurent JC, Brandley M, Boutin C. Intrapleural IL-2 in passive immunotherapy for malignant pleural effusion. *Chest* 1993; **103**: 209–13.

67. Astoul P, Picat-Joossen D, Viallat J, Boutin C. Intrapleural administration of interleuken-2 for the treatment of patients with malignant pleural mesothelioma: a phase II study. *Cancer* 1998; **83**: 2099–104.

68. Boutin C, Viallat J, VanZandwijk N, *et al.* Activity of intrapleural recombinant gamma-interferon in malignant mesothelioma. *Cancer* 1991; **67**: 2033–7.

69. Boutin C, Nussbaum E, Monnet I, *et al.* Intrapleural treatment with recombinant gamma-interferon in early stage malignant pleural mesothelioma. *Cancer* 1994; **74**: 2460–7.

70. Robinson B, Bowman R, Manning L, Musk A, Van Hazel G. Interleukin-2 and lymphokine-activated killer cells in malignant mesothelioma. *Eur Respir Rev* 1993; **3**: 220–2.

71. Goey SH, Eggermont AM, Punt CJ, *et al.* Intrapleural administration of interleukin-2 in pleural mesothelioma: a phase I–II study. *Br J Cancer* 1995; **72**: 1283–8.

72. Mukherjee S, Haenel T, Himbeck R, *et al.* Replication-restricted vaccinia as a cytokine gene therapy vector in cancer: persistent transgene expression despite antibody generation. *Cancer Gene Ther* 2000; **7**: 663–70.

73. Rochlitz C, Jantscheff P, Bongartz G, *et al.* Gene therapy study of cytokine-transfected xenogeneic cells (Vero-interleukin-2) in patients with metastatic solid tumors. *Cancer Gene Ther* 1999; **6**: 271–8.

74. Caminschi I, Venetsanakos E, Leong CC, Garlepp MJ, Scott B, Robinson BWS. interleukin-12 induces an effective antitumor response in malignant mesothelioma. *Am J. Respir Cell Mol Biol* 1998; **19**: 738–46.

75. Caminschi I, Venetsanakos E, Leong CC, Garlepp MJ, Robinson BW, Scott B. Cytokine gene therapy of mesothelioma. Immune and antitumor effects of transfected interleukin-12. *Am J Respir Cell Mol Biol* 1999; **21**: 347–56.

76. Lukacs KV, Nakakes A, Atkins, CJ, Lowrie DB, Colston MJ. *In vivo* gene therapy of malignant tumors with heat shock protein-65 gene. *Gene Ther* 1997; **4**: 345–50.

77. Lanuti M, Rudginsky S, Force S, *et al.* Cationic lipid: bacterial DNA complexes elicit anti-tumor effects and adaptive immunity in murine intraperitoneal tumor models. *Cancer Res* 2000; **60**: 2955–63.

78. Lukacs KV, Porter CD, Pardo OE, *et al.* *In vivo* transfer of bacterial marker genes results in differing levels of gene expression and tumor progression in immunocompetent and immunodeficient mice. *Hum Gene Ther* 1999; **10**: 2373–9.

79. Rudginsky S, Siders W, Ingram L, Marshall J, Scheule R, Kaplan J. Antitumor activity of cationic lipid complexed with immunostimulatory DNA. *Mol Med* 2001; **4**: 347–55.

80. Rosso R, Rimoldi R, Salvati F, *et al.* Intrapleural natural beta interferon in the treatment of malignant pleural effusions. *Oncology* 1988; **45**: 253–6.

81. Odaka M, Sterman DH, Wiewrodt R, *et al.* Eradication of intraperitoneal and distant tumor by adenovirus-mediated interferon-β gene therapy is attributable to induction of systemic immunity. *Cancer Res* 2001; **61**: 6201–12.

82. Frizelle SP, Rubins JB, Zhou JX, Curiel DT, Kratzke RA. Gene therapy of established mesothelioma xenografts with recombinant p16INK4a adenovirus. *Cancer Gene Ther* 2000; **7**: 1421–25.

83. Frizelle SP, Grim J, Zhou JX, *et al.* Re-expression of p16INK4a in mesothelioma cells results in cell cycle arrest, cell death, tumor suppression, and tumor regression. *Oncogene* 1998; **16**: 3087–95.

84. Yang C, You L, Yeh C, *et al.* Cell cycle arrest and induction of apoptotic death in mesothelioma cells by the adenovirus-mediated p14ARF expression. *J Natl Cancer Inst* 2000; **92**: 636–41.

85. Yang C, You L, Yeh C, *et al.* p14ARF modulates the cytolytic effect of ONYX-015 in mesothelioma cells with wild-type p53. *Cancer Res* 2001; **61**: 5959–63.

86. Giuliano M, Catalano A, Strizzi L, Vianale G, Capogrossi M, Procopio A. Adenovirus-mediated wild-type p53 overexpression reverts tumourigenicity of human mesothelioma cells. *Int J Mol Med* 2000; **5**: 591–6.

87. Pataer A, Smythe WR, Yu R, *et al.* Adenovirus-mediated Bak gene transfer induces apoptosis in mesothelioma cell lines. *J Thorac Cardiovasc Surg* 2001; **121**: 61–7.

88. Cicala C, Pompetti F, Carbone M. SV40 induces mesothelioma in hamsters. *Am J Pathol* 1993; **142**: 1524–33.

89. Carbone M, Rizzo P, Grimley PM, *et al.* Simian virus-40 large-T antigen binds p53 in human mesotheliomas. *Nat Med* 1997; **3**: 908–12.

90. Schrump DS, Waheed I. Strategies to circumvent SV40 oncoprotein expression in malignant pleural mesothelioma. *Semin Cancer Biol* 2001; **11**: 73

91. Imperiale MJ, Pass HI, Sanda MG. Prospects for an SV40 vaccine. *Semin Cancer Biol* 2001; **11**: 81–5.

Chapter 20

Supportive and palliative care in mesothelioma

S. H. Ahmedzai and H. Clayson

Prevalence and manifestation of mesothelioma

Mesothelioma is an increasingly important malignant disease affecting all developed and developing countries. The vast majority of cases are linked to occupational exposure to asbestos, whether directly in men and women who worked in industrial environments or indirectly in their wives who washed their contaminated clothing [1]. The proportional mortality ratios of those dying from mesothelioma are highest in metal plate workers, vehicle body builders, plumbers, and gas fitters [2]. Mesothelioma was first recognized as a specific malignant tumour in the 1960s, and it is estimated that the incidence of new cases will rise over the next two decades, reaching a peak in Europe around 2020 [3]. It could eventually account for up to 1 per cent of all deaths of men born in the 1940s [1,3].

The clinical significance of mesothelioma lies in its extremely poor prognosis and heavy burden of physical symptoms and other types of morbidity. The median survival in various series ranges from 5–9 months for the sarcomatoid variety to 13–16 months for the epitheloid form [4,5]. These statistics alone dictate that supportive and palliative care should be regarded as an essential part of its management from the time of diagnosis, even more so than in some forms of lung cancer. The disease arises mostly in the pleura (95 per cent of cases), with a minority starting in the peritoneum (5 per cent) [6]. Mesothelioma can readily spread to the pericardium but, rarely, it has also been described as starting there (<1 per cent of cases). In the chest, the right side is affected more commonly than the left (the ratio of right to primary site left is 1.6:1) [5].

It used to be thought that mesothelioma does not readily metastasize. However, a large post-mortem series showed that it had spread from one hemithorax to the other lung, peritoneum, or more distally in 55 per cent of cases [5]. True distant metastases have been described in individual cases. A patient with epitheloid type mesothelioma, who had partially responded to courses of chemotherapy and radiotherapy over 2 years, was found to have soft tissue metastases in his buttock and psoas muscles [7]. Another male with epitheloid type mesothelioma presented with pain in the left leg 10 months after chemotherapy and was found to have a metastasis in the vastus lateralis muscle [8]. A man with a previous pleural mesothelioma diagnosed and treated with radiation therapy 9 months earlier developed multiple skin lesions on his lip, leg, and groin. Histological and immunohistochemical testing revealed these to be metastatic mesotheliomas rather than primary squamous cell cancer [9]. Interestingly, bone metastases which are common in other forms of lung cancer, as opposed to direct bony invasion in the thorax, have not been described with mesothelioma.

Central nervous system (CNS) metastases, presenting early in the disease, have also been described. A male with recently diagnosed mesothelioma, who developed a bizarre mental disturbance with features of depression, was found on CT scanning to have multiple cerebral metastases [10]. In another case, a male patient presented with a history suggestive of transient ischaemic attacks and was found to have a single cerebral metastasis. He concurrently developed a soft tissue lesion on the chin and was found to have pleural disease, and all these were confirmed histologically to be arising from a primary sarcomatoid mesothelioma [11].

Mesothelioma is one of the malignant diseases that are associated with increased venous thrombosis. A male being investigated for left-sided pleural effusion was found to have epitheloid type mesothelioma. Soon after the diagnosis, he developed enlargement of the neck with ultrasound evidence of extensive thrombosis of the left jugular and subclavian veins [12]. Another case has been reported of portal vein thrombosis arising in a patient with pleural and peritoneal mesothelioma [13]. Overall, 40 per cent of patients may have thrombocytosis at diagnosis and up to 90 per cent later in the course of the disease [14].

Physical symptom burden

Mesothelioma is associated with a heavy burden of physical symptoms and other forms of psychosocial, spiritual (existential), and financial distress. The main symptoms experienced by nearly all patients include pain, dyspnoea, and weight loss. A study of 495 patients with mesothelioma which used a modified form of the Lung Cancer Symptom Scale (LCSS) to measure morbidity found that over 85 per cent reported pain, dyspnoea, fatigue, and loss of appetite [15].

Pain

Chest pain, which arises primarily from tumour infiltration of intercostal nerves, is nearly always present by the advanced stages. The pain is usually described as diffuse and encircling the affected hemithorax. Tenderness is not a common feature, unless tumour has extended onto the skin through a diagnostic port in the chest wall. The patient may also describe the pain as having a burning quality [16]. Although there is usually a component of neuropathic pain arising from actual nerve damage, it is unusual to observe the full set of classical features of hyperalgesia (increased pain after a pain-inducing stimulus), allodynia (pain after a non-painful stimulus such as light touch), and paraesthesia. Numbness may occur in a dermatomal distribution either because of intercostal nerve damage by tumour or after surgical intervention. Mesothelioma was the most common diagnosis in a series in 1000 patients reviewed for the presence of post-thoracotomy neuropathic pain, and affected 43 per cent of patients at 2 months [17].

A review of 142 cases of mesothelioma was subjected to univariate and multivariate regression analyses to determine factors predictive of survival [18]. The presence of chest pain at diagnosis was associated with a significantly raised survival hazard ratio of 1.70 (95 per cent confidence interval (CI) 1.08–2.68) which was highly significant for a poor outcome ($P = 0.017$).

Dyspnoea

Dyspnoea usually arises initially because of recurrent pleural effusions which affect 95 per cent of patients in the early stages of disease, but breathlessness continues to be a major symptom later, even when effusions are no longer present. This is partly because of loss of volume in the hemithorax, fixation of the chest wall due to encroaching pleural disease, and in some cases because of pericardial constriction. A review of 28 published cases of mesothelioma associated with pericardial involvement showed that all histological types were implicated, but males were twice as likely to have this association [19]. The most commonly cited symptoms in these patients were dyspnoea (affecting 46 per cent), fever (32 per cent), chest pain (32 per cent), and weight loss (21 per cent). Pericardial mesothelioma is associated with a particularly poor prognosis.

A recent study of 53 mesothelioma patients undergoing chemotherapy with cisplatin and gemcitabine examined the responses to questions in the European Organization for Research and Treatment of Cancer (EORTC) quality-of-life questionnaires [20]. Using the EORTC core questionnaire (QLQ-C30), the authors found the mean scores for symptoms to be as follows: fatigue 42/100, dyspnoea 39/100, pain 38/100, insomnia 37/100, cough 33/100, and anorexia 33/100. All these scores were higher, i.e. worse, than reference scores for lung cancer. The lung cancer module (LC-13) gives more detailed scores for chest-related symptoms. The scores for pain were higher for chest pain (28/100) than for arm pain (25/100), but pain from other sites was even higher (33/100). Another troublesome symptom was constipation (21/100). Nowak *et al.* [20] used the symptom scores in Cox regression analyses to determine their predictive value for estimating survival. They found that fatigue, pain, and dyspnoea had significant prognostic value.

Weight loss

The mechanism of weight loss is of interest as it probably arises from several causes. Cancer cachexia is a well-described syndrome consisting of anorexia, weight loss, and fatigue [21]. It is now acknowledged to be largely due to the production of inflammatory cytokines such as tumour necrosis factor 1α (TNF-1α) and interleukins (ILs), especially IL-6, by macrophages as part of the host response to tumour invasion. These factors have been well described in both lung and pancreas cancer [22,23]. The cytokines and other peptides associated with the host response to malignancy induce weight loss by activating metabolic pathways which lead to proteolysis, adipolysis, and loss of liver energy stores. They are also responsible for some of the symptoms experienced by patients with lung cancer or mesothelioma (e.g. anorexia, fatigue, sweating, and fever).

Another cause of weight loss in some patients may be oesophageal compression leading to dysphagia and reduced ingestion. A pseudo-achalasia syndrome has been described in a group of mesothelioma patients found to have dysphagia. They had radiological features of achalasia but on further investigation were seen to have tumour infiltration of the oesophageal wall, which could extend from the pleura into the peritoneal cavity [24,25]. In one series of 13 cases of different cancers associated with pseudo-achalasia, histological evidence of involvement of the myenteric plexus was seen in only a few and was absent in the one patient with mesothelioma.

Regardless of the cause, weight loss is a poor prognostic sign in mesothelioma, as it is in many other solid tumours. Patients with weight loss at presentation had an increased survival hazard ratio of 1.89 (95 per cent CI 1.27–2.82) which was highly significant ($P = 0.002$) [18].

Miscellaneous

Peritoneal mesothelioma frequently causes abdominal pain and distension with ascites [14]. Patients also complain of nausea and vomiting and have signs of abdominal or pelvis masses, bowel obstruction, leg oedema, obstructive uropathy, and fever.

Mesothelioma may cause paraneoplastic syndromes, the most common of which is related to the thrombocytosis and increased tendency to the thrombotic complications mentioned above. It is thought that the increased amounts of platelet-derived growth factors and thrombocytosis may be related to the excess production of interleukins including IL-6. Other haematological complications include disseminated intravascular coagulation and autoimmune haemolytic anaemia. Rarely, biochemical abnormalities such as syndrome of inappropriate antidiuretic hormone secretion (SIADH), hypoglycaemia, and hypercalcaemia may occur. The latter may be caused by the secretion of parathyroid-hormone-like peptide, which has been identified in mesothelioma cells [14].

Understanding symptoms and their rational management

The use of anticancer therapies, such as radiotherapy and chemotherapy, and the role of surgery are not discussed here as they are covered in detail elsewhere in this volume. It is assumed that

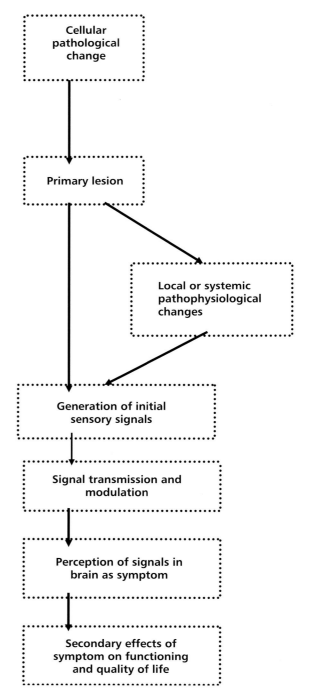

Figure 20.1 Generic model of symptom generation.

these options have been pursued if appropriate. This chapter will focus on the palliation of symptoms using pharmacological, anaesthetic, and other supportive treatments.

A model of symptoms has recently been proposed [26]. It aims to improve the understanding of how symptoms are first generated, perceived by the individual, and then impact on his or her functioning, and finally how palliative treatments can intervene at these different stages. Figure 20.1 shows this model, which emphasizes the following sequential steps of symptom production.

1. Initial cellular pathological change.

2. Development of a primary lesion.

3. Local or systemic pathophysiological effects.

4. Production of a symptom by:

    (a) initial generation of sensory signals

    (b) transmission and modulation of signals on the way to the brain

    (c) perception of those messages in the brain as a symptom

    (d) secondary effects of the symptom on functioning and quality of life.

In the case of mesothelioma, the steps leading to pain, as shown in Figure 20.2, could consist of the following.

1. Induction of malignant change in pleural mesothelial cells by asbestos fibres.

2. Established mesothelioma and its infiltration into the pleura.

3. Lesions extending into intercostal spaces, chest wall diagnostic intervention tracks, pleural or pericardial spread, metastases, thrombocytosis, and prothrombotic tendency.

4. Pain production by:

    (a) infiltration of intercostal nerve fibres and sensitization of pain-transmitting C-fibres.

    (b) transmission and modulation of pain sensory signals in dorsal horn of spinal cord.

    (c) pain perception and processing in primary and secondary somatosensory cortex, anterior cingulate gyrus, and prefrontal cortex.

    (d) inhibition of chest wall movement and restriction of general mobility, psychological stress leading to depression, and impaired sleep leading to daytime drowsiness and fatigue.

It is now becoming possible, as we learn more about the pathophysiology of other symptoms such as dyspnoea and anorexia, to map out the steps in their generation and effects. The main benefit of this classification comes when we examine the therapeutic options in a similarly logical stepwise manner. Thus it can be seen from Figure 20.2 that symptom palliation also has four main steps.

1. Prevention of the initial cellular pathology, for example by elimination of asbestos fibres from inhaled air in working environments.

2. Surgical removal of initial mesothelioma, followed by best combination of radiation and chemotherapy.

3. Radiotherapy to video-assisted thorascopy surgery (VATS) or pleural biopsy sites, pleurectomy, radiation therapy for painful metastases, and anti-coagulant therapy.

4. Pain reduction by:

    (a) peripheral intercostal nerve blockade or radiofrequency ablation, non-steroidal anti-inflammatory drugs (NSAIDs) to reduce sensitization of pain fibre nerve endings.

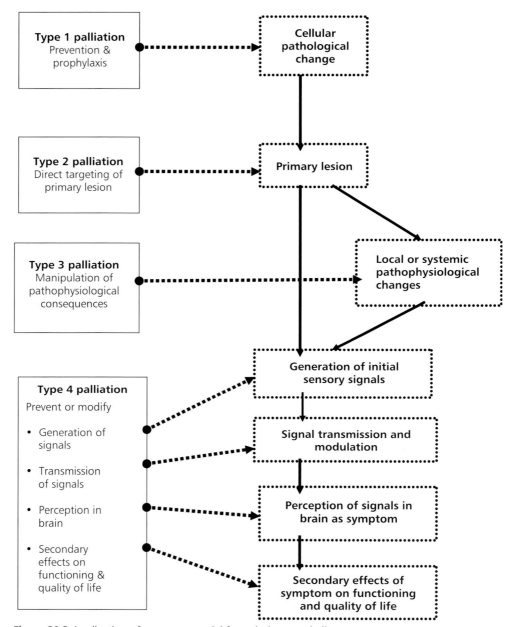

Figure 20.2 Application of symptom model for pain in mesothelioma.

    (b) opioids to reduce spinal dorsal horn synaptic transmission and hyperexcitability of central projection of pain neurons, and ion-channel blockers to reduce spontaneous firing of damaged and collateral nerves and subsequent sensitized dorsal horn synapses.

    (c) opioids or benzodiazepines to reduce cerebral consciousness of pain, and distraction therapies or relaxation to modify awareness of pain.

(d) physiotherapy to aid mobilization, anti-depressants (for depression and to reduce pain through 4(b)), and psychostimulants to raise arousal and reduce depression.

It is hoped that the exploration and testing of this model for symptom production and its palliation could lead to more rational strategies for prevention and targeted therapies. These are clearly needed, because the current state of symptom control in mesothelioma, as in many other solid tumours, is far from ideal.

WHO cancer pain programme

It is worth reviewing briefly the considerable importance of the WHO cancer pain programme, which was initiated in 1986 [27]. The main tenets of the WHO approach were revolutionary at the time, and have now become incorporated into the general management of pain. They are as follows:

- pain control by the clock (meaning anticipating pain and giving medications regularly according to their known pharmacodynamic profiles, not waiting until the patient complains)
- pain control by mouth (avoiding, where possible, the previous reliance on intramuscular or intravenous injections)
- pain control by a three-step ladder approach
- the drug of choice, in 1986, was morphine.

In combination, these principles have been greatly influential in improving pain control for millions of patients throughout the world, particularly in developing countries where potent oral medications were not available. However, the relevance of these statements has been called into question in the past decade because of technological and pharmacological advances. Whereas the original oral morphine solution has an effective half-life of 4 h, most strong opioids currently available are manufactured with modified-release oral formulations offering pain relief for 12 h or even 24 h. The exploitation of transdermal drug absorption from patches containing lipophilic opioids (fentanyl or buprenorphine) has taken sustained drug delivery to a higher level of patient convenience, as these can last for 72 h. However, it is true to point out that short-acting medications are still necessary for 'breakthrough' pain (e.g. movement-induced pain in a patient with bone metastases).

The introduction of transdermal patches for pain control has also reduced the need to emphasize the oral route. Other routes that are currently available and being increasingly exploited include the oral or nasal transmucosal route (for fentanyl) or the spinal route (e.g. intrathecal morphine or bupivacaine for axial or lower limb pain). The subcutaneous route is now preferred if opioid drugs have to be given parenterally, as it is reliable and more comfortable for both single injections and 24 h infusions than the former intramuscular or intravenous routes. The subcutaneous route only becomes problematic in patients with very poor peripheral circulation or those with thrombocytopaenia and other bleeding tendencies.

The WHO three-step ladder has been an important teaching aid and simple rubric for the application of opioids.

- Step 1 for mild pain: paracetamol.
- Step 2 for moderate pain: 'weak opioids' such as codeine or dihydrocodeine.
- Step 3 for severe pain: 'strong opioids' such as morphine, oxycodone, hydromorphone or fentanyl.

One problem with this approach has arisen with the increased availability, at least in Western countries, of a wider range of opioids in different formulations than were envisaged in 1986. For example, current useful drugs such as tramadol and buprenorphine do not fit well in the three-step model as they lie somewhere between 'weak' and 'strong' opioids. Furthermore, the use of small doses of modified-release oral morphine or oxycodone has effectively made step 2 redundant for many patients. A randomized controlled trial comparing the standard WHO three-step ladder approach with starting patients directly on strong opioids (step 3) has been conducted [28]. The latter led to significantly better pain control with fewer changes in therapy and greater satisfaction with treatment than in those who went through step 2 and then step 3. There was no increase in adverse effects in those going straight to step 3 opioids.

A systematic review of the published studies which allegedly 'validated' the WHO analgesic ladder found that none of the studies to date were methodologically sound as prospective validation trials and many had weaknesses such as poor follow-up or documentation [29]. As the authors of the review stated [29]:

> Eight studies purporting to evaluate the effectiveness of the WHO ladder were included in the review. Meta-analysis was not performed because the studies were case series with no control groups. The studies had other limitations: none provided information on the conditions in which pain was assessed; two were retrospective; one had short follow-up periods; three had high withdrawal rates; and one had variable follow-up periods ... the evidence they provide is insufficient to estimate confidently the effectiveness of the WHO analgesic ladder for the management of cancer pain ... Despite the widespread dissemination of the WHO ladder, most cancer patients around the world still appear to have inadequate analgesia ... Other factors that could explain, at least in part ... are that either the WHO analgesic ladder is not as applicable and as effective as the existing evidence suggests, or that achieving adequate pain relief is more difficult that we think. The limited effectiveness of the ladder as a management tool is rarely, if ever, acknowledged.

As a response to this lack of validation and also the apparent lack of progress in cancer pain following the introduction of the WHO ladder in 1986, an alternative model was recently proposed. Building on the original WHO concept, it takes a three-dimensional view and thus employs the metaphor of a pyramid rather than a ladder [30,31]. Figure 20.3 shows how the pyramid approach includes drugs such as opioids on one face, but also stresses other important approaches to cancer pain, including surgical and neurolytic techniques, anticancer therapies, and psychological or nursing approaches. A useful extension of the pyramid model is that each

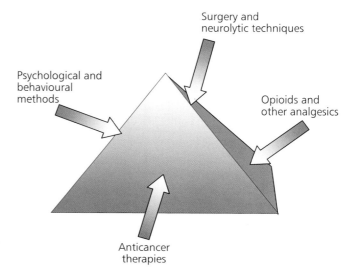

Figure 20.3 Pyramid model for pain control.

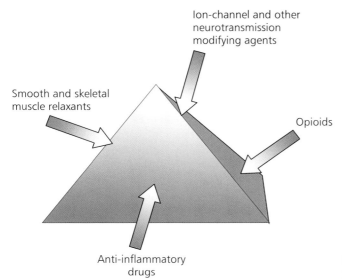

Ion-channel and other
neurotransmission
modifying agents

Smooth and skeletal
muscle relaxants

Opioids

Anti-inflammatory
drugs

Figure 20.4 Meta-pyramid for
pain control in cancer.

face of the pyramid can give rise to new 'meta-pyramids'; for example, the drug therapy face
yields a new pyramid with its four faces displaying anti-inflammatory drugs, opioids, ion-channel and other neurotransmission modifying agents; and smooth or skeletal muscle relaxants (Fig.
20.4) [31]. It is true that the updated published WHO pain programme mentions these pharmacological approaches, but as they are sometimes only referred to in the ladder as 'adjuvants', their
potential contribution is buried. The highly visual pyramid model, in contrast, makes therapeutic alternatives more explicit and encourages a multimodal attack on symptoms from the outset.

The fourth basic principle of the WHO cancer pain programme, namely that oral morphine is
the 'drug of choice', has also recently been called into question. With the development of new
modified release preparations of alternative oral opioids such as oxycodone or hydromorphone,
or transdermal delivery of fentanyl, randomized controlled trials have repeatedly shown that the
new synthetic agents are as effective as morphine, but carry advantages in terms of better side-
effect profile and/or improved convenience. The reason for the reduced adverse effects of some
opioids compared with morphine can be understood partly in terms of the differential effects of
opioid receptors. Whereas morphine is a pure μ-opioid agonist, oxycodone is mainly a κ-opioid
agonist. This confers advantages in terms of reduced CNS toxicity such as sedation and hallucinations [32]. Fentanyl is a predominantly μ-opioid agonist like morphine, but it has an intrinsi-
cally lower inhibitory effect on smooth muscle and thus causes significantly less constipation at
equi-analgesic doses compared with morphine [33]. The extremely stable flat pharmacokinetics
provided by the transdermal delivery method may also help to account for its reduced sedative
and nausea-producing effects [34].

In a large systematic review of randomized controlled trials comparing oral morphine with
transdermal fentanyl in both cancer and non-malignant pain, the latter emerged as having many
advantages for patients in terms of improved pain control, reduced side effects, and convenience
[35]. Indeed, when patients are asked for their preference between oral modified-release morphine or transdermal fentanyl in cross-over trials, every study so far has shown the superiority of
fentanyl. Therefore it is increasingly difficult to argue that oral morphine is still the 'drug of
choice'. Although the newer agents and routes are generally more expensive, it has been shown in
rigorous health economic studies that when the cost of side-effect management (e.g. for

constipation) is taken into consideration alongside drug acquisition cost, the differences are greatly reduced [36]. Furthermore, taking side effects and their management into consideration, transdermal fentanyl can be associated with a higher number of quality-adjusted life days compared with oral morphine or oxycodone.

Pain control in mesothelioma

The preceding discussion has shown that the management of pain in cancer patients is far from simple, and even two decades after WHO launched its cancer pain programme there is still much to be done. Pain control in mesothelioma is especially difficult because the primary lesion and subsequent pathophysiological changes (steps 2 and 3 in the symptom model in Fig. 20.1) have profound pain-generating potential. The pain arising in mesothelioma can be of inflammatory, neuropathic or bony origin. The soft tissue inflammatory element comes from the bulky tumour which grows in the pleural and sometimes the pericardial or peritoneal spaces. Tumour cells growing in soft tissue interact with host macrophages, resulting in the local production of cytokines, prostaglandins, and other kinins. These can directly sensitize the unmyelinated small C-fibre endings which are responsible for deep pain signal transmission [37]. Thus there is a high probability of mesothelioma generating pain signals as it grows and invades healthy pleural, pericardial, or peritoneal spaces. Inflammatory pain tends to settle down when the inflammatory process subsides or is modified, for example with anti-inflammatory drugs or radiotherapy.

There are many ways of relieving inflammatory pain. Radiotherapy can be very effective, as discussed in Chapter 15. NSAIDs such as ibuprofen and diclofenac may be valuable but are limited by their gastric and renal toxicities. It is interesting to note that the recently introduced class of cyclo-oxygenase (COX)-2 anti-inflammatory agents may have a special advantage in mesothelioma, as this tumour type is known to over-express COX-2 protein directly [38]. However, the COX-2 NSAIDs are liable to cause increased cardiovascular risk.

Opioids are also very useful for inflammatory pain at two levels. First, they act centrally in the spinal cord and brain to reduce the sensitivity of pain-conducting ascending pathways [39]. Secondly, it is now known that opioid receptors are expressed peripherally in inflamed tissues [40]. Thus, theoretically, peripherally applied opioids may be helpful and there is early evidence that topical formulations of morphine in gel placed directly on open sores or fungating cancers can add to pain control with minimum side effects [41].

Neuropathic pain arises when there is damage either to peripheral nerves or to nerve structures in the CNS (e.g. in the spinal cord or thalamus). Unlike inflammatory pain, neuropathic pain can be self-perpetuating as the nerve damage leads to long-term trophic changes via adjacent undamaged nerves and can also cause plastic changes in the synaptic connections in the dorsal horn of the spinal cord. These changes all lead to neuronal hyperexcitability and a special pain state known as central sensitization [37]. This term refers to the condition in which the whole pain-conducting pathway from the lesion to the brain is set to a lower threshold point. This in turn leads to greater pain perception in response to the same or lesser noxious stimuli (hyperalgesia). Hyperalgesia may extend to a much wider area of skin than the innervation of the original lesion. If the damage continues, the sensitivity of pain-transmitting nerves increases further, and a situation arises when even non-noxious stimuli such as a light touch induces a painful response that is felt in the area being stroked. This phenomenon is known as allodynia. Figure 20.5 explains how these phenomena arise in terms of the stimulus–response curve. Paradoxically, both these conditions often arise in the presence of reduced touch sensation or numbness in the dermatome of the damaged nerves.

In mesothelioma, the malignant growth of tumour into the intercostal spaces leads to early damage and destruction of sensory nerve fibres, thus readily leading to the generation of neuro-

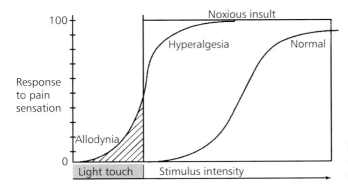

Figure 20.5 Stimulus–response curves for pain and the effects of hyperalgesia and allodynia.

pathic pain. Unfortunately, incisions made in the same spaces for thoracotomy and sometimes even the tracks made for VATS can damage nerves not invaded by tumour and lead to iatrogenic neuropathic pain [16,17].

Recent studies of neurotransmission and structural changes in the spinal cord in chronic pain states have shown that central sensitization and the accompanying hyperalgesia and allodynia have a common mechanism. Central to this is the N-methyl-D-aspartate (NMDA) receptor channel in the postsynaptic membrane of dorsal horn ascending nerve fibres [37,39]. The NMDA channels are normally closed by magnesium ions. If stimulated by repeated arrival of presynaptic pain signals, mediated by the synaptic neurotransmitter glutamate, they open and allow the ingress of calcium ions into postsynaptic nerves. This initiates a sequence of events culminating in the intracellular induction of nitric oxide. This has the effect of increasing postsynaptic nerve membrane sensitivity, which in turn leads to increased pain signal transmission.

At present the NMDA receptor channel can only be blocked in humans by a few drugs. The most potent is ketamine, an anaesthetic induction agent which, in subanaesthetic doses, powerfully blocks NMDA channels and so produces profound analgesia. Unfortunately, the drug is associated with significant psychotropic toxicities such as visual hallucinations and sedation, which limit its usefulness. However, it has been found that some opioid drugs can also exert an action on the NMDA receptor. These include dextromethorphan, ketobemidone, and methadone. The latter has long been associated with the rehabilitation of heroin (diamorphine) addicts, but has the advantage of being a widely available and cheap synthetic μ-opioid agonist. It has moderate NMDA receptor channel-blocking potency and thus is a useful drug when both inflammatory and neuropathic pain coexist. Its drawback is a long elimination phase that can be a problem in older people, but in skilled hands it is a safe and predictable analgesic [42].

There are many other ways of interfering with the production and maintenance of central sensitization which do not directly involve the NMDA receptor channel mechanism [43]. Many anticonvulsant drugs are ion-channel modulators, and these can reduce neuropathic pain although sedation can be a limiting toxicity. Examples in current use for pain management include gabapentin, valproate, and carbamazepine. Gabapentin is unusual in being an anticonvulsant that is free from drug interactions, although its absorption is reduced by concomitant administration of antacids [44]. It's analogue, pregabalin, is not affected in this way. Despite its name, it does not work via the inhibitory γ-aminobutyric acid (GABA) pathway but rather through calcium ion channel blockade in neuronal membranes. Serotonin and norepinephrine reuptake inhibitors (SNRIs) such as tricyclic antidepressants and venlafaxine have spinal actions as well as central antidepressant effects. These actions can reduce synaptic transmission and thus downregulate the pain pathways.

Bony pain arises in many malignant conditions, including mesothelioma, when there is destruction of bones by locally advancing or metastatic tumour. In mesothelioma this nearly always occurs in the ribs and often in the vertebral bodies. Bones are now known to possess rich nerve supplies not only in the periosteum, but also in the cortex and medullary regions [45]. When these are invaded by tumour, the release of cytokines and kinins referred to above again causes early and long-term sensitization of the C-fibres. Thus, just as in neuropathic pain, bone tumours can cause central sensitization and its sequelae of hyperalgesia and allodynia. There is an added problem when the bones are weight bearing or required for important body movements, as these stresses can aggravate the pain intensely. Thus bone pain readily leads to restricted movement and loss of limb function and affects the whole person.

NSAIDs and opioids are useful for bone pain because of the inflammatory element. Radiotherapy is also very effective for the same reason. When central mechanisms are involved, it also makes sense to use the drugs described above which reduce central sensitization. A further approach specific to bone pain is the use of bisphosphonates. These agents work by several mechanisms at the site of bone destruction by tumour cells [46]. They reduce the activation of osteoclasts which are responsible for the normal remodelling and resorption of bone, which becomes accentuated when cancer is present in bony tissues. They also prevent activated osteoclasts from reaching bone surfaces. Zolendronate is a potent bisphosphonate that has been shown to have activity in a range of solid tumours, but data on mesothelioma are still lacking. Bisphosphonates may also possess specific anticancer activity in some tumours, notably breast cancer, but this has also not yet been demonstrated in mesothelioma [47]. If bone destruction is sufficient to release significant amounts of free calcium, leading to the syndrome of hypercalcaemia, bisphosphonates further act by increasing calcium excretion and reducing blood levels.

A multifaceted approach to pain management

It is clear from the preceding discussion that effective pain management in mesothelioma needs to be based on a rational multifaceted approach, especially if side effects are to be kept to a minimum [31]. Table 20.1 summarizes the drug approaches which can be employed in this situation. It shows at which level of the initiation of the pathological changes and the generation or transmission of pain signals the agents are working, using the model shown in Figure 20.1.

Non-pharmacological methods are also listed in Table 20.1. These include local anaesthetic and neurolytic blocks, radiotherapy, and complementary approaches such as acupuncture or psychological therapies. Treatments apart from radiotherapy are discussed below.

Side effects of analgesics

One of the important aspects of the recent advances in pain management has been the recognition and prevention of treatment side effects. In the past, these may have been underestimated as it was assumed that maximum pain control was the goal, and in unskilled hands this would undoubtedly have been at the expense of serious adverse effects. Patients are now more vocal in complaining about these and other inconveniences of pain medication. A large interview study involving nearly 1000 terminally ill patients in the USA showed that 52 per cent of those with cancer had significant (i.e. moderate/severe) pain. Of these, 34 per cent had seen a pain specialist but 29 per cent were not seeking further medication for pain control [48]. The reasons for avoiding analgesics included fear of physical side effects (33 per cent), fear of mental side effects (34 per cent), fear of taking more pills or injections (29 per cent), and fear of addiction (34 per cent). Correspondingly, a recent survey of physicians in Israel showed that poor outcome of pain control in cancer patients was associated by 43 per cent of respondents with excessive CNS side

Table 20.1 Approaches used for pain management in mesothelioma

Type of palliation	Example of intervention
1. Prevention and prophylaxis	Primary prevention: removal of asbestos from working environment Secondary prevention: compliance with health and safety regulations when working with existing asbestos
2. Direct targeting of primary lesion	Surgical: extra-pleural pneumonectomy, decortication Radiation therapy for primary lesion Chemotherapy
3. Manipulation of pathophysiological consequences	Pleural effusion: paracentesis; pleurodesis; pleurectomy Irradiation of chest wall surgical ports to prevent seeding Radiotherapy for metastases Anticoagulant therapy for thrombosis
4(a) Prevent generation of signals	Peripheral neuropathic pain from nerve destruction: intercostal nerve local anaesthetic block; radiofrequency nerve destruction Peripheral nerve-ending sensitization: NSAIDs; topical opioids on fungating lesion
4(b) Prevent or modulate transmission of signals	Spinal dorsal horn synaptic transmission: reduce NMDA receptor channel activation Post-synaptic ascending nerve hyperexcitability (central sensitization): opioids; ion-channel receptor blockers (e.g. carbamazepine; gabapentin); tricyclic antidepressants and SNRIs (e.g. venlafaxine)
4(c) Modify perception in brain	Reduce awareness and subjective response to pain: opioids Reduce conscious level and general subjective awareness: benzodiazepines Reduce anxiety and conscious level: neuroleptic (e.g. haloperidol, levomepromazine)
4(d) Prevent or modify secondary effects on functioning and quality of life	Prevent mood change: antidepressants; benzodiazepine for anxiety. Raise mood, arousal and reduce fatigue, drug-induced sedation: psychostimulant (eg. methylphenidate) Prevent immobility and de-conditioning of muscles: physiotherapy; exercise programme Reduce family anxiety and tension: attention to carers' needs

NSAIDs, non-steroidal anti-inflammatory drugs; SNRIs, serotonin and norepinephrine re-uptake inhibitors.

effects such as drowsiness and confusion, and by 26 per cent with excessive gastrointestinal side effects such as nausea, vomiting, and constipation [49].

Therefore modern management of cancer pain is very much centred on the balance for each individual between therapeutic benefit and minimization of side effects. It is important to discuss potential side effects openly with patients, and to elicit their previous experiences and specific fears. Table 20.2 lists the more common side effects associated with the medications described above and suggests useful strategies to prevent or reduce these. In the case of opioids, it is our view that oral morphine can no longer be defended as the sole 'drug of choice' because of its troublesome side-effect profile, and the evidence-based first-line alternatives are oxycodone for oral use and fentanyl by transdermal patch.

Specific problems with opioids

Because of the central place of the opioid drugs in the management of pain it is worth considering in more detail other specific problems associated with their use. One issue that has barely

Table 20.2 Side-effects of symptom palliation drugs and their management

Palliative drug	Side effect	Minimization and control
Opioid	Nausea	Tolerance usually develops, so may settle spontaneously in few days Use opioid with less emetogenic potential (e.g. fentanyl) Treat with anti-emetic (e.g. for delayed gastric emptying use metoclopramide; for central effect use haloperidol)
	Constipation	Tolerance does not develop Use opioid with less constipation effect (e.g. fentanyl) Ensure roughage in diet, bowel stimulant, stool softener
	Sedation	Tolerance may develop Dose-related More likely with methadone in patients with renal impairment Use opioids with reduced sedation potential (e.g. oxycodone, fentanyl) Reverse with psychostimulant (e.g. methylphenidate, modafinil)
	Hallucinations, delirium	Tolerance does not develop More likely with morphine, methadone in patients with renal impairment Ensure hydration Use opioids with reduced CNS toxicity (e.g. oxycodone) Manage with neuroleptic (e.g. haloperidol, levomepromazine) For severe agitation, sedate with benzodiazepine
NSAIDs	Dyspepsia	Ensure NSAID taken after food Protect with proton pump inhibitor (e.g. omeprazole) or H2 antagonist (e.g. ranitidine) Consider COX-2 inhibitor (caution: coronary and stroke risk)
Tricyclic antidepressant (for neuropathic pain)	Muscarinic anti-cholinergic effects (e.g. dry mouth, blurred vision, bladder retention)	Use antidepressant without muscarinic effects (e.g. venlafaxine – caution in heart disease) Use alternative approach for neuropathic pain (e.g. gabapentin)
Neuroleptic	Parkinsonian dystonia	Use minimum effective dose Control dystonia with anticholinergic (e.g. benztropine)
	Sedation	Use minimum effective dose Use single dose at night Manage with psychostimulant (e.g. methylphenidate, modafanil)

NSAIDs, non-steroidal anti-inflammatory drugs.

reduced over the past two decades, despite education of professionals and the public, is the misconception regarding addiction. It is true that most opioids are potentially very addictive and indeed are misused in most countries where they are available. However, in therapeutic use, especially when the prescriber is experienced and works as part of a team, addiction rarely becomes a problem. Indeed, if pain is substantially reduced because of a procedure such as a neurolytic block, opioid drugs can be cut back and in some cases stopped without physical or psychological signs of addiction behaviour. One of the advantages of being under the care of a specialist palliative care service (SPC) is that opioid usage is kept under constant review and is often reduced with no detriment to pain control. In a review of 970 advanced cancer patients attending a range of services, 15 per cent of those referred to SPCs had their opioid dose reduced and 7 per cent had opioids stopped altogether [50].

On the other hand, tolerance has probably been underestimated and, until recently, poorly managed. It is likely that tolerance to most opioids does develop over weeks and months, but because in therapeutic settings this occurs against the background of malignant disease progression and increasing number and size of painful lesions, it is masked by a 'true' need for higher doses of opioids. However, if the disease is stable, in some cases it can be observed that patients will gradually need increasing doses. This should not be regarded as addiction or psychological craving for more opioid, and the patient should be reassured accordingly. Two strategies can be used: either small stepwise increases in the opioids, or switching to an alternative opioid. The reason for the second approach is that there is good evidence that incomplete cross-tolerance exists between different opioids even if they are working on the same receptor type. Thus, if a patient is becoming tolerant to morphine, it may be helpful to switch to fentanyl, even at an equianalgesic dose. This effect is more marked when the new opioid has a different receptor activity (e.g. using oxycodone which works predominantly on κ-receptors [51]). Similarly, switching a patient from morphine, oxycodone, or fentanyl to methadone, which has both opioid and NMDA activity, can be helpful. It should be emphasized that opioid switching in this manner should be done only by experienced practitioners such as pain or palliative medicine specialists.

A recently recognized issue with opioids is that, paradoxically, they can induce a form of centrally mediated hyperalgesia [52]. This arises because of intracellular interaction between opioid and NMDA receptors in postsynaptic neurons in the dorsal horn. In both acute and chronic pain situations, there may be a measurable increase in pain sensitivity after initial successful opioid dosing. Usually, this is masked in normal therapeutic situations because of the WHO principle of pain management by giving pain control 'by the clock'. Thus, if patients are given free access to regular medication according to the pharmacodynamic profiles of the drug and formulation being used, it is unlikely that there will be an opportunity to unmask opioid hyperalgesia. However, if patients are only given as-required medication and required to wait until pain builds up before being given access to the next dose, this may be a factor in apparently increasing demands. Occasionally, a patient who has been on a single opioid drug for several weeks or months may be seen to require rapidly escalating doses without apparent reason, i.e. no obvious increasing pathology. Such patients may end up on very high doses of morphine (e.g. several hundred or thousand milligrams per day). Often the patient remains alert and agitated and continues to complain of pain, and indeed may exhibit signs of hyperalgesia and allodynia as described above.

The first step of managing established or suspected central opioid-induced hyperalgesia is to recognize the problem and refer to a specialist. The main therapeutic manoeuvre is usually an opioid switch (e.g. from morphine or oxycodone to methadone). Often, it will be possible to reduce the opioid dose drastically in a few days, ending up on around one-tenth of the original morphine-equivalent dose [53].

Another problem that sometimes occurs in the terminal stage of illness when a patient has been on long-term opioids, usually morphine, is the development of confusion, generalized irritability, and myoclonic jerking of limb muscles. This is believed to be mediated by the hyperstimulation of the CNS and muscles by escalating morphine and its metabolites, often in the context of dehydration and renal impairment. One of the metabolites of morphine is morphine-6-glucoronide, which has been shown experimentally to cause CNS hyperexcitability. Thus caution should be observed with morphine (or its analogue precursor diamorphine) infusions with patients in renal failure or who are slipping into unconsciousness at the end of life. The treatment of opioid-induced myoclonus and hyperexcitability is based on opioid switching, correction of dehydration, and the use of benzodiazepines to reduce muscle irritability [54]. In severe renal failure, it is safer to use fentanyl or methadone, which do not give rise to toxic metabolites.

Breakthrough pain

Even if a patient is well controlled for the greater part of the day by 'around the clock' (ATC) pain medication (e.g. using 12-hourly oxycodone or a fentanyl patch), very often there will be brief episodes of breakthrough pain. In a study of 164 cancer patients with stable background pain, it was found that breakthrough episodes occurred in 51 per cent, with a median of six episodes per day [55]. The median duration from onset to peak intensity was 3 min. In 13 per cent pain was related to the end of fixed dose schedules, i.e. when the blood level of background opioid had fallen too low, and in 20 per cent it was related to movement ('incident pain'). Patients who had breakthrough pain had more intense background pain than those without breakthrough episodes. The latter finding was confirmed by a large international survey of pain experience in 1095 patients with cancer pain, which found with a multivariate model that the presence of breakthrough pain, somatic pain, and lower performance status were the most important predictors of more intense pain [56].

The significance of breakthrough pain in mesothelioma is that these episodes can seriously impair quality of life. In the study by Portenoy *et al.* [55], patients who had episodes of breakthrough pain had significantly higher depression and anxiety scores and reduced scores for activity and enjoyment of life. The management of these episodes depends on trying to identify and correct predictable causes, for example reducing end-of-dose failures by increasing background doses or sometimes increasing frequency. If the pain is movement related, education and aids for the patient on how to mobilize with the minimum of strain on the chest wall or spine can be helpful. The medical interventions include normal-release opioids that usually work within 20–30 min or, more recently, oral transmucosal fentanyl lozenges which are more rapidly absorbed and can give a better degree of pain relief, compared with oral morphine, within 15 min [57].

Non-pharmacological methods

It is important to consider the use of non-pharmacological methods in pain control because most patients want to minimize the number of medications and are increasingly wary of side effects [48]. Referral to a specialist pain clinic for the early consideration of neurolytic blocks is recommended for mesothelioma patients. The blocks can be short term, using local anaesthetics, or may be longer lasting if alcohol, phenol, or radiofrequency ablation are used. In skilled hands, percutaneous cervical cordotomy can be useful and may reduce the need for the analgesic drug treatments described above [58,59]. There is a small but significant risk of loss of function or dysaesthesia in the ipsilateral upper limb and patients should be counselled about this.

Acupuncture has been used successfully for pain control in chronic benign conditions and may also be tried in cancer patients. There are no published trials of its use in mesothelioma. Similarly, trancutaneous electrical nerve stimulation (TENS) may theoretically work for moderate and fairly superficial pain, but it is unlikely to be effective on its own for the severe inflammatory and neuropathic pain of established chest wall mesothelioma. However, TENS may provide the patient with an element of control over the pain as it can be switched on and off at will. Encouraging patients to control their lifestyle and factors that influence pain is part of a comprehensive pain-management programme. Teaching patients to relax using music or specially prepared audiotapes can also be helpful for some.

Dyspnoea management

Breathlessness or dyspnoea is very common in mesothelioma, especially in the advanced stages when a whole hemithorax may be obliterated and the situation is complicated by pericardial constriction and/or ascites. If pulmonary thromboembolism is added to this scenario, it is easy to see why dyspnoea is almost universal in the terminal stage. A recent review of current understanding of dyspnoea in disease has been provided by Gillette and Schwartzstein [60]. The anticancer treatments using chemotherapy and radiation are described in Chapters 14, 15, and 16 of this volume. Surgical interventions such as pleurectomy may assist by reducing the recurrence of pleural effusion. The use of bronchodilators for airflow obstruction and management of heart failure or anaemia, which may contribute to dyspnoea, are beyond the scope of this chapter.

The palliative management of dyspnoea can be viewed, as with pain, in terms of a three-dimensional pyramid (Fig. 20.6). The four faces that represent the main therapeutic modalities are as follows: opioids; benzodiazepines and other sedatives; oxygen and airflow; psychological and behavioural methods.

Opioids

Opioids have a special place in the relief of dyspnoea because they have multiple potential benefits. They can act directly on the medullary respiratory centre to reduce sensitivity to retained carbon dioxide (lowered blood pH) which arises when the ventilatory pump is failing for any reason. They can also reduce pain in the chest or spine, which may be hindering respira-

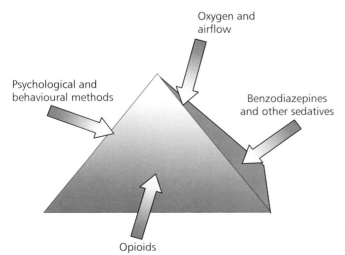

Figure 20.6 Pyramid for control of dyspnoea.

tory movements, and they reduce cough that may produce paroxysms of pain. Although they are not used primarily as anxiolytics or sedatives, this may be a beneficial side effect for some patients. In others, especially morphine, confusion or hallucinations may have the opposite effect of raising anxiety and causing agitation.

There is very little research on the best opioids to use for dyspnoea, and the best methods for delivery and dosing. Several small controlled studies have shown that morphine given orally or parenterally can relieve dyspnoea in cancer or chronic obstructive pulmonary disease (COPD) [61,62]. There are no good studies with other potent opioids. There have been several randomized trials comparing nebulized morphine with saline and, apart from one study in COPD, all, including studies of cancer patients, have failed to show significant benefit over 'placebo' [62]. However, it may be that nebulized saline, partly because it can act as an aid to expectoration, may be an 'active' intervention in itself.

It is recommended that an opioid-naive patient, i.e. one who is not currently on strong opioid for pain control, is started at 5–10 mg of morphine (or 2.5–5 mg of oxycodone) every 4 h if using normal release formulations; or a total daily dose of 30–60 mg of morphine (or 15–30 mg of oxycodone) if using modified-release preparations.

Only one study has attempted to clarify the dosing to use in the common scenario of patients who are already on a stable dose of strong opioid for pain and then develop dyspnoea [63]. This trial compared the effect of 25 per cent of the four-hourly equivalent of the daily opioid dose with 50 per cent of the dose. For example, for patients already taking 60 mg of morphine daily, the study compared 2.5 mg with 5 mg. Both regimens gave an almost identical significant reduction in dyspnoea intensity and respiratory frequency, which lasted for up to 4 h. Thus it is reasonable to start at the lower dosing level and increase it if there is no response.

Benzodiazepines and other sedatives

Because of the strong association of anxiety and panic with dyspnoea, it is reasonable to consider the role of centrally acting sedatives such as benzodiazepines or neuroleptic agents (e.g. haloperidol, levomepromazine). These agents are used extensively in palliative care of patients in the advanced stages of cancer who are anxious or delirious. However, there are no good randomized studies of these agents in cancer patients. In the absence of research evidence, it is considered safe initially to use small as-required doses of a benzodiazepine (e.g. 0.5 mg lorazepam every 6 h). Haloperidol can be given as a single night-time dose, starting at 1.5–3 mg. For a patient who is still agitated with constant or intermittent breathlessness, a subcutaneous infusion of midazolam can be used with a starting dose of 10–20 mg/24 h [62]. Similarly, haloperidol can be given by infusion over 24 h, starting at 5 mg; alternatively, the more potent neuroleptic levomepromazine can be used, starting at 12.5 mg/24 h [54]. All these agents can be titrated upwards by 50 per cent every 24 h until the patient becomes calmer. They can be mixed with opioids, either orally or in a syringe driver for subcutaneous infusion. Extra doses of these drugs can be given, using about 25 per cent of the total daily dose and preferably subcutaneously, for 'breakthrough' episodes of breathlessness.

Oxygen and airflow

A full description of the role of oxygenation and the therapeutic use of supplementary oxygen is not possible here, and the reader is recommended to study the comprehensive review by Booth *et al.* [64]. In summary, there is a place for short-burst supplementary oxygen for patients who have been demonstrated to have desaturation on exertion or at rest. A cut-off of 90 per cent oxygen saturation is a considered reasonable level at which to add supplementary oxygen. For patients who are constantly below this level, for example those with obliteration of a hemithorax or significant pericardial constriction and consequent low lung perfusion, it is justifiable to offer continuous oxygen.

Some patients with exercise-induced desaturation and dyspnoea may gain additional benefit over conventional 28 per cent inhaled oxygen with nitrogen by using a combination gas consisting of 28 per cent oxygen in helium (Heliox28). A recent randomized blinded study in lung cancer patients showed that Heliox28 was able to give such patients faster relief of dyspnoea and, when breathed continuously, allowed them to walk further in a 6 min walking test [65].

Schwartzstein et al. [66] have shown that cooling the facial areas innervated by the second and third divisions of the trigeminal nerve can produce significant reduction in the sensation of dyspnoea. This may be a reason for the frequently observed 'placebo' response to oxygen delivery by mask in patients who are not actually hypoxaemic. It is possible to reproduce this effect by employing a small portable bedside fan and, together with ensuring that patients can gain access to fresh moving air by opening a nearby window, such simple measures can give reassurance as well as actual relief.

Psychological and behavioural approaches

There is a significant body of research on the role of psychological and behavioural techniques for the management of dyspnoea. Many of these rely on encouraging the patient to take more control over his or her own lifestyle and pattern of breathing both to prevent breathless attacks and to cope with them once they have started. These methods include a cyclical feedback model of goal-setting, pacing, and breathing control, learning to reduce breathing rate and adopt the most advantageous positions during an attack, and making the best use of aids and adaptations around the house and for going out. Other approaches which may be helpful for selected patients are music therapy and art therapy, which allow the patient to pursue non-energetic activities to bring distraction and restore a feeling of self-control [67].

In a chest clinic or oncology service, it may be possible to recruit the assistance of a physiotherapist or occupational therapist to help the patients with these methods. Bredin et al. [68] have described a nurse-led approach with a range of these psychological and behavioural techniques being taught to patients with lung cancer and mesothelioma. This has led to the development of nurse- and physiotherapist-led breathlessness clinics which have increased the therapeutic possibilities for cancer patients. Ideally, there should a full multidisciplinary team including occupational therapists and physicians, as is more common in the area of pulmonary rehabilitation [69].

Cachexia syndrome

Weight loss is a major type of morbidity and source of other complaints in mesothelioma. As stated above, the presence of weight loss at presentation is a poor prognostic sign. The causes of the anorexia–cachexia syndrome that lead to weight loss and fatigue are complex, and thus the management response needs to be multimodal. Figure 20.7 shows a pyramid of approaches for this topic: its four therapeutic faces cover drugs to reduce the cytokine and inflammatory response, agents that stop proteolysis, nutritional supplementation, and fatigue and exercise management.

Reduction of cytokine and inflammatory response

Most of the currently used methods fall into this category, and although they come from pharmacologically distinct groups of drugs, their modes of action overlap. Corticosteroids

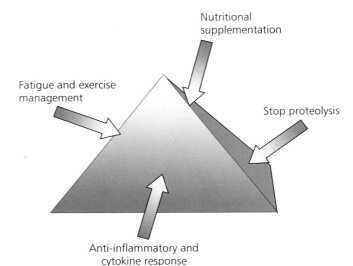

Figure 20.7 Pyramid for management of cachexia.

(prednisolone, dexamethasone) are potent inhibitors of acute and chronic inflammation. Progestogens (megestrol, medroxyprogesterone) have anti-inflammatory effects but may also work by reducing levels of procachectic cytokines such as IL-6. There are many published trials of these agents and, on balance, it is best to use the progestogens as although they are slower to act than steroids, they have reduced systemic toxicities and a longer duration of action [70]. Thus, for a quick 'boost' to appetite and wellbeing, it is reasonable to use a 5 day course of prednisolone or dexamethasone, and to follow this with a long-term course of megestrol. It is important to be aware that megestrol in doses higher than 480 mg/day could add to the pre-existing thrombotic tendency present in mesothelioma patients. Doses of 160 mg twice daily are safe, and can be tolerated with minimal fluid retention and without the myopathy associated with long-term corticosteroids.

Recently, thalidomide has been shown to be effective in quickly improving appetite and weight [71]. It is a potent blocker of TNF-1α which, like IL-6, is a major cause of cachexia. Antibodies to TNF-1α are being tested for this indication but no results are currently available. Another recently introduced pharmacological approach is the use of an angiotensin-converting enzyme (ACE) inhibitor. Although much is known about the role of ACE in the production of angiotensin II, which is crucial in fluid and blood pressure regulation, recent studies have shown that, at the cellular level, ACE can block the production of IL-6 [72].

Inhibition of proteolysis

As well as their action in blocking IL-6 production, ACE inhibitors are also now believed to act by blocking the action that angiotensin II has on directly upregulating cellular proteolysis by activating the ubiquitin-proteasome system [72]. An international study using low doses of the ACE inhibitor imidapril is presently testing the importance of this mechanism in lung and pancreatic cancer patients with cachexia [73].

Eicosapentaenoic acid (EPA) is an omega-3 fatty acid that is found in oily fish. When purified and given in large doses, it has been shown to act as a competitor for arachidonic acid in lipoxygenase and cyclo-oxygenase pathways, reduce circulating leukotrienes and prostaglandins, and block proteolysis-inducing factor (PIF) [22]. Thus EPA has both anti-inflammatory and antiproteolysis actions. It has been shown to reverse weight loss in pancreatic cancer, which has one of the highest rates of cachexia of all solid tumours. Unfortunately, to obtain a therapeutic level of EPA, patients have to consume large numbers of capsules or take the oily liquid, which many find unacceptable.

Nutritional supplementation

It used to be thought that simply increasing nutritional intake could prevent weight loss and possibly increase survival in solid cancer patients. The evidence from many studies is that this manoeuvre alone is ineffective [74]. However, when combined with anti-inflammatory agents or inhibitors of proteolysis such as EPA, increased nutritional intake can give positive results [75]. There is a large range of dietary supplements and ideally a dietician experienced in the care of cancer patients should first assess the patient for current deficiencies and then prescribe the best combination of nitrogen, carbohydrate, and fat sources. There is one form of liquid nutritional supplement that contains EPA, and if patients can tolerate the therapeutic dose of this, it can slow down weight loss in pancreatic cancer [76].

Fatigue and exercise management

One of the first consequences of anorexia–cachexia syndrome is the reduction in energy level that leads to a more sedentary lifestyle. Cytokines such as TNF-1α and IL-6 also directly cause fatigue, as well as initiating muscle breakdown. Pain and exercise-induced dyspnoea aggravate this situation, leading to an increasingly debilitated patient who is experiencing rapid loss of skeletal muscle bulk and power.

A major feature of pulmonary and cardiac rehabilitation programmes is that they address this spiralling decline by introducing graded exercise at an early stage [69]. Recently, there have been attempts to introduce a similar approach into the rehabilitation of cancer patients (e.g. breast cancer patients after mastectomy) to allow earlier return to work [77]. Exercise programmes have not yet been introduced into the management of lung cancer or mesothelioma. Even without a formal programme, patients should be encouraged to take regular exercise and, in particular, to maintain the use of both upper and lower limbs. Walking is probably the safest form of exercise, preferably outside the house and at a steady pace that does not induce dyspnoea or pain. Exercise programmes are particularly important if patients are on long-term corticosteroids.

It is possible to reverse the sense of fatigue and drowsiness that accompanies cachexia and is also an adverse effect of many of the drugs used for pain or dyspnoea control. Opioids, benzodiazepines, and neuroleptics may be prescribed for good indications and tailored to reduce symptoms, but may still cause unacceptable sedation. Psychostimulants have long been used in this situation in North America [78]. European practitioners have been more cautious, perhaps concerned about the risk of addiction to amphetamine analogues or cardiac toxicity. However, with appropriately titrated and supervised doses of methylphenidate, these potential risks are hardly ever seen.

The starting dose for methylphenidate is 10 mg in the morning and 10 mg at noon. This can be increased every 2–3 days in 10-mg increments until the patient reports useful wakefulness. Many patients also report elevation of mood, and indeed in North America psychostimulants may be used as quick-acting antidepressants. Recently, modafinil has been introduced; it is less potent but safer than the amphetamine analogues for patients at risk of cardiac over-stimulation [79]. By using methylphenidate or modafinil it should be possible to minimize or prevent the constant lethargy and consequent low mood that exists, often iatrogenically, in cancer patients.

Psychological distress

Psychosocial distress, like physical symptom load, is a common experience in mesothelioma patients. In an Australian study of 53 patients formally evaluated using the EORTC QLQ-C30, it was possible to compare the scores of mesothelioma patients with those of a lung cancer (stage IV non-small cell) and a normal (Norwegian) population reference group [20]. Psychological functioning, which includes questions on anxiety and depression, in mesothelioma was intermediate between normal people and lung cancer patients who scored worst. However, mesothelioma patients reported a worse experience in social and role functioning than both the other groups. On overall global health and quality of life, mesothelioma patients scored the same as lung cancer patients and were worse than the normal population. Emotional functioning and role functioning emerged as independent prognostic factors for survival in a multivariate Cox model in this study.

Mesothelioma patients may have already lived for many years with a kind of 'anticipatory anxiety' as they hear about coworkers who have succumbed to fatal asbestos-related diseases [80] This can feel like the 'sword of Damocles' hanging over their heads for some time. Depression is a known psychological consequence of having a cancer diagnosis and may be partly related to the knowledge of the very poor outcome. It is more likely to occur in advanced cancer patients with poor social support systems [81]. However, it has also been shown in colorectal cancer that depression was associated with levels of the circulating soluble cytokine receptor sIL-2rα [82]. By analogy, the known high incidence of the cytokine-related inflammatory response in mesothelioma may predispose patients to depressive symptoms.

Cognitive impairment may be a feature in advanced disease, possibly because of the cumulative effect of opioids and other drugs used in symptom control. It is recognized that long-term use of corticosteroids can result in episodes of depression, even mania, and a measurable degree of cognitive impairment such as memory loss [83]. These changes with corticosteroids are dose dependent, and may occur with both prednisolone and dexamethasone.

Management of psychological distress

It is not possible here to go into details of the management of anxiety and depression; this can be found in many standard medical and psychiatric texts. Despite the high prevalence of depression in cancer patients, there have been no well-designed large trials of antidepressants in this situation. However, when cancer patients were referred to a specialist psychological consulting service, 67 per cent were prescribed antidepressants and there was a good clinical response of 80 per cent [84].

It is worth pointing out that, of the antidepressants, venlafaxine has a specific advantage for use in mesothelioma because of its effectiveness against neuropathic pain without the troublesome anticholinergic side effects of traditional tricyclics [85]. Its use is limited, however, in patients with cardiac disease. Because of the 2–3 weeks it requires for even modern antidepressants to have their full effect, the use of psychostimulants to provide a quicker boost should be considered. The use of methylphenidate has been described above.

Anxiolytics that are helpful in cancer patients include lorazepam (starting at 0.5–1.0 mg twice daily) or haloperidol (starting at 1.5–3.0 mg at night). For patients who are very agitated, especially in the terminal stages, subcutaneous boluses and/or an infusion of midazolam are very helpful. Dosing of midazolam has been described above under the management of dyspnoea.

Non-pharmacological interventions are worth considering to minimize the adverse effects associated with psychotropic medication. Many palliative care services, and increasingly cancer units, provide massage and guided relaxation. Although unproven claims are often made for complementary therapies such as aromatherapy, a recent Cochrane review identified that massage itself could be helpful for anxiety reduction [86]. The additional benefit of aromatherapy was not proven and there was no effect on depression. A recent randomized controlled trial in primary care of massage compared with relaxation by means of a tape-recording showed similar positive results with both interventions [87].

Spiritual/existential distress

Although chest physicians, oncologists, and specialist nurses working with mesothelioma patients may have become more comfortable with asking about and intervening with psychological distress, it is still much less common for them to address spiritual or existential matters that may be troubling patients. Yet it is evident that spiritual concerns are very important to patients with cancer and those facing any serious illness. It is important to distinguish spiritual from religious matters: the latter refers to aspects of organized faiths, whereas the former applies to all people, be they believers, agnostics, or atheists [88].

Patients with a diagnosis of mesothelioma may have many reasons to question their faith systems or previous 'macho' lifestyles which become challenged with increasing debility, or to harbour uncertainties over the future [80]. The stigma, shame, self-blame, and blame of others experienced by lung cancer patients may be heightened in mesothelioma patients, who have an occupational risk factor to consider [89].

A detailed interview study in Sweden has highlighted the linkage between constant unrelieved pain and existential forms of distress [90]. Patients with higher overall pain scores expressed significantly more fears about the future and lifestyle, and worries about the progression of pain, and generally had more worries and anxieties that interfered with daily living. In general, younger patients expressed higher levels of existential distress in response to chronic pain.

More so than physical or psychological aspects of distress, spiritual or existential distress can be shared by, or contribute to suffering of, a family member [91]. It is important to give voice to carers' own spiritual concerns. The fact that death from mesothelioma is classed as an 'unnatural death' can also add to the distress of bereaved relatives.

Management of spiritual/existential distress

The National Institute for Clinical Excellence (NICE) guidance on supportive and palliative care for adults with cancer has stressed the importance of recognizing and offering support to those with spiritual concerns [92]. If the issues are connected with religion and faith systems, it is crucial that an appropriate religious adviser is available for inpatients at all times. In many European countries, people from smaller minority ethnic groups may pose a challenge if they are not represented in the local services' team of professionals.

However, not all spiritual concerns need to be addressed by religious professionals. Specialist nurses, counsellors, and psychologists may be able to help patients explore their deep fears and uncertainties. Doctors are often ill-prepared by their training and have little time to explore these issues in busy hospitals and outpatient clinics. However, it is important for them to be able to recognize when such issues may exist and to refer them to an appropriate colleague. The right person may not be in the hospital cancer service, but in the local specialist palliative care team. Referral to such a service could also ensure that attention is paid to unrelieved pain and other symptoms which could aggravate spiritual distress.

What are supportive care and palliative care?

Supportive care and palliative care are increasingly bracketed together as an entity, especially since the publication in 2004 of the guidance from NICE which was called *Guidance on Cancer*

Services: Improving Supportive and Palliative Care for Adults with Cancer" [92]. However, in reality, these two terms represent a radical shift in health care thinking over the past 30 years and it is likely that their meanings will mature and evolve further over time.

Palliative care is really the extension of 'terminal care' for cancer patients as pioneered in the modern hospices starting in the UK and North America in the 1960s and 1970s. The historical explanation for this relatively new use of 'palliative' is the reluctance of the newly developing terminal care services in French-speaking Canada in the 1970s to use the term 'hospice', which had already been accepted in the UK. In Montreal, the word 'hospice' implied a residential system for elderly people, with strongly negative connotations. It is said that Balfour Mount, a surgeon working in the Royal Victoria Hospital who had been inspired by Dame Cicely Saunders to establish the first terminal care service in Canada, started to use the term 'palliative care' as an alternative to both hospice and terminal care. This new usage rapidly gained currency on both sides of the Atlantic and is the favoured expression worldwide today to describe what are essentially 'end-of-life' healthcare services. However, it is somewhat regrettable that the term 'palliative', which is used to describe the *relief of symptoms*, has also been used to describe the *health care system*, since this has only added to the confusion about what the former has tried to achieve.

One of the driving influences behind the hospice and subsequently palliative care movements is recognition that terminally ill patients, usually identified as having incurable cancer, have a need to receive good quality care at the end of life. In the words of the preamble of the Poznan Declaration [93]:

> It is a human right to receive effective cancer pain relief and palliative care. It is unethical to tolerate unnecessary and unacceptable suffering.

The most recent attempt to clarify what palliative care is, as a health care system, arose from a European Union funded workshop in Milan, whose purpose was to propose a new programme of activities and priorities for harmonizing and improving palliative care across Europe. The workshop published the following new definition [94]:

> Palliative care is the person-centred attention to physical symptoms, psychological, social and existential distress and cultural needs in patients with limited prognosis, in order to optimize the quality of life for the patients and their families or friends.

The workshop also agreed that it is essential to separate palliative care interventions that can and should be undertaken by *any healthcare professional* from those which should fall within the responsibility of *specialists with postgraduate training*. This view gave rise to the following further definitions of how palliative care could be implemented:

> **Basic palliative care** is palliative care which should be provided by all health care professionals, in primary or secondary care, within their duties to patients with life-limiting disease.

> **Specialized palliative care** is palliative care provided at the expert level by a trained multiprofessional team, who must continually update their skills and knowledge in order to manage persisting and more severe or complex problems and to provide specialized educational and practical resources to other non-specialized members of the primary or secondary care teams.

'Basic' is usually called 'generic' and 'specialized' is called 'specialist' in the UK. These secondary definitions are helpful in that they make explicit an issue that until recently had still not been openly accepted, namely that some aspects of palliative care are the domain of a specialty. The Milan statement expanded on what it meant by 'basic palliative care' but, in practice, each country has to decide for itself where the dividing line lies between basic and specialized, as most European countries still do not recognize the medical specialty of palliative medicine.

It should be noted that the Milan definition states 'limited prognosis' and not, as in previous definitions, 'incurable' or 'unresponsive to curative treatment'. Thus patients should be deemed eligible for palliative care even if they are at the very beginning of a malignant disease, possibly undergoing radical life-extending treatment. In reality, patients still tend to be referred to palliative care specialists when it is thought that they are approaching the end of life, usually conceived as the last few months.

Specialist palliative care (SPC) services in the UK are highly developed, and can be found in the acute sector as part of hospital support teams, in the community, and as stand-alone palliative care units or hospices, including day hospices. Uniquely for an integral part of British health care, the voluntary sector, including local and national charities, has a major role in funding and staffing palliative care teams in all but the hospital services.

The NHS Cancer Plan and its implementation through the NHS Modernization Agency have led to more explicit structures for palliative care services within the acute hospital sector. Thus all hospitals in the UK which serve cancer patients must now have a core palliative care team—at least a specialist nurse and doctor—and cancer centres should have good access to a broader range of professionals such as a social worker, a psychologist, and a physiotherapist.

What new services or facilities are added by the term 'supportive care'? This embraces a much wider range of issues than palliative care, which emphasizes end-of-life care, could or should respond to. These issues include information resources for all cancer patients and carers, rehabilitation services including nutritional support as well as occupational therapy, speech and language therapy, and psychological support services, going up to consultant psychologist or psychiatrist level. Some of the other prescribed elements of supportive care are often well represented within hospices and their outreach teams (e.g. spiritual care, complementary therapies, services for families and carers including bereavement support). However, the message of the new guidance is that these should be available to *all* cancer patients and their carers, not just those who are, often arbitrarily, considered to be approaching the end of life. Thus the real challenge for cancer and other acute hospital departments, such as respiratory medicine, is to integrate supportive care into their own work, whilst clarifying whom and when to refer to specialist palliative care.

Sheffield model of supportive care

In Sheffield, UK, a model has been evolving which aims to clarify how the relationships between acute hospital departments, palliative care services, and primary care can be made explicit and operational [95]. Figure 20.8 shows how it is first useful to dissociate the elements of care that are directed to the disease process from those directed to the patient and to the family carers. The patient may have significant needs beyond those expressed by the new disease, for example comorbidity from other chronic illnesses and informational, financial, or existential concerns. In a US study of 301 cancer patients, it was found that, overall, 83 per cent of those with lung cancer had other significant comorbid issues (e.g. 52 per cent cardiovascular, 34 per cent arthritis, 24 per cent pulmonary) [96]. The family often has other pressing needs, such as financial support, psychological stress, and bereavement support after the patient dies [97].

Putting these three elements together, the Sheffield model displays how supportive care runs alongside the disease-directed therapies at all stages, and even begins before there may be a histological diagnosis. Therefore it does not matter whether the patient is currently receiving disease-directed treatment aimed at cure, prolonging life, or just maintaining life. Furthermore, in this model supportive care applies to patients who are (temporarily or, increasingly, permanently) in remission or 'cured'. The supportive care needs of these patients and their carers may focus rather

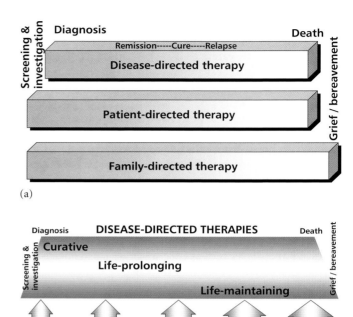

Figure 20.8 Sheffield model of supportive care.

(b)

more on rehabilitation and social or financial support, but control of symptoms arising from surgical or other therapeutic interventions may also be necessary.

Supportive and palliative care for mesothelioma

What is the ideal supportive and palliative care package for patients with mesothelioma and their family carers? From the preceding discussion, it should be clear that mesothelioma patients are best served in an environment where they are regularly reviewed by a multidisciplinary cancer service which includes respiratory, oncology, and surgical specialists. A nurse or medical member of the local specialist palliative care team should be present at the team meetings, but in addition it should be possible to refer patients to other specialists offering aspects of supportive or palliative care at all times. In most large hospitals, there will be good access to a dietician, physiotherapist, occupational therapist, social worker, and psychologist. In smaller hospitals, where these professionals are not readily available, it may be appropriate to refer the patient, regardless of the stage of disease, to the local hospice where it is likely that they will be present.

Most patients, even with a poor prognosis disease such as mesothelioma, spend the majority of their lives at home. The primary care team, essentially the general practitioner and district nurse, should be kept informed about the patient's condition, planned investigations and treatments, and expected complications of these. Even if palliative care specialists can visit at home or the patient is attending a day hospice for social support, it is important for the primary care team to remain in overall control [98].

It is helpful and reassuring for both patient and family, and also for the primary care team, that vulnerable patients should have free or open access to the hospital team which is currently actively pursuing their disease-directed care. A pilot scheme for an 'open-access' lung cancer clinic in a moderate-sized district general hospital gave good results for satisfaction of users [99]. There were actually fewer visits than predicted, suggesting that open-access clinics are reassuring but unlikely to be misused. In localities where the local chest service or cancer service is unable to provide such a scheme, the next challenge for the ever-evolving palliative care teams may be to take on and develop this patient-centred model of care.

Bibliography

Ahmedzai SH, Muers MF. *Supportive Care in Respiratory Disease*. Oxford: Oxford University Press, 2005.

Doyle D, Hanks G, Cherny N, Calman K (eds). *Oxford Textbook of Palliative Medicine*, 3rd edn. Oxford: Oxford University Press, 2004.

Twycross R, Wilcock A, Charlesworth S, Dickman A. *Palliative Care Formulary* (2nd edn). Oxford: Radcliffe Medical Press, 2002.

References

1. British Thoracic Society Standards of Care Committee. Statement on malignant mesothelioma in the United Kingdom. *Thorax* 2001; **56**: 250–65.

2. Peto J., Hodgson JT, Matthews FE, Jones JR. Continuing increase in mesothelioma mortality in Britain. *Lancet* 1995; **345**; 535–9.

3. Peto J, Decarli A, La Vecchia C, Levi F, Negri E. The European mesothelioma epidemic. *Br J Cancer* 1999; **79**: 666–72.

4. Parker C, Neville E. Lung cancer 8. Management of malignant mesothelioma. *Thorax* 2003; **58**: 809–13.

5. Yates DH, Corrin B, Stidolph PN, Browne K. Malignant mesothelioma in south east England: clinicpathological experience of 272 cases. *Thorax* 1997; **52**: 507–12.

6. Clayson H. Mesothelioma and asbestos—from magic mineral to public health disaster. *Eur J Palliative Care* 2003; **10**:

7. Parra HS, Zucali PA, Colombo P, Balzarini L, Santoro A. Uncommon manifestations of common malignancies. Case 1: soft-tissue metastases from malignant pleural mesothelioma. *J Clin Oncol* 2004; **22**: 3191–5.

8. Akyurek S, Nalca Andrieu M, Hicsonmez A, Dizbay Sak S, Kurtman C. Skeletal muscle metastasis from malignant pleural mesothelioma. *Clin Oncol (R Coll Radiol)* 2004; **16**: 585.

9. Cassarino DS, Xue W, Shannon KJ. Widespread cutaneous and perioral metastases of mesothelioma. *J Cutan Pathol* 2003; **30**: 582–5.

10. Davies MJ, Ahmedzai S, Arsiwala SS, Leverment JN. Intracranial metastases from malignant pleural mesothelioma. *Scand J Thorac Cardiovasc Surg* 1995; **29**: 97–9.

11. Krishnaraj N. Malignant mesothelioma presenting as stroke—a case report. *Eur J Cancer Care* 2003; **12**: 365–8.

12. Schattner A, Kozack N. A 47 year old man with mesothelioma and neck swelling. *Can Med Assoc J* 2004; **170**: 465.

13. Isildak M, Guven GS. Mesothelioma and venous thrombosis. *Can Med Assoc J* 2004; **171**: 11.

14. Kufe D, Pollock R, Weichselbaum R, *et al*. Section 27: The thorax. 93: Malignant mesothelioma. Clinical features. *Holland–Frei Cancer Medicine 6*. Hamilton, Ontario: BC Decker, 2003.

15. Hollen PJ, Gralla RJ, Liepa AM, Symanowski JT, Rusthoven JT. Adapting the Lung Cancer Symptom Scale (LCSS) to mesothelioma. *Cancer* 2004; **101**: 587–95.

16. Ripamonti C, Fulfaro F. Mechanisms of pain associated with respiratory disease. In: Ahmedzai SH, Muers MF (eds). *Supportive Care in Respiratory Disease*. Oxford: Oxford University Press, 2005; 413–25.

17. Richardson J, Sabanathan S, Mearns AJ, Sides C, Goulden CP. Post-thoracotomy neuralgia. *Pain Clinic* 1994; **7**: 87–97.

18. Edwards JG, Abrams KR, Leverment JN, Spyt TJ, Waller DA, O'Byrne KJ. Prognostic factors for malignant mesothelioma in 142 patients: validation of CALGB and EORTC prognostic scoring systems. *Thorax* 2000; **55**: 731–5.

19. Thomason R, Schlegel W, Lucca M, Cummings S, Lee S. Primary malignant mesothelioma of the pericardium. *Texas Heart Inst J* 1994; **21**: 170–4.

20. Nowak A, Stockler MR, Byrne MJ. Assessing quality of life during chemotherapy for pleural mesothelioma: feasibility, validity, and results of using the European Organization for Research and Treatment of Cancer Core Quality of Life Questionnaire and Lung Cancer Module. *J Clin Oncol* 2004; **22**: 3172–80.

21. MacDonald N, Easson AM, Mazurak VC, Dunn GP, Baracos VE. Understanding and managing cancer cachexia. *J Am Coll Surg* 2003; **197**: 143–61.

22. Inui A. Cancer anorexia–cachexia syndrome: current issues in research and management. *CA Cancer J Clin* 2002; **52**: 72–91.

23. Tisdale MJ. Clinical trials for the treatment of secondary wasting and cachexia. *J Nutr* 1999; **129**: 243S–6S.

24. Seki H, Matsumoto K, Ohmura K, *et al.* Malignant pleural mesothelioma presenting as achalasia. *Intern Med* 1994; **33**: 624–7.

25. Lui W, Fackler W, Rice TW, Richter JE, Achkat E, Goldblum JR. The pathogenesis of pseudoachalasia: a clinicopathological study of 13 cases of a rare entity. *Am J Surg Pathol* 2002; **26**: 784–8.

26. Ahmedzai SH. The nature of palliation and its contribution to supportive care. In: Ahmedzai SH, Muers MF, eds. *Supportive Care in Respiratory Disease.* Oxford: Oxford University Press, 2005; 3–38.

27. World Health Organization. Cancer pain relief and palliative care: report of a WHO expert committee. *Tech. Rep. Ser. 804.* Geneva: WHO, 1990.

28. Marinangeli F, Ciccozzi A, Leonardis M, *et al.* Use of strong opioids in advanced cancer pain: a randomized trial. *J Pain Symptom Manage* 2004; **27**: 409–16.

29. Jadad AR, Browman GP. The WHO analgesic ladder for cancer pain management. Stepping up the quality of its evaluation. The WHO analgesic ladder for cancer pain management. Stepping up the quality of its evaluation. *JAMA* 1995; **274**: 1870–3.

30. Ahmedzai SH. Window of opportunity for pain control in the terminally ill. *Lancet* 2002; **357**: 1304–5.

31. Lübbe AS, Ahmedzai SH. A new approach for cancer pain management—the pyramid model. *Prog Palliat Care* 2004; **12**: 287–92.

32. Mucci-LoRusso P, Berman BS, Silberstein PT, *et al.* Controlled-release oxycodone compared with controlled-release morphine in the treatment of cancer pain: a randomized, double-blind, parallel-group study. *Eur J Pain* 1998; **2**: 239–49.

33. Megens AA, Artois K, Vermeire J, Meert T, Awouters FH. Comparison of the analgesic and intestinal effects of fentanyl and morphine in rats. *J Pain Symptom Manage* 1998; **15**: 253–7.

34. Ahmedzai S, Brooks D. Transdermal fentanyl versus sustained-release oral morphine in cancer pain: preference, efficacy, and quality of life. *J Pain Symptom Manage* 1997; **13**: 254–61.

35. Clark AJ, Ahmedzai SH, Allan LG, *et al.* Efficacy and safety of transdermal fentanyl and sustained-release oral morphine in patients with cancer and chronic non-cancer pain. *Curr Med Res Opin* 2004; **20**: 1419–28.

36. Neighbors DM, Bell TJ, Wilson J, Dodd SL. Economic evaluation of the fentanyl transdermal system for the treatment of chronic moderate to severe pain. *J Pain Symptom Manage* 2001; **21**: 129–43.

37. Bridges D, Thompson SWN, Rice ASC. Mechanisms of neuropathic pain. *Br J Anaesth* 2001; **87**: 12–26.

38. DeLong P, Tanaka T, Kruklitis R, *et al.* Use of Cyclooxygenase-2 inhibition to enhance the efficacy of immunotherapy. *Cancer Res* 2003; **63**: 7845–52.

39. Dubner R, Gold M. The neurobiology of pain. *Proc Natl Acad Sci USA* 1999; **96**: 7627–30.

40. Sawynock J. Topical and peripherally acting analgesics. *Pharmacol Rev* 2003; **55**: 1–20.

41. Zeppetella G, Paul J, Ribeiro MDC. Analgesic efficacy of morphine applied topically to painful ulcers. *J Pain Symptom Manage* 2003; **25**: 555–8.

42. Davis MP, Walsh D. Methadone for relief of cancer pain: a review of pharmacokinetics, pharmacodynamics, drug interactions and protocols of administration. *Support Care Cancer* 2001; **9**: 73–83.

43. Sindrup SH, Jensen TS. Efficacy of pharmacological treatments of neuropathic pain: an update and effect related to mechanism of drug action. *Pain* 1999; **83**: 389–400.

44. Rose MA, Kam PCA. Gabapentin: pharmacology and its use in pain management. *Anaesthesia* 2002; **57**: 451–62.

45. Mach DB, Rogers SD, Sabino MC, *et al*. Origins of skeletal pain: sensory and sympathetic innervation of the mouse femur. *Neuroscience* 2002; **113**: 155–66.

46. Conte P, Coleman R. Bisphosphonates in the treatment of skeletal metastases. *Semin Oncol* 2004; **31**(Suppl 10): 59–63.

47. Jagdev SP, Coleman RE. The bisphosphonate, zoledronic acid, induces apoptosis of breast cells: evidence for synergy with paclitaxel. *Br J Cancer* 2001; **54**: 1126–34.

48. Weiss SC, Emanuel LL, Fairclough DL, Emanuel EJ. Understanding the experience of pain in terminally ill patients. *Lancet* 2001; **357**: 1311–15.

49. Sapir R, Catane R, Kaufman B, *et al*. Cancer patient expectations of and communication with oncologists and oncology nurses: the experience of an integrated oncology and palliative care service. *Support Care Cancer* 2000; **8**: 458–63.

50. Brooks D.J., Gamble W., Ahmedzai S. A regional survey of opioid use by patients receiving specialist palliative care. *Palliat Med* 1995; **9**: 229–38.

51. Nielsen CK, Ross FB, Smith MT. Incomplete, symmetric, and route-dependent cross-tolerance between oxycodone and morphine in the dark Agouti rat. *J Pharmacol Exp Ther* 2000; **295**: 91–9.

52. Carroll IR, Angst MS, Clark JD. Management of perioperative pain in patients chronically consuming opioids. *Reg Anesth Pain Med* 2004; **29**: 576–91.

53. Davis PD, Walsh D. Methadone for relief of cancer pain: a review of pharmacokinetics, pharmacodynamics, drug interactions and protocols of administration. *Support Care Cancer* 2001; **9**: 73–83.

54. Twycross R, Wilcock A. *Symptom Management in Advanced Cancer*, 3rd edn. Oxford: Radcliffe Medical Press, 2001; 259–89.

55. Portenoy RK, Payne D, Jacobsen P. Breakthrough pain: characteristics and impact in patients with cancer pain. *Pain* 1999; **81**: 129–34.

56. Caraceni A, Martini C, Zecca E, *et al*. Breakthrough pain characteristics and syndromes in patients with cancer pain. An international survey. *Palliat Med* 2004; **18**: 177–83.

57. Portenoy RK, Payne R, Coluzzi P, *et al*. Oral transmucosal fentanyl citrate (OTFC) for the treatment of breakthrough pain in cancer patients: a controlled dose titration study. *Pain* 1999; **79**: 303–12.

58. Jackson MB, Pounder D, Price C, Matthews AW, Neville E. Percutaneous cervical cordotomy for the control of pain in patients with pleural mesothelioma. *Thorax* 1999; **54**: 238–41.

59. Zuurmond WWA, de Lange JJ. Pain in association with respiratory disease. Neurolytic procedures. In: Ahmedzai SH, Muers MF, eds. *Supportive Care in Respiratory Disease*. Oxford: Oxford University Press, 2005; 453–60.

60. Gillette MA, Schwartzstein RM. Mechanisms of dyspnoea. In: Ahmedzai SH, Muers MF, eds. *Supportive Care in Respiratory Disease*. Oxford: Oxford University Press, 2005; 93–122.

61. Ahmedzai SH. Palliation of respiratory symptoms. In: Doyle D, Hanks GW, MacDonald N, eds. *Oxford Textbook of Palliative Medicine*, 2nd edn. Oxford: Oxford University Press, 1998.

62. Davis C. Management of dyspnoea. Drug therapies. In: Ahmedzai SH, Muers MF, eds. *Supportive Care in Respiratory Disease*. Oxford: Oxford University Press, 2005; 147–64.

63. Allard P, Lamontagne C, Bernard P, Tremblay C. How effective are supplementary doses of opioids for dyspnea in terminally ill cancer patients? A randomized continuous sequential clinical trial. *J Pain Symptom Manage* 1999; **17**: 256–65.

64. Booth S, Wade R, Johnson M, Kite S, Swannick M, Anderson H. The use of oxygen in the palliation of breathlessness. A report of the expert working group of the Scientific Committee of the Association of Palliative Medicine. *Respir Med* 2004; **98**: 66–77.

65. Ahmedzai SH, Laude E, Robertson A, Troy G, Vora V. A double-blind, randomised, controlled phase II trial of Heliox28 gas mixture in lung cancer patients with dyspnoea on exertion. *Br J Cancer* 2005; **90**: 366–71.

66. Schwartzstein RM, Lahive K, Pope A, Weinberger SE, Weiss JW. Cold facial stimulation reduces breathlessness induced in normal subjects. *Am Rev Respir Dis* 1987; **136**: 58–61.

67. MacLeod R. Management of dyspnoea. Psychosocial therapies. In: Ahmedzai SH, Muers MF, eds. *Supportive Care in Respiratory Disease*. Oxford: Oxford University Press, 2005; 229–38.

68. Bredin M, Corner J, Krishnasamy M, Plant H, Bailey C, A'Hern R. Multicentre randomised controlled trial of nursing intervention for breathlessness in patients with lung cancer. *Br Med J* 1999; **318**: 901–6.

69. Lindsay J, Goldstein R. Management of dyspnoea. Rehabilitation and exercise. In: Ahmedzai SH, Muers MF, eds. *Supportive Care in Respiratory Disease*. Oxford: Oxford University Press, 2005; 189–214.

70. Loprinzi CL, Kugler JW, Sloan JA, *et al.* Randomized comparison of megestrol acetate versus dexamethasone versus fluoxymesterone for the treatment of cancer anorexia/cachexia. *J Clin Oncol* 1999; **17**: 3299–306.

71. Peuckmann V, Fisch M, Bruera E. Potential novel uses of thalidomide: focus on palliative care. *Drugs* 2000; **60**: 273–92.

72. Tisdale MJ, Saunders PM. Effects of angiotensin II on protein synthesis and degradation in murine myotubes. *Support Care Cancer* 2004; **12**: 369–70.

73. Gagnon B, Ahmedzai SH, Grunberg S, Murray N. Phase III trial of imidapril (Vitor™)—a novel pharmacological intervention for cancer cachexia. *Support Care Cancer* 2004; **12**: 368–9.

74. Kotler DP. Cachexia. *Ann Intern Med.* 2000; **133**: 622–34.

75. Barber MD, McMillan DC, Preston T, Ross JA, Fearon KCH. Metabolic response to feeding in weight-losing pancreatic cancer patients and its modulation by a fish-oil-enriched nutritional supplement. *Clin Sci* 2000; **98**: 389–99.

76. Fearon KCH, von Meyenfeldt MF, Moses AGW, *et al.* Effect of a protein and energy dense n-3 fatty acid enriched oral supplement on loss of weight and lean tissue in cancer cachexia: a randomised double blind trial. *Gut* 2003; **52**: 1479–86.

77. Campbell A, Mutrie N, White F, McGuire F, Kearney N. A pilot study of a supervised group exercise programme as a rehabilitation treatment for women with breast cancer receiving adjuvant treatment. *Eur J Oncol Nurs* 2005; **9**: 56–63.

78. Bruera E, Driver L, Barnes EA, *et al.* Patient-controlled methylphenidate for the management of fatigue in patients with advanced cancer: a preliminary report. *J Clin Oncol.* 2003; **21**: 4439–43.

79. Webster L, Andrews M, Stoddard G. Modafinil treatment of opioid-induced sedation. *Pain Medicine* 2003; **4**: 135–40.

80. Clayson H. Suffering in mesothelioma: concepts and contexts. *Prog Palliat Care* 2003; **11**: 251–5.

81. Lloyd-Williams M, Friedman T. Depression in palliative care patients—a prospective study. *Eur J Cancer Care* 2001; **10**: 270–4.

82. Allen-Mersh TG, Glover C, Fordy C, Henderson DC, Davies M. Relation between depression and circulating immune products in patients with advanced colorectal cancer. *J R Soc Med* 1998; **91**: 408–13.

83. Brown ES, Chandler PA. Mood and cognitive changes during systemic corticosteroid therapy. *Prim Care Companion. J Clin Psychiatry* 2001; **3**: 17–21.

84. Lloyd-Williams M. Are antidepressants effective in cancer patients? *Prog Palliat Care* 2004; **12**: 217–19.

85. Lusier D, Huskey AG, Portenoy RK. Adjuvant analgesics in cancer pain management. *Oncologist* 2004; **9**; 571–91.

86. Fellowes D, Barnes K, Wilkinson S. Aromatherapy and massage for symptom relief in patients with cancer. *Cochrane Database Syst Rev* 2004; CD002287.

87. Hanley J, Stirling P, Brown C. Randomised controlled trial of therapeutic massage in the management of stress. *Br J Gen Pract* 2003; **53**: 20–5.

88. Speck P, Higginson I, Addington-Hall J. Spiritual needs in health care. *BMJ* 2004; **329**: 123–4.

89. Chapple A, Ziebland S, McPherson A. Stigma, shame, and blame experienced by patients with lung cancer: qualitative study. *BMJ* 2004; **324**; 1470.

90. Strang P. Existential consequences of unrelieved cancer pain. *Palliat Med* 1997; **11**: 299–305.

91. Murray SA, Kendall M, Boyd K, Worth A, Benton TF. Exploring the spiritual needs of people dying of lung cancer or heart failure: a prospective qualitative interview study of patients and their carers. *Palliat Med* 2004; **18**: 39–45.

92. NICE. *Guidance on Cancer Services. Improving Supportive and Palliative Cafe for Adults with Cancer.* London: National Institute for Clinical Excellence, 2004.

93. The Poznan Declaration (1998). *Eur J Palliat Care* 1999; **6**: 61–3.

94. Ahmedzai SH, Costa A, Blengini C, *et al*. A new international framework for palliative care. *Eur J Cancer* 2004; **40**: 2192–200.

95. Ahmedzai SH, Walsh TD. Palliative medicine and modern cancer care. *Semin Oncol* 2000; **27**: 1–6.

96. Ko C, Chaudhry S. The need for a multidisciplinary approach to cancer care. *J Surg Res* 2002; **105**: 53–7.

97. Emanuel JE, Fairclough DL, Slutsman J, Emanuel LL. Understanding economic and other burdens of terminal illness: the experience of patients and their caregivers. *Ann Intern Med* 2000; **132**: 451–9.

98. Borg-Bortolo P, Simmonds P, Ahmedzai SH. Conflicting advice in the care of a dying patient. *Practitioner* 2000; **244**: 672–7.

99. Adlard JW, Joseph J, Brammer CV, Gerrard GE. Open access follow-up for lung cancer: patient and staff satisfaction. *Clin Oncol* 2001; **13**: 404–8.

Chapter 21

The treatment of mesothelioma cases in the US and UK legal systems

A. Budgen and J. N. Lipsitz

Introduction

Mesothelioma patients must deal not only with their debilitating and fatal disease, but also, in many cases, with the legal system. This system includes workers' compensation laws, which provide no-fault benefits for industrial accidents and diseases, as well as the traditional lawsuit, in which the mesothelioma patient sues asbestos manufacturers, and suppliers, and sometimes landowners. While numerous medical doctors frequently testify as experts in asbestos litigation, many more see an occasional mesothelioma patient in the usual course of their medical practice. In this chapter we provide the legal framework of the mesothelioma case from which the asbestos or occupational disease expert, as well as the medical practitioner, may approach the mesothelioma patient.

Because mesothelioma patients are, by definition, short-term patients and because the time available for collecting information important to their legal claims is brief, their doctors must act quickly in deciding whether to refer the patient to an attorney. Often, the patient will have died by the time his case is resolved by either settlement or jury verdict. Once the mesothelioma patient decides to bring a lawsuit and after he has hired an attorney, he and his attorney must next decide whether to arrange for the new client to testify while he is still well enough to do so.

The plaintiff's testimony is given in two stages. The first stage is the discovery deposition during which lawyers for the defendants do most of the questioning. Before submitting the deposition, the plaintiff meets with his attorney to prepare for questions that cover background (prior addresses, education, marital status, children, etc.); work history, with an emphasis on asbestos exposure, job assignments, and work sites; medical history, and personal knowledge of the hazards of exposure to asbestos, including warnings and the use of masks and respirators. Depending on the complexity of the plaintiff's work history and the progress of the disease, the deposition may last for one or two days. The deposition process may occupy the client and their family for a number of precious remaining days. The decision to go forward with the deposition is based on the client's objectives, relative level of comfort, clarity of mind, and whether the effort required will enhance the size of the recovery.

Once the deposition is complete, the plaintiff's attorney will usually proceed, within a day or two, to take the client's *in extremis* trial testimony. Like the deposition, the trial testimony is recorded and transcribed, but it is also videotaped for later presentation to a jury in the event that the case does not settle before trial and the plaintiff is no longer available to testify in person. Trial testimony unfolds in a narrative fashion and is usually accomplished in less than 2 hours.

The purpose of this chapter is to provide physicians with a practical analysis to help patients decide whether to pursue a lawsuit. This chapter should also assist doctors in preparing themselves in the event that they are called to testify about a patient's diagnosis, the cause of his disease, and damages, including pain and suffering. The sections below provide a brief history of asbestos, the development of knowledge of the health risks of asbestos, the legal background of asbestos claims, and the legal issues surrounding a mesothelioma lawsuit.

Asbestos: a brief history

The basic dangers relating to asbestos have been recognized since the end of the nineteenth century. The 'evil effects' of asbestos manufacture and 'the sharp, glass-like jagged nature of the particles' were first described in a report by Her Majesty's Lady Inspectors of Factories as early as 1898 [1], a century before the mineral fibre was finally banned in the UK.

In 1899, a 33-year-old man was admitted to Charing Cross Hospital, London, suffering from breathlessness caused by his job. He told his physician, Dr Montague Murray, that he had worked for 14 years in the asbestos industry and that he was the only survivor from amongst 10 others in his place of work. Within a year, the asbestos worker (whose identity is not known) had died. At the subsequent post-mortem, Dr Murray found that the unfortunate gentlemen's lungs were blackened and stiff with fibrosis caused by inhaling asbestos dust. However, the death of Dr Murray's patient aroused almost no interest at the time.

It was not until 1924 that the first clear case of death due to an asbestos-related disease appeared in the medical literature. In that year, Dr William Cooke, an English physician, performed a post-mortem examination on the body of a 33-year-old woman, Nellie Kershaw, who had started working at the age of 13 in an asbestos textile factory in Rochdale, Lancashire. After 14 years in this factory, she moved to Turner Brothers Asbestos (TBA) in 1917 where she worked in the spinning room on machines that twisted the strands of asbestos. Meanwhile, she had married and had one child. After 14 years of exposure, this young woman had developed a persistent cough and was in poor health. Her physician told her that she was suffering from 'asbestos poisoning'. Nellie Kershaw's health declined steadily and she died, 2 years after giving up work, in March 1924. The autopsy showed lung scarring and dense strands of abnormal fibrous tissue connecting the lungs and the pleural membranes surrounding them. The subsequent inquest was the first on an asbestos worker in the UK.

Dr Cooke's discovery, which was published in the *British Medical Journal* [2], was the point of departure for an intensive study of asbestos-related illness in England over the next 7 years. Cooke published the results in 1927 [3,4]. He called the scarring of the lungs from asbestos dust 'pulmonary asbestosis' (or more simply 'asbestosis'). Cooke also identified the 'curious bodies', which were later termed asbestos bodies.

Development of knowledge of the health risks associated with asbestos

Asbestos has been killing and disabling people since we began to use it well over 100 years ago, and by the mid-1920s real concern had begun to grow about the rising death toll. Even so, asbestos continued to be used with little or no regard for the health of workers or anyone else who came into contact with it. In 1929, a case of asbestos disease was reported in a person living next door to an asbestos factory in the North of England. Therefore there is nothing new in the concept of 'neighbourhood victims'.

Nevertheless, it was not until 1995 [5] that British claimants won the right to sue for (so-called) 'environmental' exposure. The late June Hancock was the first mesothelioma sufferer in the UK to be compensated as a result of neighbourhood exposure to asbestos, when she won a landmark case. Incidentally, June Hancock's mother, Maie Gelder, had also suffered from

Table 21.1 Historical events

1898	Report of Her Majesty's Lady Inspector of Factories
1899	Montague Murray's case
1924	Nellie Kershaw dies of asbestosis in England
1927	William Cooke coins the term 'asbestosis'
1931	First claim for compensation for asbestosis in the USA
1931	The UK establishes health laws regulating exposure to asbestos
1936	Asbestosis becomes a compensable disease in Germany. A. J. Lanza writes 'Asbestosis' article
1960	Wagner et al. publish the link between asbestos exposure and mesothelioma in the British Journal of Industrial Medicine [8]
1964	Irving Selikoff begins publishing results of epidemiological research on the effects of exposure to asbestos; caution labels begin to appear on some products
1967	Seven English asbestos workers file suit for negligent exposure and disease
1969	Asbestos insulator Clarence Borel files lawsuit in Texas against manufacturers. He later dies of mesothelioma
1972	Occupational Safety and Health Administration begins to regulate exposure to asbestos in industry and construction in the USA
1979	Workers' compensation ('no-fault') statute enacted in the UK
1982	The Johns–Manville Corporation and related companies file for bankruptcy reorganization
1986	New York passes the Toxic Tort Reform Act, opening courts to previously time-barred claims
1995	UK claimants win the right to sue for environmental exposure

mesothelioma following similar exposure whilst living in the immediate vicinity of a former asbestos factory (owned by J W Roberts Ltd, Armley, Leeds).

Beginning in 1933, doctors started to record that workers with asbestosis were also suffering from cancer. In 1933, S. R. Gloyne wrote of the damage to the pleura and lungs in asbestosis and reported having seen a case of 'squamous carcinoma of the pleura' with asbestosis. In Germany, asbestosis became a compensable disease in 1936. Germany also began providing compensation to victims of asbestos-induced lung cancer in 1939, the first country to do so. In many other countries, in particular the USA, this did not happen until much later.

Asbestos manufacturing companies (Turner & Newall and Johns–Manville being two notable examples) were well aware of the hazards of asbestos from the early part of the twentieth century (in Turner & Newall's case 'long before' 1925) [6]. Indeed by 1918, many US and Canadian insurance companies had started declining insurance to asbestos workers. One large insurer, Metropolitan Life, actually began a conscious policy of declining insurance to asbestos-exposed workers or increasing premiums to account for the increased cost due to their shortened lifespan.

In 1931, the UK became the first country to establish health laws regulating exposure to asbestos. This followed the publication in 1930 of a report by Merewether and Price [7], who showed that chronic exposure to high concentrations of asbestos fibres could lead to asbestosis. The research undertaken for this report was mentioned in the Annual Reports of the Chief Inspector of Factories for 1928 and 1929. In the Margereson and Hancock judgement (at first instance), the trial judge cited the first page of the report by Merewether and Price which spoke of local effects following the inhalation of dust, including pulmonary and bronchial catarrh, asthma, bronchitis, and fibrosis, and secondary changes such as local or diffuse emphysema. The report pointed out that fibrosis was recognized to be the most important lesion. This seminal piece of work led to the introduction of the Asbestos Industries Regulations 1931, which came into force on 1 March 1932. These were intended to regulate asbestos exposure levels for factory workers and to protect their health, but Merewether and Price also recognized that users of asbestos products, such as laggers and ship builders, were also heavily exposed to asbestos fibres and could be at risk.

However, knowledge of health effects did cause companies to take precautions—not to protect the health of their workers, but against legal action from them. At meetings in the 1930s, many of the asbestos companies got together and took 'concerted' action to create a strategy for defending future claims. The strategy included the establishment of 'standards', later called 'threshold limit values' (TLVs), for exposure to asbestos and silica products which, if complied with, could serve as a 'defence' to claims. They were false.

In 1939, Edmund Pilling, an employee of Turner Brothers, died. He was employed in the cheese-winding and disintegration department. Post-mortem examination revealed cancer of the pleura (i.e. mesothelioma) and no naked-eye evidence of asbestosis. The inquest verdict was death due to carcinoma of the lung. However, mesothelioma's link with asbestos did not emerge fully until the 1950s, in South Africa [8].

In 1952, Dr Christopher Sleggs, a physician in a hospital in Kimberley, Cape Province, became aware of a number of unusual pleural cancers. In 1955, he began work in a clinic situated in the heart of the asbestos mining territory where he found more pleural malignancy cases. Sleggs and a colleague (Paul Marchand) passed biopsies to Dr Christopher Wagner, as they were unsure about the nature of the disease. Dr Wagner was then a young pathologist in Johannesburg, working as an asbestos research fellow. In 1956, Wagner had diagnosed a single case of mesothelial tumour where asbestos bodies had been found in the lung. A connection with asbestos was made after the three doctors had examined the patients' life histories in detail. The industrial and residential case histories revealed that many of the individuals had lived near, but not necessarily worked in, the asbestos mines and mills in the Northwest Cape.

In 1959, Wagner and Sleggs publicized their findings at the International Pneumoconiosis Conference in Johannesburg. Then, in 1960, came the bombshell as the South African doctors published their research in the *British Journal of Industrial Medicine*. They had found 47 cases of mesothelioma and had established a possible association with exposure to blue asbestos (crocidolite) in all but two. News of the disease and its link with asbestos gradually spread around the world, and the article became the most cited paper in industrial medicine.

In the Margereson and Hancock case [5], Turner & Newall argued that it was impossible to have known of the mesothelioma risk before 1960. However, this view was not endorsed by the Court of Appeal, as Lord Justice Russell, in his judgement, said:

> We take the view that liability only attaches to these defendants if the evidence demonstrated that they should reasonably have foreseen a risk of some pulmonary injury, not necessarily mesothelioma … We reject therefore, as did the Judge, that the plaintiffs failed to show culpability on the part of the defendants by virtue of their knowledge of the risk prior to 1933. The information which should have operated upon the defendant's corporate mind was in existence long before Mr. Margereson's birth date [1925].

After the publication of the classic paper by Wagner *et al.* in 1960 [8], a number of letters and papers dealing with asbestos-induced diseases were published in the medical and scientific literature, culminating in the paper by Newhouse and Thompson in 1965 [9]. These authors reported on 83 mesothelioma cases in the East London area, including nine patients whose exposure was 'domestic' as a result of asbestos fibres being brought into the home environment from workplaces where asbestos fibres or materials were handled or used, and 11 patients who had 'neighbourhood exposure', having lived within half a mile of Cape's asbestos factory in Barking (in the East End) at some stage during the course of their lives. Newhouse and Thompson showed that mesothelioma could be caused by much lower exposures to asbestos fibres than had previously been thought to be hazardous to health. It was this paper that initiated the subsequent explosion of concern, information, and interest about asbestos in the media (e.g. *The Sunday Times*, 31 October 1965) and in government departments, which led to the setting up of the Senior Medical Inspectors' Advisory Panel.

American cases: background

The first claim for compensation for asbestosis in the USA was made in 1927 [10]. The disability claim was filed by the foreman in the weaving department of a Massachusetts asbestos plant and was upheld by that state's Industrial Accident Board. In his 1936 article, A.J. Lanza wrote that 'asbestosis figured in the extraordinary occupational disease litigation that has spread over the country ...' [10]. If there was something extraordinary about it, the phenomenon was apparently eclipsed for three decades by the Second World War and its aftermath. However, by 1985 the litigation was described as 'a flood' and was rightfully attributed to the former widespread use of asbestos products, the tendency of the dust to spread, and the dramatic effects of asbestos-related diseases [11].

In the late 1940s and early 1950s, American insulation workers were filing no-fault claims for asbestosis against their employers. Most state worker compensation statutes have strictly prohibited workers from suing their employers for negligence. When asbestos insulator Clarence Borel filed a lawsuit in the Federal District Court for the Eastern District of Texas in 1969, this signalled the contemporary beginning of asbestos-related personal injury litigation in the USA. Borel directly handled asbestos-containing insulation products at numerous jobsites between 1936 and 1969. He became disabled as a result of asbestosis in 1969, and was diagnosed with malignant mesothelioma in 1970. Borel's lawsuit, based on the theory of strict products liability, initiated the spread of similar lawsuits throughout all 50 states and the District of Columbia, and set the stage for the thousands of mesothelioma lawsuits that followed.

Borel's lawsuit named 11 manufacturers of asbestos-containing insulation products and charged that they failed to warn him of the dangers which were known to them or knowable at the time their products were manufactured. Failure to provide adequate warning of such hazards renders the products unreasonably dangerous. The jury awarded monetary damages in favour of the plaintiff implicitly finding that, had adequate warnings been provided, Borel would have chosen to avoid the danger. Although American jurisdictions already allowed victims of occupational disease, including dust diseases, to file workers' compensation claims for wage replacement and related medical expenses, the *Borel* case brought the issues of liability for fault and recovery for pain and suffering before a civil jury.

Jury trials to determine both fault and damages quickly became a regular feature of the pursuit of claims for asbestos disease in the American legal system. A notable feature of mesothelioma litigation has been the size of awards made in certain jurisdictions where juries have reacted with horror to the ravages of the disease and with outrage at the failure of some asbestos producers to provide an adequate warning, or any warning at all. Apart from those jurisdictions which place limits on non-economic awards for pain and suffering, American juries are free to deliver verdicts with no restraints apart from the facts presented at trial. However, as lawyers are well aware, huge verdicts are often reduced by trial judges and appellate courts and are seldom collected in full.

Trials of mesothelioma cases often pit large and profitable corporations against struggling workers and their families. However, from the defendant's perspective, mesothelioma cases illustrate the unintended costs and consequences of social and economic progress. American juries not only assess economic and non-economic damages, but are also capable of imposing punitive (or exemplary) damages. The ability to impose punitive damages expands the competence of American juries even further.

The *Borel* case featured the major issues that were to surface in most or all of the litigation that has followed. Those issues include latency and time limitations on bringing civil actions (statutes of limitations), the adequacy of warnings, proof of exposure, medical causation, and, implicitly, the effects of mass tort litigation on industry and society. These issues are discussed more fully in the following sections.

Latency and time limitations

Legal time limits can still cause problems. In the UK, court proceedings have to be commenced within 3 years of the claimant becoming aware that he or she is suffering from an asbestos-related disease.

If at all possible, court proceedings should be commenced within 3 years from the date that the disease manifested itself, i.e. when the claimant becomes symptomatic. In any event, proceedings should be commenced within 3 years from the date when the claimant was first advised that he or she was suffering from an asbestos-related illness, usually the date of diagnosis. Section 33 of the Limitation Act 1980 allows the court, in certain circumstances, to exercise discretion and to waive the limitation period. Inevitably, each case will turn on its own facts, but limitation is rarely a problem in mesothelioma cases because of the serious nature of the condition and the poor prognosis. Where a person suffering from the disease dies within 3 years, his or her estate (personal representatives) and dependants have a further 3 years in which to start a court action.

In the USA, time limitations and their application to specific cases vary from jurisdiction to jurisdiction.

Clarence Borel's occupational exposure lasted until 1969, the year he became disabled by asbestosis. When Borel brought suit, he did so within a short period of time after his last exposure. As recognized by the US Court of Appeals for the Fifth Circuit, which affirmed the judgement of the trial court, the period of latency for asbestosis

> may vary according to individual idiosyncrasy, duration and intensity of exposure and the type of asbestos used. In some cases, the disease may manifest itself in less than 10 years after initial exposure. In general, however, it does not manifest itself until 10 to 25 or more years after initial exposure. [12]

The court also recognized that the effect of the disease is cumulative and that, as a practical matter, it would be impossible to determine which exposure or exposures to asbestos dust were the particular cause of the disease. As for Borel's mesothelioma, the court also recognized a long period between initial contact and manifestation, and the inherent difficulty in determining which exposure to asbestos dust was responsible for the disease in a particular individual.

The *Borel* court, writing in 1973, did not make much of a distinction between asbestosis and mesothelioma. Rather, it emphasized the cumulative nature of the plaintiff's condition, observing that each exposure to asbestos dust can result in additional tissue changes. Borel's mesothelioma was attributed to his asbestosis, and there was no discussion of the relationship between brief low-level exposure and the development of mesothelioma.

Soon after the *Borel* decision, claims for mesothelioma began to enter the legal system. The disease was most frequently diagnosed long after the victim was last exposed to asbestos or had retired from the trade. The sequence of events-cessation of exposure, followed by an interval of latency and then manifestation of disease—provided asbestos companies in many American jurisdictions with a defence based upon the statute of limitations because courts often equated the period of exposure with the period of injury.

Although massive unregulated exposure to asbestos in the USA was over by the 1980s, millions of workers had been exposed in the shipbuilding industry in the 1940s, during the construction boom after the Second World War, and in heavy industry. Under these circumstances, new cases of mesothelioma, with or without accompanying asbestosis, generally manifested themselves several years after the last exposure, and in some cases decades later. In jurisdictions such as New York State, victims of asbestos-related disease were denied access to the courts because of the application of the statute of limitations, generally a 3 year period running from the date of the alleged injury (or wrong) rather than the discovery of the harm. The need for legal reform became clear.

In the *Borel* case, the defendant asbestos manufacturers argued that the plaintiff's claims were untimely, either because he must have contracted asbestosis long before he brought suit, having been first exposed to asbestos dust in 1936, or because it was too late for him to pursue damages for injuries occurring prior to Texas's 2 year period of limitations, on the theory that each exposure constituted a separate injury or wrong. The Court of Appeals rejected this alternative argument and adhered to an earlier decision by the US Supreme Court in a silicosis case brought under a federal statute. In 1949, the Supreme Court held that the limitations period began to run when the plaintiff either knew or had reason to know of the disease, because any other rule would deprive him of his day in court [13].

Although the Fifth Circuit refused to deprive Borel of his day in court, there was no national consensus on this point. In fact, the traditional exposure rule was alive and well in a number of important jurisdictions, including New York State. Under the exposure rule, the statute of limitations begins to run at the moment the potential plaintiff is exposed to a harmful substance that gives rise to the possibility of the future manifestation of a latent disease. Under a New York Court of Appeals decision in 1936, the statute began to run when the plaintiff was exposed to the harmful substance, in that case free silica, or on the last day of employment at the exposure site. New York's highest court determined that the injury occurred when the wrongful or negligent act was committed, while acknowledging that 'the statutory period of limitations begins to run from the time the liability for wrong has arisen even though the injured party may be ignorant of the existence of the wrong or injury' [14]. The Court of Appeals reaffirmed this rule and its application in a mesothelioma case brought by an asbestos insulator in 1975 [15].

As with most personal injury litigation in the USA, the evolution of legal rules was uneven and varied from one jurisdiction to another. In fact, there are no uniform laws or court rules that apply across state jurisdictional lines.

In 1986, New York fell into line with those jurisdictions that applied the discovery rule when its legislature passed the Toxic Tort Reform Act, overruling the state's judicial precedent. The new law opened a window for a period of 1 year for filing previously time-barred claims and provided a 3 year limitations period in which to bring suit for recently discovered cases, running from the date of discovery of the injury. In the 1970s, more liberal jurisdictions had already begun to apply a variation of the discovery rule in latent disease cases under which the statute of limitations does not begin to run until discovery of the disease as well as its cause, i.e. exposure to a particular toxic substance having latent effects [16–18].

Today, the statute of limitations rarely presents an immediate dilemma. If the victim's jurisdiction applies a variation of the discovery rule, he or she can usually begin legal action within the applicable period. On the other hand, if the jurisdiction imposes an exposure rule, the lawsuit will probably be long barred unless there are grounds to bring it in a discovery jurisdiction. In any event, health care professionals should assume that the mesothelioma patient does have legal recourse, even if the only discernible exposure occurred in the distant past.

Obviously, latency is not only a problem of conceptual importance for the courts to resolve, but also has implications for the role of health care professionals. Where malignant mesothelioma is a diagnostic consideration, the importance of taking a detailed exposure history cannot be overstated. Special emphasis should be placed on the possibilities of exposure occurring 20 or even 50 years earlier, including household exposure and neighbourhood exposure.

Dr Irving Selikoff

By the mid-1960s large-scale epidemiological research on the effects of exposure to asbestos-containing insulation products in the construction industry was under way. These studies were performed under the auspices of the Mount Sinai School of Medicine, New York City, and involved the asbestos insulators' union, the government, and asbestos manufacturers. This research prompted some companies, such as Johns–Manville, to place caution labels (or warnings) on their products. As claims for mesothelioma and other asbestos diseases began to accelerate in the mid-1970s, asbestos companies were able to employ another defence, based upon the presence of the warnings themselves, alongside the statute of limitations. Whether the warnings were adequate for the purpose, and indeed whether they appeared on the products at all, became issues of fact for juries to decide. The warnings became more prevalent as research on asbestos disease became more public and the pace of litigation increased.

Beginning with the publications of Dr Irving Selikoff of the Mount Sinai Medical Center in the mid-1960s, knowledge of the hazards of exposure to asbestos became more generally widespread. Between 1964 and 1973, Selikoff authored or co-authored nine published articles dealing with the health hazards of exposure to asbestos, and another ten between 1974 and 1980. By 1972, the Occupational Safety and Health Administration (OSHA), established by statute in 1970, was regulating exposure to asbestos at the local level and severely restricted workplace exposure. In December 1971 OSHA imposed a standard that limited exposure to 5 fibres/cm^3. In 1976 OSHA lowered the standard to 2 fibres/cm^3. By the end of the 1970s, although American workers continued to be exposed to asbestos fibres through the deterioration of asbestos-containing building materials and the demolition of old structures, there was virtually no more exposure to new asbestos-containing materials.

Court success in the UK at last

In the UK the possibility of successfully taking court action for compensation only opened up after the passing of the Limitation Act 1963. Previously, the time limit rules had made it impossible.

On 6 October 1967, proceedings were commenced by seven English asbestos workers in the case that became known as *Smith* v. *Central Asbestos Company*. All had developed moderate to severe asbestosis. The claims were pursued through the civil courts (Queen's Bench Division) and came to trial together. The seven men were successful, but the defendant company appealed. After a 4 day hearing in the Court of Appeal, on 26 May 1971, the men again won their case [19]. For the very first time in the UK, victims of negligent exposure to asbestos, at long last, recovered damages through the courts.

Compensation today in the UK

There are three main routes to securing compensation in the UK today.

State social security

A prescribed industrial disease system, administered by the Department of Work and Pensions, entitles sufferers to claim Industrial Injuries Disablement Benefit (IIDB), which covers those suffering from asbestosis, mesothelioma, lung cancer (with or without pleural thickening or asbestosis), and bilateral diffuse pleural thickening. The amount of benefit paid depends on the level of the sufferer's disability, provided that the injury has occurred as a result of exposure at work since 5 July 1948. All qualifying mesothelioma sufferers now receive the top payment (currently slightly over £120 per week based on an automatic 100 per cent disability assessment). The requirement for an independent medical assessment was removed on 29 July 2002. IIDB is also a passport to certain other injury-related benefits, in particular Constant Attendance Allowance. These benefits can usually be claimed on top of any amount of savings and whilst working full time. It is also possible to claim IIDB after the sufferer has died, but the widow/widower (or dependant) will need to submit a claim within 12 months of the date of death.

State 'no-fault' compensation scheme

Under the Pneumoconiosis etc. (Workers' Compensation) Act 1979, a state 'no-fault' scheme, payments can be obtained if no relevant employer is still in operation (and provided that IIDB has also been paid to the applicant in respect of the prescribed disease). The intention of the Act is to provide payments to sufferers of certain dust-related diseases, or their dependants, who are unable to claim compensation from the employers who caused the disease, for example because those employers have gone out of business. One of the conditions of entitlement is that neither the sufferer, nor any relative, has brought any court action or received compensation from an employer in respect of the injury complained of. For the purposes of the 1979 Act, 'brought an action' means that a claim form has been issued for damages against an employer.

Civil claims for damages

Common law claims for 'damages' (compensation) can be prosecuted through the civil courts with the assistance of a suitably qualified solicitor (or lawyer). Claims can be pursued for all of the (so-called) 'prescribed' diseases referred to above and, until very recently, symptom-free pleural plaques [20].

For people with benign pleural disease, provided there is some level of disability UK claimants are entitled to claim 'provisional damages'. This allows a relatively modest sum to be accepted in settlement (i.e. immediate payment) with the opportunity to reopen the case if a more serious disease (e.g. mesothelioma) develops at a later date. Provisional damages can also be awarded in asbestosis cases, bearing in mind the increased risk of lung carcinoma in particular.

Civil claims

Until the year 2000, there was a false perception in the UK that asbestos-related claims were fairly routine. Difficulties that arose mainly concerned the liquidation of a potential defendant and the problem of tracing an insurer for the relevant exposure period. While this remains a major problem, a number of important recent court decisions demonstrate that these claims are complex and far from straightforward.

Proof of actual asbestos exposure is needed. The claimant must also prove negligence (i.e. 'guilty exposure') and foreseeability with specific evidence, thus giving rise to the popular axiom 'no blame: no claim'.

The claimant needs to find the right company, or companies, to sue. In most cases they also need to find the relevant insurer, or insurers, to have a realistic chance of recovering a payment.

Causation must also be established medically. Without causation, there is no case. A detailed medical report must be obtained from a respiratory physician who is an expert in occupational lung disorders and, in less clear-cut cases, from a histopathologist. In some cases, defendants have argued that the claimant's mesothelioma is spontaneous (or idiopathic) if the fibres identified in the lung tissue are 'below background levels'. However, a European Respiratory Society paper [21] is helpful to claimants because the authors acknowledge that a positive occupational history is to be preferred over a negative fibre count.

Unfortunately, in December 2001, the Court of Appeal, in the conjoined cases of *Fairchild*, *Fox*, and *Matthews* [22], held that a claimant cannot recover damages in cases where he or she has suffered asbestos-induced mesothelioma after being exposed to asbestos dust whilst working for more than one employer. Why? The reason, the Appeal Court Judges said, is that mesothelioma, unlike asbestosis, is a single 'indivisible' disease and a claimant 'cannot establish, on the balance of probabilities, when it was that he inhaled the asbestos fibre, or fibres, which caused a mesothelial cell in his pleura to become malignant'. As the three claimants (all of them sadly deceased) had been employed, and exposed to asbestos inhalation, by more than one employer, the Court of Appeal held that because scientific knowledge is not available to determine from which source this suppositious 'guilty fibre' came (i.e. which defendant exposed the victim to the specific fibre(s) which caused the illness), it was impossible to say whether any of the employers were liable. Therefore, in those circumstances, the Court found that *no* employer was liable. The Lord Justices of Appeal observed that, in these circumstances, claimants may have a claim under the state administered Pneumoconiosis etc. (Workers' Compensation) Act 1979 scheme (see above), in which event they accepted that the cost to the Treasury 'may run into tens of millions of pounds each year'. If they did not, the Appeal Court Judges said that 'these cases have revealed a major injustice crying out to be righted either by statute, or by an agreed insurance industry scheme'. The Court of Appeal judgement in the *Fairchild* cases (as they collectively became known) was widely perceived as an injustice. Tony Blair, the Prime Minister, was even moved to comment on the case in the House of Commons on 13 February 2002, expressing his dismay at the decision.

In a joint letter published in *Thorax* [23], the three medical experts in the original Fairchild case [24] (Dr Robin Rudd, Dr John Moore-Gillon, and Dr Martin Muers) stated:

> The medical evidence presented to the Court made it clear that the risk of mesothelioma increases in relation to the [amount] of asbestos and that it is not possible to identify the particular fibre or fibres involved in the genesis of a particular mesothelioma. … From an epidemiological viewpoint, it is therefore appropriate to regard [all] sources of significant exposure as having contributed to causation of the disease, in the same way that all cigarettes smoked would be considered as having contributed to the causation of lung cancer.

Permission was given by the House of Lords (the highest court in the UK) to appeal the causation issue alone in the cases of *Fairchild*, *Fox* and *Matthews*, and the appeals were heard on 7–10 May 2002. The result was announced on 16 May 2002, and the full written reasons (judgement) were handed down on 20 June 2002 [25]. The five Law Lords are to be congratulated for righting the 'major injustice' (acknowledged by Lord Justice Brooke in the Court of Appeal) and demonstrating that the common law was up to the challenge of doing so.

In *Fairchild*, the House of Lords extended the principle recognized by the Lords in *McGhee* v. *National Coal Board* [26], namely that in certain circumstances the claimant need not prove on the balance of probabilities that the defendant's tortious (wrongful) conduct caused (or materially contributed to) the claimant's injury, but can jump the evidentiary gap concerning cause-in-fact merely by proof on the balance of probabilities that the defendant materially contributed to the risk of the injury the claimant suffered.

Major questions left open by the House of Lords decision in *Fairchild* concern the issues of causal apportionment and contribution. First, when a claimant sues a defendant and the Court applies the *McGhee/Fairchild* 'material contribution to risk' principle, should the defendant only be liable to the claimant for a portion of the total injury on the basis that there had been other sources of risk, i.e. can the defendant successfully argue for some form of apportionment of responsibility to the claimant? Secondly, if the defendant can raise the apportionment issue, what basis of apportionment should be used? Thirdly, if the principle does not allow the defendant to raise the apportionment point against the claimant, because the principle leads to joint and several liability, what basis of contribution should be used between tort feasors (wrongdoers)? This latter issue also arises where a court accepts that a mesothelioma victim was only exposed to asbestos during the period of employment with a single careless employer (so that the victim can recover fully from that party), but the employer then seeks a contribution from a number of negligent parties who had supplied asbestos to the employer during this period. In the USA, virtually all mesothelioma claims brought by asbestos workers are against those who supplied the asbestos to their employers. Claims against employers are typically barred by the rule that workers' compensation is 'the sole remedy'.

UK courts have been faced with a wave of contribution claims following *Fairchild* [27], although, in *Fairchild*, the Lords had been told that apportionment was not in issue in the case because 'no such assessment, even on a rough basis, was possible' (including, perhaps, account being taken of the different levels of risk posed by different forms of asbestos). These contribution claims were inevitable, and some basis for contribution will have to be crafted. This basis may be built on factors such as relative length/intensity of exposure or market share. However, it will necessarily be artificial because, since the aetiology of mesothelioma is unknown, the extent of a defendant's contribution to the total risk is, as a matter of science, also unknown. This means that the relative culpability, which will include a consideration of the defendant's contribution to the total risk, is unknown. As a matter of scientific logic, we cannot, for example, equate quantity of dust inhaled with the extent of contribution to risk.

Damages

The assessment of damages always comes last after all other points have been dealt with. Furthermore, litigation can take a long time (more than 12 months in a significant number of cases), although there has been a marked improvement since the civil justice reforms introduced by Lord Woolf in 1999. Expedited (speedy) trials are now frequently ordered in mesothelioma cases where the prognosis is particularly poor, and many claims can be concluded within a year.

What sort of compensation is paid to asbestos victims in the UK? In most cases, the damages paid are very modest. For example, a mesothelioma victim might be awarded between £45 000 and £70 000 for 'general damages' (to compensate for pain and suffering and loss of enjoyment of life), plus care costs and financial losses. The largest award, to date, in a mesothelioma case in the UK is £4.37 million, paid to the widow of Anthony Farmer, a very successful entrepreneur. Sadly he was only 47 when he died, leaving a widow and 2 dependent children.

Awards for asbestosis are less common now. The largest award to date was made in February 1998 to Bryan Ward, a very successful Yorkshire-based businessman. Although the total amount was just under £750 000, only £40 000 was awarded for pain and suffering. It was, in fact, very much in line with other cases, as the vast majority of the damages were for financial loss (loss of income).

Awards in pleural disease cases, paid on a provisional damages basis as opposed to a once and for all basis, are much lower still. A typical award for symptomatic pleural thickening is between £10,000 and £40,000. Perhaps if we had juries, not judges, assessing damages, things might be different.

In the USA, by contrast, a jury in California awarded the sum of $33 million in damages to a former electrician who claimed he was exposed to asbestos whilst working on ship boilers during the 1970s. Such awards are not uncommon and go some way to explaining the recent wave of Chapter 11 bankruptcies in the USA, Federal Mogul (Turner & Newall's parent company) being a notable 'casualty'.

Proof of exposure: American cases

American plaintiffs must meet basic requirements in order to establish a civil claim for asbestos-related disease. These requirements sometimes involve overlapping concepts of factual, medical, and legal causation. The issue of causation is particularly critical because every case of asbestos-related disease potentially involves multiple concurrent causes. The injured worker tends to sue every company that made asbestos-containing products to which he may have been exposed throughout the latency period for his disease. Typically, American plaintiffs seeking damages for mesothelioma or other asbestos-induced diseases bring suit against 20 or more potentially responsible asbestos manufacturers and distributors, as well as site owners whose premises were contaminated by asbestos dust.

The minimum prerequisite for keeping any potential defendant in the lawsuit is proof of the injured person's exposure to dust emanating from one or more products for which a particular defendant was responsible [28]. Proof of exposure requires evidence that the defendant's asbestos was present and that the injured person was in close enough proximity to inhale it. The facts alleged by the plaintiff must be sufficient to allow a reasonable inference that the injured person inhaled dust for which an individual defendant was legally responsible. For the plaintiff to prevail against a defendant at trial, he must demonstrate a causal relationship between exposure to that defendant's products and the injury, either asbestosis or mesothelioma.

In proving the required connection to a particular defendant's products, a potential plaintiff must provide and document as much evidence as possible of the details of his exposure history. This documentation includes the names of coworkers, the locations of work sites, and the identities of individuals who personally and directly handled asbestos products. Exposure evidence is particularly crucial where the injured person was merely a bystander to the use and application of products. Exposure, of course, is not limited to the particular trades handling asbestos-containing materials [29].

An occupational history should also elicit details about the duration of particular exposures and their intensity. Consideration should be given to the type or types of asbestos fibres to which the injured person was exposed, because most experts hold the opinion that amphibole fibres (including crocidolite, amosite, and tremolite) have a substantially greater potential to induce mesothelioma than do serpentine (or chrysotile) fibres. All information of this type is potentially useful in proving both exposure and a causal relationship to the products of individual defendants.

American courts have uniformly rejected attempts by plaintiffs to impose group theories of liability upon defendants in asbestos litigation. These theories include market-share and enterprise liability, and depend upon a judgement that the defendants and the asbestos industry as a whole derived substantial benefits from the sale of asbestos products. Manufacturers of asbestos-containing insulation materials commonly rebranded or relabelled one another's products for sale. Courts give various reasons, usually cast in terms of fairness, for rejecting these theories. Because asbestos products and their uses are not fungible, and because the products of some manufacturers differ in their degree of harmfulness from those of others, the courts have consistently required that the injured person produce proof of identification of the particular products of each defendant for each defendant to be held liable [28]. This is a difficult problem, since by 1965 there were already more than a thousand documented uses of asbestos [30]. In addition, American courts have not welcomed the use of the class action device because each plaintiff's case presents its own peculiarities of proof as to causation and damages [31,32]. However, some jurisdictions have allowed the consolidation of numerous claims for presentation before one jury [33].

In the *Borel* case, the court upheld the jury's finding that each defendant was the cause-in-fact of some injury to the plaintiff, as the plaintiff was exposed on many occasions to the products of all of the defendants at trial and the effect of this exposure was cumulative. Of course, Borel had personally identified the products with which he had worked and testified to their dustiness. However, over the course of the next decade, a more restrictive rule was developed for judging the adequacy of proof of exposure. This new rule grew out of cases of shipyard workers suffering from asbestosis and mesothelioma.

Some courts began to look at the frequency, regularity, and proximity of exposure in determining whether the injured party's exposure to an identified defendant's asbestos products was a substantial factor in causing the alleged injury. The frequency, regularity, and proximity test for product identification was rooted in the desire of the courts to ensure that exposure to a particular defendant's asbestos was indeed probable and more than some vague possibility of an isolated and indeterminate nature [34], especially where the injured plaintiff did not personally handle asbestos products in his work.

The application of this proof of exposure test has been criticized, especially in mesothelioma cases, and has not been adopted in every jurisdiction.

> The inquiry for the trial judge should be whether there is evidence of exposure and evidence tying that exposure to the disease. Whether that evidence is strong enough to prove causation is an issue for the jury. [35]

New York courts have never applied the test, relying instead on a requirement that the plaintiff simply prove exposure to the defendant's product, i.e. that the defendant's product was capable of being inhaled when it was in the zone of the plaintiff's exposure [36]. Whether the test is applied in a particular jurisdiction or not, the courts tend to take a more flexible approach in dealing with mesothelioma cases, primarily because of the belief that exposure to asbestos dust for 2 or 3 months may be sufficient to cause mesothelioma. At the same time, the courts recognize that asbestos-induced diseases are cumulative and that all exposures that fall within the broad period of latency may be causative.

The question as to whether a particular defendant's product was a cause-in-fact of the plaintiff's injuries is a question for the jury, but one which may be informed by expert scientific or medical testimony while not necessarily depending upon it. Substantial evidence of the required cause-in- fact can consist of proof that the plaintiff was present at a contaminated workplace (or neighbourhood) coupled with proof of the aerodynamic qualities of asbestos dust and the competence of minimal exposure to cause mesothelioma.

The frequency, regularity, and proximity test may be more suitable for assessing the sufficiency of proof of exposure in an asbestosis case than in a mesothelioma case, given that the degree of severity of asbestosis is tied to the cumulative dose. A prolonged intense exposure to the products of an identified defendant would clearly be a substantial factor in an asbestosis claim. On the other hand, a brief low-level exposure may have no medical or legal relevance. In contrast, in a mesothelioma case, there are no meaningful gradations in the severity of disease, the damage may be considered indivisible, and any inhalation tied to the products of a particular defendant may be causative. To require frequency or regularity of contact would be unscientific. The requirement of proximity must be modified in light of testimony that asbestos dust remains in the air for many hours even after it is no longer visible and that low-level concentrations of dust migrate over considerable distances from the point of use.

While American courts do not necessarily require expert scientific or medical testimony to prove the fact of exposure to asbestos, most courts require that the alleged exposure constitutes a substantial factor in the development of the plaintiff's disease. In other words, the evidence offered to prove exposure must be meaningful in relation to the production of disease. Therefore expert testimony may provide evidence for the jury and the court to consider that minimal exposure to asbestos dust above urban background levels can contribute to the development of mesothelioma. Such testimony may also bear on the potency of even a brief low-level exposure and necessarily encompasses evidence that most, if not all, cases of mesothelioma are the result of some exposure to asbestos. Expert testimony may also provide evidence that the effect of exposure above background levels is cumulative in increasing the risk of disease, thus establishing the predicate for keeping in the case a defendant whose overall involvement may otherwise be characterized as minor. Additionally, where there is a question about the proximity of the injured person to the source of asbestos dust at a given jobsite, expert testimony can explain the aerodynamic qualities of asbestos dust which allow it to remain suspended in the air for hours and drift from its point of origin [37].

Medical causation

Expert testimony is indispensable in proving the diagnosis of mesothelioma and its medical cause. The mesothelioma victim must present competent medical testimony establishing the diagnosis of malignant mesothelioma to a reasonable degree of medical certainty. Although the expert's opinion may rest on clinical evidence, it is preferable to present the testimony of a pathologist as the clinical course of the disease may not be sufficient to distinguish it from other conditions. Where there is a dispute over the diagnosis, the opinion of the pathologist will be crucial. In all cases, the basis of the doctor's opinion should be placed before the court. This consists of the doctor's report of his findings based upon special stains, microscopic examination, and other techniques.

There is no precise line demarcating the role of the medical expert from that of the fact witness when it comes to the requirement that the plaintiff prove that his exposure to the products of a particular defendant was a substantial factor contributing to the development of his mesothelioma. In any event, where the medical expert is called upon to offer his opinion, it must be offered to a reasonable degree of medical certainty, just as his opinion about diagnosis.

After establishing the diagnosis of malignant mesothelioma, the core of the medical expert's testimony is the causal connection between the history of exposure, as proven by the plaintiff and other fact witnesses, and the plaintiff's mesothelioma. Thus the medical expert must be familiar with a reliable history of the plaintiff's exposure to asbestos and with the epidemiology proving that mesothelioma is generally caused by exposure to asbestos above background levels. The plaintiff will also offer testimony through an expert that the only established environmental cause of mesothelioma is exposure to asbestos and that mesothelioma has been shown to develop in individuals with relatively brief or light exposures. In this regard, the plaintiff must prove through medical expert testimony that asbestos exposure in general was more likely than not the cause of his or her disease [38].

Other evidence relevant to prove that the plaintiff's mesothelioma was caused by asbestos exposure (and which itself tends to prove that exposure) is evidence of underlying asbestos disease of the chest in the form of asbestosis or bilateral pleural plaques. An asbestos burden above background levels in the injured person's lung tissue is also relevant to exposure and cause. In addition, a fibre burden analysis will distinguish fibre types found in the lung. The relative amounts of amphibole and serpentine asbestos fibres found in the lung tissue may have a bearing on the degree, if any, to which a particular defendant is held liable. Because it is commonly estimated that chrysotile fibres account for 95 per cent of all asbestos used in manufacturing in the USA, defendants whose products were free of amphiboles typically contend that their asbestos products were incapable of causing mesothelioma. Plaintiffs counter this argument with evidence of mesothelioma arising from chrysotile exposures and evidence of tremolite contamination of chrysotile [39].

The medical expert will also be called upon to testify about the latent nature of the disease and whether an appropriate period of time has elapsed between exposure and manifestation. This testimony is crucial in proving the cause-and-effect relationship between the exposure (as proven by other evidence) and the mesothelioma.

The plaintiff must present evidence justifying an inference of probability that the defendant's product (or the products of each individual defendant) caused or contributed to the cause of his disease [40]. However, the American cases do not appear to allow the defendant to escape liability simply because the degree to which an alleged exposure to a particular defendant's products contributed to the disease could not be determined with medical exactitude. The plaintiff is not required to prove that certain fibres identified in time and space and inhaled by the plaintiff from particular products for which the defendant was responsible were those or among those 'that actually began the cellular process of malignancy' [41]. Courts tacitly accept expert testimony that one asbestos fibre can cause mesothelioma, while at the same time accepting testimony that each exposure increases the risk that one fibre will initiate the cancer. Nonetheless, a medical expert should be prepared to testify in response to questions concerning the significance of the timing of exposures (whether early or late), the duration and intensity of exposures, and the type of fibre or contaminant involved.

Asbestos manufacturers have attempted to introduce evidence that an individual's mesothelioma has no known cause, or that it was possibly caused by radiation therapy for another tumour or even by poliovaccine contaminated with simian virus 40 (SV40). The contention that some mesotheliomas either occur spontaneously or are unrelated to exposure to asbestos may be supported by studies that document the disease in the absence of any history of exposure. One such study claims no evidence of exposure in 15 per cent of cases in England, Wales, and Scotland for the period 1967–1968 [42]. In 1998, in a case involving alleged exposure to insulation materials during the summer of 1955, an American asbestos producer attempted to introduce expert medical testimony that SV40 virus was present in the tissue of the decedent and was a possible cause of his mesothelioma. The court refused to allow the defendant to introduce the testimony because a cause-and-effect relationship could not be proven to a reasonable degree of scientific certainty [43].

In order to suggest that there are other causes of mesothelioma, apart from exposure to asbestos, defendants have attempted to introduce indirectly, by cross-examining plaintiffs' experts, discussion of the incidence of mesothelioma among Turkish villagers which is believed to be caused by exposure to dust from naturally occurring mineral rock used as building material

[44, 45]. Although studies of Turkish villagers may prove that occupational and environmental exposure to asbestos is not the only cause of mesothelioma, it proves little else in a court of law trying the claims of someone who is not a Turkish villager.

Lawsuits for mesothelioma have been pursued in American courts against the manufacturers of Kent cigarettes who utilized crocidolite fibres as a component of their filters between 1952 and 1956. Asbestos manufacturers have used this fact to raise doubt about the causal relationship between occupational exposure to their products and the plaintiff's mesothelioma.

Evidence of other suggested causes of mesothelioma is more likely to be introduced in a case where the plaintiff's proof of exposure to asbestos is less than substantial, for example where the period of alleged exposure is very brief or a coworker's testimony is very vague. It is unlikely that a court would allow expert medical testimony about a competing possible cause solely to cast doubt upon a probable cause.

Legal causation

Even where the plaintiff produces evidence that asbestos dust for which a particular defendant is responsible was the cause-in-fact of his or her disease, thus allowing the case to move forward to trial, it does not necessarily follow that the defendant's negligent conduct was a legal cause of the plaintiff's injury. Neither does such a conclusion follow from evidence that the exposure was a medical cause.

The law imposes upon the plaintiff the burden of demonstrating the existence of legal (or proximate) cause, a concept that embodies cause-in-fact, medical causation, and a connection to the alleged wrongful conduct of the individual defendant or, in the case of a product allegedly defective owing to the absence of an adequate warning, a connection to that defect. First, the plaintiff must prove exposure to the products of a particular defendant and that such exposure was a substantial factor in bringing about his disease. Without proof of actual exposure, there can be no proof of proximate cause. Then the plaintiff must prove, as a matter of social policy, that the defendant should be held legally responsible for his injury. In law, the concept of proximate cause imposes a limitation on the scope of liability based on economic and political considerations.

In a failure-to-warn case, the plaintiff must prove that the alleged absence or inadequacy of the warning carried by the defendant's product at the time it entered the stream of commerce was itself a cause of the injurious exposure suffered by the plaintiff. Therefore, at trial, the jury will be asked to assess the warning, its adequacy, and whether the product, as sent to market, was a substantial factor in causing the exposure that resulted in the disease. In this way, for example, the plaintiff's social history, particularly his smoking habits, become factually relevant even if they have no scientific relationship to the development of his mesothelioma. The defendants will try to use whatever facts they can to prove that a warning, if applied, would have made no difference to this plaintiff.

Funding arrangements

In the UK, unlike the USA, costs 'follow the event', i.e. the winning party's costs are (usually) paid by the losing party (subject to a test of reasonableness).

Legal Aid (or state financial assistance) is no longer available for mainstream personal injury claims in England and Wales, and this includes respiratory disease claims. However, Legal Aid has been retained for certain categories of cases, for example group/multi-party actions and 'test' cases. A Public Funding Certificate was issued in the *Matthews* case, referred to above, because the appeal raised a point of public interest. However, such cases are few and far between. Apart from trade union funding, the normal method of funding will be by way of a Conditional Fee Agreement, rather crudely called a 'no win–no fee agreement'. Unfortunately, until recently, such cases have not been without cost to the claimant, as claimants have been obliged to take out 'after the event' insurance policies to guard against the risk of paying the other side's costs if the case is lost. However, new rules came into force when the Access to Justice Act was introduced in July 2000, and now, provided that due notice has been given, both the after the event insurance premium and the lawyer's 'success fee', in addition to reasonable legal costs, will be recoverable from the other side in the event of a successful claim. Therefore the claimant's damages ought not to be diminished.

This is a better system for claimants, provided that they can find a competent specialist lawyer who is prepared to take a risk and that adequate opponent's costs cover can be obtained.

Mass tort litigation: the American phenomenon

The lengthy and elegant opinion by the US Court of Appeals in 1973 affirming the decision of the trial court in favour of Clarence Borel implicitly recognized the looming massive scope of asbestos litigation. The court's first reference to the history of asbestos claims in the USA is Lanza's article 'Asbestosis', published in 1936 [10]. According to Lanza, of course, occupational disease litigation had already spread over the country.

The problem of fairly compensating the victims of asbestos-related diseases through the American legal system has been resistant to any workable solution since attempts began in the mid-1970s. The system has been marked by delays in resolving serious cases, unnecessary transactional costs, and a failure to treat like cases in a like manner. This has resulted in grossly disproportionate recoveries, depending on geographical location and other factors including the bargaining position of the parties and their attorneys. The litigation has also had a major impact on the financial position of liability insurance companies and has placed a strain on the continuing business operations of companies formerly involved with asbestos, arguably resulting in dozens of bankruptcy filings.

In 1982, the Johns–Manville Corporation and related companies filed for bankruptcy reorganization. Johns–Manville was an industry leader, dominating the manufacture, mining, and supply of asbestos. Although bankruptcy effectively took Johns–Manville, which had an estimated 30 per cent share of the market for asbestos-containing products, out of the nationwide asbestos litigation, the pace of filing asbestos lawsuits, including mesothelioma lawsuits, continued to grow.

There may be disagreement over whether the bankruptcy was necessary or inevitable because Johns–Manville had more assets than liabilities when it filed for bankruptcy. However, there should be no disagreement that the company failed to protect workers against known dangers. In fact, it was company policy not to tell its own workers that their medical examinations revealed asbestosis because Johns–Manville saved money by letting them work until they dropped dead [46].

The Johns–Manville bankruptcy was the first and the largest. It preceded and may have helped to precipitate an expansion of asbestos litigation to include other kinds of defendants, including owners of fixed sites such as oil refineries, chemical plants, and power plants where plaintiffs claimed that they were knowingly and carelessly exposed to hazardous conditions. Over the following two decades the litigation continued to expand to take in claims against local distributors of asbestos products, the manufacturers of products with asbestos-containing components, the producers of friction products, and certain products that are ordinarily non-friable in nature. As indicated earlier in this chapter, there were over a thousand different uses for asbestos in industry.

The enormous size of the litigation becomes even clearer considering that the approximate number of new cases of mesothelioma every year in the USA is 2200 and that most claims in litigation involve either non-malignant conditions or lung and other cancers.

Since 1982, about seventy companies have filed for bankruptcy protection, alleging current and projected liabilities related to asbestos business activities. There were fifteen filings in the 1980s, almost an equal number in the 1990s, and about forty since 2000. The industry alleges that with each new filing the pressure on the remaining companies increases, as settlement demands and new filings against the surviving companies climb.

In mid-1985 approximately 25,000 lawsuits were pending in the state and federal courts, with 500 new cases being filed every month. In an attempt to address the situation, 34 asbestos producers and 16 insurers were brought together to sign a pact known as the Wellington Agreement, after its architect, Harry Wellington, the Dean of the Yale Law School. The Agreement ended disputes over insurance coverage and created the Asbestos Claims Facility to provide injured persons with an efficient and more equitable alternative to the courts. The original concept limited compensation to persons suffering an impairment or dysfunction and provided a deferral mechanism for other claims. As one member company after another dropped out during the second half of the 1990s, the entire scheme fell apart on 31 January 2001, when the Center for Claims Resolution, formerly the Asbestos Claims Facility, stopped settling claims on behalf of its remaining members.

During the 1970s and 1980s, a few plaintiffs' law firms based in major US cities and in locations where shipbuilding activities and heavy industry were concentrated began representing large numbers of asbestos victims. Soon attorneys with specialized knowledge of asbestos litigation began to establish themselves in almost every US jurisdiction. Some larger firms drew clients from jurisdictions throughout the country and used large numbers of cases as leverage to negotiate out-of-court settlements for their clients. As this mass tort litigation phenomenon continued to expand, the manufacturers of asbestos-containing insulation materials faced rapidly increasing numbers of claims.

By the mid-1980s there was major competition among law firms for new cases. At the same time, labour unions and community activists were engaged in establishing occupational health clinics and area councils on occupational safety and health. Unions and community activists viewed asbestos exposure and disease as public health issues, and in some contexts established medical screening programmes for large worker cohorts along the lines of those set up by Selikoff for the asbestos workers of New York and New Jersey.

However, some lawyers viewed asbestos disease screening as an opportunity to attract business. The screening of members of the sheet metal workers union was a positive example of a union-sponsored effort to educate workers about the risk of disease, to detect disease at an early stage, and to generate useful information about the incidence of cancer among members of the trade. Even this screening was done with guidance from and in conjunction with a large plaintiffs' law firm with a national presence [47]. Unfortunately, some lawyer-sponsored asbestos screening programmes were predisposed to find disease, provided no follow-up, and were conducted primarily, if not solely, for the purpose of generating legal claims. Some unions eventually allowed law firms to use them solely for business purposes.

Criticism has been directed at the practice of lawyer-sponsored screenings for two reasons. First, they advertised in a sensational way to exploit the fears of workers who may or may not have had significant asbestos exposure. Secondly, they encouraged workers to bring claims for asymptomatic conditions, which would not otherwise be revealed to the would-be plaintiff. The ethics and tactics of the lawyers sponsoring these screenings have also been called into question because they hold out the prospect of 'free screenings' when in fact the costs are passed on to the plaintiffs to be recouped from future settlements. Also, the screenings have very limited diagnostic value, do not involve a detailed occupational history or a physical examination by a qualified doctor, and result in relatively small settlements for large numbers of individuals. This process allows attorneys to earn large amounts in fees with very little risk or investment of time or money. Not surprisingly, there have been allegations of fraud and abuse against the companies taking the screening radiographs and arranging for them to be read because they have an incentive to produce positive results for the lawyers who hire them.

In the mid-1980s, well before the latest round of bankruptcies which began in 1999, American lawyers and judges were already proposing a variety of solutions for the increasing number of asbestos claims, including the establishment of case-management orders with uniform and streamlined discovery procedures. A common feature of these local case-management orders was the establishment of an inactive docket for unimpaired cases. However, the definition of impairment and the appropriate criteria by which to judge it were often matters of contention among the parties.

At least one state court system, the Commonwealth of Pennsylvania, has barred the filing of cases for non-disabling asbestos-related pleural disease, presumably to control the size of court dockets and to ensure the availability of resources to compensate seriously disabled and fatally ill plaintiffs [48]. This decision also recognized, as have other court decisions through the country, the ability of a plaintiff to file suit for mesothelioma within the statutorily prescribed time, notwithstanding the failure of the plaintiff to file an earlier lawsuit for a diagnosed non-disabling or non-malignant condition. The two-disease rule was intended to ameliorate the hardships of the statute of limitations by allowing an unimpaired claimant to chose not to file suit without sacrificing the availability of a remedy should he or she later develop mesothelioma or another cancer. However, the rule may have caused an overall increase in the number of lawsuits: a single plaintiff may sue twice, initially for asbestosis and later for cancer.

More recently, legislators, judges, and even some plaintiffs' lawyers have advocated a complete end to litigation and recovery for cases of asymptomatic non-malignant asbestos-related disease. However, in most jurisdictions, plaintiffs asserting these claims retain the right to a jury trial, if only on the claim for damages for fear of cancer based on the objective manifestation of asbestos-related scarring of the pleura or lungs. While in some cases such claims may be highly speculative, they are quite compelling when they arise out of fixed locations involving high numbers of mesotheliomas among coworkers.

In March 1991, the Report of the Ad Hoc Committee on Asbestos Litigation, chaired by the Chief Justice of the US Supreme Court, called for a legislative solution to a problem

> becoming a disaster of major proportions … which courts are ill-equipped to meet effectively … In the final analysis, the committee has concluded that congressional action is necessary to enable the courts to meet the unique problems presented by asbestos litigation. [49]

No solution has been adopted. In July 2002, the US Court of Appeals for the Third Circuit designated the present situation 'a crisis' and suggested the desirability of 'a nationwide class action' to resolve issues of general importance for all litigants but that 'such proposals frequently made have not passed both houses of Congress' [50].

Despite the large volume of asbestos litigation in the USA, one of the foremost publications chronicling American asbestos litigation reported on 40 verdicts in asbestos litigation for the year 2003 [51]. Many, but not all, involved multiple plaintiffs, and not all the plaintiffs sued for mesothelioma. The verdicts were reported from 13 states, including a subtotal of 27 from Texas, Pennsylvania, California, New York, and Ohio. Cumulative subtotals for these states for the period 1997–2002 were 86 for Texas, 66 for Pennsylvania, 82 for California, 28 for New York, and

16 for Ohio. These figures are notable for the fact that asbestos litigation is concentrated in relatively few jurisdictions. The same leading publication reported on 44 verdicts for 2005.

As the legal system is ever-changing, federal legislation in the USA may alter some of the dynamics of mesothelioma litigation. Regardless of these inevitable changes, the historical overview and description of the shape of litigation given in this chapter is still instructive as a blueprint for mass tort litigation.

Asbestos is still out there

The real crime is that asbestos is still out there. Dust-covered workers were a common sight as recently as 25 years ago, or even less. It is a worldwide problem. Who is at risk today? Asbestos product manufacturing workers. Asbestos product users. Facility workers. Those exposed domestically and those exposed in the environment. The youngest mesothelioma victim the authors are aware of is just 32 years old.

What of the future? Worldwide, the number of victims can only be guessed at. At present, the number of people pursuing civil claims for compensation, in the UK and the USA combined, is well in excess of 600 000.

The scale of the asbestos tragedy is like the substance itself, literally breathtaking. Asbestos has been called the 'the grand-daddy of all occupational killers—not one amongst equals, but the leader of the pack' (Laurie Kazan-Allen, Editor, *British Asbestos Newsletter*). No-one can do more than guess at how many lives, worldwide, will be claimed in the end. The only thing which is certain about the future is that the legacy will be here for decades to come.

Conclusion

It is difficult to conceive of a mesothelioma case today that does not have its roots in an asbestos manufacturer's or user's wrongful actions. Such warnings as may have been issued at the time of exposure would not have fairly reflected the magnitude of the risk and the gravity of the harm known or knowable to asbestos businesses. The widespread use of asbestos and its extreme carcinogenicity have combined to make recovery for mesothelioma as much of a social as a legal problem, and whether the American legal system has the creative potential to deal fairly with the next generation of mesothelioma victims remains to be seen.

References

1. Chief Inspector of Factories and Workshops. *Annual Report for the Year 1898*. London: HMSO, 1899; ii, 172
2. Cooke WE. Fibrosis of the lungs due to the inhalation of asbestos dust. *BMJ* 1924; ii: 147.
3. Cooke WE Pulmonary asbestosis. *BMJ* 1927; ii: 1024–5.
4. Selikoff I, Greenberg M. A landmark case in asbestosis. *JAMA* 1991; **265**; 898–901.
5. *Margereson & Hancock* v. *J. W. Roberts Ltd: Holland J*, 27.10.95 (Leeds High Court).
6. *Per Russell LJ: Margereson & Hancock* v *J. W. Roberts Ltd*, CA: 3.04.96.
7. Merewether ERA, Price CW. *Report on Effects of Asbestos Dust on the Lungs and Dust Suppression in the Asbestos Industry*. London: HMSO, 1930.
8. Wagner JC, Sleggs CA, Marchand P. Diffuse mesotheliomas and asbestos exposure in north western Cape Province. *Br J Indust Med* 1960; **17**: 260–71.
9. Newhouse ML, Thompson H. Mesothelioma of pleura and peritoneum following exposure to asbestos in the London area. *British Journal of Industrial Medicine* 1965; **22**: 261–9.

10. Lanza AJ. Asbestosis. *JAMA* 1936; **106**: 368–9.

11. *Jackson* v. *Johns–Manville Sales Corporation*, 750 F. 2d 1314 (5th Cir., 1985).

12. *Borel* v. *Fibreboard Paper Products Corporation*, 439 F. 2d 1076, 1083 (5th Cir. 1973).

13. *Urie* v. *Thompson*, 337 U.S. 163 (1949).

14. *Schmidt* v. *Merchants Dispatch Transport Co.*, 270 N.Y. 287 (1936).

15. *Steinhardt* v. *Johns–Manville Corporation*, 54 N.Y. 2d 1008 (1981).

16. *Nolan* v. *Johns–Manville*, 74 Ill. App. 3d 778 (1979) (applying Illinois law);

17. *Harig* v. *Johns–Manville Corporation*, 284 Md. 70 (1978) (applying Maryland law).

18. *Louisville Trust Co.* v. *Johns–Manville Corporation*, 580 S.W. 2d 497 (1979) (applying Kentucky law).

19. *Smith, Dodd, Sampson, Drake et al.* v *Central Asbestos Co.* Times Law Reports: 27.05.1971.

20. *Rothwell, Grieves et al.* (2006) EWCA civ 27.

21. De Vuyst P, Karajalainen A, Dumortier P, *et al.* Guidelines for mineral fibre analyses in biological samples: report of the ERS Working Group. *Eur Respir J* 1998; **11**: 1415–26.

22. *Fairchild* v. *Glenhaven Funeral Services Ltd & Others*: *Fox* v. *Spousal (Midlands) Ltd*: *Matthews* v. *Associated Portland Cement (1978) Ltd & Others*, CA: 11.12.02.

23. Rudd R, Moore-Gillon J, Muers M. Mesothelioma. *Thorax* 2002; **57**:187.

24. *Fairchild* v. *Glenhaven Funeral Services Ltd & Others*, Curtis J: 1.02.01.

25. *Fairchild* v. *Glenhaven Funeral Services Ltd & Others*: *Fox* v. *Spousal (Midlands) Ltd*: *Matthews* v. *Associated Portland Cement (1978) Ltd & Others*, [2002] 3 WLR89; [2002]3 All ER 305.

26. *McGhee* v. *National Coal Board*, (1973) 1 WLR 1: (1972) 3 All ER 1008.

27. *Barker* v. *Corus (UK) Plc, Murray* v. *British Shipbuilders (Hydrodynamics) Ltd & Others, Patterson* v. *Smiths Dock Ltd and Another* – Mouse of Lords, Times Law Reports 04.05.06.

28. *Blackston* v. *Shook and Fletcher Insulation*, 764 F.2d 1480 (11th Cir. 1985).

29. Selikoff IJ. Asbestos exposure and neoplasia. *JAMA* 1964; **188**: 22–6.

30. Hendry NW. The geology, occurrences, and major uses of asbestos. *Ann NY Acad Sci* 1965; **132**: 12–22.

31. *Amchem Products* v. *Windsor*, 521 U.S. 591 (1997).

32. *Ortiz* v. *Fibreboard Corporation*, 527 U.S. 815 (1999).

33. *Hopeman Bros Inc.* v. *Acker*, 537 U.S. 1083 (2002).

34. *Lohrmann* v. *Pittsburgh Corning Corporation*, 782 F.2d 1156 (4th Cir. 1986).

35. *Horton* v. *Harwick Chemical Corporation*, 73 Ohio St. 3d 679 (1995).

36. *Reid* v. *Georgia–Pacific Corporation*, 212 A.D. 2d 462 (N.Y. App. Div. 1995).

37. *Robertson* v. *Allied Signal Inc.*, 914 F. 2d 360 (3rd Cir. 1990).

38. *Maiorana* v. *United States Mineral Products Co.*, 52 F. 3d 1124 (2nd Cir. 1995).

39. Smith AH, Wright CC. Chrysotile exposure is the leading cause of mesothelioma. *Am J Ind Med* 1996; **30**: 252–66.

40. *Harris* v. *Owens–Corning Fiberglas Corporation* 102 F. 3d 1429 (7th Cir. 1996).

41. *Rutherford* v. *Owens-Illinois Inc.*, 16 Cal. 4th 953 (1997).

42. Greenberg M, Lloyd Davies TA. *Br J Ind Med* 1974; **31**: 91–104.

43. *John M. Stiner, Personal Representative of the Estate of Chester S. Kucinski* v. *A.P. Green Industries Inc. et al.* (N.Y. Sup. Ct.).

44. Pelnar PV (1988). Further evidence of nonasbestos-related mesothelioma. *Scand J Work Environ Health* **14**, 141–4.

45. Wagner JC, Berry G, Pooley FD (1980). Carcinogenesis and mineral fibres. *Br Med Bull* 1980: **36**: 53–6.

46. Castleman BI. *Asbestos: Medical and Legal Aspects*. Frederick, MD: Aspen Law & Business, 1996; 581.

47. Michaels D, Zoloth S, Lacher M, Holstein E, Lilis R, Drucker E. Asbestos disease in sheet metal workers. II: Radiologic signs of asbestosis among active workers. *Am J Ind Med* 1987; **12**: 595–603.

48. *Simmons* v. *Pacor Inc.*, 543 Pa. 664 (1996).

49. *Report of the Ad Hoc Committee on Asbestos Litigation.* Washington, DC: Administrative Office of the US Courts, March 1991; 26.

50. *In re Federal-Mogul Global Inc.*, 300 F. 3d 368 (3rd Cir. 2002).

51. *Mealey's Litigation Report: Asbestos. Special Report.* King of Prussia, PA: LexisNexis, 2004.

Index